The New Psychology of Pandemics

The New Psychology of Pandemics

Uncertainty, Fear, Control, and Conflict

Steven Taylor

Foreword by
Gordon J. G. Asmundson

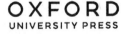

OXFORD
UNIVERSITY PRESS

Oxford University Press is a department of the University of Oxford.

It furthers the University's objective of excellence in research, scholarship, and education by publishing worldwide. Oxford is a registered trade mark of Oxford University Press in the UK and in certain other countries.

Published in the United States of America by Oxford University Press
198 Madison Avenue, New York, NY 10016, United States of America.

© Oxford University Press 2025

All rights reserved. No part of this publication may be reproduced, stored in a retrieval system, transmitted, used for text and data mining, or used for training artificial intelligence, in any form or by any means, without the prior permission in writing of Oxford University Press, or as expressly permitted by law, by license or under terms agreed with the appropriate reprographics rights organization. Inquiries concerning reproduction outside the scope of the above should be sent to the Rights Department, Oxford University Press, at the address above.

You must not circulate this work in any other form
and you must impose this same condition on any acquirer.

CIP data is on file at the Library of Congress

ISBN 9780197810972

DOI: 10.1093/9780197811009.001.0001

Printed by Integrated Books International, United States of America

The manufacturer's authorized representative in the EU for product safety is Oxford University Press España S.A., Parque Empresarial San Fernando de Henares, Avenida de Castilla, 2 – 28830 Madrid (www.oup.es/enor product.safety@oup.com). OUP España S.A. also acts as importer into Spain of products made by the manufacturer.

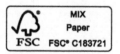

For Meeru, Alex, and Anna

Contents

Foreword — ix
Preface — xi
Acknowledgments — xiv
Glossary — xv
About the Author — xix

PART I. PSYCHOLOGICAL PHENOMENA AND PANDEMIC-MITIGATION METHODS

1. The Psychological Footprint — 3
2. Pandemic-Related Stressors — 24
3. Pandemic-Mitigation Methods: An Overview — 36
4. Risk Communication — 44
5. Face Masks and Vaccines — 50
6. Social Distancing: Impact, Objections, and Alternatives — 60
7. Politics and Protests — 72
8. Coping During Disease Outbreaks — 83
9. Fleeing: Urban Exodus from Contagion — 99

PART II. PSYCHOLOGICAL PROCESSES AND MECHANISMS

10. Exposure to News and Social Media — 111
11. Heuristics and Biases in Threat Evaluation — 122
12. Rumors and Conspiracy Theories — 133
13. Beliefs About Health and Disease — 149
14. Death Anxiety — 162
15. Diseases, Disgust, and Xenophobia — 171
16. Magical Thinking and Superstitious Behavior — 179
17. The Illusion of Control and Other Self-Serving Biases — 189

18. Personality and Pandemics — 199

PART III. MENTAL HEALTH

19. Pandemics and Mental Health — 215
20. Infection-Induced Psychopathology — 235
21. Immunization Stress Reactions — 245
22. Managing Mental Health During Pandemics — 253

PART IV. AFTERMATH AND FUTURE

23. Life in the Aftermath — 267
24. Future Pandemics — 275

References — 289
Index — 408

Foreword

The COVID-19 pandemic was a stark reminder of the significant interplay between infectious diseases and human cognitions, emotions, and behaviors. Indeed, despite the incredibly devastating loss of life and still-lingering medical challenges related to the SARS-CoV-2 virus and its variants, the psychological footprint was substantially larger. Recent experiences stemming from COVID-19 have revealed how uncertainty, fear, anxiety, and various forms of disruptive behavior are, themselves, contagious, and ripple through societies. While prior infectious outbreaks have harkened some of these issues, it is the COVID-19 pandemic that thrust them into the global spotlight. In response, Dr. Steven Taylor's *The New Psychology of Pandemics: Uncertainty, Fear, Control, and Conflict* not only illuminates the psychological complexities of widespread outbreaks of infectious disease but also provides a roadmap for navigating their challenges.

This book is an extension of Dr. Taylor's *The Psychology of Pandemics: Preparing for the Next Global Outbreak of Infectious Disease*, which, published in October 2019 just prior to the onset of the COVID-19 pandemic, was seemingly prophetic in its coverage of issues that were observed by the world in the months and years that followed. Yet, while deeply insightful, Dr. Taylor's work stemmed from his astute observations of the limited literature on psychological responses to infectious outbreaks available at the time, rather than prophecy. His ability to draw from historical and cultural contexts and integrate these observations with the lessons from the considerably expanded body of research on human responses to infectious outbreaks emerging from opportunities afforded by COVID-19 positions this new book as the ultimate source for understanding the psychology of pandemics. Readers will gain a clear understanding of how and why people think, feel, and behave the way they do in the face of widespread contagion and in response to public health strategies to mitigate spread of disease.

As a long-time collaborator and colleague, I have been consistently impressed by Dr. Taylor's capacity to synthesize research into practical frameworks. In this book, he bridges the gap between science and society, ensuring that readers—whether psychologists, public health professionals, policymakers, or members of the public—gain an enriched understanding of, and a global perspective on, the factors influencing our reactions to pandemics.

One of the most compelling aspects of this book is its actionable recommendations. While pandemics inevitably bring distress and disruption, they also offer opportunities for growth, resilience, and innovation. Dr. Taylor adeptly captures this duality, emphasizing how understanding psychology can better equip us to address the challenges of future pandemics which, as he aptly discloses, are not once-in-a-lifetime events and will inevitably occur within the next few years or decades.

It is my sincere hope that this book reaches the hands of those who shape the world's response to public health crises and, importantly, that it is read prior to another global outbreak of infectious disease. In these pages lies not only a deep exploration of pandemic-related psychological phenomena but also a guide for proactive actions that will enhance mental health outcomes and adherence to pandemic mitigation strategies in the face of future global outbreaks of infectious disease.

I commend Dr. Taylor for his dedication to advancing the field and for providing a resource that will undoubtedly inspire meaningful change moving forward. This work is a testament to his expertise, and I am honored to have been invited to introduce it to you.

Gordon J. G. Asmundson,
OC, SOM, PhD, RD Psych, FRSC, FCAHS
Professor and Head of Psychology, University of Regina
Editor-in-Chief, *Clinical Psychology Review*

Preface

Global outbreaks of infectious disease—pandemics—are not once-in-a-lifetime phenomena. Outbreaks of emerging or re-emerging infectious diseases will likely become more prevalent in the years ahead due to climate change and other reasons. Psychology plays an essential role in pandemics. The psychology of pandemics concerns how people perceive, think, feel, and behave during pandemics and how these factors influence the spreading versus containment of infection, distress, and societal disruption.

In October 2019, a few weeks before the onset of the COVID-19 pandemic, I published a book titled *The Psychology of Pandemics: Preparing for the Next Global Outbreak of Infectious Disease*. At the time, no previous book had brought together findings from diverse fields of psychology and related disciplines to understand the vital role played by psychology in pandemics. The psychological phenomena described in the 2019 book were remarkably similar to those later observed in the course of COVID-19, including panic buying, xenophobia, conspiracy theories, protests about wearing protective face masks, anti-vaccination attitudes, lockdown protests, and increases in mood and anxiety disorders.

Psychologists like myself were participant observers during COVID-19, investigating and experiencing various aspects of the pandemic, such as lockdowns and mandates regarding masks and vaccines. The present volume arose from a series of seminars on various aspects of the psychology of COVID-19 and other pandemics. This book is an exercise in applied psychology, in which psychological principles and findings are used to understand three vital concerns associated with widespread infectious outbreaks:

- Mental health problems arising or worsening due to the disease threat
- Nonadherence to disease control measures
- Societal discord and conflict

The book consists of interlinked seminar-like chapters covering significant topics and central issues concerning the psychology of pandemics. Readers will note that pandemic mitigation methods, such as social distancing, face masks, and vaccines, are explored in detail. Detailed discussions are necessary because pandemic mitigation measures are sources of many psychological phenomena reviewed in this volume.

This book builds and expands on the 2019 publication in several ways. The new book identifies four major themes in the psychology of pandemics: uncertainty, fear, control, and conflict. The themes are cross-cutting—that is, associated with many pandemic-related psychological phenomena and evident across diverse disease outbreaks. Uncertainty pervades pandemics from onset to end. Fear is a common response to infectious threats—too much or too little fear leads to problems during pandemics. Various measures are used to control pandemics, often leading to conflicts over their efficacy, necessity, and adverse effects.

The current volume reviews and integrates the copious research on the psychology of COVID-19 with existing knowledge on the psychology of pandemics. The amount of psychological research on pandemics from 2020 to 2024 vastly exceeds all previous research on the topic. Accordingly, many new findings and insights have emerged since 2019. The current volume also expands on the previous book by presenting additional findings from archival investigations into historical outbreaks of infectious diseases, including yellow fever, cholera, and encephalitis lethargica. Historical and contemporary case examples are provided to give readers a close-up view of how people experienced and reacted to infectious outbreaks.

In many fields of psychology, research is mainly based on Western samples, typically college-educated young adults. While informative, such research provides an incomplete picture, especially concerning global problems such as pandemics. In addition to reviewing findings from modern Western countries, the present volume draws extensively on findings from numerous cultures, nations, and historical epochs. Examples include research from Asia (China, Hong Kong, Taiwan, Korea, Thailand, and Japan) concerning COVID-19, SARS, and swine flu. Also reviewed are findings from India and Pakistan concerning COVID-19 and the plague. Russian findings concerning cholera and plague are discussed, along with African studies of Ebola virus disease, HIV/AIDS, COVID-19, and the Spanish flu. South American case material—from Argentina, Brazil, and Venezuela—is surveyed concerning riots arising from smallpox, yellow fever, and cholera outbreaks. Findings from Mexico and Caribbean countries (Haiti, Barbados) concerning COVID-19 and cholera are discussed. The book also reviews multinational COVID-19 mega-studies comparing dozens of countries on psychological variables such as anxiety and depression.

Understanding the causes of pandemic-related psychological phenomena can help us prepare for the inevitable pandemics in the years or decades ahead. The present volume explores promising avenues for maintaining and improving mental health and for enhancing adherence to pandemic mitigation measures. This book is intended for those working in psychology, healthcare, public health, and related fields—clinicians, researchers, policymakers, and students—as well as the general reader. To prepare for future global outbreaks of infectious diseases, we all would benefit from a better understanding of the psychology of pandemics.

Acknowledgments

Several people contributed directly or indirectly to the completion of this book. I want to single out two individuals for special thanks: Thanks to my wife, Meeru Dhalwala, for her interest, encouragement, and support throughout the writing of this volume. Thanks also to my friend, colleague, and research collaborator, Professor Gordon J. G. Asmundson. Gord and I have been research collaborators for many years. Our investigations into the psychology of COVID-19 provided the impetus for this book.

Glossary

Anxiety: An emotional response to anticipated threat, characterized by apprehension, worry, vigilance for future danger, increased muscle tension, and avoidance and escape behaviors. Anxiety overlaps with fear—the two are similar phenomena. Anxiety is a response to future threat whereas fear is a response to imminent or immediate threat (see *Fear*).

Behavioral immune system: A psychological system that detects disease cues, thereby eliciting disgust and fear, which motivate escape and avoidance behavior.

Burnout: A state of emotional, mental, and physical exhaustion arising from prolonged stress. Features include irritability, cynicism, and perceived meaninglessness of one's activities. Burnout is experienced by frontline healthcare workers and the general public during pandemics. For the latter, burnout arises from prolonged social distancing restrictions (see *Pandemic fatigue*).

Conspiracy theories: A set of loosely connected, sometimes illogical, and largely unsupported beliefs centering on ideas that malevolent and shadowy individuals or organizations conspire to exploit the population or cover up some misdeed. Conspiracy theories may be based on a grain of truth (e.g., young people are less prone to complications from COVID-19) from which conspiratorial beliefs are constructed (e.g., COVID-19 is a hoax to control the population).

Cordon sanitaire: A restriction on the movement of people in or out of a geographic region to stem the spread of infection. Cordon sanitaire may involve placing entire communities in seclusion. An example is a guarded perimeter around a town, preventing ingress and egress.

Disgust sensitivity: A trait representing a person's tendency to readily and intensely experience disgust.

Distress (emotional distress): A general term referring to the experience of aversive emotions, particularly anxiety and depression.

Endemic: Constant circulation of an infectious disease in a region or community, maintained without new infectious cases entering the area.

Face mask: A mask made from cloth or paper intended to cover the nose and mouth, used to protect people from droplet and airborne infections. Masks may be medical grade (e.g., N95) or homemade.

Fear: An emotional response to real or perceived imminent threat, involving surges of autonomic arousal, thoughts of imminent danger, and escape behaviors. Fear and anxiety overlap considerably in features (see *Anxiety*).

Fomites: Objects or surfaces, such as handrails, furniture, and utensils, likely to become contaminated with infectious agents such as virus particles.

Germ theory: The currently predominant scientific model of infectious disease, proposing that some diseases are caused by microorganisms invading the body, such as viruses and bacteria. Germ theory came to prominence in the late 19th century, gradually displacing miasma theory.

Hygiene theater: Excessive, unnecessary sanitization of fomites, involving frequent and conspicuous cleaning of high-touch public surfaces (e.g., handrails, doorknobs, touchscreen cash registers). These performative sanitization activities, intended to reassure the public, can provide a false sense of security.

Infodemic: A neologism referring to a massive amount of rapidly disseminated information on a given topic, consisting of a mix of reliable and unreliable material circulated in news reports and on social media. The immense volume of information and uncertainty about its accuracy leads to confusion and conflict over important issues.

Intolerance of uncertainty: A trait defining the extent to which a person is anxious about uncertainties in daily life. People scoring high on this trait tend to frequently worry and strive to avoid or eliminate uncertainties by recurrent checking and reassurance-seeking.

Lockdown: A neologism referring to restrictions on public mobility. Lockdown involves stay-at-home or shelter-in-place orders in which people are encouraged or required to remain at home as much as possible to reduce the spread of infection, being allowed out only under specific circumstances, such as shopping for groceries or performing jobs designated as essential services.

Long COVID: Persistent symptoms after a person has recovered from acute SARS-CoV-2 infection. Long COVID, also known as Post-Acute COVID-19 Syndrome, is a post-viral syndrome or multiple syndromes characterized by various symptoms and may resemble chronic fatigue syndrome.

MERS: Middle Eastern Respiratory Syndrome, caused by the MERS-CoV coronavirus.

Miasma theory: An obsolete theory stating that infectious diseases are caused by miasma, which consists of vapors or mists, particularly foul-smelling nocturnal emissions from rotting plant or animal matter.

Nudges: Health-promotion strategies that subtly guide or encourage people toward particular choices or behaviors without forbidding options, forcing people to do things, or significantly changing a person's economic or other incentives. Nudges involve prompts to perform simple, low-effort behaviors. An example of a nudge is when employees hand out free face masks at store entrances, encouraging but not requiring shoppers to wear these protective coverings.

Pandemic fatigue: A burnout-related syndrome that emerges from prolonged pandemic-related restrictions on socialization. Pandemic fatigue is associated with emotional exhaustion and an increasing disregard for social distancing and other restrictions.

Panic buying: The urgent purchasing of large quantities of food or other supplies, arising from fear of impending shortages or perceived need for supplies in preparation for an impending lockdown.

Plague: A disease generally attributed to the bacterium, *Yersinia pestis*. Plague is subtyped according to how the person is exposed to the pathogen, with the most common types being bubonic, pneumonic, and septicemic.

Polarization: A marked disparity between groups concerning beliefs, emotions, behaviors, or social conditions. Beliefs about the seriousness of a disease threat may be polarized, with some people becoming alarmed while others dismiss the threat as exaggerated. Compliance with mitigation measures can be polarized (e.g., pro- vs. anti-mask groups). Socioeconomic hardships may also be polarized, with greater hardships experienced by some groups than others.

Psychological reactance: A trait defined by the extent to which a person values personal freedom. For people scoring high on this trait, perceived threats to personal autonomy evoke anger, resistance, and rebellion.

Quarantine: A restriction on the movement of people, goods, and animals, intended to prevent the spread of disease. Travelers arriving in a country might be required to remain in isolation for a specified time in a dedicated quarantine facility. People are quarantined because they may have been exposed to a communicable disease, even if they do not show signs or symptoms.

Resilience: The capacity to withstand or quickly recover ("bounce back") from adversities. Resilient people might become anxious or depressed during a pandemic but rapidly recover once the threat has passed.

Risk communication: Public messages from health authorities or other leaders concerning the degree of risk associated with a disease outbreak and what the public can or should do to mitigate the risk. Good risk communication is unambiguous, concise, practical, and evidence-based.

SARS: Severe Acute Respiratory Syndrome caused by the SARS-CoV-1 coronavirus.

SARS-CoV-2: The virus causing COVID-19.

Social distancing: A method better described as "physical distancing," in which people are required to keep a safe distance apart in public places to limit the spread of infection. Social distancing is used for infections spread by airborne transmission, fomites, and direct physical contact. Examples of social distancing include closures of schools and workplaces, lockdown, quarantine, cancellation of mass gatherings, cordon sanitaire, travel restrictions, and maintaining a set distance from one another (e.g., 3 or 6 feet apart) in lines.

Social end of a pandemic: An ending defined by the resumption of pre-pandemic social and commercial activities even though infection is still prevalent in communities. The social ending is associated with a mindset that the pandemic is essentially over. This contrasts with the physical ending of a pandemic, defined by disease-related criteria such as the decline or elimination of infection.

Stress reaction: Increased arousal in response to a stressor, involving increased muscle tension, agitation, nervousness, irritability, and a tendency to be easily upset. Stress reactions, anxiety, and fear substantially overlap with one another.

Stressor: A disruptive force, event, or condition requiring some form of adaptation or adjustment. Pandemic-related stressors include threats to one's health, well-being, and livelihood.

Superspreaders: People who disproportionately contribute to the spreading of infection.

Superspreading events: Events in which an unusually large number of people become infected.

Test-trace-isolate approach: A targeted social distancing approach in which an infected person's contacts are traced (e.g., via digital phone tracing) and asked to self-isolate for a given period (e.g., days or a week or two).

Vaccination hesitancy: Indecision, reluctance, or frank refusal concerning vaccination.

Xenophobia: Dislike, fear, or prejudice against strangers or members of an outgroup—that is, a group to which one does not belong.

About the Author

Steven Taylor, Ph.D., is a professor and clinical psychologist in the Department of Psychiatry at the University of British Columbia, Canada. He received his B.Sc. (Hons.) and M.Sc. at the University of Melbourne, and Ph.D. at the University of British Columbia. Dr. Taylor's work focuses on the psychology of pandemics and anxiety-related clinical phenomena such as anxiety disorders, obsessive-compulsive disorder, health anxiety, and post-traumatic stress disorder. He has authored over 300 scientific publications and over 20 books, translated into several languages. His books include *Understanding and Treating Panic Disorder* (2000), *Treating Health Anxiety* (2004, coauthored with Gordon J. G. Asmundson), and *Clinician's Guide to PTSD* (2017). His most recent book, published a few weeks before the outbreak of COVID-19, was *The Psychology of Pandemics: Preparing for the Next Global Outbreak of Infectious Disease* (2019). Dr. Taylor served as a member of several expert panels on COVID-19, including the Canadian federal government's expert advisory panel, the Royal Society of Canada's task force on mental health during COVID-19, and a WHO panel on future pandemics. Dr. Taylor has received awards for his research from the Anxiety Disorders Association of America, the Canadian Psychological Association, and the Association for Advancement of Behavior Therapy. In 2023 and 2024, Dr. Taylor was recognized as a *Clarivate Highly Cited Researcher* in psychology and psychiatry, based on his work on the psychology of pandemics.

PART I
PSYCHOLOGICAL PHENOMENA AND PANDEMIC-MITIGATION METHODS

1
The Psychological Footprint

Introduction

Pandemics are global epidemics of emerging or re-emerging infectious diseases for which people have little or no preexisting immunity. Pandemics reveal aspects of humanity rarely seen in calmer times. Pandemics are not simply about some microbe "going viral." Pandemics are largely psychological events in which people's beliefs, emotions, and behaviors play a vital role in spreading and containing disease, distress, and societal disruption.

Psychology plays a crucial role in every aspect of pandemic management and is essential for understanding pandemic-related mental health problems. The purpose of this book is to examine the three major classes of psychological phenomena associated with pandemics—mental health problems, nonadherence to disease-mitigation measures, and societally disruptive reactions such as protests and conflicts. By studying the psychology of pandemics and other, more minor epidemics, we are better equipped to prepare for future outbreaks. The present chapter provides an introduction and overview.

Pandemics arise when animal pathogens mutate and spread to humans. Some re-emerging bacterial diseases, like cholera and plague, are concerning because they have caused pandemics and continue to represent threats (Primrose, 2022; WHO, 2023a). In fact, at the time of writing, the seventh cholera pandemic was still ongoing, as was the HIV/AIDS pandemic (Ramamurthy & Ghosh, 2021; WHO, 2023a, 2024a).

Five virus families are of special concern because of their pandemic potential (CDC, 2024; Chan-Yeung & Xu, 2003; Dixon & Schafer, 2014; Kelly et al., 2011; Lycett et al., 2019; National Collaborating Centre for Infectious Diseases, 2024; WHO, 2021, 2024b).

- Flaviviruses, including the yellow fever, Zika, West Nile, and Dengue viruses.
- Filoviruses, such as the Ebola and Marburg viruses.

- Coronaviruses, including those causing Severe Acute Respiratory Syndrome (SARS), Middle East Respiratory Syndrome (MERS), and Coronavirus Disease 2019 (COVID-19).
- Influenza viruses.
- Paramyxoviruses, such as measles, mumps, and human parainfluenza viruses.

This book uses common or conventional names for historical disease outbreaks because the labels will be familiar to most readers (e.g., Spanish flu, Russian flu, plague). However, names matter, particularly for ongoing pandemics, as discussed later in this volume.

Tables 1.1 to 1.3 summarize the pandemics and other major outbreaks surveyed in this book. The data in the tables were derived from the following sources: (Ahmad & Anderson, 2021; Berche, 2022; CDC, 2024; Chan-Yeung & Xu, 2003; Dawood et al., 2012; Eisenberg & Mordechai, 2019; Elliott, 2024; Fenner et al., 1988; Glatter & Finkelman, 2021; Halani et al., 2021; Hoffman & Vilensky, 2017; Honigsbaum, 2020b; Kanungo et al., 2022; Littman, 2009; Mathieu et al., 2024; Michaelis et al., 2009; Mordechai et al., 2019; National Collaborating Centre for Infectious Diseases, 2024; Ramamurthy & Ghosh, 2021; Tomori, 2004; WHO, 2023b, 2024a, 2024b). Other infectious outbreaks are also considered, but in lesser detail (e.g., measles, mpox, syphilis, typhus, and typhoid).

Over the past 60 years (1965–2025), there have been seven pandemics: The 1968 and 1977 influenza pandemics and the HIV/AIDS, Zika, Swine flu, cholera, and COVID-19 pandemics. Tables 1.1 to 1.3 show that for over 2,000 years, there have been many additional large-scale outbreaks of high-mortality diseases. Most lasted years or longer, often occurring in waves. At the height of the second plague pandemic in the 14th century, for example,

Table 1.1 Plague, Cholera, Smallpox, and Yellow Fever Outbreaks.

Period	Outbreak	Description	Reference
430–426 BC	Plague of Athens	An epidemic in the city-state of Athens, killing about 25% of the inhabitants (75,000–100,000 estimated deaths), and spreading to the eastern Mediterranean. Unknown etiology, possibly typhus or smallpox.	Littman (2009)
165–180 AD	Antonine Plague	Considered by some to be the world's first pandemic, likely smallpox, afflicting much of the Roman Empire, with millions of fatalities.	Elliott (2024)

Period	Outbreak	Description	Reference
6th–20th centuries, and sporadic outbreaks since	The Plague	Attributed to *Yersina pestis* and classified according to route or primary site of infection (e.g., pneumonic, bubonic, septicemic). In addition to numerous sporadic outbreaks, there have been three plague pandemics: 1. 541–767 AD, consisting of 15 or more major waves, with millions of deaths, although the exact figures are disputed. The Plague of Justinian (541–750 AD) formed part of the first plague pandemic. 2. 1347–1771, including the Black Death (1347–1353), which eradicated over a third of the European population (more than 25 million deaths), and the Great Plague of London (1665–1666), which killed about a quarter of London's citizens. 3. 1855–1950s, resulting in an estimated 15 million deaths, worldwide.	Eisenberg & Mordechai (2019), Glatter & Finkelman (2021), Mordechai et al. (2019)
17th century–present	Cholera pandemics	Caused by *Vibrio cholerae*. In the past 200 years, there have been 7 cholera pandemics resulting in tens of millions of deaths: 1817–1823, 1829–1851, 1852–1859, 1863–1879, 1881–1896, 1899–1923, and 1961–present. Recent outbreaks are mostly in developing countries.	Kanungo et al. (2022), Ramamurthy & Ghosh (2021)
17th century–present	Yellow fever epidemics	Recurrent outbreaks caused by the yellow fever flavivirus. The disease is endemic in parts of sub-Saharan Africa and Central and South America, although epidemics have occurred in the United States and Europe. Currently, there are about 200,000 infections and 30,000 deaths annually.	Tomori (2004)
6th–20th centuries, and likely earlier	Smallpox pandemic and epidemics	Caused by forms of variola virus. A smallpox pandemic (1870–1875) and smaller epidemics (e.g., 735–737, 1520–1527, 1862) were associated with several million deaths. Smallpox was eliminated by vaccination in 1977.	Fenner et al. (1988)

Table 1.2 Influenza and Coronavirus Pandemics and Epidemics

Period	Outbreak	Description	Reference
1889–1890	Russian flu pandemic	Attributed to either the H2N2 or H3N2 influenza viruses or possibly the OC43 coronavirus. Led to an estimated 1 million deaths.	Berche (2022)
1918–1920	Spanish flu pandemic	Arising from a strain of the H1N1 influenza virus. Infected about a third of the world's population, with up to 100 million deaths.	Snowden (2019)
1957–1958	1957 flu pandemic	Due to the H2N2 influenza virus, resulting in over a million deaths.	Honigsbaum (2020)
1968–1969	1968 flu pandemic	Arising from the H3N2 influenza virus, leading to 1–4 million deaths.	Honigsbaum (2020)
1977–1979	1977 flu pandemic	Due to a strain of the H1N1 virus, leading to 0.7 million deaths.	Michaelis et al. (2009)
1997–present	Avian flu outbreaks	Sporadic outbreaks caused by strains of H5N1 and other influenza viruses. From 2003–2019, there have been over 880 human infections and more than 460 deaths from at least 19 countries.	National Collaborating Centre for Infectious Diseases (2024)
2002–2004	SARS epidemic	An epidemic of Severe Acute Respiratory Syndrome afflicting over a dozen countries, caused by the SARS-CoV-1 coronavirus. There have been over 8,000 cases and over 900 deaths. No cases have been reported since 2004.	Chan-Yeung & Xu (2003)
2009–2010	Swine flu pandemic	Arising from a strain of the H1N1 influenza virus. Infected 11–21% of the global population, with an estimated 284,000 deaths.	Dawood et al. (2012)
2012–present	MERS outbreaks	Periodic outbreaks of Middle East Respiratory Syndrome, caused by the MERS-CoV coronavirus. As of April 2024, there had been 2,613 cases and 941 deaths, mostly in Saudi Arabia.	WHO (2024)

Period	Outbreak	Description	Reference
2020–2023	COVID-19 pandemic	Coronavirus disease 2019, due to the SARS-CoV-2 coronavirus. In 2023, the World Health Organization declared that the COVID-19 global public health emergency was over, although the coronavirus continued circulating at low levels in communities. In 2020, COVID-19 was the third leading cause of death in the United States. By 2021, about a third of Americans knew someone who had died from the coronavirus disease. As of 2024, over 7 million deaths worldwide were attributed to COVID-19.	Ahmad & Anderson (2021), Mathieu et al. (2024), WHO (2023)

Table 1.3 Other Pandemics and Epidemics

Period	Outbreak	Description	Reference
1915–1927	Encephalitis lethargica pandemic	The first neuropsychiatric pandemic. Etiology unknown. Afflicted over a million people worldwide. Low mortality rate but possibly linked to subsequent Parkinsonism.	Hoffman & Vilensky (2017)
1976–present	Ebola outbreaks	Sporadic outbreaks of Ebola virus disease in sub-Saharan Africa. From 1976–2022, there were more than two dozen outbreaks. The largest outbreak was from 2013–2016, resulting in 28,000 infections and 11,000 deaths. There have been several outbreaks since then.	CDC (2024)
1981–present	HIV/AIDS pandemic	Arising from the human immunodeficiency virus. As of 2022, over 40 million deaths have been attributed to HIV/AIDS.	WHO (2024)
2015–2016	Zika virus pandemic	Caused by the Zika virus. A generally mild infection (0.1% mortality) but was linked to neurological problems and birth defects.	Halani et al. (2021)

waves of plague swept Europe about once a decade (Byrne, 2006). Today, plague is rare but remains a health threat. From 2010 to 2019, there were 4,547 plague cases worldwide, of whom 17% died (Butler, 2023).

The Psychological Footprint Is Bigger Than the Medical Footprint

In pandemics, more people are affected psychologically compared to the number infected. Fear and anxiety are common reactions to pandemics. Fear is an emotional response to imminent threats, whereas anxiety is a response in anticipation of future threats. Worry is a central cognitive component of anxiety, consisting of future-oriented thinking ("What if X happens?"). Fear and anxiety overlap phenomenologically, and one blends into the other. As the threat looms closer, anxiety morphs into fear.

The psychological significance of pandemics is underscored by the psychological effects of sickness, bereavement, and socioeconomic hardships, as well as mental health problems and effects on society and culture. The psychological footprint is substantial in terms of the number of people losing friends and family. For every COVID-19 fatality in the United States in 2020, there was an average of five bereaved immediate family members: parents, spouses, siblings, and children (Verdery et al., 2020). The psychological impact can be substantial for survivors of infection. Some develop persistent post-infection psychological problems—such as post-traumatic stress disorder and anxiety disorders—as well as post-viral syndromes such as Long COVID (Taylor, 2022; Tzeng et al., 2020).

The psychological impact of a disease can be felt even before it arrives in one's community. Anticipatory anxiety commonly arises when the threat of infection looms large. This is illustrated by the following examples concerning Ebola, Swine flu, and COVID-19. Throughout the 2014 outbreak of Ebola virus disease in West Africa, there was widespread anxiety in the United States; "the American public reacted to Ebola with a level of fear and panic that was disproportionate to the actual risk to the U.S. population" (Paules et al., 2017, p. 809). There was only a handful of cases of Ebola in America, mostly acquired from travel to afflicted countries.

When Swine flu broke out in 2009, researchers in Utah documented a surge in hospital emergency visits, in which people worried about influenza even though there were few or no cases in their community (McDonnell et al., 2012). Most of the surge was due to pediatric visits. Young children commonly catch infections with flu-like features (e.g., fever, cough, congestion), which parents likely misinterpreted as signs of Swine flu.

Early in the COVID-19 pandemic, fear of infection was prevalent even in places where infections were rare. A study of 6,800 U.S. and Canadian adults in the early months of COVID-19 found that 28% had elevated anxiety associated with worries about the coronavirus, even though infections were scarce; only 2% of the sample had acquired COVID-19, and only 6% personally knew anyone who had been infected (Taylor et al., 2020).

The Human Faces of Pandemics

The following personal accounts provide readers with a sampling of how people experienced and responded to pandemics. The descriptions illustrate many of the psychological phenomena described later in this book. The first account is an excerpt from the diary of Miquel Parets, a master tanner who wrote in Barcelona in 1651 during the second plague pandemic.

Plague, 1651, Barcelona

The authorities initially tried to deny the arrival of the plague in Barcelona; "they covered it up by saying that those who died were all poor people and that it all came from the bad food they ate last winter" (Parets, 1651, p. 43). As deaths accumulated, denial by city officials was no longer possible. There was widespread fleeing from the city but also crowded religious processions and ceremonies seeking divine intercession.

> The streets were constantly full of people, many greatly devout and carrying candles and crying out "Lord God, have mercy!" . . . There was not a single church nor monastery which did not carry out processions both inside and outside their buildings. But Our Lord was so angered by our sins that the more devotions were carried out, the more the plague spread. . . . This disease does not favor gatherings of people. (pp. 44–45)

We will return to Miquel Paret's diary periodically throughout this book as we examine various pandemic-related psychological phenomena.

Cholera and Yellow Fever, 1832–1833, New Orleans

Reverend Theodore Clapp provided a detailed account of his experiences ministering to the sick and dying during the 1832–1833 cholera and yellow fever outbreaks in New Orleans. His account revealed widespread death.

People were frequently "found dead all along the streets, particularly early in the mornings" (Clapp, 1857, p. 131). Almost every house he visited contained the sick, dying, and dead; many crowded in the same room. Stores, banks, and businesses were closed due to illness or fleeing.

Corpse disposal was a significant undertaking: "All the drays, carts, carriages, hand and common wheelbarrows, as well as hearses, were employed in the transportation of corpses, instead of cotton, sugar, and passengers" (p. 125). Reverend Clapp recounted "the awful sight of carts driven in the graveyard, and there upturned, and their contents discharged as so many loads of lumber or offal, without a single mark of mourning or respect, because the exigency rendered it impossible" (p. 125).

To purportedly purify the air against diseases, people burned tar and pitch on street corners, and cannons were fired. "Often, walking my nightly rounds, the flames from the burning tar so illuminated the city streets and river, that I could see everything almost as distinctly as in the daytime" (pp. 132–133).

The unpredictability of cholera was among its most frightening aspects. Seemingly healthy people suddenly and unexpectedly expired. Reverend Clapp described several encounters with seemingly healthy people who unexpectedly perished hours or a day later. In one instance, he married a young couple. The bride unexpectedly died of cholera a few hours later. The reverend was summoned to perform a final service as she lay in her coffin. The bride "had on her bridal dress, and was very little changed in the appearance of her face" (p. 130).

Spanish Flu, 1918, North Carolina

When the Spanish flu struck in 1918, Daniel Tonkel was seven years old, living with his family in the small town of Goldsboro, North Carolina (Barry, 2018; Iezzoni, 1999). Doctors had little to offer for the Spanish flu, so people turned to folk preventives and other remedies. It was commonly believed that strong interventions (e.g., awful-tasting medicines) were needed to fight off powerful diseases. One folk preventive involved wearing a bag around one's neck containing the foul-smelling plant, asafetida. As Daniel recalled, "People thought the smell would kill germs . . . so, we all wore a bag . . . and smelled like rotten flesh" (Iezzoni, 1999, p. 119).

As influenza spread, people became increasingly frightened, avoiding public places and keeping their children indoors. Young Daniel was terrified: "You never knew from day to day who was going to be next on the death list . . . that was the horrible part, people just died so quickly" (Barry, 2018, p. 346). But despite widespread distress during the Spanish flu, Daniel later reflected on how quickly most people returned to their previous lives once the pandemic had passed. People grieved their losses, but eventually, "everyone just went back to their normal way of living" (Iezzoni, 1999, p. 206).

COVID-19, 2020, Texas

Tony Green, a 43-year-old man from Texas, used to call COVID-19 a "scamdemic," an overblown media hoax (Green, 2020). He used to make fun of people who wore masks. In 2020, Tony had been in lockdown for months as part of community-wide efforts to stem the spread of infection. Tony was bored, isolated from his family, worried about finances, and depressed and angry about the situation. As the summer of 2020 arrived, he persuaded himself that the worst was over. Disregarding social distancing guidelines, Tony hosted a family get-together consisting of himself, his partner, and their four parents. The gathering was a long-awaited respite. They cooked meals, talked, watched movies, and had a good time. Although it was nothing special, it felt like a welcome return to normalcy.

Tony awoke feverish and sweating the following day, with aches, pains, and breathing difficulties. He tried to assure himself that it was just the flu, but the symptoms worsened. Tony had acquired COVID-19 and was hospitalized. The others attending the gathering were also infected. They passed the disease on to at least eight other people. Tony's 52-year-old father-in-law was hospitalized, placed on a ventilator, and died after several weeks on life support. Tony was devastated, unable to stop thinking about the ordeal. He described persistent feelings of guilt, punctuated by periods of intense grief; "the grief comes in waves, but that guilt just sits" (Green, 2020, p. 1).

Sequences of Events

How do pandemics generally unfold? As we will see in later chapters, in the initial stages of an outbreak of a novel, potentially lethal disease, rumors abound about causes and cures, along with anxiety and fleeing for some people, while others deny or downplay the threat. As infection spreads, people seek ways of protecting themselves and loved ones, so there is widespread use of folk preventives, quack cures, and other nostrums. Panic buying may occur initially and sporadically thereafter in response to threatened lockdowns or rumored threats to the supply chain (Taylor, 2021).

A state of exception or emergency may be declared to stem the spread of infection, involving the temporary suspension of everyday rules and rights. This may involve curfews, travel restrictions, and business closures. Some people resist the restrictions, fearing the loss of freedom may become permanent once the emergency is over (Agamben, 2005; Swenson, 1988; Zinn, 2020). Others become more accepting or welcoming of authoritarian, restrictive government interventions when faced with collective threats—trading privacy and freedom for greater security (Altemeyer, 2009; LeHardy, 1888; Wnuk et al., 2020).

Anxiety levels tend to rise in pandemics, especially early in an outbreak (Chapter 19). Over time, people generally adapt or acclimate to threats, becoming less concerned, even while acknowledging the danger is real (Collinson et al., 2015; Garfin et al., 2020). For pandemics where lockdowns are implemented, pandemic fatigue emerges as restrictions are drawn out (Chapter 6). Tiring of constraints, people increasingly behave as if the pandemic is over, flouting guidelines about social distancing and other health precautions.

Pandemics do not end neatly (Honigsbaum, 2020a). One can distinguish between two types of endings—social and physical—with the former arising before the latter. The social ending is defined by the resumption of pre-pandemic social and commercial activities, even though infection is still prevalent in communities. The social ending is associated with a mindset that the pandemic is essentially over. People become less concerned about the outbreak, focusing on other issues. For COVID-19, the social ending began in 2022 as the pandemic took a back seat to other world concerns such as climate change, social injustices, and geopolitical events.

The physical endings of pandemics are typically uneven and gradual, with declining rates of infection interspersed with sporadic, localized outbreaks. Usually, there is no sudden cessation and much uncertainty about whether a pandemic is over. The pathogens causing pandemics may become endemic.

How Do Pandemics Spread?

Animals, Crowds, and Travel

Pandemics arise from human-wildlife interactions. People living at the urban-wildland interface and people who frequently interact with domestic animals (e.g., poultry farmers) or deal in exotic animal products sold at wet markets are at risk of being infected by animal pathogens that have mutated to infect humans (Aguirre et al., 2020; Almagro-Moreno, 2022; Morens et al., 2008).

Pandemics spread through human populations in various ways. Depending on the pathogen, infection can spread via direct person-to-person contact (e.g., coughs, sneezes, transfer of bodily fluids), insects (e.g., fleas, mosquitos), or contaminated food or water.

Crowds and travel networks propagate pandemics. Networks include trade routes, transportation hubs that concentrate people (e.g., train stations, seaports, and airports), and military operations involving the mass aggregation and transportation of troops. Global, rapid mass transit (e.g., air travel) and crowded city living conditions facilitate the spreading of infections, especially those diseases spread by aerosols or droplets (e.g., sneezing or coughing), such as influenza and COVID-19.

Superspreaders

Many diseases spread according to an 80/20 rule, where 80% of infections arise from 20% of people (Stein, 2010). Individuals who infect unusually large numbers of people are known as superspreaders (Galvani & May, 2005). Superspreaders tend to disregard health guidelines (e.g., neglect hand hygiene) and interact with many people due to social activities or occupational roles (Galvani & May, 2005; Temime et al., 2009).

Superspreaders have been linked to the proliferation of many diseases, including measles, tuberculosis, mpox, smallpox, HIV/AIDS, Ebola virus disease, SARS, and COVID-19 (Mohindra et al., 2021; Shin et al., 2020). There were many documented superspreaders throughout COVID-19. One of the first was in February 2020 in South Korea, where 544 infections were linked to a single contagious individual attending a church gathering (Mohindra et al., 2021).

Historically, the most famous superspreader was Mary Mallon, whom the media dubbed "Typhoid Mary" (Soper, 1939). Mary was an asymptomatic carrier of the bacterium *Salmonella typhi*. She infected more than 50 people from 1902 to 1909 while working as a domestic cook, while showing no signs or symptoms herself. Every time Mary moved to a new household to work as a cook, the family came down with typhoid. She vigorously denied being infected and insisted on working as a cook despite orders from health authorities to desist. Mary was involuntarily detained by authorities, spending her final two decades in a New York quarantine hospital (Brooks, 1996).

Superspreading Events

Superspreading events are those leading to unusually large numbers of infections. These events occur in conditions conducive to spreading disease, regardless of whether superspreading individuals are present. Superspreading events are most likely when (1) diseases have incubation periods of several days to a week or more, so people may be asymptomatic (unaware of being infected) but contagious, and (2) people attend social events that are held under conditions favoring disease spread (Chen et al., 2021; Lewis, 2021; Lloyd-Smith et al., 2005). People flouting restrictions on social gatherings led to numerous superspreading events throughout COVID-19, some involving police intervention and arrests (Cha, 2021; Lewis, 2021; Walker, 2021).

For infections spread by droplets and aerosols, superspreading events typically occur in crowded, poorly ventilated spaces where social distancing isn't possible and masks aren't worn. Schools and preschools are superspreading hotspots for influenza and other respiratory infections (Cauchemez et al., 2009; CDC, 2007).

In countries throughout the world, religious services, such as prayer services, funerals, and choir practices, were identified as superspreading hotspots during COVID-19 (Alsharif & Almasy, 2020; Aschwanden, 2020; Becker, 2020; DeFranza et al., 2021; LaGrassa, 2020; Spinney, 2020). In the course of the Spanish flu, one of the largest superspreading events occurred in the Spanish town of Zamora. The Catholic Bishop Álvaro y Ballano defied health authorities by convening a novena, consisting of nine consecutive evenings of crowded church services in honor of St. Rocco, the patron saint of plague. In one service, the congregation queued to kiss the saint's relics. Zamora had the highest influenza mortality rate in Spain and among the highest in Europe (Spinney, 2017).

Superspreading may also occur at sporting events, family gatherings, parties, business conferences, gym classes, festivals, bars, and clubs (Majra et al., 2021). Parades and political rallies can become superspreading events (Arnold, 2018; Davis, 2018). In the final year of World War I, which overlapped with the 1918 Spanish flu, morale-boosting marches were organized in the United States. In one parade in Philadelphia, 200,000 people jammed the streets, creating a superspreading event that infected thousands and filled hospitals (Davis, 2018).

In the first year of the COVID-19 pandemic, U.S. President Trump conducted 18 political campaign rallies, leading to an estimated 30,000 cases of COVID-19 (Bernheim et al., 2020). India's Prime Minister Modi faced criticism during COVID-19 for permitting events with superspreading potential, such as political rallies, cricket matches, and the Kumbh Mela religious festival (Associated Press, 2021; Cagnassola, 2021).

Over 9,000 COVID-19 infections were linked to the Euro football games in 2021 (Walker, 2021). Even greater superspreading was associated with the Sturgis motorcycle rallies. Each year, the annual rally draws hundreds of thousands of motorcyclists to the small town of Sturgis, South Dakota. Rallies were held in 2020 and 2021, with over 400,000 and 500,000 attendees, respectively. Masks were largely absent, and there was little or no little effort at social distancing (Brittany et al., 2021). Both rallies were associated with dramatic increases in COVID-19 infections, with the larger (2021) rally associated with a 700% increase in COVID-19 in South Dakota (Brittany et al., 2021; McEvoy, 2021). A rally organizer dismissed concerns about superspreading as "baloney" (Brittany et al., 2021, p. 1).

Pandemics Are Dynamic Events

Pandemics are dynamic events, with infections often coming in waves. Fluctuating patterns of human aggregation can create waves of infection. Examples include the seasonal movements of crowds, such as when schools close for the summer, dispersing students, and then reopen in the fall (Caley et al., 2008; Herrera-Valdez et al., 2011).

Pandemics are dynamic in the exponential spread of infection. Humans have a cognitive bias to expect linear rather than exponential (accelerating) growth (Stango & Zinman, 2009). People often express fearful surprise at what appears to be a sudden, dramatic increase in infection, failing to see that this happens with exponential growth—"There were hardly any cases last week and now everyone is sick!" Failure to appreciate the need for social distancing for COVID-19 was linked to people's difficulty in understanding the exponential spread of infection (Lammers et al., 2020).

Pandemics are dynamic in their psychological reactions. Anxiety may rise and fall in concert with the prevalence of infection (Angus Reid Institute, 2020; Asmundson & Taylor, 2020; Penninx et al., 2022; Robinson & Daly, 2021). Vaccination hesitancy can fluctuate throughout disease outbreaks. From 2020 to 2021 in the United States, willingness to be vaccinated against COVID-19 declined until vaccines became available, after which willingness gradually rose as vaccination programs were implemented and shown to be safe (Daly et al., 2021; Daly & Robinson, 2021).

Pandemics Evoke Extremes

Pandemics evoke a range of responses, including extremes. Pandemics bring out the best and worst in people. The diversity of reactions includes panic buying, fleeing, selfishness, opportunism, altruism, frivolity, piety, and crime (Fiquepron, 2018; Garza, 2008; Gowen, 1907; Hirst, 1953; Honigsbaum, 2010; McGee, 2022; Procopius, 551 AD; Reynolds, 2022; Steel, 1918; Taylor, 2022; Taylor et al., 2020; Thucydides, 431 BC). The extremes may represent only a fraction of the community but have a disproportionate impact on pandemic management and significant mental health implications.

Pandemics can polarize, evoking or exacerbating divergent attitudes, emotions, and behaviors. Polarization is a process in which people (or groups) move toward opposite extremes on some variable, such as beliefs about the seriousness of a disease threat (McCoy et al., 2018; Wu et al., 2022). Polarization can take many forms, including the emergence of extreme reactions to a crisis or the progressive widening of preexisting divisions. Polarized thinking is the tendency to think in terms of opposites (black-and-white thinking). Emotionally, polarization may be characterized by positive feelings toward one's in-group and distrust or hatred for out-groups (Gestefeld et al., 2022).

Most research on polarization has focused on political attitudes, but the range of polarized phenomena is broader. As we will see throughout this book, polarized extremes include the following:

- Excessive anxiety versus lack of concern (over- vs. under-reactions)
- Polarized attitudes about mitigation measures (pro vs. contra attitudes about masks, vaccines, and social distancing)
- Widening ideological and socioeconomic divisions (e.g., the wealthy vs. people living in poverty; liberals vs. conservatives)
- Increases in both religiosity and the wanton pursuit of pleasure
- Increases in both authoritarianism (e.g., insistence on regulations and strong leaders) and insistence on freedom from government control

There are many examples of over- and under-reactions to infectious threats (Honigsbaum, 2010; Taylor, 2022; Taylor et al., 2020). In the 1832 outbreak of cholera in London, many people became alarmed, while others denied the existence of the disease, dismissing concerns as "cholera humbug" promulgated by the government to divert public attention away from pressing social issues (Burrell & Gill, 2005, p. 479). In the course of the Russian flu, some people were excessively anxious—"they are so fully alive to the prospects of the spread of this ailment that they have almost passed into a state of panic where, after all, no panic is warranted" (London St. James Gazette, 1890, p. 19). Other people reacted oppositely, regarding the pandemic as "something almost too trivial for serious consideration" (p. 19).

Regarding the balance between over- and under-responding in the course of the Spanish flu, Dr. J. B. Anderson, a city health officer in Spokane, Washington, cautioned that people needed to recognize the difference between "wholesome fear of influenza" versus "morbid dread of the disease" (Spokane Daily Chronicle, 1918, p. 1). People were advised to "take every possible care to keep from getting the disease and to prevent its spread" without getting "hysterical over the problems of the epidemic" (p. 1).

As we will see in the chapters ahead, COVID-19 was associated with several kinds of extreme reactions. Some people became highly alarmed, while others thought the danger was exaggerated. Some sought safety from infection, while others sought freedom from restrictions. Various pro and contra groups emerged concerning masks, lockdowns, and vaccines, leading to conflicts and protests. There were acts of altruism and opportunism, along with the rise of piety (religious coping) and the pursuit of diverting pleasures. As discussed in later chapters, uncertainty and controversies about mitigation measures enabled and perpetuated some types of polarization.

Disease Characteristics That Trigger Public Alarm

Pandemics commonly evoke widespread fear, especially when the disease kills in painfully gruesome ways and afflicts all segments of society, including children and young adults (Snowden, 2019). However, disease virulence by itself—disease severity, debility, and lethality—is often insufficient to trigger widespread public alarm. Consider, for example, cancer and heart disease, which are highly prevalent and frequently lethal but rarely trigger widespread panic (Humphreys, 2002).

Several factors contribute to public alarm about infectious outbreaks, particularly the extent to which the disease is unfamiliar, unpredictable, swift-acting, and uncontrollable (Fung et al., 2011; Shryock, 1960; Taylor, 2022). Virulent infectious diseases are most likely to trigger widespread public fear when the following conditions are met:

- *Unfamiliar*: Diseases are more likely to be feared if they are associated with uncertainties about their course, mode of transmission, prevention,

and treatment (Chapter 2). Diseases with mild, familiar symptoms (e.g., cough, fever, runny nose) are less frightening than novel diseases producing unusual or dramatic signs or symptoms (e.g., suppurating lesions). But even familiar symptoms may be feared if they resemble those of pandemic infections, creating uncertainty about once-familiar bodily reactions ("Do I have a cold or is it COVID-19?").
- *Volatile and unpredictable*: Volatile, unpredictable diseases are frightening. These diseases are highly contagious, spreading swiftly with exponential growth, striking people suddenly and unexpectedly.
- *Uncontrollable*: People become alarmed when there are no sure ways of protecting themselves or loved ones, often resorting to quack cures and superstitious coping (Chapters 8, 16, and 17).
- *Lack of clear boundaries between danger and safety*: Diseases are frightening when there are no clear boundaries between safety and danger. Formerly safe places feel unsafe. All groups feel vulnerable, not just high-risk groups such as the elderly, poor, and infirm.
- *Disgusting*: Diseases elicit disgust by their signs or symptoms (e.g., diarrhea, vomiting, external hemorrhaging) and by their mode of transmission (e.g., transfer of fluids from sexual intercourse, drinking water contaminated with fecal matter). Disgust evokes a range of responses, including xenophobia, which amplifies the societally disruptive effects of pandemics (Chapter 15).
- *Stressful mitigation measures*: Stressful measures such as lockdowns adversely impact livelihoods and well-being (Chapters 6 and 19), adding a further layer of stress to the accumulating burden of adversity associated with pandemics.
- *Newsworthy*: Public alarm is amplified when the above-mentioned features are widely reported in the news media and social media (Chapter 10).

Widespread public alarm occurs more often when these factors are present. Some disease outbreaks, such as cholera, are associated with all these factors. COVID-19, which evoked widespread anxiety, was associated with most factors but without the degree of disgust seen in cholera and some other diseases. Diseases differ in their disgust value. Cholera and yellow fever are particularly disgusting. Cholera is associated with profuse vomiting and diarrhea. Yellow fever is associated with black vomit, consisting of foul-smelling, partially digested blood. Smallpox and mpox are characterized by prominent slimy, crusty, and fluid-filled skin lesions. Respiratory illnesses, such as influenza and COVID-19, are less dramatic in their disgust value, with coughing and sneezing being more common than vomiting and diarrhea.

Some pandemics were associated with few of the factors mentioned above and correspondingly low levels of public alarm. The 1968 influenza pandemic, for example, had few of these risk factors. The 1968 outbreak was more virulent than seasonal influenza. People from all social classes succumbed, and there was some media sensationalism (Economist, 1969; MacCarthy, 1969; Peckham, 2020). However, other risk factors for public alarm were largely absent. The disease (influenza) was not unfamiliar or unusually disgusting, and stressful mitigation methods such as lockdowns were not implemented. There was little evidence of public alarm (Honigsbaum, 2020b) and only scattered reports of panic buying of pharmacy supplies and food staples (Wilson et al., 2009).

Psychological Reactions to COVID-19 Versus Other Pandemics

Each pandemic or outbreak has distinctive characteristics, defined by the nature of the disease and its historical, scientific, sociocultural, and geopolitical context. Broad differences between COVID-19 and past pandemics, reviewed in detail in later chapters, are as follows:

- Differences in the scientific understanding of how infections are spread (e.g., miasma theory in which diseases were believed to be disseminated via "bad air" vs. modern germ theory).
- Prevailing views on protective measures (e.g., need to avoid night air vs. need for social distancing).
- The effects of the 24/7 news cycle and social media.
- Differences in medical management. Life-saving measures available for COVID-19 were absent in historical pandemics, such as intensive care hospitalization involving mechanical ventilation and treatments for secondary pneumonia.

Despite these differences, there were many similarities between COVID-19 and past pandemics, including the following: initial efforts of governments to downplay the seriousness of the outbreak to calm the populace and keep the economy running; the rise of anticipatory anxiety ahead of the arrival of infection in one's community; xenophobia, rumors, and conspiracy theories; panic buying and fleeing from infection hotspots; emotional disorders (e.g., anxiety, depression) arising or worsening; protests over pandemic-mitigation restrictions and related mandates; quack cures and profiteering; and sporadic protests and riots, but also acts of altruism as people come together to help one another.

Pandemic-related psychological phenomena—contemporary and historical—are characterized by four cross-cutting themes: uncertainty, fear, control, and conflict. The themes are associated with important issues, variables, concepts, and phenomena related to pandemics.

The first theme concerns uncertainty, which is an inherent aspect of pandemics from inception to end. People with high scores on particular personality traits tend to become highly distressed by uncertainty (Chapter 18). Central to understanding the effects of uncertainty are the concepts of prediction and control, which are relevant for understanding various pandemic-related psychological phenomena (e.g., reliance on quack cures, superstitious coping behaviors, and hygiene rituals).

The second theme concerns fear (and anxiety; the two overlap conceptually and phenomenologically). Fear is expressed in various ways, including fleeing, panic buying, and xenophobia. Fear extremes—too much or too little—each create problems. Some people develop excessive, debilitating fears. Others deny or downplay the threat and neglect health guidelines. Fear of death is prominent in pandemics, leading to increases in religious observances, nationalism, and other phenomena (Chapter 14). In infectious outbreaks, fear co-occurs with disgust, motivating people to escape or avoid disease cues (Chapter 15). Anxiety disorders may be triggered or worsened by pandemics (Chapter 19).

The third theme concerns control. When faced with novel pathogens, individuals cope with these invisible, uncertain threats in various ways, including coping strategies providing only an illusion of control (Chapter 17). Some people "disinfected" their groceries with sanitary towelettes during COVID-19, believing it kept them safe from the coronavirus. Wiping down groceries provided an illusion of control—a calming behavior of no protective value. Other personal protective measures—for example, handwashing with soap and water—offer better protection. The theme of control is further illustrated by pandemic-mitigation methods involving compulsory or strongly encouraged behaviors (e.g., wearing a mask, getting vaccinated). Nudges, mandates, and fear-evoking messages induce public adherence to mitigation measures (Chapter 5). Interventions for dealing with one problem (e.g., nonadherence) may worsen others (public anxiety) (Chapter 4).

The fourth theme concerns conflict. Two kinds of conflicts are discussed in this book: (1) internal conflicts, particularly the approach-avoidance conflict, which occurs when a person desires to help others but also fears infection; and (2) external conflicts between people over mitigation measures. External conflicts can arise from polarized attitudes concerning the necessity and safety of protective measures such as masks, vaccines, and social distancing. Conflicts can lead to protests and sometimes rioting. Most of the conflicts discussed in this book are the external type.

The themes are linked in various ways. Generally speaking, uncertainty exacerbates fear; fear leads to increasing demands for control measures; control measures lead to conflicts about their efficacy, necessity, and adverse effects; and conflicts can fuel uncertainty about the correct course of action. These and other links are explored in the chapters ahead.

Overview of the Following Chapters

This book is divided into four sections. Part I, comprising Chapters 1 to 9, covers pandemic-related psychological phenomena and the contexts in which they arise. Pandemic-mitigation measures are reviewed in detail because many of the psychological phenomena observed in pandemics emanate from the mitigation measures. The chapters in Part I describe the various psychological reactions to pandemics, including how people cope when threatened with infection and how people respond to government mandates concerning masks, vaccines, and social restrictions. These chapters highlight the many uncertainties associated with pandemics and how uncertainty is linked to fear, control efforts, and conflict.

Part II, comprising Chapters 10 to 18, focuses on the processes and mechanisms underlying the psychological phenomena seen in pandemics. Although there is no unified theory of the psychology of pandemics, theories from personality and social psychology, cognitive science, and allied disciplines have long been used to investigate and explain health-related phenomena. Cognitive and social processes and personality traits are surveyed concerning their relationship to emotions, beliefs, and behaviors during disease outbreaks. The effects of news and social media are reviewed, along with considerations of how information exposure can lead to attitude polarization. Also reviewed are cognitive decision-making mechanisms—heuristics and biases—which influence how people appraise and respond to disease threats. Rumors, conspiracy theories, and beliefs about sickness, health, and death are also discussed.

An entire chapter is devoted to death anxiety. Strategies for coping with death anxiety are somewhat different from other types of coping. When confronted with death, people often cope by affiliating themselves with groups or social institutions that are larger, more powerful, and more enduring than themselves. Thus, dealing with death anxiety leads to increases in nationalism, xenophobia, and religious observances (Chapter 14).

Some coping strategies, such as those based on magical thinking or self-serving cognitive biases, can alleviate anxiety while providing little or no protection against infection. Such strategies make people calmer but not safer. Chapters 16 and 17 discuss superstitious behavior and the illusion of control. Chapter 18 investigates the relationship between personality traits and pandemic-related psychological phenomena.

Part III (Chapters 19 to 22) focuses on mental health problems and their treatments. Of the four themes in this volume—uncertainty, fear, control, and conflict—Part III mostly concerns fear and associated problems. Anxiety disorders and other fear-related reactions are common in pandemics, along with other problems such as mood disorders, grief reactions, and substance abuse. There are various ways in which pandemics can worsen preexisting mental health problems and trigger new ones, including exposure to pandemic-related stressors (Chapter 19), the direct effects of infection (Chapter 20), and immunization-related stressors (Chapter 21). The final chapter in Part III explores important and innovative methods for preserving and strengthening the mental health of communities and healthcare workers during pandemics.

Part IV reviews the aftermath of pandemics and explores how we can prepare for future ones. Preparing for future disease outbreaks involves developing predictions, constructing scenarios, and recognizing and countering cognitive biases that can undermine pandemic preparation.

The present volume applies contemporary psychological concepts and empirical research to understand modern and historical pandemics. COVID-19 served as a major impetus for research into the nature and management of pandemic-related psychological problems—including issues concerning nonadherence and mental health—and for looking at ways of boosting the resilience of individuals and communities. These and other advances, placed in historical perspective, are examined in the following chapters, along with recurring challenges for pandemic mitigation, such as rumors, conspiracy theories, and polarized attitudes and behaviors. Armed with new insights, we can better prepare for future outbreaks of emerging and re-emerging infectious diseases.

2
Pandemic-Related Stressors

Introduction

To understand the psychological reactions to pandemics, we must consider the stressors people endure. A stressor is a disruptive force, event, or condition that requires some form of adjustment or adaptation. This chapter surveys the types of stressors arising in pandemics. The most apparent pandemic-related stressors involve exposure to infection and death, as well as socioeconomic hardships. Other, less-obvious stressors are also important to consider. Stressors can co-occur or pile up, forming an accumulating burden of adversity. Given the additive impacts of stressors, it is important to consider even mild stressors, especially if they are chronic.

Pandemic-related stressors differ in type, duration, and intensity. Some are low-grade and prolonged, such as lockdowns, while others are severe and sudden, such as infection-triggered emergencies. New stressors may emerge, and existing ones may worsen. Pandemics can disrupt routines significantly, posing challenges in adapting to changing circumstances. Additional stressors include extremes of social isolation and crowding, separation from loved ones, and the stress of chronic disease for people with post-viral syndromes.

In the following sections, we discuss particular types of stressors, beginning with uncertainty—a pervasive, abstract stressor. We then survey stressors that arise when societal infrastructures falter due to widespread illness, death, and fleeing. Trauma-related stressors are reviewed in addition to less apparent stressors such as stigma and disrupted social rituals. The chapter concludes by discussing the effects of stress on physical health. Pandemic-related stressors can dampen the immune system, potentially increasing one's risk of infection.

Uncertainty: A Pervasive, Abstract Stressor

People generally find uncertainty to be aversive, especially uncertainties concerning threats (Keren & Gerritsen, 1999). Pandemics entail all kinds of uncertainties. There is uncertainty about whether a disease outbreak will become a pandemic, how bad it will be, whether there are effective protective measures, how long it will last, who is infected (e.g., who is an asymptomatic carrier), and when to decide that the pandemic is over. Given that pandemics often come in waves, there is uncertainty about whether a pandemic has run its course.

The uncertainty of sickness and death pervades pandemics. Numerous historical examples illustrate the unpredictability of sudden infection-related death. In Paris in 1832, cholera-related deaths were seemingly random and often grotesque—"people fell down and died in the streets, their faces turned a frightening blue-violet from sudden massive circulatory collapse" (Morens, 2011, p. 528). Similarly, the plague could strike unexpectedly: "Some retired at night, apparently well, and were found dead next morning; some fell into a deep sleep from which they could not be roused; some were struck suddenly and died within a few hours" (Gowen, 1907, p. 7). The unpredictability of a swift, lethal infection was also a source of dread in the Spanish flu (Graves, 1969). Seemingly healthy young adults suddenly and unexpectedly perished from the flu (Pettigrew, 1983).

Messages from community leaders and health authorities influence uncertainty. Uncertainties are exacerbated when community leaders, health authorities, and experts are inconsistent or seemingly unreliable in their recommendations. Consider that the World Health Organization (WHO) recommended in early 2020 that asymptomatic people out in public should *not* wear masks because of COVID-19. For people without respiratory symptoms, the WHO stated that "a medical mask is not required, as no evidence is available on its usefulness to protect non-sick persons" (WHO, 2020a, p. 1). The WHO offered additional reasons for not wearing masks: Mask-wearing by the public would create a shortage of masks for healthcare workers (HCWs), and wearing masks would "create a false sense of security that can lead to neglecting other essential measures such as hand hygiene practices" (WHO, 2020a, p. 1).

Neither reason proved true. The public's wearing of cloth masks did not create a shortage of N95 or other medical-grade masks for HCWs. Individuals and small businesses manufactured cloth masks as needed. Wearing masks did not increase the rate at which people touched their faces (Chen et al., 2020). Mask-wearing did not lead to risk compensation, which is when doing one safe behavior (e.g., mask-wearing) leads to the reduction in other safety behaviors (e.g., handwashing, social distancing) (see Chapter 17).

Based on accumulating research, the WHO reversed its position later in 2020, strongly recommending mask-wearing (WHO, 2020b). However, uncertainties about masks persisted throughout the COVID-19 pandemic. A controversial review of the research found little clear evidence in support of mask-wearing by the general public, suggesting that the beneficial effects were uncertain (Jefferson et al., 2023). The use of masks is further discussed in Chapter 5.

Pandemics Strain the Fabric of Society

Pandemics strain societal infrastructures because of worker shortages due to sickness, death, and fleeing. Failing infrastructures give rise to a host of stressors. Healthcare systems may falter or collapse as clinics and hospitals become overwhelmed with the sick and dying. To illustrate the scope of the problem during COVID-19, a survey of 625 American hospitals found that most emergency departments (63%) experienced overcrowding, and 12% of hospitals had ventilator shortages, which impaired the ability to provide intensive care to severely ill patients (Sandhu et al., 2022).

As a result of sickness, death, and fleeing, there may be insufficient personnel for public sanitation, to care for the sick and dying, or to perform funeral services (Cohn, 2018; D'Irsay, 1927; Moote & Moote, 2004; Shryock, 1960; Slack, 1985). There may be coffin shortages and insufficient mortuary workers to prepare and inter the bodies (Johnson, 2006). Garbage may pile up in the streets due to shortages of sanitation workers (Schoch-Spana, 2004). In disease-depopulated towns, looting may occur (Lee, 1869; Nohl, 1926; Parets, 1651). Stores and markets may be shuttered—because of fleeing, sickness, death, or supply shortages—leading to food insecurity (i.e., insufficient or uncertain access to nutritious meals).

Pandemic-related food insecurity afflicts some groups more than others. During COVID-19, people in high-income countries such as the United States and Canada tended to gain weight while in lockdown, and many increased their consumption of recreational drugs and alcohol (Taylor et al., 2021). Meanwhile, people in developing countries such as Bangladesh experienced worsening food insecurity because of business closures and unemployment (Bhuiyan et al., 2020; Lin et al., 2021).

In other outbreaks, including the Spanish flu and the plague, there were reports of people starving because they were either too sick to procure food, lacked help in obtaining food, or because of food shortages (Barry, 2018; Cameron, 1996; Lee, 1869; Moote & Moote, 2004; Pettigrew, 1983; Slack, 1985; Thucydides, 431 BC). Food shortages arise in various ways, including panic buying, which creates short-term shortages even though the supply chain is intact. In other instances, food shortages are supply chain problems; worker absenteeism due to illness or fleeing may stall food production, and transportation workers may refuse to convey goods to infected regions.

Exposure to Death

Historical descriptions of pandemics and other outbreaks, including eyewitness accounts of plague, cholera, and influenza, make it clear that people were exposed to gruesome horrors (Anonymous, 1849; Butcher, 1855; Clapp, 1857; Lyon et al., 1919; Morens et al., 2008; Parets, 1651; Pearse, 2017; Schoch-Spana, 2004; Thucydides, 431 BC). The following are some examples.

When cholera swept Paris in 1832, thousands of bodies filled mass graves, sending a sickening stench over the city. Wagons carrying corpses were so hastily and shoddily constructed that they "spilled corpses, viscera, and putrid fluids into the streets" (Morens et al., 2008, p. 715). Furniture vans were requisitioned to remove thousands of bodies. Onlookers were "horrified to see layers of corpses piled upon them, claiming they heard cries and sobs coming from still-living victims" (p. 715).

In Constantinople, during the years 541–549 AD, graveyards overflowed due to the Plague of Justinian. City fortification towers were used to warehouse the bodies. Tower roofs were torn off, and the bodies were tossed inside:

> They piled them up just as each one happened to fall, and filled practically all the towers with corpses, and then covered them again with their roofs. As a result of this an evil stench pervaded the city and distressed the inhabitants still more, and especially whenever the wind blew fresh from that quarter. (Procopius, 551 AD, p. 126)

The massive rise in mortality led to the abandonment of previous socially prescribed methods of handling the dead. Necessity required that the dead be treated like objects to be processed in large-scale disposal operations. The diarist Miquel Parets, whom we met in Chapter 1, provided the following description from Barcelona in 1651, amid the second plague pandemic:

> For many days now eight or ten carts have travelled throughout Barcelona with the sole purpose of removing corpses from houses, which are often thrown from the windows to the street and then carried off in the carts by the grave diggers, who go about playing their guitars, tambourines, and other instruments in order to forget

> such great afflictions.... These grave diggers stop their carts at a street corner in the city and cry out for everyone to bring the dead from their houses, sometimes taking two from one house, four from another, and often six from another, and after filling their carts they would take the bodies to be buried in a field near the monastery.... Apart from these, some forty to fifty stretchers were used to carry those bodies which didn't fit in the carts, and it often happened that the grave diggers would carry dead babies or other children gravely ill with the plague on their backs. (Parets, 1651, pp. 106–107)

Attempts were made to protect the living from the sight of so much death. Efforts included removing the sick or dead from their homes and transporting them to pesthouses (plague hospitals) or burial grounds at night (Parets, 1651). When the dead were removed in daylight hours, attempts were made to conceal the corpse-laden carts from public view:

> Each cart was accompanied by a deputy of the plague warden whose job was to keep people out of the streets when the carts passed by. It was terrifying to see the carts.... To see them move through the streets filled with the dead, some fully dressed and others naked, some wrapped in sheets and others with only their shifts on, was a terrifying sight, and there were so many of them that anyone going through the streets constantly ran into them. (Parets, 1651, p. 55)

Caring for sick and dying loved ones is a further source of pandemic-related stress, as evident in Miquel's description of the difficulties tending to his wife, who was infected with the plague:

> When anyone fell sick, he lost all touch with friends and relatives, as there was no one who would risk contact with him, just the person nursing him.... My wife fell ill with a plague boil on her leg and another on her thigh, from which she died. And although she had two sisters in Barcelona, neither was willing to come to nurse her.... She wanted to talk with them and see them before she died, [but] there was no way to convince them to come, as everyone fled from the plague.... The sick had to find someone, man or woman, who would nurse them for pay ... all this could be accomplished only by paying money. (Parets, 1651, p. 55)

People adapt or grow accustomed—to some extent—to daily exposure to mass mortality (Butcher, 1855; Olson, 2002). In an 1883 cholera outbreak in Jacksonville, Illinois, an observer remarked that "to meet a man at night and attend his funeral in the morning has ceased to alarm, much less to surprise" (Olson, 2002, p. 9). However, not everyone grows accustomed to widespread, unpredictable death.

Pandemics Are Extended Hazardous Periods

The examples in the previous section describe disease outbreaks at their grisly worst. Observers and historians chronicled these dramatic examples. Less often documented were relatively more mundane periods in pandemics when people tried to go about their daily lives despite the constant threat of lethal disease. Pandemics per se are not traumatic stressors—not everyone is exposed to death or severe hardship. A pandemic is "an extended hazardous period" in which the risk of trauma is heightened (American Psychiatric Association, 2022, p. 306). The situation is analogous to military deployment to a conflict zone. Deployment in itself is not traumatizing but entails a heightened risk of encountering a life-threatening situation or witnessing injury and death. The longer the hazardous period—for example, the longer the pandemic or the more time spent in a combat zone—the greater the chances of experiencing trauma.

If pandemics are extended hazardous periods, then what counts as a pandemic-related traumatic stressor? The question is relevant for diagnosing post-traumatic stress disorder, which is discussed in later chapters. To diagnose the disorder, the person must be exposed to a traumatic stressor, as defined in the *Diagnostic and Statistical Manual of Mental Disorders*, Fifth Edition (DSM-5; American Psychiatric Association, 2022).

DSM-5 traumatic stressors are those involving exposure to actual or threatened death, serious injury, or sexual violence. A life-threatening illness or debilitating medical condition is "not necessarily considered a traumatic event" (American Psychiatric Association, 2022, p. 305). Traumatic medical events include "life-threatening medical emergencies (e.g., an acute myocardial infarction, anaphylactic shock) or a particular event in treatment that evokes catastrophic feelings of terror, pain, helplessness, or imminent death (e.g., waking in the midst of surgery, debridement of severe burn wounds, emergency cardioversion)" (p. 305).

For people exposed to pandemic-related deaths of close friends or loved ones, only a fraction of those experiences would meet DSM-5 criteria for trauma. If you learned that a loved one had passed away from an infectious disease, the event would be diagnosed as traumatic only if the death was violent, accidental, or "unnatural" (American Psychiatric Association, 2022, p. 305). A beloved elderly grandparent quietly slipping into a coma and peacefully passing away would be a sad loss for those left behind, but not a DSM-5 trauma.

The following example illustrates pandemic-related trauma, as experienced by the family members of COVID-19 patients. In Delhi, 2020, medical staff in one hospital ran out of medical oxygen and allegedly abandoned patients in an intensive care unit, leaving six to die. When family members arrived, the ward was deserted apart from the bodies of their loved ones. Videotape footage showed family members wandering about the unit, trying to rouse the patients. "Dead," said a man in one video, "dead—everyone" (Khare, 2021, p. 1). Meanwhile, doctors hid elsewhere in the hospital, fearing violence from distraught family members (Khare, 2021). The experience of discovering dead family members in an abandoned intensive care unit qualifies as a DSM-5 trauma.

Does vicarious exposure count as trauma? It depends. Watching the nightly television news of pandemic-related deaths may be upsetting, but it usually does not qualify as vicarious trauma unless one was personally involved in the news story. Personal involvement may be work-related. Vicarious exposure for emergency first responders counts as traumatic, as per DSM-5 criteria. Vicarious trauma exposure occurs when these workers experience repeated or extreme exposure to disturbing details of traumatic events from secondhand sources—for example, from co-workers, supervisors, the news, and social media.

Additional stressful events exacerbate the impact of traumatic stressors—that is, an accumulating burden of adversity (Taylor, 2017). For example, a person might be traumatized by a life-threatening illness requiring hospitalization and then, post-discharge, experience a slew of compounding stressors such as medical bills, unemployment, stigma because of being infected, and, in some cases, the stress of chronic disease—that is, the ongoing stressful effects of a post-viral syndrome or other residual illness.

Disrupted Rituals

Health-related threats are the most obvious stressors associated with pandemics. Many other, less-apparent stressors must be considered to appreciate what people go through during widespread disease outbreaks. Disrupted rituals are a source of distress. Social order is rooted in rituals, which may be religious or otherwise. Rituals are characterized by formality, pattern, sequence, and repetition (Kumar, 2013). Rituals provide a sense of meaning and social cohesion. Breakdown of society is evident in the loss or curtailment of social roles and rituals. In pandemics, people may be unable to attend religious festivals, birthday parties, graduation ceremonies, weddings, or funerals. They may be unable to bury or cremate the dead according to their cultural or religious customs.

Funeral rituals impart meaning and continuity to personal existence, provide social support, and ease the pain of losing loved ones. Such rituals may not always be possible when death is widespread. During COVID-19, India's crematoria were forced to skip individual ceremonies and religious rituals due to the unprecedented number of dead: "We are just burning bodies as they arrive," said one crematorium worker; "it is as if we are in the middle of a war" (Associated Press, 2021, p. 1). Elsewhere, funeral rituals were curtailed but not entirely suspended, as people attended services virtually via videoconferencing.

Stigma as Stressor

Disease-related stigma is a pervasive but under-appreciated stressor during infectious outbreaks. Stigma is a mark of social disgrace (Goffman, 1963). Disease-related stigma is blame-related, where specific people or groups are blamed for supposedly starting or spreading the infection. Disease-related stigma can be a widespread problem. According to a recent meta-analysis, a third of people experience some form of disease-related stigma or discrimination during infectious outbreaks (Yuan et al., 2022).

The nature of the infectious disease influences stigmatization, with some illnesses attracting more stigma than others. Diseases are more likely to be stigmatizing when they are highly contagious and potentially dangerous, have noticeable, disgusting lesions (e.g., large boils, weeping sores), and are seen as the victim's fault due to some action or inaction (Vega, 2016).

Infection-related stigma is likely greatest in situations where there are relatively few cases, as compared to situations in which almost everyone is infected. Ethnic minorities are commonly stigmatized in disease outbreaks, along with HCWs and people who have recovered from infection (Cohn, 2012; Markel, 2004). People may be blamed for their supposedly "dirty habits." For people who blame others, scapegoating provides an illusion of safety—a comforting but deceptive belief that one can stay safe by identifying and avoiding particular others.

Stigma has several harmful effects (Barrett & Brown, 2008; Crocker et al., 1998; Jäger et al., 1988; Schibalski et al., 2017). Stigma is stressful and alienating. People infected with a stigmatizing disease are liable to be shunned, avoided, and blamed. These individuals may be reluctant to disclose that they have a stigmatizing disease, thereby undermining their medical care. Stigma can be internalized; people may feel unduly guilty or ashamed if they or their social group have been blamed for spreading some infection (Cameron, 2014).

Examples of stigmatization include blaming people from Wuhan for COVID-19, blaming Jews in the Middle Ages for spreading the plague, and blaming the poverty-stricken for spreading cholera in the 19th century (Cohn, 2018; Rosenberg, 1987; Taylor, 2022). Stigma is not simply a matter of one ethnic group blaming another; it occurs within groups. Non-Wuhan Chinese stigmatized Wuhan residents during COVID-19 (Xu et al., 2021). At the outset of COVID-19, people in China sometimes referred to COVID-19 as "Wuhan pneumonia," attributing the disease (and stigma) to people specifically from Wuhan (Chang et al., 2020).

The problem of HCW stigmatization was highlighted during the 2003 SARS outbreak. At the time in Singapore, 49% of HCWs reported being stigmatized because of their potential contact with SARS patients (Koh et al., 2005). Meanwhile, in Taiwan, 20% of HCWs reported feeling stigmatized and rejected by their neighbors for the same reason (Bai et al., 2004). Survivors of SARS were also shunned, even though they had fully recovered (Cheng, 2004).

Early in the COVID-19 pandemic, fear of infection led to worldwide discrimination against HCWs, including ostracism by neighbors and friends, denial of access to shops and public transport, and verbal and physical abuse. A survey from Italy, for example, found that 25% of HCWs reported at least one episode of discrimination involving themselves, family members, or colleagues, and 11% reported more than 10 episodes (Cabrini et al., 2020). A community survey of over 3,500 adults from communities in Canada and the United States in the early months of COVID-19 found that 28% held stigmatizing attitudes toward HCWs, believing that these workers should not be allowed out in public because they could be infected (Taylor et al., 2020).

In the opening years of the HIV/AIDS pandemic—the mid-to-late 1980s—infected individuals were morally condemned for having the disease. They lost their jobs, were barred from attending schools, evicted from their homes, shunned by friends and family, and verbally or physically harassed (Bishop et al., 1991; Herek & Capitanio, 1993; Jäger, 1988; Nardi & Bolton, 1991; Sander, 1988; Tomes, 1999).

The ordeal of 13-year-old Ryan White is an egregious example of disease-related stigmatization (White & Cunningham, 1991). Ryan acquired HIV in 1984 after a blood transfusion for hemophilia. When people in his hometown of Kokomo, Indiana, learned of his HIV status, Ryan and his family were shunned. Rumors abounded, blaming Ryan's disease on poor home hygiene. Rumormongers claimed that Ryan deliberately spat on produce in the grocery store to spread the disease. Over 100 parents and 50 teachers signed a petition to ban Ryan from attending school. At church, Ryan and his family were asked to sit in a separate pew so the congregation could avoid his coughs. In the local diner, the owner reportedly made a waitress throw away the dishes Ryan and his family had used. Eventually, "the only people who would spend time with him were the reporters sent to cover his story for the national media" (Tomes, 1999, p. 256). Harassment and abuse persisted and intensified when Ryan insisted on attending high school. After a bullet was fired through the family's living room window, they moved to another town. Ryan's tragic life ended a few years later when he passed away from complications of HIV/AIDS.

Education programs are promising methods for reducing disease-related stigma (Chenneville et al., 2019; Frye et al., 2017; Gronholm et al., 2021; Lohiniva et al., 2016). Increased social contact with HIV-positive individuals tends to reduce the stigma regarding the disease (Chan & Tsai, 2017). Mental health professionals can help people cope with the stigma of disease (Prasad et al., 2020). For further details on pandemic-related stigma reduction, see Gronholm et al. (2021).

Stress and the Immune System

Stress has far-reaching effects, impacting emotional well-being and physical health. Pandemic-related stressors, especially protracted or severe stressors, can impair one's health even without getting infected with the pandemic pathogen. Research in psychoneuroimmunology shows that stressors can (1) increase susceptibility to infection by suppressing innate immunity responses, such as decreasing the function of T and B cells, (2) increase inflammation and associated responses, and (3) dampen the beneficial effects of vaccines (Bower et al., 2022; Irwin & Slavich, 2017; Kiecolt-Glaser, 2009). Conversely, social support is associated with enhanced T and B cell activity and lower inflammation. In other words, social support may buffer the adverse impact of stress on the immune response (Bower et al., 2022).

Immune responses to vaccines, including influenza vaccines, are delayed, substantially weakened, or shorter-lived in people exposed to stress (Glaser & Kiecolt-Glaser, 2005; Kiecolt-Glaser, 2009). These effects tend to be strongest in people prone to experiencing intense negative emotions in response to stressors—that is, people scoring high on a personality trait known as negative emotionality (Phillips et al., 2005). This personality trait is considered in more detail in Chapter 18.

Psychological interventions such as cognitive behavior therapy can reduce negative emotionality and increase stress resilience, potentially offsetting stress-related immunosuppression (Bower et al., 2022; Moraes et al., 2017). Yoga, tai chi, and mindfulness meditation may have similarly beneficial effects (Bower & Kuhlman, 2023). By countering the effects of stress, cognitive behavioral and other interventions might improve the immune response to vaccination (Bower et al., 2022)—that is, psychological interventions could help make vaccines more effective. Research is needed to investigate this theoretical possibility.

Conclusions

Pandemics entail a range of stressors, including widespread exposure to sickness and death. Dysfunctions or breakdowns in societal functioning—as indicated by strained or failing infrastructures—are further sources of stress. Other stressors include stigma and the disruption of social rituals. Uncertainty is a significant stressor that permeates pandemics. Uncertainty impacts people differently, although most find it aversive, especially concerning threats. Health authorities and other leaders can ease or worsen uncertainties, depending on their communications with the public.

In dealing with pandemic-related stressors, a robust pre-pandemic healthcare system is essential—one that can cope with large volumes of infection-related cases. With a robust healthcare system, health-related stressors can be reduced. In future pandemics, we can expect to see some or all of the stressors described in this chapter. Some stressors may be difficult to avoid. Business closures may be necessary, and social rituals may be unavoidably curtailed. Some of the uncertainties associated with pandemics can be reduced via risk communication, in which health authorities provide clear, consistent advice.

There is a two-way relationship between vaccination and the occurrence of stressors: Stressors can undermine vaccine efficacy, and community-wide vaccination programs can reduce the prevalence of stressors. Stress exposure can weaken immune responses, but much remains to be learned about how much stress affects the effectiveness of vaccination programs during large-scale outbreaks. That is, the magnitude of stress-related effects on vaccine efficacy needs to be determined. Also needed are investigations of whether stress reduction programs can facilitate vaccine efficacy.

Although stress can attenuate the effects of vaccines, some stressors can be subverted via vaccination. Vaccines are effective ways of reducing the odds of traumatic death-related events, including personally life-threatening experiences and the deaths of loved ones. When the risk of severe illness is reduced, hospitals and other healthcare services are less likely to be overwhelmed. Vaccination can also reduce illness-related worker absences, easing a disease outbreak's strain on societal infrastructure. At a societal level, vaccination may reduce or attenuate many of the pandemic-related stressors described in this chapter.

3
Pandemic-Mitigation Methods
An Overview

Introduction

There are two major, sometimes conflicting, goals of pandemic management: controlling infection while keeping the populace calm. This chapter presents an overview of contemporary and historical pandemic-mitigation methods. This discussion provides a foundation for subsequent chapters because many of the psychological phenomena described in this book are caused or amplified by pandemic-mitigation methods.

The chapter begins with germ and miasma theories of infectious diseases, illustrating how beliefs about diseases influence the types of mitigation measures used. The chapter then summarizes contemporary and historical methods for controlling pandemics. We conclude by examining which countries fared best regarding the COVID-19 pandemic. The relevant findings and expert consensus guidelines are used to identify promising and problematic methods for managing future pandemics.

Germ Theory and the Rise of Modern Methods

The distinction between germ theory and miasma theory illustrates how beliefs about diseases influence what people fear and the protective measures they take. Miasma theory has existed for centuries in one form or another (Tomes, 2010). The theory proposes that many diseases are caused by miasma—vapors and foul-smelling "bad air"—emanating from putrefying organic matter, particularly at night in the form of mists or fog (Baldwin, 2003; Cohn, 2008; Karamanou et al., 2012). Once exposed to miasma, a person might infect others by breath or touch—hence the use of lockdowns, quarantine, and cordon sanitaire in disease outbreaks. However, according to miasma theory, exposure to miasma rather than person-to-person contact was the primary source of infection. According to the 18th century physician

Richard Mead, "A corrupted state of air is without doubt necessary" (Mead, 1744, p. XXII).

Miasma theory was embedded in folk and religious beliefs about diseases (Byrne, 2006; Cohn, 2018; Elliott, 2024; Slack, 1985). Although miasma was seen as the main driver of infection, people also believed that other factors, including poor diet and intemperate (morally dissolute) habits, could directly cause infectious diseases.

Folk beliefs about diseases involve distal and proximal causal factors. Miasma, poor diet, and intemperate habits are proximal factors—factors thought to cause diseases directly. Distal factors are remote or indirect causes of proximal factors. Distal factors include the wrath of god(s) and celestial events such as the atmospheric disturbances caused by comets and other celestial bodies. In sum, before germ theory, it was commonly believed that miasma was an important proximal factor causing diseases, influenced by the distal actions of deities and astronomical or atmospheric events.

For people who believed in miasma theory, safety lay in avoiding or extirpating the sources of miasma and appeasing deities through religious supplication. Miasma theory led people to think that pleasant-smelling substances such as perfumes and aromatic herbs kept one safe by countering the effects of foul smells. Even some unpleasant smells from folk remedies were thought to drive away the miasmatic threat (Chapter 15). Social distancing was used—such as lockdown, quarantine, and cordon sanitaire—based on observations that once a person was affected by miasma, they could pass the disease on to others.

Today, pandemic-mitigation measures are based on germ theory, which states that microbial pathogens are the agents of infection and that diseases can be managed by neutralizing, removing, or avoiding the pathogens. Robert Koch's seminal work on germ theory became prominent in the 1880s, eventually replacing miasma theory as a scientific explanation for infection and disease.

Germ theory, like miasma theory, co-occurs with cultural and other folk beliefs about the causes of diseases. Germ theory explains proximal causal factors. Distal factors linked to germ theory include the actions of deities, such as beliefs that a disease outbreak is a divine punishment for collective sins. The religiously devout may believe in germ theory but see divine action as the distal driving force.

Germ and miasma theories were competing explanations when the Russian flu emerged in the late 19th century. Germ theory led to the search for the pathogen causing the Russian flu. Miasma theory had a greater impact on what people did to limit their risk of getting sick. Physicians recommended the avoidance of miasma and prescribed medications for symptomatic relief (e.g., quinine, antipyrine) (Charles River Editors, 2020; Tomes, 2010). Based on beliefs about the harmful effects of night air, people kept their windows closed, preferring to live in stuffy quarters rather than open their windows to the night air. This view on how infection spreads differed significantly from those expressed a couple of decades later in the Spanish flu, where the importance of fresh air was emphasized (Baldwin, 2003).

Compared to miasma theory, germ theory places greater emphasis on person-to-person contagion. Accordingly, germ theory led to greater emphasis on social distancing, handwashing, and covering coughs as essential interventions. Based on germ theory, public health authorities during the Spanish flu and COVID-19 implemented social distancing at unprecedented scales and made great efforts to get people to cover their coughs and sneezes (CDC, 2020; Tomes, 2010; WHO, 2021a). Although scientifically discredited, miasma theory continues to influence how people react to disease outbreaks, as discussed in Chapter 15 regarding olfactory cues to safety and danger.

Contemporary Mitigation Methods

Several contemporary methods are used to control disease outbreaks (Aiello et al., 2010; WHO, 2008, 2012, 2021b; WHO Writing Group, 2006). The methods, some used historically, are introduced here and discussed in more detail in subsequent chapters. When used alone, the interventions may be insufficient, so they are typically combined to manage pandemics (Haug et al., 2020).

- *Risk communication* from health authorities, informing the public about what they can do to stay safe.
- *Testing* people for infection, with results used for disease surveillance and statistical modeling of disease trends. Testing and surveillance enable health authorities to track and predict the progress of infection under various scenarios (e.g., with or without border closures). Testing also allows individuals to gain certainty about whether they are infected: Personal testing kits reduce uncertainty, at least temporarily, especially for diseases with ambiguous (nonspecific) symptoms.
- *Hygiene measures*, particularly hand hygiene, which includes handwashing with soap or hand sanitizer, covering sneezes and coughs (e.g., sneezing into the crook of one's arm), and hand awareness (i.e., refraining from touching one's eyes, nose, or mouth).

- *Face masks* worn in clinical and public settings.
- *Vaccines*, antiviral therapies, and other pharmacologic agents.
- *Social distancing*—social restrictions on movement and public congregation (e.g., remaining 6 feet apart in lines, closures of schools and businesses, quarantine, lockdowns, cordon sanitaire, border restrictions).
- *Measures to increase adherence* to the mitigation measures, such as nudges and mandates.

These methods are discussed in further detail in Chapters 4 to 6. Some measures have long been used in managing disease outbreaks, particularly social distancing and risk communication. The use of quarantine, lockdowns, and cordon sanitaire, for example, dates back to the second plague pandemic (Chapter 6). Masks and vaccines have been used for over a century (Chapter 5). Hygiene measures such as handwashing rose to prominence with the emergence of the modern hygiene movement early in the 20th century (Tomes, 1999). Testing and surveillance using digital technology are more recent endeavors, although these methods have their origins in efforts centuries earlier to determine whether a person was liable to infect others, as discussed in later chapters concerning acclimation and immunity passports.

According to an extensive review of non-pharmaceutical interventions for managing outbreaks of infectious respiratory diseases, the most effective methods are various kinds of social distancing, such as small gathering cancellations and closures of educational institutions (Haug et al., 2020). Lockdowns of entire communities were rated as moderately effective. The efficacy of masks and vaccines is discussed in Chapter 5.

Regarding handwashing, a meta-analysis found that handwashing reduced the incidence of respiratory infections by 14%, "suggesting a probable benefit" (Jefferson et al., 2023, p. 2). For everyday handwashing outside medical settings, there is no compelling evidence that alcohol-based hand sanitizers are more effective than plain soap and water in preventing respiratory or diarrheal diseases (Hoffmann et al., 2021; Jefferson et al., 2023; Wolfe et al., 2017).

People often neglect to follow hygiene recommendations, especially if no one else is watching (Pfattheicher et al., 2018). A systematic review of 96 studies found that 40% of people fail to wash their hands after toilet use (Erasmus et al., 2010). A British study of rail and bus commuters found that 28% had fecal bacteria on their hands (Judah et al., 2010). During the swine flu pandemic and COVID-19, people who viewed themselves as having a low risk of infection were less likely to wash their hands (Gilles et al., 2011;

Taylor et al., 2020). Nonadherence is a common problem in managing infectious diseases. Accordingly, various strategies for boosting adherence, such as nudges and mandates, are frequently used, as discussed in later chapters.

The mitigation methods described above have been applied mainly to outbreaks of respiratory infections, such as influenza and coronavirus diseases. The methods can be modified for other diseases, depending on how infection is spread. Infections spread by contaminated water (e.g., cholera) can be managed by public sanitation, hand awareness (e.g., keeping hands away from one's mouth), and oral rehydration therapy. Diseases transmitted via bodily fluids (e.g., HIV, syphilis, and Zika) can be prevented by practicing safe sex, using prophylactic drugs, and other ways. Protective measures for insect-borne infections (e.g., Zika and yellow fever) include insect repellants, insecticides, and protective clothing and coverings (CDC, 2024).

Dual Goals of Pandemic Management

The broad goals of pandemic management are (1) to encourage people to take the pandemic seriously and follow the recommended pandemic-mitigation methods and (2) to implement these measures without precipitating mass panic, adverse mental health effects, or widespread protest. Mitigating pandemics involves balancing public safety with individual freedom. Keeping people safe involves temporarily curtailing personal liberties.

Health authorities often emphasize the first goal over the second. When nonadherence becomes a problem, governments and health authorities have responded in various ways, including nudges, shaming, mandates, threats, and fines. In the course of the Spanish flu in Chicago, Police Commissioner Robertson announced that officers would "arrest thousands if necessary to stop sneezing in public" (Chicago Herald and Examiner, 1918, p. 11). Dr. J. B. Anderson, city health officer for Spokane, Washington, also during the Spanish flu, declared that "the man or woman who allows himself or herself to contract influenza when the disease might have been prevented ... is a menace to the community and should be treated as such" (Spokane Daily Chronicle, 1918, p. 1).

In the same pandemic, Dr. Royal S. Copeland, New York City health commissioner, offered a different perspective, emphasizing the importance of keeping people calm amid a public health crisis. Dr. Copeland believed that one of his primary responsibilities was "to prevent panic, hysteria, [and] mental disturbance" (New York Times, 1918, p. 42). Although social distancing was implemented, he wanted people "to be able to go about their business without constant fear and hysterical sense of calamity" (p. 42). Copeland emphasized the importance of not closing places of entertainment, such as movie theaters, despite the risk of superspreading: "I found that movies kept the minds of the people off the subject of flu and death" (Robins, 2005, pp. 153–154). According to Copeland, "To combat sickness successfully, a doctor has to be something of a psychologist" to preserve the public's mental health and to maintain hope (p. 154).

The goals of reducing mortality while protecting mental health are sometimes at odds with one another. To illustrate, if many people are not taking a disease outbreak seriously—for example, not adhering to social distancing guidelines—health authorities might resort to fear-evoking messages to increase compliance. This approach is commonly used in health promotion campaigns such as anti-smoking initiatives. The problem is that fear-evoking messages can exacerbate fears in people already terrified of infection (Chapter 4). Tackling one problem (nonadherence) can exacerbate another (distress).

Stemming the spread of infection and managing mental health are also at cross-purposes when social restrictions are implemented over long periods (e.g., weeks or months). Humans are social animals. Social distancing and related methods require people to inhibit their inclinations to socialize. As social-distancing mandates are drawn out over time, a form of burnout known as pandemic fatigue can emerge, and adherence to social distancing tends to deteriorate (Chapter 6).

COVID-19: Which Countries Fared Best?

Pandemic mitigation can be done in various ways, involving some mix of the measures described above. What are the most promising combinations? We can look to COVID-19 for insight. There have been several attempts to determine which countries did well or poorly throughout COVID-19. Most were piecemeal efforts, looking at only a subset of relevant variables (e.g., case fatality rates across countries at a given time). The most comprehensive attempt to chart the relative progress of countries was conducted by the Bloomberg media company. Their COVID Resilience Ranking, published monthly from November 2020 to June 2022, amid the worst of the pandemic, scored the largest 53 economies on their success at containing COVID-19 with the least amount of social and economic disruption (Bloomberg, 2022a, 2022b).

Eleven indicators (variables) were constructed for each country based on data from various sources. The indicators were summed to form the Bloomberg Resilience Scale, whereby countries were ranked according to their score. The indicators assessed three domains:

- *Reopening progress*: Four indicators (e.g., vaccine uptake, lockdown severity).
- *COVID-19 status*: Three indicators (e.g., number of COVID-19 deaths per million since the start of the pandemic).
- *Quality of life*: Four indicators, including measures of economic growth and strength of the healthcare system.

Consistently low-ranking (poor outcome) countries were Indonesia, the Philippines, Pakistan, Mexico, and Brazil. While China was not low-ranking, it was criticized because its stringent restrictions to drive COVID-19 cases to zero had the effect of "paralyzing economic growth and fomenting social unrest" (Bloomberg, 2022a, p. 1).

Consistently high-ranking countries throughout the survey were the United Arab Emirates, South Korea, Canada, Finland, and Norway. Top-ranking countries tended to accept the coronavirus as being here to say—that is, they avoided the stringent lockdowns characteristic of China's zero-COVID policy—and successfully implemented vaccination programs. South Korea avoided stringent lockdowns by using a test-trace-isolate approach involving digital surveillance.

The Bloomberg survey has strengths and weaknesses. The survey provided a detailed longitudinal picture of how COVID-19 played out from 2020 to 2022. However, the methodology has been criticized, including objections that economic impacts were overemphasized and mental health was given insufficient weighting (Ruikang, 2021). Accordingly, the findings must be interpreted with caution. Nevertheless, the Bloomberg results are consistent with a consensus survey on the management of COVID-19 from 386 experts in healthcare and related fields (Lazarus et al., 2022).

The consensus survey emphasized the importance of risk communication, building public trust, and encouraging community involvement in decision-making while also implementing established measures, particularly vaccines, as part of a comprehensive approach involving testing and surveillance, masks, and social distancing. Reliance on vaccines alone was not recommended because of various limitations, including problems of waning immunity, inequitable access, and vaccination hesitancy

(Lazarus et al., 2022). These recommendations underscore the importance of understanding and engaging the public in pandemic management.

Conclusions

Pandemic-mitigation methods are based on prevailing beliefs about how diseases spread. Based on germ theory, contemporary strategies for managing pandemics include disease testing and surveillance, risk communication, vaccines, face masks, hygiene practices, and social restrictions. None of these methods is sufficient alone, so they are typically combined. Highly restrictive measures such as lockdowns are moderately effective but unpopular and subject to nonadherence.

Pandemic mitigation highlights the four cross-cutting themes of this volume: uncertainty, fear, control, and conflict. Risk communication reduces uncertainty and can increase or decrease fear, depending on the message (Chapter 4). Public nonadherence to mitigation measures is a common problem, undermining control efforts (Chapters 5–6). Conflicts commonly arise concerning the necessity and efficacy of pandemic control measures, such as face masks and vaccinations (Chapter 5). Unpopular mitigation measures are especially prone to nonadherence and can lead to protests and sometimes riots (Chapter 7). Governments often respond to nonadherence and protests by redoubling their control efforts, including threats, fines, and incarceration (Chapter 7). These issues are examined in further detail in the chapters ahead.

4
Risk Communication

Introduction

The purpose of this chapter is to discuss the uses and effects of risk communication. A vital part of pandemic mitigation, risk communication is when health authorities and other community leaders inform the public, via news reports or public announcements, about the degree of risk posed by an infectious outbreak and what precautions should be taken. Risk communication involves giving people the information they need to make informed decisions about protecting their health and safety. Relevant information may include advice about hygiene practices, social distancing, mask-wearing, and vaccination, and advisories about strategic closures of places of congregation such as bars, restaurants, places of amusement (e.g., cinemas), schools, and churches.

The chapter begins by discussing guidelines for risk communication. The use of fear-evoking messages is then reviewed, including concerns about their adverse effects. The chapter then considers the psychological implications of the names given to diseases. The names we give to diseases influence how people perceive and respond to infectious threats. The adverse effects of disease names are considered, and recommendations for naming diseases are reviewed.

Guidelines for Risk Communication

The following risk communication guidelines were developed by the World Health Organization (WHO, 2005, 2008):

1. Announce the outbreak early, even with incomplete information, to limit the spread of rumors and misinformation.
2. Provide specific information about what the public can do to stay safe.
3. Maintain transparency to ensure public trust. Acknowledge uncertain and controversial issues and assure the public that efforts are being made to resolve these problems.

4. Demonstrate that efforts are being made to understand the public's views and concerns about the outbreak.
5. Evaluate the impact of communication programs to ensure the messages are correctly understood, and advice followed.

A review of the risk communication literature, including studies of Ebola, Zika, and yellow fever outbreaks, shows that a one-size-fits-all approach to messaging is not optimal and that community input is vital (Toppenberg-Pejcic et al., 2019). Local communities should be involved in crafting and disseminating risk communication messages. Messages can be devised for particular demographic groups to address specific issues—for example, messages targeting young people about the importance of social distancing. Over time, the public may tune out often-repeated messages. Periodically revised messages may be needed to maintain public engagement and cooperation. Social media is also a venue for risk communication, but the impact must be monitored.

Fear-Evoking Messages

Governments may be reluctant to announce the arrival of a dangerous disease or even fail to disclose an impending outbreak for fear that the news could lead to mass panic (Tomes, 2010; WHO, 2005). Mass panic refers to widespread public anxiety, as seen in episodes of panic buying and sudden bursts of fleeing from infection hotspots (Chapters 8 and 9). Governments and health authorities in several pandemics—the Russian flu, Spanish flu, and COVID-19—also expressed concern that while some people were overreacting to the outbreak, others were underreacting by not taking it seriously (Taylor, 2022; Tomes, 2010). Essentially, the message that governments sought to convey was "don't panic but take the outbreak seriously." However, the result was often confusion. Throughout the Spanish flu, it made sense to urge people to remain calm and not misinterpret cold symptoms as incipient influenza, yet this "don't panic" message "surely contributed to public confusion about exactly how scared people should be" (Tomes, 2010, p. 53).

Despite concerns about causing undue alarm, governments and health authorities continue to use fear-evoking messages in measured doses to influence health-related behaviors. Fear-evoking messages were used during COVID-19 to encourage people to adhere to social distancing, mask-wearing, and other guidelines. Some critics claimed the messages frightened people excessively (Dodsworth, 2021). For fear-evoking messages to be effective, the risk must be perceived as credible—not over- or understated—and should contain a balance of reassuring and fear-inducing information (Nerlich & Halliday, 2007). Messages evoking fear are most likely effective in promoting health behaviors if the threat is perceived as high *and* the person believes they can do something to deal with it (Peters et al., 2013).

Frightening people without giving them any means of protecting themselves leads to defensive reactions such as denying the severity of the threat—for example, disparaging government health warnings (Goldenberg & Arndt, 2008). Messages should be pilot-tested because they can backfire. For example, panic buying may be triggered by informing people to stock up because of an impending lockdown (Chapter 8).

Naming Diseases: Labels Matter

Risk communication about a disease threat requires that the disease has a name. Giving a novel disease a name makes it seem more familiar, knowable, and potentially controllable. Successfully managing pandemics involves the careful choice of names. Past outbreaks were routinely named after animal vectors (e.g., swine flu, avian flu), demographic groups, or places where the pathogen was first identified. The Zika virus was named after the Zika Forest in Uganda. The Ebola virus was named after the Ebola River in the Democratic Republic of the Congo. Lassa virus was named after the Nigerian town of Lassa. Lyme disease was named after the Connecticut town of Lyme. The Hendra virus was named after the suburb of Hendra, in Brisbane, Australia. According to an article published in *Science*, Dr. Linfa Wang, the infectious disease expert who named the Hendra virus in 1994, "still gets angry calls from residents complaining that the name hurts property values" (Kupferschmidt, 2015, p. 745).

Sexually transmitted diseases are sometimes given ill-advised names, either by the public, health researchers, or health authorities. Examples include monkeypox—renamed mpox in 2022—and early terms for HIV/AIDS, such as "gay-related immunodeficiency disease" and "gay compromise syndrome" (Altman, 1982; Brennan & Durack, 1981; Nick, 2021; WHO, 2022). Early terms for syphilis provide further examples. Emerging in the late 15th century, syphilis did not acquire its current name until the mid-19th century. Before that, it was commonly named after foreigners or enemy nations—that is, naming as blaming. Eponymously naming syphilis after an enemy nation became a universal trope, at least among the public (Abel, 2018). The French named it after the Italians (e.g., the "Neapolitan evil"), the English called it the "French disease," and the Polish called it the "German disease." In Russia, it was called the "Polish disease." Among the Portuguese, it was called the "Castilian disease," and the Moors in North Africa called it the "Spanish evil" (Abel, 2018).

Names such as swine flu and Spanish flu have become standard labels for pandemics. However, such terms should be used with caution. Naming diseases after groups of people, places, or specific animals can have unintended consequences in a disease outbreak, including impacts on trade, travel, tourism, food consumption, and animal welfare. Naming diseases after animals has led to the needless culling of livestock (Taylor, 2019).

Poorly chosen disease names can lead to public misconceptions, discrimination, and conflict. Consider, for example, the diplomatic incident over the naming of what came to be called swine flu. The early cases originated in Mexico. According to a report in *The Guardian*, an Israeli health minister raised objections to the label "swine flu" because of Jewish and Muslim sensitivities over pork. The alternative "Mexican flu" was suggested by the Israeli minister, claiming "the advantage of sparing Jews and Muslims discomfort" (Pilkington, 2009, p. 1). Not surprisingly, Mexico's ambassador to Israel vehemently protested, pointing out the potentially harmful effects of the proposed name on Mexico and Mexicans. The idea was dropped—the outbreak became known to the public as swine flu.

The problem did not end there. Pork sales in the United States and China declined amid fears of swine flu, and pork imports were banned in some countries (Business North Carolina, 2010; Kupferschmidt, 2015; Wilson, 2009). Misconceptions were widespread, particularly the erroneous belief that swine flu could be acquired by eating pork (Kanadiya & Sallar, 2011; Kaur et al., 2015; Singh et al., 2013; Viveki et al., 2012).

A similar situation arose in a 2005 avian flu outbreak, due to the name given to the disease. Poultry sales plummeted in the United States because of the misguided belief that preparing and eating chicken caused avian flu (Evans & Bartholomew, 2009). Kentucky Fried Chicken, the National Chicken Council, and the US Poultry and Egg Association reassured consumers that chicken and eggs were safe to eat (MacArthur & Thompson, 2005; National Chicken Council, 2021).

Given the concerns about the names given to diseases, readers may ask why this book uses the following disease names: Spanish flu, Russian flu, swine flu, avian flu, Zika virus disease, and Ebola virus disease. Several factors determined the choice. The terms are widely used, well-known, and standard in some fields. The alternatives would be unfamiliar and potentially confusing to readers. Names could be replaced with dates—for example, relabeling the Russian, Spanish, and swine flu outbreaks as the 1889, 1918, and 2009 pandemics—but the profusion of dates would likely make the text difficult to follow.

A further problem is that sometimes we need to know the common names—for example, "swine flu"—to understand the ensuing psychological effects (e.g., fear and aversion to pork). There are no widely used alternatives for some diseases that refer to places (e.g., Ebola and Zika virus diseases). Sticking with these original names seemed easier for reader comprehension, at least for the historical outbreaks reviewed in this volume. However, caveats remain concerning the naming of future or ongoing disease outbreaks.

Naming the Next Pandemic

In 2015, the WHO released guidelines to "minimize unnecessary negative impact of disease names on trade, travel, tourism or animal welfare, and avoid causing offence to any cultural, social, national, regional, professional or ethnic groups" (WHO, 2015, p. 1). According to the guidelines, names should use (1) generic descriptors of symptoms or signs (e.g., terms such as respiratory or hemorrhagic), (2) specific terms describing patients, epidemiology, or the environment (e.g., seasonal, juvenile, coastal), and (3) pathogen names (e.g., H1N1).

The WHO recommended that disease names should not include strongly fear-evoking terms such as "unknown" or "fatal," although the term "severe" is acceptable (WHO, 2015). Pathogen novelty influences the degree of perceived threat; newly discovered pathogens (e.g., SARS-CoV-2) tend to be perceived as more threatening than well-known pathogens (e.g., measles virus) (White et al., 2014). Accordingly, pandemics and their causative agents are more likely to be perceived by the public as threatening if their name emphasizes the newness of the threat; for example, "novel coronavirus" is a more threatening label than mere "coronavirus."

When the next pandemic arrives, health authorities must assess the implications of disease labels. If the pandemic is mild and mostly harmless, give it a benign name (e.g., "Three-Day Fever"). If the pandemic is severe, a fear-evoking name could be used, but if the label is too dramatic, some people will become unduly anxious, while others might dismiss the threat as overblown.

For some types of severe disease, giving it a fear-evoking label has little or no value. Consider the encephalitis lethargica (EL) pandemic (1915–1927), the world's first neuropsychiatric pandemic. EL typically began with flu-like symptoms followed by stupor, persistent sleepiness, oculomotor disturbances, and other symptoms (Giordano et al., 2020). The pathogen was never discovered. There was no cure or apparent means of protecting oneself from the disease. To the public, EL was known by the innocuous epithet "sleeping sickness." Dr. Royal S. Copeland, well-known for his role in managing the Spanish flu, proposed that EL be called "epidemic coma," implying a severe disease (Copeland, 1923). Indeed, EL was serious, but what was the point in highlighting the threat of a serious, uncontrollable, and largely unpredictable disease? Renaming EL as "epidemic coma" did nothing for pandemic mitigation but could cause public anxiety. "Sleeping sickness" was a widely used label that understated the seriousness of the affliction but did not put people in danger or hamper pandemic mitigation—because EL could not be mitigated. Dr. Copeland's proposal did not catch on. EL is discussed in further detail in Chapter 20.

Conclusions

Risk communication is essential for encouraging people to perform protective behaviors during pandemics, such as social distancing, mask-wearing, and vaccination. Good risk communication is clear, specific, and balanced. It alerts people to infectious dangers and informs them of ways of avoiding harm. Risk communication is vital to pandemic mitigation but fraught with challenges, including issues concerning fear-evoking messages and the naming of diseases.

Fear-evoking messages are commonly used in health promotion campaigns and during disease outbreaks. Evoking fear to induce compliance can backfire, making some people excessively anxious while others dismiss the threat as overstated. Health authorities sometimes worry about mass panic—that is, panic buying or fleeing—when people learn of a dangerous infection sweeping the community. Accordingly, it may be necessary to pilot-test some messages to avert unintended effects. There are also ethical concerns about frightening people excessively to compel their cooperation. Fear-evoking messages are most likely to work if the threat is perceived as credible and tied to protective behaviors that the person believes they can perform.

5
Face Masks and Vaccines

Introduction

Vaccination and protective face masks are widely used contemporary methods for limiting the spread of infection. However, vaccines and masks are also sources of contention, nonadherence, and conflict. This chapter examines the nature of opposition to mask-wearing and vaccination in disease outbreaks. Our focus is on nonclinical settings, such as mask-wearing in public places where people congregate.

The chapter begins with a historical discussion of face masks, including comparisons between COVID-19 and the Spanish flu. Although separated by over a century, these pandemics were remarkably similar in terms of objections to mask-wearing. We then consider vaccines and related pharmacologic measures, followed by a review of vaccination hesitancy and anti-vaccination attitudes. Vaccine hesitancy is one of the world's leading health threats (WHO, 2019; Yaqub et al., 2014). The chapter concludes by reviewing methods for improving adherence to masks and vaccines.

Face Masks

Protective facial and body coverings have long been used to safeguard wearers from disease. The iconic 17th-century plague doctor costume is a widely known historical example. The garb—essentially a HAZMAT suit from the early modern period—consisted of an ankle-length protective cloak, leather gloves, wide-brimmed leather hat, goggles, boots, cane, and beak-shaped full-face mask. The pointed beak, containing aromatic herbs to counter the effects of miasma, gave rise to the epithet *Dr. Schnabel* ("Dr. Beak"). According to 17th-century satirists, the costume did nothing but terrify people (Townsend, 1965). Some historians doubt whether doctors ever wore the experimental garb (Mattie, 2023). If used, it may have offered some protection as it shielded the user from the aerosol expectorate, bodily fluids, and fleas.

Modern personal protective equipment for healthcare workers—scrubs, gloves, face shield, and mask—bears little resemblance to the 17th-century beaked costume. Contemporary hospital-grade face masks (e.g., N95 masks) are essential for stemming the spread of infection in clinical settings. However, scientific evidence is mixed concerning the efficacy of cloth and N95 masks for everyday use by the public (Jefferson et al., 2023).

Jefferson and colleagues concluded that "compared with wearing no mask in the community studies only, wearing a mask may make little to no difference in how many people caught a flu-like illness/COVID-like illness ... and probably makes little or no difference in how many people have flu/COVID confirmed by a laboratory test" (p. 4). However, given the limitations of the research studies, the authors acknowledged that "there is uncertainty about the effects of face masks" (p. 3). The effectiveness of masks for COVID-19 was hotly debated, partly because of the equivocal evidence (Taylor & Asmundson, 2021).

The empirical research on face masks worn by people in public spaces can be interpreted in two ways. Either the research is flawed, as some critics suggest (MacIntyre et al., 2023), or the studies indicate that masks provide limited protection when used in public—possibly effective in some situations but not others. Logically, mask-wearing in congested, ill-ventilated public places should confer some protection from respiratory infections. In situations where the risk of infection is low—such as shopping in an empty store, walking down a deserted street, or driving solo in one's car—mask-wearing offers no benefit beyond an illusion of protection.

The Anti-Mask League

Adherence to wearing protective face masks is influenced by the meaning people attach to them. Positive attitudes include mask-wearing as a sign of safety and civic virtue. Negative beliefs include misgivings about the efficacy of masks and unfavorable attitudes toward mask-wearers. Mask-wearing may be interpreted as a sign of fear, weakness, conformity, or possible infection (Siu, 2016; Taylor & Asmundson, 2021). People with predominantly negative views are reluctant to wear masks. Social factors influencing mask-wearing include peer pressure, nudges, and mandates (Taylor & Asmundson, 2021).

Mask-wearing in public places was a prominent part of pandemic mitigation in the Spanish flu and COVID-19 (and, to a lesser extent, in SARS).

Opposition to mask-wearing from a vocal minority arose in the course of the Spanish flu in San Francisco when authorities attempted to make mask-wearing mandatory in public places. People failing to don masks—"mask slackers," as they were called—were threatened with fines or jail (Oakland Tribune, 1918; San Francisco Chronicle, 1918; San Francisco Examiner, 1918). In 1919, the Anti-Mask League was formed, a short-lived protest movement in which proponents argued that masks were inconvenient and ineffective and that mandatory mask-wearing violated their civil rights (Dolan, 2020).

During COVID-19, most people complied with guidelines about wearing masks in public places. However, there was also attitude polarization, with people tending to align themselves with either the pro-mask majority or the anti-mask minority (Lang et al., 2021). In their analysis of mask-related Twitter hashtags relating to COVID-19, Lang and colleagues found "stark rhetorical polarization in terms of semantic antagonism between pro- and anti-mask hashtags" (p. 1). In other words, the most prevalent mask-related hashtags were emotionally charged and tended to be either strongly in favor—for example, #MaskItOrCasket—or adamantly against—#MasksAreForSheep—with the pro group being the largest.

Conflicting attitudes about masks sometimes led to verbal or physical altercations between "maskers" and "anti-maskers" during COVID-19. The reasons identified for refusing to wear masks in the coronavirus pandemic were much the same as those expressed by the Anti-Mask League a century earlier: objections that masks are uncomfortable, perceived to be inefficacious, and that mandatory mask-wearing violated one's rights concerning personal freedom (Taylor & Asmundson, 2021). People with particular personality traits are especially likely to object to compulsory mask-wearing and other mandates, as discussed in Chapter 18.

Vaccines, Antivirals, and Antibiotics

Developing vaccines for infectious diseases is costly and time-consuming. Most experimental vaccines are ineffective, with a 90% failure rate (Gouglas et al., 2018). Vaccines conferring lifelong immunity have been developed for smallpox but not for coronaviruses or influenza. In the Spanish flu, experimental vaccines were developed on the erroneous assumption that the infection was bacterial (Pettigrew, 1983). Many of these vaccines were available to the public, creating confusion as to which, if any, might be beneficial (Heagerty, 1919).

Later vaccines—targeting viruses—were used in subsequent influenza outbreaks. These vaccines offered valuable but incomplete protection, with benefits waning over time. Vaccines were not available for SARS. For COVID-19, the coronavirus will likely never be globally eradicated because of incomplete vaccination coverage, viral variants that elude vaccines, and the widespread presence of the coronavirus, which has been documented in many animals, including domestic dogs and cats (Skegg et al., 2021). Just like seasonal influenza, annual shots are required for COVID-19.

In addition to vaccines, antiviral medications are used to treat influenza and other infections and to provide prophylaxis for exposed individuals. Antivirals, particularly neuraminidase inhibitors such as oseltamivir (Tamiflu), may be effective against the next strain of pandemic influenza because of the track record of these drugs in previous influenza outbreaks (Beard et al., 2018). However, their efficacy is not guaranteed because of the possible emergence of resistant strains. Population-based simulation studies suggest that, under certain conditions, neuraminidase prophylaxis could have paradoxical effects, promoting the occurrence and transmission of neuraminidase-resistant strains of influenza (Eichner et al., 2009).

People hospitalized for viral infection sometimes develop secondary, hospital-acquired bacterial pneumonia. The latter complicates treatment and increases mortality (Morens et al., 2010). Most (95%) postmortem samples from the Spanish flu revealed bacterial infection, and most deaths likely resulted from secondary pneumonia caused by common upper respiratory tract bacteria (Morens et al., 2008). Therefore, antibiotics will likely be critical in managing future viral pandemics. An issue of concern is the rise of antibiotic-resistant bacteria. The growing prevalence of such bacteria could increase the death toll of future pandemics, even if those pandemics are viral in origin (Megiddo et al., 2019).

Vaccines are essential for reducing morbidity and mortality for seasonal and pandemic influenza (Alcalde-Cabero et al., 2016; Babcock et al., 2014; CDC, 2018; WHO, 2012). Vaccines might not be suitable for everyone, and there is a risk of adverse effects such as Guillain Barré syndrome. However, such complications are rare. It has been estimated that only one or two new cases of Guillain Barré syndrome occur for every million vaccine doses for seasonal influenza (CDC, 2018). Complications from COVID-19 vaccines were rare despite more than 12.7 billion doses administered worldwide (Bloomberg, 2022; CDC, 2023b). Vaccination stress-related reactions are surveyed in Chapter 21.

Vaccination Hesitancy

"Vaccination hesitancy" is a broad term encompassing indecision, reluctance, and refusal to receive vaccination despite evidence of vaccine safety and efficacy. Vaccination-hesitant people include adamant refusalists and those who are amenable in principle but, for various reasons, are reluctant or slow to accept vaccination. In many pandemics and outbreaks—including the plague, cholera, Russian flu, and the SARS epidemic—vaccination hesitancy was not an issue because there were no vaccines. For diseases for which vaccines are available, vaccination hesitancy is a significant obstacle to infection control and eradication. Objections against vaccination raised in the past are similar to those today, with the main reasons being as follows (Hornsey et al., 2018; Taylor et al., 2020; Wolfe & Sharp, 2002):

- Concerns that the risks outweigh the benefits.
- Belief that vaccination is unnecessary or unimportant.
- Preference for natural immunity.
- Belief in vaccination conspiracy theories (e.g., the belief that vaccination is a money-making scam perpetrated by the pharmaceutical industry).
- Concerns that mandatory vaccination is a threat to personal autonomy and civil rights.

Cost is a further consideration when individuals must pay for vaccination. People dislike uncertainty, especially about potential hazards, so unsurprisingly, vaccine uncertainty heightens vaccine hesitancy. People tend to be wary of vaccines lacking a track record of safety and efficacy (Han et al., 2018).

For some people, vaccination elicits an approach-avoidance conflict: The decision to get vaccinated can evoke an internal conflict between a person's desire to be protected from disease versus their desire to avoid adverse vaccine effects (Du et al., 2022). The conflict may be especially pronounced for vaccines without an extensive track record, as is often the case for vaccines designed to target novel pathogens such as the coronavirus causing COVID-19. Approach-avoidance conflicts are associated with procrastination (Lewin, 1935; Vandenbos, 2007)—for example, delaying one's decision about whether or not to be vaccinated.

Attitudes about vaccines can become polarized, increasing the odds of conflicts among people over issues such as mandatory vaccination. Polarization was found in a longitudinal survey of vaccination attitudes in 15 countries during COVID-19 (Macdonald, 2021). For the unvaccinated, the proportion of people uncertain or undecided about getting the vaccine shrank from 18%

in January 2021 to only 1% in February 2022. Thus, almost all the undecided became either for or against vaccination. Over this period, the proportion of people unvaccinated and unwilling to be vaccinated fell from 47% to 17%, while the proportion of people vaccinated or willing to be vaccinated rose from 36% to 82%. Thus, from 2021 to 2022, two major, polarized groups emerged: a pro-vaccine majority (82%) and an unwilling minority (17%).

Vaccines have aroused mistrust and nonadherence since the earliest vaccination procedures for smallpox in the 18th century, known as "variolation" or "inoculation" (Henderson, 1965; Wolfe & Sharp, 2002). Measles was eliminated through vaccination in the United States in 2000, only to re-emerge some years later, mainly due to parental opposition to vaccines (Leibovitch & Jacobson, 2016). Wakefield et al. (1998) claimed that vaccination for measles, mumps, and rubella increased the risk of autism. Their research paper was fraudulent and later retracted, but it garnered much media attention and heightened vaccination hesitancy (Godlee et al., 2011).

Smallpox is the only infectious disease to be eradicated through vaccination. Systematic vaccination programs were initiated in the late 19th century (Rolleston, 1933). When some countries tried to make smallpox vaccination compulsory, anti-vaccination protests arose, along with courtroom challenges and the emergence of anti-vaccination groups such as the British Anti-Compulsory Vaccination League (1867), the Anti-Vaccination League of New York City (1885), the Liga Contra Vacina Obrigatória in Brazil (1904), and the Anti-Vaccination League of Canada (1900) (Berman, 2021; Needell, 1987; Wolfe & Sharp, 2002).

Riots over mandatory smallpox vaccination occurred in England, Canada, Brazil, and elsewhere in the 19th century (Berman, 2021; Bliss, 1991; Needell, 1987; Wolfe & Sharp, 2002). The smallpox antivaccination riots in Montreal (1885) and Rio de Janeiro (1904) were attributable, in part, to tensions between the government and people in poverty, with the latter objecting to the way the government was managing smallpox and other infectious diseases, such as by forcible vaccination and by demolishing tenement housing as part of urban modernization (Bliss, 1991; Needell, 1987).

While mandatory vaccination may give rise to protest and conflict, voluntary programs suffer from low uptake. For example, most people do not seek vaccination for seasonal influenza. A meta-analysis of 522 studies from 68 countries or regions found that globally, in a given year, only 25% of people get vaccinated against seasonal flu (Chen et al., 2022). People are more likely to be vaccinated if they regard the flu as a severe threat, perceive the vaccine as efficacious, and vaccination is free and recommended by healthcare workers (Chen et al., 2022).

Low vaccination rates were a problem in the 2009 swine flu pandemic. The vaccination rate was only 23% in the United States and less than 40% in the United Kingdom, Canada, and Switzerland (Bangerter et al., 2012; CDC, 2023a; Statistics Canada, 2010; SteelFisher et al., 2012; Taha et al., 2013). The vaccination rate for COVID-19 was substantially higher, with 72% of people worldwide receiving at least one vaccine dose (Holder, 2023). To encourage people to be vaccinated against COVID-19, governments used a combination of reassuring information about the safety and efficacy of vaccines, nudges, appeals to altruism, and mandates. Public health messaging strategies were widely used to target different sources of vaccination hesitancy. For example, campaigns appealing to altruism (e.g., "Do it for your community") encourage vaccination among people who regard it as unnecessary for themselves.

Vaccinating 72% of the world's population was an impressive feat. But given the considerable efforts at global vaccination, including the widespread availability of free vaccines, why wasn't the vaccination rate even higher? Vaccination disincentives include vaccine-related adverse events, which are rare but draw media attention and fuel hesitancy (Clements, 2003). Entrenched negative attitudes about vaccines, including beliefs in conspiracy theories, further contribute to vaccination hesitancy, as discussed in Chapter 12.

Immunity Documentation

Classifying people as safe—that is, uninfected or previously infected and now immune—or dangerous (infected or possibly infected) has long been used to determine who should be quarantined or restricted in their movements. For plague outbreaks in the 15th to 18th centuries, many European cities issued health passes attesting that the bearer was traveling from a city free from plague or had completed 40 days of quarantine (Bamji, 2019). The passes—considered by some to be vital for plague control—were required for travelers to gain entry to some cities or countries (Bamji, 2019). People lacking passes were liable to be denied entry or quarantined.

A similar system was used for yellow fever in 19th-century Gibraltar, where people who had survived yellow fever were issued official "fever passes" to assert their "non-liability" (immunity), permitting freedom of movement while much of the community was in quarantine (Sawchuk & Tripp, 2021). Health passes enabled the fulfillment of economic and social needs for travel while mitigating health risks to others. During COVID-19, documents attesting that one had been vaccinated—"vaccine passports"—were commonly required for travel and to gain access to social venues such as restaurants, clubs, and stadium events.

Nudges and Mandates

Nudges and mandates were used extensively in COVID-19 to encourage adherence to mask-wearing, vaccines, social distancing, and hygiene. This chapter discusses nudges and mandates because of their particular relevance to vaccination. Nudges are used when traditional messages are insufficient to improve adherence. Nudges are subtle attempts to encourage particular behaviors without forbidding options, forcing people to do things, or significantly changing a person's economic or other incentives (Thaler & Sunstein, 2008). Nudges involve prompts to perform simple, low-effort behaviors. Pandemic-related examples of nudges are as follows:

- *Product placement in stores*: Hand sanitizer placed on an eye-level shelf in the check-out aisle is more likely to be purchased than sanitizer placed on less visible, hard-to-reach shelves.
- *Handwashing*: Touchless washroom faucets, where you can wash your hands simply by placing them under the tap.
- *Social distancing*: Stickers spaced 6 feet apart on pavements where people line up, with notices on the stickers asking people to maintain social distancing.
- *Vaccination*: Readily available, free vaccination walk-in services offered by pharmacies.

Text messages can be used as nudges, prompting people to get vaccinated. Some messages work better than others. In a study of 19 different text messages for seasonal flu vaccination, the most successful were ones that (1) reminded people twice to get their flu shot, (2) indicated that the shot was explicitly reserved for them, and (3) contained a web link for booking an appointment (Milkman et al., 2021).

The effects of nudges may be modest, but at a population level, they can be significant. Even small increases in vaccine uptake may correspond to millions of extra vaccinations (Huang et al., 2023). Some nudges work better than others, and some can backfire, underscoring the importance of pilot-testing. People might not be aware of being nudged. Accordingly, some nudge interventions may need ethical safeguards. Guidelines for developing and implementing nudges are discussed elsewhere (Murayama et al., 2023; Thaler & Sunstein, 2008).

Governments resort to mandates when adherence remains a problem. Performing particular health-related behaviors (e.g., getting vaccinated or wearing a mask) may be required to access specific goods and services, such as stores, restaurants, clubs, and schools. Vaccine passports may be required to enter these venues. Many workplaces, particularly healthcare settings, require workers to be vaccinated. During COVID-19, most people adhered to vaccine mandates, although there were also many protests (Chapter 7).

The pros and cons of mandatory vaccination have been discussed extensively in the healthcare literature (e.g., Behrman & Offley, 2013; Born et al., 2015; Lukich et al., 2018). Mandatory programs infringe on personal liberty and autonomy, but such programs also reduce morbidity and mortality (Antommaria & Prows, 2018; Born et al., 2015; Frederick et al., 2018; Wang et al., 2017). Mandates are effective but unpopular. Less-restrictive options should be pursued where possible.

Conclusions

Across historical eras and cultures, mask-wearing and vaccination have been sources of objection, nonadherence, and conflict. Anti-vaccination attitudes are as old as vaccination itself. Anti-mask attitudes today resemble those voiced over a century ago by the Anti-Mask League. In the course of COVID-19, attitudes toward masks and vaccines were polarized into pro and contra groups, with the latter representing a small but vocal minority.

Despite arousing opposition and mistrust among some, face masks and vaccines will likely play a vital role in managing future outbreaks of influenza, coronavirus disease, and other infections spread by aerosols, droplets, and fomites. There is no guarantee that vaccines will be available for the next pandemic, as vaccine development requires time. However, vaccines for COVID-19 were produced remarkably swiftly. The U.S. vaccination program was named Operation Warp Speed, emphasizing the urgent need. This program and others produced safe, effective vaccines within a year of the pandemic's onset.

Adherence to mask-wearing and vaccination can be improved with nudges and mandates. Adherence to masks can also be enhanced by further researching the efficacy of mask-wearing in public places. The available research provides mixed support and is open to interpretation. We need studies using large, representative community samples and robust methodologies to provide definitive answers about the efficacy of masks worn by the public. If the scientific support is unequivocally strong, this should improve adherence to some degree. Presumably, masks are more helpful in preventing infections in some public or social situations than others. Research is needed to develop evidence-based guidelines about situations where mask-wearing would most benefit the public.

Adherence can be further improved by better understanding the beliefs and other factors associated with opposition to masks and vaccines. Later chapters explore these issues, including the effects of political beliefs (Chapter 7), the roles of rumors and conspiracy theories (Chapter 12), and the influence of personality traits (Chapter 18).

6
Social Distancing
Impact, Objections, and Alternatives

Introduction

Keeping people apart from one another has been an infection control strategy for centuries, even before humans knew of the existence of viruses and bacteria. The purpose of this chapter is to review the efficacy and adverse effects of various forms of social distancing, with particular attention to how these interventions psychologically affect communities.

Social distancing, more accurately called physical distancing, is a pandemic-mitigation strategy in which people are asked to keep apart from one another to slow and contain the spread of infection (Finkelstein et al., 2010). Social distancing is used primarily for infections spread by airborne transmission, fomites, and direct physical contact. Accordingly, social distancing has been used to control influenza, coronavirus diseases, and the plague. For water-borne diseases such as cholera, public sanitation is a more effective means of disease control.

Social distancing can involve lockdown, in which people are requested or required to remain at home for a given period, being allowed to leave home only under specific circumstances (e.g., to purchase supplies). Quarantine is a targeted form of social distancing where potentially infected people are physically kept apart from others for some fixed period (e.g., two weeks) in a dedicated isolation facility. Quarantine of new arrivals at ports and borders has long been used in disease management, dating back to the plague control strategies of 14th-century Venice and earlier (Mackowiak & Sehdev, 2002).

Other forms of social distancing include cordoning towns or cities (cordon sanitaire), closures of workplaces and schools, canceling mass gatherings such as sporting events and concerts, closing recreational facilities and community centers, closing nonessential businesses (e.g., restaurants, clubs, and bars), border closures, and travel restrictions (Pan-Canadian Public Health Network, 2016; WHO, 2010b). Increasing interpersonal space in public places is a further social-distancing strategy; for example, keeping 6 feet apart from one another (Pan-Canadian Public Health Network, 2016; WHO, 2010a).

The following sections review the controversies associated with social distancing, including the common objections concerning lockdowns and business closures. Adverse effects such as pandemic fatigue are discussed. Alternatives to social distancing are reviewed, including controversial options. We conclude by discussing proposals concerning surveillance-based, targeted social distancing.

Recurrent Controversies

Lockdowns, quarantine, cordon sanitaire, and closures of schools, churches, and businesses have long been used to manage pandemics and other outbreaks. Lockdowns were used extensively in plague outbreaks, even in small villages. For example, in a 1604 plague outbreak in Salisbury, England, 20% of villagers were shut in, corresponding to 1,300 people confined to 411 homes (Byrne, 2006).

The experience of lockdown and quarantine has shifted over the centuries. In plague outbreaks in 17th-century England, people suspected of being infected and their co-inhabitants were involuntarily confined to their homes, with doors nailed shut and guards posted when possible (Slack, 1985). In plague outbreaks and the Spanish flu, unlike today, people in lockdown had little entertainment—no radio or television, for example—and limited communication with the outside world. Quarantine and lockdown for COVID-19 differed markedly from past pandemics in that physically isolated people were able to remain in social contact with others via electronic means (internet, cell phones), which also provided entertainments unavailable in past pandemics (e.g., streaming movies).

Despite variations in lockdown and quarantine over the centuries, the necessity and efficacy of these methods continue to be debated, with contentious issues concerning individual freedom and economic interests versus contagion management (Tognotti, 2013). Objections to lockdown were raised in treatises concerning the management of plague in the 17th century and reiterated in other outbreaks, such as cholera in the 19th century (Anonymous, 1665, 1721; Boghurst, 1666; Rosenberg, 1987; Slack, 1985). The objections were succinctly articulated in a 17th-century monograph titled *The Shutting Up Infected Houses as It Is Practised in England Soberly Debated* (Anonymous, 1665). These arguments—reiterated centuries later concerning COVID-19 lockdowns—can be summarized as follows:

- Lockdowns are inhumane and impose undue hardships, especially when people are confined in cramped or crowded quarters.
- Locking up the healthy with the sick is unfair to the healthy, creating undue distress.
- In addition to their human toll, lockdowns disrupt commerce and create financial hardships. The closure of businesses and confinement of healthy workers to their homes lead to labor shortages and economic strain.
- The efficacy of lockdown is doubtful as a disease-control strategy.

How effective is lockdown in stemming the spread of infection? According to the 17th-century apothecary William Boghurst in his treatise on the plague, lockdown was "oft enough tried and always found ineffectual" (Boghurst, 1666, p. 57). Modern research suggests that lockdowns are effective but only moderately so, with "mild impacts" on disease transmission—that is, useful but insufficient as stand-alone measures (Haug et al., 2020, p. 1308). As such, the effects of lockdown on disease prevalence are probably too small to be detected by casual observers like William Boghurst, leading to disagreements as to the value of the intervention.

Similar objections were raised about quarantine (Carmichael, 1986). Even today, quarantine can be stressful, sometimes leading to lasting psychological problems (Brooks et al., 2020). Stressful effects include uncertainty, boredom, financial loss, stigma, and the looming threat of infection (Brooks et al., 2020).

Objections to Closing Churches, Schools, and Businesses

Pandemic-related closures have long been controversial, with much uncertainty about whether or when to close shops, schools, places of worship, and other public venues (Becker, 2020; Tomes, 2010). Closures were widely implemented in COVID-19 and the Spanish flu. In both pandemics, common objections were that the economic impact due to closures was excessive, given the perceived severity of the disease (Taylor et al., 2020; Tomes, 2010). Concerns about socioeconomic consequences were sometimes predominant in plague outbreaks, with fear of poverty trumping fear of infection. In the plague of 1630 in Bologna, Italy, the fear of contagion was not enough to dissuade city residents, who continued trading with outsiders despite government prohibitions against outside contact (Rose, 2018).

Business closures throughout COVID-19 and the Spanish flu led to debates about what constitutes an essential service that should remain open (Storr et al., 2021; Tomes, 2010). In some places during COVID-19, liquor stores were classified as essential services, prompting criticism. While keeping liquor stores open prevents withdrawal symptoms in people dependent on alcohol, it also enables increased consumption as people try to cope with lockdown and other pandemic stressors (Neufeld et al., 2020).

Perceived inequity of closures was a common complaint in COVID-19 and the Spanish flu. These complaints were of the form "why close X and not Y?" Examples include complaints about the unfairness of (1) closing churches while allowing schools and bars to remain open, (2) closing schools while allowing churches and theaters to stay open, and (3) closing restaurants while allowing stores to remain open (Atlanta Constitution, 1918; Baltimore Sun, 1918; Charleston News and Courier, 1918; Cleveland Plain Dealer, 1918; New Orleans Times-Picayune, 1918; Newark Evening News, 1918; Nicholson & Martins, 2021; Philadelphia Inquirer, 1918; Rocky Mountain News, 1918; Salt Lake Tribune, 1918; Weisgarber, 2021; Worcester Evening Post, 1918).

Arguments raised by church leaders and churchgoers for keeping places of worship open throughout COVID-19 were essentially the same as those raised a century earlier in the Spanish flu. It was argued that banning or limiting services violated civil rights, that churches were well-ventilated and safe and that churches were essential for maintaining hope, morale, and equanimity (Alonso & Hackney, 2020; CBC News, 2020; CBS News, 2020; Evening Star, 1918a, 1918b; New Orleans Times-Picayune, 1918; Newark Evening News, 1918; Quinn, 2020). These claims notwithstanding, church services are sources of superspreading (see Chapter 1).

School closures are widely used but contentious methods of stemming the spread of infection. For COVID-19, schools closed and online learning was implemented via videoconferencing in many countries. In planning for school closures in disease outbreaks, the main concerns are whether the benefits outweigh the costs and whether there are viable alternatives. Adverse effects of school closures include (1) loss of access to school nutrition programs (breakfast and lunch), (2) income loss if parents have to look after their children when schools are closed, and (3) disrupted learning and socialization (Berkman, 2008).

These concerns are moot if schools cannot remain open because of illness-related staff absences. Nevertheless, if schools must be closed, it is necessary to plan to mitigate the adverse effects on students and caregivers. Timing is critical. Closing schools early rather than later in an outbreak is more effective in stemming the spread of infection (Davis et al., 2015; House et al., 2011; Kawaguchi et al., 2009; Wu et al., 2010).

Nonadherence to Social Distancing

Social distancing must be applied immediately, rigorously, and consistently to be effective (Maharaj & Kleczkowski, 2012). Nonadherence is common. In plague outbreaks, healthy people sometimes refused to be locked in their homes with sick household members. In the second plague pandemic in the 17th century, if people broke out of their homes when locked down, they were arrested, fined, and locked back in their homes or sent to a pesthouse (Byrne, 2006; Slack, 1985). Despite these measures, nonadherence was widespread. In London, Exeter, Bristol, and other towns and villages, "people refused to be shut up, or broke out of their homes when they were, hurling abuse at constables and aldermen as they did so" (Slack, 1985, p. 298). Rebellion against lockdown led to redoubled government efforts to enforce the restrictions, leading to further protest in a "vicious spiral in which public disturbances and efforts at control chased one another" (Slack, 1985, p. 303).

Restrictions were similarly unpopular in COVID-19 and the Spanish flu—people wanted to resume everyday life despite active, widespread infection (Cincinnati Enquirer, 1918; Kovac, 2020; Miljure, 2021). Governments met nonadherence with threats, fines, and sometimes incarceration (CBC News, 2020; Chicago Herald and Examiner, 1918; Chicago Tribune, 1918; Cincinnati Enquirer, 1918; Kovac & Greig, 2021; Labine, 2021; Salter, 2020; Spokane Daily Chronicle, 1918; St. Paul Daily News, 1918).

Lockdowns and closures were not implemented in the 2009 swine flu pandemic, but the sick were asked to avoid unnecessary contact with others. Adherence was poor under this light form of social distancing. A study of faculty and students from the University of Delaware found that very few people (6% to 9%) with acute respiratory infections stayed home when ill, and many sick people (45%) attended social events, even though they were contagious (Mitchell et al., 2011). A multinational study in the same pandemic found that many respondents from the United Kingdom and the United States (79% and 44%, respectively) made no effort to avoid being near someone who had influenza-like symptoms (SteelFisher et al., 2012). Most respondents (89% and 72%) did not attempt to avoid crowded public places such as shopping centers or sporting venues.

Pandemic Fatigue

For some people, lockdown during COVID-19 meant job loss and financial hardship. For others, it required working from home, which can be stressful if the home environment is not conducive to this arrangement, such as working from home while caring for young children. Some people in lockdown experienced crowding in small dwellings, while others were isolated in their single-occupant homes.

With the prolonged stress of lockdowns and other social restrictions, pandemic fatigue sets in. Pandemic fatigue is a burnout-related syndrome characterized by emotional exhaustion and declining motivation to follow health guidelines (WHO, 2020). People suffering from pandemic fatigue report exhaustion, tiredness, or feeling worn out due to the pandemic and associated restrictions. As the pandemic drags out, the perceived costs of complying with the constraints, such as daily inconveniences and socioeconomic losses, feel increasingly burdensome. The perceived costs of compliance begin to outweigh the perceived risks of infection (WHO 2020). People become increasingly lax about staying safe from infection, disregarding social-distancing guidelines and even flouting guidelines by holding covert social gatherings or engaging in nonessential travel (e.g., holiday trips). Compliance with health guidelines may decline even if infections continue to rise (Crane et al., 2021; Duca et al., 2020).

According to the World Health Organization, pandemic fatigue was a significant obstacle in managing COVID-19 (WHO, 2020). About 8% to 10% of people showed signs of pandemic fatigue, as indicated by a gradual deterioration in adherence to social distancing (Kleitman et al., 2021; Taylor et al., 2022). A survey of over 7,700 U.S. adults found that pandemic fatigue was mainly expressed by (1) nonadherence to remaining at home, (2) increased socialization with non-household members in one's home (e.g., having visitors over), and (3) socializing outside the home (Crane et al., 2021). Mask-wearing was not subject to pandemic fatigue, possibly because mask-wearing in places like stores and public transit was widely mandated (Crane et al., 2021).

People experiencing pandemic fatigue during COVID-19, compared to the adherent majority, tended to be younger, saw themselves as more affluent than others, tended to have greater levels of narcissism, psychological entitlement, and sociability, and were more likely to report having been previously infected with the coronavirus, which they regarded as an overstated threat (Taylor et al., 2022). Narcissism, psychological entitlement, and other personality traits are discussed in more detail in Chapter 18.

Controversial Alternatives to Lockdowns and Closures

Are lockdowns something we must endure in future pandemics, or are there viable alternatives? Since humans are inherently social beings, and lockdowns aim to limit social interactions, lockdowns are not feasible as long-term interventions. Brief lockdowns may be tolerated reasonably well by most people, but protracted or recurrent lockdowns harm mental health and spark protest (Chapters 7 & 19).

An alternative is to lift all restrictions. During COVID-19, an American group called the Urgency of Normal proposed immediately lifting many social distancing restrictions based on the argument that closing economies, restaurants, gyms, schools, and so forth is not sustainable (Blackwell, 2022). The Urgency of Normal group pushed for, among other things, a rapid return to unrestricted in-person learning for children. The group comprised several hundred signatories, including dozens of physicians and other healthcare professionals. The group disputed evidence for the efficacy of school closures and keeping students in face masks. Critics objected that the group's website was rife with misleading and false claims (Blackwell, 2022).

Another controversial alternative to lockdown was proposed in an online petition called the Great Barrington Declaration (Kulldorff et al., 2020). By the fourth year of COVID-19 (November 30, 2023), the petition had been endorsed by nearly a million signatories, including 63,767 scientists and medical practitioners.

The declaration outlined a "focused protection" plan in which only vulnerable individuals (e.g., the medically frail and elderly) would be encouraged to go into lockdown or receive special protections. The rest of the community would roam free without constraints, getting infected and gradually building immunity. The virus would burn through the community until herd immunity is attained, conferring protection to everyone (Kulldorff et al., 2020). Herd immunity, also known as community immunity, occurs when a large proportion of the community becomes immune to infection, thereby conferring indirect protection to those who are not immune.

There were many criticisms of the Great Barrington Declaration, including (1) no pandemic has ever been effectively controlled with focused protection, (2) focused protection discriminates against particular demographic groups (e.g., older adults would be actively discouraged from venturing out of their homes), (3) it is not clear that it would be possible to protect vulnerable people because immunity wanes over time and virus variants may escape immunity, and (4) achieving herd immunity in this way is unethical because it increases the rate of morbidity and mortality (Barry, 2020; Hart, 2020; Yamey, 2020). More promising, although not without problems, are methods involving targeted isolation.

Test-Trace-Isolate Approaches

Targeted Isolation

Test-trace-isolate approaches involving targeted isolation are promising alternatives to community-wide lockdowns (Ferretti et al., 2020). A test-trace-isolate approach involves tracing an infected individual's recent physical contacts—for example, using digital phone tracking. Those contacts are then directed to self-isolate for a certain period, such as several days. For instance, if an infected individual visited a restaurant on a specific evening, all patrons and staff would be contacted and instructed to self-isolate for several days.

An advantage of a test-trace-isolate approach compared to lockdown is that fewer people tend to be affected. With low infection levels, the number of people in self-isolation will be small. If infection is widespread, most people will be in self-isolation until their risk of infecting others diminishes. This approach differs from lockdown because everyone has their self-isolation period instead of being confined to their homes for some uniform, fixed period.

Based on computer modeling, Nuzzo et al. (2020) argued that community-wide lockdown could be replaced, without loss of efficacy, with a test-trace-isolate approach called "advanced automated contact tracing and targeted isolation" (Nuzzo et al., 2020). This method uses an application on GPS-enabled phones that alerts people about the need for self-isolation based on an individual's likely exposure to infected others.

Surveillance Methods

A disease-detection system is required for targeted isolation. Modern methods utilize digital surveillance, stemming from technological advancements and the necessity to assess disease patterns and prevalence in increasingly large numbers as the global population expands.

Surveillance, based on cellphone data, can be used to track the spread of infection (trend forecasting), to track adherence (e.g., compliance with stay-at-home orders), and to guide the deployment of targeted interventions (e.g., to identify hot spots to plan closures). These data can be obtained by a variety of means, including cellphone applications, social media, surveillance cameras in public spaces using facial-recognition software, drones, and thermal (infrared) cameras at airports (Wnuk et al., 2021). Surveillance data can be integrated with other types of information, such as infection history, vaccination status, travel history, and credit card transaction history.

In China, tracking systems using location data plus facial-recognition software were used to identify infected people and those not wearing masks (Wnuk et al., 2020). Several countries implemented aerial drone surveillance in the course of COVID-19 to enforce compliance with lockdown and mask-wearing. Drones equipped with loudspeakers were used in China to break up public gatherings, such as to disperse people from public parks (D'Amore, 2020).

China's Surveillance-Based Health Code System

In China during COVID-19, the technological giant Alibaba developed a health-tracking cellphone application that used data about personal health, location, and other information to generate a colored QR (quick reader) code on one's phone. Code green allowed its owner to travel freely, yellow imposed some restrictions on mobility (e.g., 7-day self-isolation), and red indicated a high risk of infection and the corresponding need for 14-day self-isolation (Tan et al., 2022). This system, which shared data with law enforcement authorities, was used to determine a person's eligibility to access public spaces and services. People had to display a green code before entering restaurants, shopping malls, buses, and subways (Xuefei, 2022). Evidence of infection, travel history in high-risk regions, or contact with infected people changed the code from green to yellow or red, barring a person from some public places.

China also implemented a national text alerting system in which citizens received daily text alerts from local governments (Yuan, 2021). When a case of infection was identified, all residents in the neighborhood received text alerts containing details of the time and location of the infected individual (Yuan, 2021). People checked these text alerts daily (Moon, 2020). Most Chinese citizens reportedly found the surveillance system acceptable for managing the pandemic (Tan et al., 2022). However, concerns were raised about the transparency of the process. Critics objected that data sources and algorithms to assign color codes were "shrouded in mystery" and thereby open to misuse (Tan et al., 2022, p. 1).

South Korea's Approach

South Korea was one of the better-performing countries throughout COVID-19 in terms of healthcare, restrictions, and economic impacts (Chapter 3). South Korea relied on a test-trace-isolate approach, while refraining from country-wide lockdowns (Bentotahewa et al., 2021). This approach enabled the rapid identification and isolation of cases (Nikolaeva & Versnel, 2022; Túri & Virág, 2021).

As with China, South Korea's approach involved tracking people's movements using GPS phone data and other information such as credit card records and video surveillance footage. People were warned via text messaging if they had come in contact with an infected individual. When a person tested positive for COVID-19, a text alert was sent to everyone living nearby, providing a detailed log of the infected person's movements (Yoon, 2021). In this process, South Korea's Center for Disease Control and Prevention Agency disclosed people's personal information, including their age, gender, neighborhood, and workplace location (Yoon, 2021). A cellphone application monitored adherence to self-quarantine for infected individuals. This approach, although efficacious, involved a deep invasion of privacy.

Concerns About Digital Surveillance

Privacy Versus Safety

Privacy entails the ability to control the visibility of personal information. The moral right to privacy is central to defining us as human beings, as opposed to animals or objects. Pandemic surveillance involves a trade-off between security and privacy, relinquishing personal privacy in the service of public health. Surveillance data, such as geolocation information, can be stripped of names, addresses, and other identifying information. However, it may be possible to re-identify people, thus highlighting privacy concerns (Bentotahewa et al., 2021). Without proper safeguards, digital surveillance technologies could be misused for discriminatory, political, or commercially exploitive purposes (Andrew & Baker, 2021; Gasser et al., 2020; Zuboff, 2019).

Surveillance Creep

One of the biggest concerns with surveillance programs has to do with surveillance creep, where methods developed for a specific, time-limited purpose (e.g., infection monitoring) become established permanently, applied broadly, and potentially misused (French & Monahan, 2020; Nay, 2020). In addition to concerns about privacy, there are concerns about the psychological effects of being constantly surveilled. Being continually observed can undermine one's sense of volition and choice, creating a sense of being controlled. The feeling of being under continual surveillance may lead people to comply with normative expectations (e.g., remaining in self-isolation) without actually being surveilled (Foucault, 1979).

Public Acceptance

According to an editorial in the journal *Nature*, South Korea's COVID-19 management system was "based on a degree of surveillance that people in many other countries would find hard to accept" (Nature, 2020, p. 536). This conclusion is likely wrong because it fails to appreciate how readily people adapt to changing circumstances. People worldwide have grown increasingly accustomed to surveillance in the form of security cameras in stores and public places, targeted advertising entailing the tracking of one's internet browsing history, and credit card companies tracking one's purchases for signs of credit card theft or fraud.

Surveys found that people in many countries generally accepted contact-tracing surveillance for COVID-19 (Hassandoust et al., 2021; Majeed, 2022; Wnuk et al., 2021). However, adoption rates for voluntary-use contact tracing applications varied widely, from low (India, Ireland, and Bahrain) to high (Singapore and Israel) (Majeed, 2022). Most countries failed to get more than 60% of citizens to voluntarily install contact tracing applications on their phones (Hassandoust et al., 2021; Majeed, 2022).

Surveillance in the course of COVID-19 tended to be more acceptable among adults who were younger, more frightened of the coronavirus, more authoritarian, had greater prosocial responsibility, and more positive attitudes toward technology (Kokkoris & Kamleitner, 2020; Wnuk et al., 2021; Wnuk et al., 2020). People scoring high on a personality trait known as psychological reactance (Chapter 18) tend to object to surveillance, asserting the moral right to be left alone (Yost et al., 2019).

Conclusions

Social distancing helps control pandemics but is also a source of contention and conflict. There may be much uncertainty about whether or when to implement closures. Disease modeling and surveillance can aid in this regard by estimating how timed closures can impact the spread of disease. Highly restrictive forms of social distancing, such as lockdown and quarantine, are moderately effective but unpopular and prone to nonadherence. Criticisms have focused on the necessity and efficacy of these interventions and the hardships they create. Nonadherence arises for a range of reasons. Sometimes, the fear of economic hardship is greater than the fear of infection, causing people to violate lockdowns, closures, cordons, and other restrictions.

Several alternatives to closures and lockdowns have been proposed. Promising methods are test-trace-isolate approaches involving targeted isolation of potentially infected individuals. The primary concern with these approaches has to do with data privacy. Digital surveillance is most likely to be accepted by the public when it is limited in scope, minimally intrusive, clearly shown to be necessary, and there is transparency concerning the collection, security, analyses, and disclosure of surveillance data. Given the invasive nature of disease surveillance programs, further research is needed to investigate whether the benefits outweigh the costs.

Even with digital surveillance methods, social distancing may be required in some form or other, especially when infection is widespread. To gain a deeper understanding of how people experience and respond to social distancing restrictions, including adherence to lockdowns and closures, we need to consider several factors discussed in upcoming chapters, including political factors (Chapter 7), personal coping strategies (Chapter 8), rumors and conspiracy theories (Chapter 12), personality traits influencing adherence (Chapter 18), and the effects of social distancing on mental health (Chapter 19).

7
Politics and Protests

Introduction

Politics and pandemics are intertwined due to the global nature of the infectious threat and the national and international measures needed to arrest the spread of disease. As the title suggests, this chapter surveys two linked domains: political factors pertaining to the psychology of pandemics and pandemic-related protests against government restrictions. Our coverage of political factors is selective, focusing on issues concerning trust in government and public acceptance of pandemic mitigation measures.

The first aim is to survey political factors that can erode public trust and cooperation with pandemic mitigation measures. We begin by considering government efforts to conceal or under-report infectious cases. Other factors linked to government mistrust are also discussed. We consider political party affiliation, which impacted the management of COVID-19 in many countries, particularly the United States. Trust in authorities—too little or too much—can lead to problems. Too little trust leads to nonadherence, whereas too much faith in one's political party can lead to political polarization over disease control measures such as masks, vaccines, and social restrictions. Political factors also extend beyond party affiliation. Pandemics reveal and exacerbate society's "fault lines," which are preexisting tensions, typically between governments and people living in poverty.

The second aim of this chapter is to investigate the nature of pandemic-related protests, including riots. Linked to government mistrust, protests complicate the management of pandemics. Demonstration rallies allow people to express their grievances, giving government leaders feedback on important issues. Protests may indicate that some pandemic-mitigation measures must be reconsidered or amended or that public messaging must be improved to address misconceptions. However, protests can also become superspreading events. Political and other factors increase the odds of demonstrations and riots. Most people follow pandemic-mitigation guidelines, but as discussed in previous chapters, there is a long history of public opposition and debate concerning face masks, vaccination, business closures, and lockdowns.

The objections raised historically are similar to those voiced today and have sometimes led to violent conflicts. Understanding the reasons for opposition and protest over mitigation measures can lead to better ways of managing pandemics.

Disease Concealment and Under-Reporting

Governments sometimes try to conceal or cover up the presence of infection. Cover-ups occur early in an outbreak. Infections become impossible to hide once a disease is widespread. Delayed disclosure and under-reporting of cases were alleged to have happened in the Russian flu, Spanish flu, SARS, COVID-19, yellow fever, plague, and cholera outbreaks (Buguzi, 2021; Cheng, 2004; Imperato et al., 2015; Parets, 1651; Pettigrew, 1983; Rosenberg, 1987; Staiano, 2008; Todd, 1909). The following are examples.

In Moscow in 1770, officials initially denied the presence of the plague, which had killed 4,000 inhabitants that year. The ostensible motive was to prevent the disruption of foreign trade (Staiano, 2008). In a cholera outbreak in Naples in 1837, officials initially under-reported the number of deaths because of concerns of triggering public panic (Imperato et al., 2015). Chinese health officials allegedly knew about the SARS outbreak long before it was publicly acknowledged (Cheng, 2004). During COVID-19, there were U.S. allegations, hotly contested by Chinese officials, that China had covered up early coronavirus outbreaks (Agence France-Presse, 2021; Ministry of Foreign Affairs of the People's Republic of China, 2020).

In the opening years of the HIV/AIDS pandemic, there were attempts to downplay or deny its seriousness in many countries (Bayramoğlu, 2021; Kalichman, 2014). In 1985, the Turkish Prime Minister Turgut Özal announced at a press conference that there was no HIV/AIDS outbreak in Turkey because the traditional Turkish family structure "did not allow for deviant sexualities" (Bayramoğlu, 2021, p. 1594). The prime minister was quickly proved wrong concerning HIV/AIDS, family structures, and homosexuality. Today, HIV/AIDs continues to be a health concern in Turkey and elsewhere (Yaylali et al., 2023).

Disease concealment and under-reporting likely occur when there is some perceived penalty or cost to disclosing cases. Concealment and under-reporting can keep the population calm and the economy running, circumvent false alarms—if the outbreak proves minor—and can be used politically to avoid blame if the outbreak spreads widely (e.g., to deny that the disease originated in one's country). However, concealment and under-reporting come with a price. Trust in government is likely eroded when concealment and under-reporting come to light, forcing authorities to acknowledge a danger they had previously denied. More empirical research is needed concerning the psychological impact of disease-related under-reporting.

Trust in Government

Trust in government, along with trust in the scientific research community, is essential for managing pandemics. Pandemic mitigation requires the public to agree to follow government guidelines about social distancing, mask wearing, vaccines, and so forth. People are less likely to be adherent if they distrust their leaders (Cohn & Kutalek, 2016; Freeman et al., 2022). To illustrate, in Monrovia, Liberia, in a 2014 outbreak of Ebola virus disease, people who mistrusted the government were more likely to flout bans on social gatherings and other restrictions and less likely to support policies concerning the safe burial of Ebola-infected bodies (Blair et al., 2017). Nonadherence was not due to a lack of knowledge about Ebola virus disease and its transmission. It was because respondents "did not trust the capacity or integrity of government institutions to recommend precautions and implement policies to slow [Ebola's] spread" (Blair et al., 2017, p. 89).

COVID-19 studies generally found that political trust was linked to increased compliance with mobility restrictions and vaccination (Blackburn et al., 2024; Cao et al., 2024; Devine et al., 2024; Skafida & Heins, 2024). However, there were exceptions, likely due to the multiplicity of factors influencing the relationship between trust and adherence, including regional cultural effects and the messages from specific leaders (Bird et al., 2023; Blackburn et al., 2024). Threat perception also plays a role; "for individuals worried about COVID-19, seeing the government respond strongly was related to higher levels of trust ... whereas, if the government was lax about COVID-19, the least concerned individuals had the highest trust" (Blackburn et al., 2024, p. 17942).

Public confidence in government is likely undermined when officials clearly underestimate or downplay the threat. Political leaders in the United States, United Kingdom, Brazil, and elsewhere initially tried to downplay the seriousness of COVID-19 (Buguzi, 2021; Falkenbach & Greer, 2021; Hier, 2021; Husna, 2021; Karimi, 2020). U.S. President Trump acknowledged that he "wanted to always play it down" because he didn't want to create a panic (Keith, 2020, p. 1). Taking it further, President Trump promoted false claims that the risks of COVID-19 were "very low" and that children were "almost immune" to the coronavirus (August, 2020; Gordon, 2020). Brazilian President Bolsonaro declared that COVID-19 was no more than "a little flu," despite 17,500 documented coronavirus deaths in Brazil at the time (Falkenbach & Greer, 2021; Walsh et al., 2020). Tanzanian President Magufuli declared in June 2020 that his country was "COVID-19 free," claiming that three days of prayer had saved the country, despite evidence of hundreds of cases of infection and countless deaths (Buguzi, 2021).

Trust in government is also likely eroded when public officials flout the rules everyone is supposed to follow. Public outrage flared during COVID-19 when political leaders flouted social-distancing and travel guidelines by holding cocktail parties and taking trips to holiday destinations (BBC News, 2022; Bensadoun, 2021; Nixon, 2022). Such exceptionalism may have prompted people in the community to violate travel restrictions as a "me too" response.

Political Polarization and Conflict

Political party affiliation and messages from party leaders influence what people believe and how they behave in disease outbreaks. Attitudes toward pandemic-mitigation measures become polarized when parties differ markedly in their positions—for example, for or against mandatory face masks in public settings. Political polarization occurs when the attitudes and behaviors of the political left and right increasingly diverge (McCoy et al., 2018). As parties become polarized, so too are politicized matters such as wearing masks and getting vaccinated. Rhetoric from political leaders can strengthen polarization on some issues (e.g., masks, vaccines, border closures).

COVID-19 was politically polarizing in many countries, including the United States, Brazil, Israel, Italy, South Korea, Canada, Sweden, and England (Flores et al., 2022; Hegland et al., 2022; Pennycook et al., 2022; Taylor & Asmundson, 2021). COVID-19 was especially polarizing in America. Mandates concerning masks, vaccination, and social distancing were proposed or implemented in some U.S. regions, only to be later overturned or litigated as political parties tussled over the necessity, efficacy, and civil rights implications of the mandated measures (Gostin, 2022).

Compared to American Democrats, Republicans were more likely to have anti-mask attitudes, stronger vaccination hesitancy, lower adherence to social distancing, and were more likely to regard the COVID-19 threat as overblown (Block et al., 2022; Christensen et al., 2020; Pennycook et al., 2022; Taylor & Asmundson, 2021). Republicans were also more likely to die from COVID-19, presumably because they were less likely to be vaccinated (Wallace et al., 2023). Compared to past pandemics, COVID-19 was especially polarizing in the political realm. Future pandemics may be associated with similar polarization, depending on political conditions when the outbreak emerges.

Regarding future pandemics in democratic nations, threats to democratic processes can undermine pandemic management during and after the outbreak. Important issues include decision-making transparency, due process, and perceived fairness and impartiality. Political polarization can complicate the process, fomenting conflict and confusion. Consider, for example, the U.S. bipartisan subcommittee on the government's handling of COVID-19. Political infighting undermined the goal of guiding future pandemic preparation (Baio, 2024). Democratic and Republican subcommittee members issued separate reports in December 2024. The Republican report, hotly disputed by Democrats, claimed that SARS-Cov-2 "likely emerged because of a laboratory or research related accident" (Select Subcommittee on the Coronavirus Pandemic, 2024, p. 1). The Republican report also baselessly accused Dr. Anthony Fauci—a key member of the White House Coronavirus Task Force—of trying to cover up the alleged laboratory origins. In response, the Democratic report concluded that "arguments for a lab origin are largely circumstantial but cannot be dismissed out of hand" (Select Subcommittee on the Coronavirus Pandemic: Democrats, 2024, p. 8). The Democratic report also disputed the claim that Dr. Fauci attempted to suppress the lab leak theory. Escaped-from-a-lab conspiracy theories are further discussed in Chapter 12.

Pandemics Reveal Society's Fault Lines

The societal effects of pandemics extend beyond political divisions. Pandemics highlight society's "fault lines," exposing and exacerbating preexisting tensions between sociodemographic groups (Aloisi & De Stefano, 2022; Charters & McKay, 2020; Evans, 1988; Gravlee, 2020; Snowden, 2019; Washer, 2010). Preexisting sources of tension or discord provide a context or backdrop, shaping how people respond to pandemic control strategies.

Amid disease outbreaks, societal fault lines are expressed in terms of blame and counter-blame. Government authorities may blame those living in poverty for high infection rates, and people in poverty may blame the authorities for inadequate public sanitation and insufficient medical care. Such blame and counter-blame occurred in many outbreaks, including cholera and smallpox (Bliss, 1991; Cohn & Kutalek, 2016). In the 1992 cholera outbreak in Venezuela, the government blamed people living in poverty for inadequate hygiene, while the latter blamed the government and multinational corporations for allegedly poisoning the food supply (Cohn & Kutalek, 2016).

Fault lines entail the inequitable distribution of stressors, where one group is impacted more than others. Contrary to a popular COVID-19 slogan, we were not "all in this together." Infectious diseases are not equal-opportunity afflictions (Washer, 2010). Cholera pandemics disproportionately affected people in poverty more than the wealthy (Cohn, 2017; Delaporte, 1986; Rosenberg, 1987). Plague in the 19th century "was radically uneven in its impact as it followed instead the international fault lines of inequality, poverty, and neglect" (Snowden, 2019, p. 38).

During COVID-19, various minority groups, including ethnic and gender minorities, were disproportionately affected in multiple ways, including adverse effects on mental health (Ayoubkhani et al., 2021; Czeisler et al., 2020; Fruehwirth et al., 2021; Le et al., 2023; Moore et al., 2021). In plague outbreaks, lockdowns impacted the poverty-stricken more than the wealthy, with the former more likely to experience overcrowding and economic hardship (Slack, 1985). There were widening inequalities between the rich and poor throughout COVID-19. According to the 2020 Bloomberg Billionaires Index, 131 billionaires doubled their net worth amid COVID-19, while 97 million people were pushed into extreme poverty (Jha, 2022). Many countries provided businesses with tax breaks and financial benefits, enabling the wealthy to improve their fortunes. Meanwhile, migrant laborers and others lost their jobs (Bhuiyan et al., 2020; Jha, 2022).

Protests and Rioting

Violent protests erupted across Europe amid 19th-century cholera pandemics. As cholera spread throughout the continent, there were protests and riots in almost every country affected by the disease (Evans, 1988). In the British Isles from 1831 to 1833, there were at least 72 cholera riots, many with crowds in the thousands, threatening physicians and attacking hospitals (Cohn, 2017). Cholera riots occur sporadically today. Contemporary examples include the 1992 riot in Venezuela and the 2010 riot in Haiti (Cohn & Kutalek, 2016; Grimaud & Legagneur, 2011).

At the outset of COVID-19 in early 2020, a panel of U.K. government advisors declared that "large scale rioting is unlikely" (Morales & Konotey-Ahulu, 2020, p. 1). The expectation proved wrong. Protests, including riots, erupted worldwide concerning COVID-19 lockdowns, vaccine mandates, and mandatory mask-wearing in public places (Akkermans, 2021a; Aljazeera, 2020; Annár, 2020; BBC News, 2020; Bloomberg, 2020, 2022a, 2022b; Bratanic & Kuzmanovic, 2020; Breeden, 2021; Bucks, 2020; Coletta et al., 2022; Connor, 2020; Davis & Macfarlane, 2021; Di Donato & Dewan, 2020; Erlanger, 2021; Farokhi, 2022; Ghitis, 2021; Hanau, 2021; Hookham, 2020; Ilsøe & Clante, 2021; Keogh & Franey, 2021; Kvetenadze, 2021; Merriman, 2021; Morton, 2021; Scott, 2021; Seputyte, 2021; Thanthong-Knight, 2020; The Guardian, 2022; The Local, 2021; Total Slovenia News, 2020; Wharton, 2021; Willems, 2021; Young, 2020; Yu & Davidson, 2022).

Despite widespread stay-at-home restrictions in the course of COVID-19, protest rallies increased worldwide by 3% in 2020 compared to the previous year (Kishi et al., 2021). The people most impacted by COVID-19 restrictions were drawn to these rallies (Bartusevičius et al., 2021). Thousands of protestors participated in dozens of rallies, even as coronavirus infections surged. Protests were organized via social media platforms such as Telegram and Facebook (Ghitis, 2021). Most demonstrations (94%) were peaceful, but numerous erupted into violence (Kishi et al., 2021). Riots in the Netherlands, for example, were the worst in over four decades, with demonstrators clashing with police over COVID-19 restrictions (Akkermans, 2021b).

Protest Motives and Triggers

Diverse Motivations

People participate in protests for all kinds of reasons. COVID-19 protests were attended by a range of groups, including anti-vaccination and anti-lockdown groups, human rights groups, far-right political groups, and anti-immigration and anti-government groups (Amarasingam et al., 2021; Kishi et al., 2021; Winter et al., 2021). Conspiracy theorists were among these groups. Many protesters expressed frustration about how closures of businesses were harming their livelihoods. Two years into COVID-19, many protesters "were simply fed up with almost two years of intermittent state controls over their lives in the name of public health" (Erlanger, 2021, p. A1).

Some COVID-19 protests were highly organized, large-scale affairs, such as the Canadian Freedom Truck Convoy. The convoy offers a glimpse into the future of pandemic-related protests. Social media facilitated its organization, and crowdsourcing supplied the funding. The protesters, consisting of thousands of people and dozens of truckers in their rigs, converged on the Canadian capital of Ottawa in early 2022 (Farokhi, 2022). On arrival, the organizers had "military-style logistics hubs keeping food, fuel and other resources flowing to the encampments, where each block has its own captain and night patrol" (Coletta et al., 2022, p. 1). The protest began as a challenge to mandatory vaccination but quickly evolved into a movement opposing all COVID-19 restrictions, including masks and lockdowns (Barrett, 2022; Farokhi, 2022). Protesters included "those who oppose vaccines, vaccine mandates and other coronavirus restrictions; anti-government groups; conspiracy theorists; and far-right extremists" (Westfall, 2022, p. 1). At the time, 90% of Canadian truck drivers were vaccinated (Barrett, 2022). The protesting truckers were a vocal minority, joined by people promoting various agendas.

Economic Hardship

The odds of protest increase when pandemic-mitigation measures create economic hardships and shortages. In the 1832 cholera outbreak in Paris, protests were incited by the introduction of sanitary measures (garbage collection), which threatened the livelihoods of people who scavenged refuse for salvageable items (i.e., rag-and-bone collectors) (Cohn, 2017). Economic hardship amid COVID-19 was a common reason for protests (Amarasingam et al., 2021). To illustrate, in November 2022, violent protests flared in the southern Chinese city of Guangzhou, which was under lockdown. At the time, China employed an unpopular zero-COVID policy involving the extensive use of lockdowns to curb the spread of infection. Protesters, mainly poor migrant laborers, objected that the lockdown led to food shortages and difficulties getting prescription medication (Bloomberg, 2022a). In a video posted on social media, hundreds of protesters were seen marching in the street and overturning police barriers (Bloomberg, 2022a). There were more than 40 other protests across 22 Chinese cities, creating "the most widespread show of dissent since the Tiananmen Square episode more than three decades ago" (Bloomberg, 2022b, p. 1).

Mounting Frustration: The Last Straw

Frustration increases the odds of anger and aggression (Berkowitz, 1989; Kruglanski et al., 2023). Protests, including violent ones, can be triggered by a "last straw" event—for example, reimposing restrictions (e.g., recurrent lockdowns) or adding new ones to a growing list of closures and constraints. Expecting something good to happen (e.g., release from lockdown) and then having it denied or taken away from you is a frustrating experience that increases the odds of protest. The omission of expected rewards—known as frustrative non-reward—has been shown in experimental studies to evoke aggression in humans and animals (Potegal, 2023).

In Europe and elsewhere in the course of COVID-19, the reimposition of pandemic restrictions, or the imposition of new ones (e.g., additional closures, curfews, adding mandatory vaccination, and mask requirements), led to protests, some violent (Akkermans, 2021a; Aljazeera, 2020; Bucks, 2020; Davis & Macfarlane, 2021; Ghitis, 2021; Keogh & Franey, 2021; Kvetenadze, 2021; Scott, 2021). Rioting broke out in the Netherlands in January 2021 when the government attempted to tighten restrictions on social congregation by imposing a curfew (Akkermans, 2021b). As the deadline for the curfew approached, "gangs of youngsters started attacking police, throwing ignited fireworks, stones and even knives" (Ghitis, 2021, p. 1). In the Dutch city of Enschede, rioters hurled rocks, smashing hospital windows. In the Dutch town of Urk, rioters burned a COVID-19 testing site. Across the country, rioters "engaged in pitched clashes with police, while looting and destroying shops" (Ghitis, 2021, p. 1). Military police were called in, and hundreds of protesters were arrested.

Another example of a last straw situation was the *Revolta Contra Vacina*—the Anti-Vaccination Revolts—consisting of five days of protests and rioting in Rio de Janeiro in November 1904 (Green & Skidmore, 2021). The threatened imposition of mandatory smallpox vaccination was the inciting factor but not the only reason for protest: "Many Rio residents viewed compulsory vaccination against smallpox as the last straw in a sanitation plan they had long opposed" (Meade, 1986, p. 308). The protestors harbored numerous grievances, including housing insecurity (forced displacement due to urban renewal), food shortages, unemployment, and chronic inflation (Green & Skidmore, 2021).

Protests, Rumors, and Conspiracy Theories

For a range of diseases—including cholera, plague, smallpox, and COVID-19—rumors and conspiracy theories have fueled protests, including violent ones (Burrell & Gill, 2005; Chandavarkar, 1992; Cohn, 2017; Cohn & Kutalek, 2016; Evans, 1988; Needell, 1987). Plague outbreaks led to rioting in India in the 1890s, arising from rumors that the British were complicit in spreading the disease (Chandavarkar, 1992). A widespread 19th-century cholera conspiracy theory was that the disease was a weapon to deal with poverty by eradicating the lower classes. Belief in the theory led to protests and rioting (Cohn, 2017; Evans, 1988). The 1832 Liverpool cholera riots were fueled by rumors that "cholera victims were being removed to the hospital to be killed by doctors in order to use them for anatomical dissection" (Burrell & Gill, 2005, p. 478).

With the cholera riots, remarkably similar conspiracy theories emerged across strikingly different cultures, economies, and regimes: "The cholera conspiracies repeated themselves in stories of elites masterminding a cull of the poor to lessen population pressures, with doctors, pharmacists, nurses, and government officials as the agents of this planned class mass murder" (Cohn, 2017, p. 162).

Conspiracy theories can contradict one another but share a common focus on some malevolent individual or group. Amid cholera outbreaks in the 19th century, one theory asserted that "cholera was a fiction designed to suppress the rights of the poor," while another declared that "the authorities had deliberately introduced cholera by poisoning as a means of attacking the poor" (Briggs, 1961, p. 88). Despite the contradiction (hoax vs. murderous plot), both theories portrayed people in poverty as unjustly harmed by elites, thereby heightening government mistrust and provoking protest.

As with cholera, COVID-19 protest rallies were composed of groups espousing contradictory conspiracy theories. To illustrate, in a 2020 protest in London, a megaphone speaker declared that COVID-19 was a "great hoax," while other protesters chanted, "Take down 5G" (Hookham, 2020). The latter refers to the conspiracy theory that COVID-19 is real and dangerous, caused by 5G telecommunication towers (Chapter 12). In future pandemics, we should not be surprised to see protest rallies composed of people promoting contradictory conspiracy theories.

Conclusions

Public trust in the government is essential for containing large-scale disease outbreaks. Past episodes show that people are likely to be nonadherent to mitigation guidelines if they don't trust their leaders. Public mistrust in government can arise in various ways, such as when governments or officials (1) try to conceal evidence of an outbreak and the cover-up is exposed, (2) severely understate the seriousness of an outbreak, (3) flout pandemic mitigation guidelines, or (4) implement inconsistent or poorly timed lockdowns and other restrictions. Fueled by rumors and conspiracy theories, mistrust of the government undermines public confidence, leading to nonadherence and protest.

In the early stages of a disease outbreak—when there is much uncertainty about how serious it might become—government leaders and officials sometimes conceal or under-report the disease. Ostensible reasons are to keep the public calm and the economy running, to avoid a false alarm—if the outbreak proves to be minor—and to avert political blame if the outbreak appears to have arisen in one's country. If the outbreak spreads widely and the initial concealment is uncovered, public trust in the government can be eroded.

Political party affiliation and messages from party leaders influence attitudes for or against masks, vaccines, and social restrictions. Preexisting societal discord—societal fault lines—can worsen in pandemics, as seen in conflicts between government authorities and people experiencing poverty. Numerous protest demonstrations took place throughout the 19th-century cholera pandemics and in COVID-19. Rumors, conspiracy theories, and growing hardships were inciting factors.

The internet and social media greatly facilitate the organization and implementation of protest rallies, which may explain why there were more protests during COVID-19 compared to previous pandemics, except for the cholera riots. Protests in the digital age have become vastly easier to organize, fund, and publicize. Pandemic-related protests may, therefore, become more frequent in the future, especially when unpopular government restrictions are announced.

The odds of protests can be reduced in various ways. Lockdowns and other restrictions should be used sparingly, and alternatives should be considered. To be avoided where possible are "catch-and-release" lockdowns—where lockdowns are imposed, removed, and reimposed. Progressively burdening people with new restrictions (e.g., adding a curfew to closures) should also be avoided if possible, as that increases the odds of protest. Threats to impose compulsory measures, such as mandatory vaccination, can also incite protests and rioting. Further insights into pandemic-related protests can be attained by understanding the psychosocial mechanisms in belief polarization and threat processing (Chapters 10 and 11) and the factors involved in rumors and conspiracy theories (Chapter 12).

8
Coping During Disease Outbreaks

Introduction

Large-scale disease outbreaks require individual and community-wide responses. This chapter focuses on individual coping responses. People learn to cope with disease outbreaks from past experiences, observing others, and the news and social media. Coping enhances one's resiliency to deal with stressors. Resilience is the ability to endure and overcome adversity, including the ability to bounce back to previous levels of psychological functioning once a stressor has passed (Bonanno & Diminich, 2013). There is debate about the prevalence of resilience after highly stressful events, mainly concerning measurement and methodological issues (Infurna & Jayawickreme, 2019). Nevertheless, research consistently shows that most people are resilient to stressful events. Even if people become highly distressed during a stressful life event, most return to their pre-stressor levels of functioning (Galatzer-Levy et al., 2018).

Coping involves more than simply following health guidelines for handwashing and so forth. Coping involves dealing with the practical and emotional costs of pandemic-related stressors, including the socioeconomic burdens arising from lockdowns and other restrictions. This chapter considers the varieties of coping seen in pandemics and other outbreaks. We begin with two broad classes of coping—emotion-focused and problem-focused coping. This is followed by discussions of social support, altruism, and approach-avoidance conflicts about risking one's health to assist others. The chapter then turns to specific types of coping, including panic buying, folk remedies and quack cures, religious coping, and coping fads. As we will see, some forms of coping are helpful, while others are more dangerous than the diseases they are supposed to prevent.

Types of Coping

There are two broad, overlapping classes of coping: problem-focused and emotion-focused coping (Lazarus, 1991). Problem-focused coping involves attempts to take action to deal with the stressor. For example, a person might use folk remedies or quack cures to stay safe or seek practical assistance from friends or medical experts. Emotion-focused coping involves attempts to dampen negative emotions through various means, such as diverting activities (e.g., hobbies), physical exercise, and the use of alcohol, or recreational drugs. Positive thinking—such as positively reappraising an aversive event—is a common form of emotion-focused coping in which people try to look on the bright side. People turn to emotion-focused coping for various reasons, such as when problem-focused coping fails to produce results.

Emotion-focused coping was widely used in historical pandemics, partly because of the widespread belief that negative emotions increased one's risk of succumbing to infections. This belief has been around for centuries. In past pandemics, it was widely believed by medical and religious authorities and by the lay community that strong negative emotions—particularly fear, anxiety, melancholy (depression), and grief—increase one's susceptibility to all kinds of diseases, including plague, cholera, yellow fever, and influenza (Anonymous, 1721, 1849; Boghurst, 1666; Butcher, 1855; Fiquepron, 2018; Honigsbaum, 2010; Luther, 1527; Mead, 1744; Milwaukee Sentinel, 1918; Rosenberg, 1987; Seeger, 1832). Commenting on cholera, one physician opined that "the greater proportional number of deaths in the cholera epidemics are, in my opinion, caused more by fright and presentiment of death than from the fatal tendency or violence of the disease" (Myer, 1912, p. 142). In dealing with the plague and other outbreaks, medical experts and religious leaders encouraged people to pursue enjoyable activities to cope, so long as they didn't do anything immoral or illegal (Boghurst, 1666; Luther, 1527; Wear, 1999).

Emotion-focused coping was widely used in COVID-19, especially while people were in lockdown. In a study of 6,854 Canadian and American adults (Taylor, Landry, Paluszek, et al., 2020), the following were common emotion-focused coping strategies used to deal with restrictions on social gatherings such as lockdown:

- Watching TV or movies (96% of respondents).
- Cooking (78%).
- Hobbies (76%).

- Playing video or computer games (56%).
- Online shopping (51%).
- Eating more than one normally would (48%).
- Practicing relaxation exercises (29%).
- Consuming more alcohol or recreational drugs than one normally would (25%).
- Searching for porn on the internet (23%).

During COVID-19, lower levels of distress were associated with problem-focused coping strategies (e.g., problem-solving about new activities to pursue while in lockdown), emotion-focused strategies (e.g., limiting exposure to distressing news media, and positive thinking), and lifestyle management such as maintaining a healthy diet, getting enough sleep and physical exercise (Cheng et al., 2024; Fullana et al., 2020; Götmann & Bechtoldt, 2021; Park et al., 2021; Pigaiani et al., 2020; Veer et al., 2021). Lifestyle management is a component of stress management programs, entailing problem- and emotion-focused coping (Lehrer & Woolfolk, 2021; Romas & Sharma, 2022).

Some coping strategies are maladaptive if overused, such as when people overspend, overeat, or consume hazardous quantities of drugs or alcohol. Good coping sometimes depends on the "dose" of the coping response. People should avoid coping strategies with hazardous potential, such as excesses of food, drink, drugs, sex, and shopping. Other emotion-focused and problem-focused coping strategies can be selected and pursued based on the person's specifics and situation.

Social Support

Emotion-focused and problem-focused coping are commonly combined, such as when one seeks social support. Social support is the experience of being cared for, held in positive regard, and having a sense of belonging (Taylor, 2011). Social support entails emotional support mixed with practical advice and other assistance. People gain social support from family, friends, co-workers, social and community ties, and even from devoted pets. Social media can facilitate a person's social support from friends and family (Gilmour et al., 2020).

The frequency and quality of one's daily social contacts, especially positive encounters, are reliably correlated with greater happiness and lower distress (Van Lange & Columbus, 2021). Accordingly, seeking social support is a common coping strategy in stressful times. In our survey of Canadian and American adults mentioned above, we found that most people (83%) sought social support amid COVID-19 (Taylor, Landry, Paluszek, et al., 2020).

There is a two-way relationship between pandemics and social support. Social support can blunt the impact of pandemics; for example, social support can ameliorate the loneliness, depression, and anxiety commonly experienced in lockdown (Chen et al., 2022; Nitschke et al., 2020; Sommerlad et al., 2021). However, pandemics also erode social support due to sickness and death in one's social circle, undermining a person's resources for dealing with adversity. Under these circumstances, additional sources of support may be needed, such as from altruistic others.

Altruism and the Approach-Avoidance Conflict

Altruistic acts are vital ways of providing social support in times of crisis. Altruism as a coping response arises from diverse motivations, including prosocial motives (e.g., desire to help others) and self-focused benefits (e.g., feeling good about oneself because you're helping others). Feeling that one is doing something can provide a sense of agency or control over at least a portion of one's life. Accordingly, affiliative, supportive, and prosocial behaviors are common amid pandemics, where widespread sickness and debility evoke acts of mutual aid (Dezecache, 2015; Pettigrew, 1983; Schoch-Spana, 2004).

Along with the rise of altruism, pandemics elicit altruism-related approach-avoidance conflicts. These are internal conflicts. A person experiences an approach-avoidance conflict when a goal (e.g., helping others) has positive and negative features, making the goal appealing and unappealing. As one approaches the goal, the negative aspects loom large, heightening the conflict between approach and avoidance (Lewin, 1935; Vandenbos, 2007).

Approach-avoidance conflicts are expressed as procrastination, hesitation, indecision, and wavering in goal pursuit. Consider the following example. In the course of the Spanish flu, food insecurity became a problem. People often could not obtain supplies because they were too sick to leave their homes. Accordingly, there was a rise in altruism in which community members planned to deliver food to the sick (New York American, 1918; Rochester Times-Union, 1918). However, people providing aid experienced mixed feelings. An approach-avoidance conflict arose: helping people by bringing food to their homes versus avoiding people because of the risk of contagion.

"Often it was an agonizing decision: go to the aid of friends and relatives, perhaps imperiling the safety of their own families, or keep away?" (Pettigrew, 1983, p. 88).

Panic Buying

Panic buying is a form of problem-focused coping where people suddenly and urgently purchase large quantities of food, pharmacy supplies, or other items. Panic buying of disinfectants and other hygiene supplies, medications (e.g., Tamiflu), quack cures, and foodstuffs has been documented in many disease outbreaks, including the Russian flu, Spanish flu, 1968 influenza pandemic, avian flu, and COVID-19 (Cheng, 2004; Cheng & Cheung, 2005; Leichtenstern, 1905; Pettigrew, 1983; Wilson et al., 2009). For example, in the course of the Russian flu, there was panic buying of antipyrin, which was widely—and misleadingly—advertised as a potent treatment for influenza (Leichtenstern, 1905). In Baltimore amid the Spanish flu, "customers ravaged drug stores in search of products to prevent influenza and relieve symptoms" (Schoch-Spana, 2004, p. 45). In the 1968 flu pandemic in Guangzhou, China, there was panic buying and hoarding of medication and other pharmacy supplies (Wilson et al., 2009).

Panic buying occurred throughout COVID-19 when people had to go into lockdown. Panic buying was driven more by the behavior of shoppers than threats to the supply chain. Medicines and food were common targets, although there was also panic buying of items with little or no protective value, such as toilet paper. Once these items were identified in the news or social media as targets of panic buying, shoppers flocked to purchase them, fearing shortages.

Episodes of panic buying are likely initiated by highly fearful people, leading other shoppers to fear that they will miss out unless they purchase the coveted items. Fear of shortages drives panic buying, fueled by rumors of threats to the supply chain and dramatic photographs and videos of frantic shoppers and empty supermarket shelves circulated on the news and social media (Jovančević & Milićević, 2020; Taylor, 2021). Fear of scarcity leads to real short-term scarcity as zealous consumers temporarily deplete supplies. Fear of scarcity creates time pressure to buy now or miss out. Time pressure increases impulsive purchasing, particularly for products that provide safety or comfort (Liu et al., 2022). "Don't panic!" messages from community leaders are ineffective or counterproductive, heightening the sense of urgency and alarm (Taylor, 2021).

Panic buying can be maladaptive, increasing one's odds of infection. During COVID-19 in Vietnam, panic buying broke out on the eve of an impending lockdown in Ho Chi Minh City, an infection epicenter. Crowds flocked to the stores, undermining efforts at social distancing (Reuters, 2021). Similar episodes occurred worldwide during COVID-19, in which frantic shoppers converged on supermarkets and drug stores, thereby increasing the odds of superspreading (ABC News, 2020; CBS News, 2020; CNN, 2020; Deutsche Welle, 2020).

Panic buying and price gouging go hand in hand. Amid a cholera outbreak in Paris in 1832, the price of patent medicines (quack cures) skyrocketed (Evans & Bartholomew, 2009). A similar situation arose in COVID-19. Some people tried to exploit the coronavirus pandemic by purchasing large quantities of hand sanitizer, resold at inflated prices. In India, there was a brisk black-market trade in dwindling medical supplies of bottled oxygen, sold at an exorbitant markup (Associated Press, 2021).

While panic buying can be self-defeating, it gives people a sense of agency—a comforting, possibly illusory sense that one is "doing something" to address the threat. Regarding COVID-19, each episode of panic buying lasted 7 to 10 days (Keane & Neal, 2020). Accordingly, if you delayed shopping by 10 days, you would hit the stores as panic buying subsided. The delay would limit exposure to infected crowds, but store shelves would be depleted to some degree. Stores can manage panic buying by placing quotas on purchases, such as daily limits on hand sanitizer purchases.

Folk Remedies and Quack Cures

Folk Remedies

People commonly turn to folk remedies and quack cures to deal with disease threats. Folk remedies are homemade treatments or preventives, typically soups or tonics, teas infused with herbs, ointments, or (historically) poultices. Poultices are soft, warmed, moist masses of plant matter affixed to the skin with a cloth.

Folk cures were widely used in historical outbreaks of plague, yellow fever, and cholera, and also used in modern outbreaks such as SARS and COVID-19 (Cheng, 2004; Fiquepron, 2018; Hymes, 2014; Rosenberg, 1987). Rhubarb was a folk cure for plague in medieval China (Hymes, 2014). Folk remedies for SARS included turnips, vinegar, and kimchee (Cheng, 2004). COVID-19 folk remedies included drinking boiled garlic water, consuming large quantities of plain water, and inhaling hot air from a hair dryer (Bauman et al., 2020; Lytvynenko, 2020; Weiss, 2020). In Tanzania amid COVID-19, the minister of health endorsed folk remedies such as covering oneself with a blanket and inhaling steam from a boiling pot of herbs (Buguzi, 2021). Folk remedies are generally harmless, providing a comforting sense of protection. Folk remedies are concerning mainly when people use them instead of evidence-based alternatives.

Quack Cures

Commercially promoted quack cures include patent medicines, which are elixirs sold as either panaceas or remedies for specific ills. Historically, patent medicines often contained alcohol or opiates, along with exotic and sometimes toxic ingredients (e.g., radium). Quack cures are usually ineffective but potentially harmful if used persistently or consumed at high doses.

In the era of the Russian flu, quack cures included opiate-infused tinctures, Turkish baths, electricity-based interventions—electrical gadgets were new and exotic at the time—and various kinds of bronchial inhalers (Freckelton, 2020; Loeb, 2005). At the time, an infamous quack cure was the Carbolic Smoke Ball, which consisted of a tube attached to a rubber bulb filled with powdered carbolic acid. The user inserted the tube into a nostril, squeezed the ball, and inhaled the powder. Advertisements offered a £100 reward—equivalent to £16,000 today—to anyone contracting influenza after using the Smoke Ball. One user, Louisa Carlill, used the product, contracted the flu, and tried to claim the reward but was denied. She successfully sued the Carbolic Smoke Ball Company for breach of contract (Lancet, 1892).

Amid the Spanish flu, quack remedies were widely advertised in newspapers and became targets of panic buying. One news report claimed that "practically every drug store in the city sold out of camphor gum as soon as word spread that to carry it hung around the neck in a tiny bag was a 'sure cure'" (Fitchburg Daily Sentinel, 1918, p. 7). There were numerous quack cures and bogus "immunity boosters" marketed during COVID-19 (Weiss, 2020). For people worried about supposed toxins in COVID-19 vaccines, one doctor recommended a special bath for "detoxing" from the vaccine (i.e., for "getting the vaccine out" of one's body). The claim was mocked in the press (Chaya, 2021).

Smoking and Drinking as Panaceas and Preventives

Smoking tobacco and drinking alcohol were used as cures and preventives in many disease outbreaks, including the plague, cholera, Spanish flu, Russian flu, SARS, and COVID-19 (Anonymous, 1721; Bauman et al., 2020; Cheng, 2004; Iezzoni, 1999; Kell, 1965; Knapp, 2020; Pettigrew, 1983; Rocky Mountain News, 1918; Taylor et al., 2021; Weiss, 2020). Tobacco gained widespread attention in medical treatises in 16th-century Europe, where it was considered by many to be a panacea that cleansed the body of impurities. Tobacco smoke was considered a fumigant against miasma (Kell, 1965). In the Spanish flu, some doctors advised train travelers to ride only in smoking cars (Kell, 1965). Since respiratory ailments were thought to result from breathing "bad air," the fumigating properties of smoking were considered to be health-enhancing.

Objectively, smoking has no protective power against infectious diseases. Indeed, the opposite is true. Compared to nonsmokers, smokers are more vulnerable to infections in general, particularly respiratory diseases. Smokers are at heightened risk for the common cold, seasonal influenza, MERS, and COVID-19 (van Westen-Lagerweij et al., 2021). Current or former smokers were at higher risk of death from COVID-19 (Patanavanich et al., 2023). Yet, beliefs persist, especially among smokers, that smoking protects against respiratory disease. Cognitive factors such as illusory correlations may perpetuate beliefs in the protective power of smoking (Chapter 17).

In the late 19th and early 20th centuries, alcohol was widely touted in the newsprint and medical journals as an invigorating supplement and analgesic (Loeb, 2005). Advertisements came with colorfully exaggerated claims. Hall's Wine, for example, was widely advertised in U.K. newspapers as a preventive and restorative for influenza. In an advertisement appearing in *The Guardian*, readers were alerted that influenza was in the air and that "the only way to fight it is by taking Hall's Wine," a "blood-food of the highest order," creating new blood need to "fight and drive out influenza" (The Guardian, 1909, p. 4). Alcohol continues to be used today in quack remedies and folk cures.

Desperate and Dangerous Measures

When threatened with a potentially lethal infectious disease, people sometimes resort to desperate and dangerous cures or preventives. The pursuit of protection led to numerous poisonings during COVID-19 when people ingested hand sanitizer, disinfectants, large quantities of alcohol, or quack cures containing sodium chlorite (Buckley, 2021; Chary et al., 2021; Cortez, 2020; Grasso et al., 2021; Le Roux et al., 2021; Lebin et al., 2021).

In the United States and other countries during COVID-19, there were reports of infection-fearful people inadvertently overdosing on hydroxychloroquine, acetaminophen, and aspirin (Busari & Adebayo, 2020; Chai et al., 2020; Henry et al., 2021; Wong, 2020). The increase in poisonings was partly attributable to misinformation on social media (Chary et al., 2021; Grasso et al., 2021; Soltaninejad, 2020). The problem was exacerbated when U.S. President Trump publicly suggested that consuming or injecting cleaning products (e.g., bleach) could protect people from COVID-19 (Clark, 2020).

In France, some people inadvertently overdosed on cocaine, believing the drug conferred protection against the coronavirus (Osikoya, 2020). In Iran and elsewhere, there were numerous alcohol poisonings amid COVID-19, arising from the misconception that people could protect themselves against COVID-19 by consuming large quantities of ethanol (Aghababaeian et al., 2020; Heidari & Sayfouri, 2022). In the opening months of COVID-19 in 2020, one Iranian province reported 797 cases of methanol poisoning and 97 deaths. These figures exceeded those of the entire country for 2018 (Sefidbakht et al., 2020). The 2020 poisonings included "several cases of methanol poisoning in children resulting from a desperate attempt by parents to prevent or cure the infection" (Sefidbakht et al., 2020, p. 416).

Poisonings arose in past pandemics when people tried to keep themselves safe from disease. In the Russian flu, antipyrin was commonly used to provide relief against flu symptoms. Antipyrin was an early non-opioid, antipyretic analgesic that was widely used before being superseded by drugs with better safety and efficacy profiles (Brune, 1997). There were reports of antipyrin overdoses amid the Russian flu (Lancet, 1890). At the onset of that pandemic, people rushed to buy the drug: "Every one who had influenza or thought he had it, and many who wanted to protect themselves from the disease, took antipyrin *ad libitum*" (Leichtenstern, 1905, p. 698).

Poisoning due to drinking hydrogen peroxide occurred amid the Spanish flu, based on the erroneous belief that if disinfectants kill germs, then people can keep themselves safe by consuming those products (Pettigrew, 1983). Also in the Spanish flu, aspirin poisonings arose from the misconception that large quantities of aspirin were protective against influenza (Robins, 2005). The cure was sometimes worse than the disease; "many persons were in bed from the prostration of the drugs taken instead of from the 'flu'" (Robins, 2005,

p. 155). Such overdoses are not specific to pandemics. Overdoses of aspirin and other antipyretics occur when people try to protect themselves against seasonal influenza (Harden et al., 2015).

Motives for Pursuing Quack Cures and Folk Remedies

Various motives drive people to seek commercial quack cures and folk remedies, including imitation, conformity, a need to feel in control of the threat, and indiscriminate reliance on authority figures such as parents or political leaders (Taylor, 2019). Some people try to cover all their bases by pursuing mainstream and fringe medicine "just to be on the safe side." The pursuit of quack cures is also influenced by magical thinking, the illusion of control, and beliefs about health, diseases, and death, as discussed in Part II of this volume.

Regulating Quackery

Authorities have sporadically tried to limit the use of potentially dangerous quack cures. In the 1832 cholera outbreak in Paris, leaflets were distributed, warning people against quacks and charlatans preying on frightened people (Evans & Bartholomew, 2009). Today, some legal scholars argue that patent medicines should be tightly regulated and that the public needs to be better educated about the hazards of these nostrums (Freckelton, 2020). To proactively identify and eliminate these threats to consumers amid COVID-19, the U.S. Food and Drug Administration launched, in early 2020, *Operation Quack Hack*, which included a website alerting consumers to quack products (McMeekin & Shah, 2020).

Religious Coping

When people can't protect themselves from invisible infectious threats, they turn to external powers—governments, gods, or other sources of potent agency—to exert control and preserve safety. Religious coping combines social support with strategies for dealing with heightened mortality salience. Disease outbreaks cause an increase in mortality salience—the heightened awareness of the inevitability of one's death. Heightened mortality salience causes an increase in religious practices such as church attendance, prayer, and other religious rituals (Bentzen, 2021; Boguszewski et al., 2020; Briggs,

1961; DeFranza et al., 2021; Fatima et al., 2022; Schuster et al., 2001; Slack, 1985). Increased religiosity is a way of coping with heightened mortality salience by providing people with membership in a collective, enduring institution that promises literal immortality in an afterlife (Greenberg et al., 2020). Mortality salience and its relationship to death anxiety is discussed in Chapter 14.

Historically, numerous deities and patron saints were dedicated to infectious diseases, to whom people prayed and made offerings. These include deities devoted to healing in general, such as the Greek god Apollo, and those dedicated to specific ailments, such as the Hindu goddess Shitala, dedicated to smallpox (Henderson, 2009). For Christians, particularly Catholics, there are many saints to petition for healing and protection, including saints devoted to the plague, cholera, HIV/AIDS, and other infectious diseases (Byrne, 2012; Doino, 2020; Henderson, 2009).

In the Antonine plague (165–180 AD), people sought various ways of protecting themselves. Supernatural solutions "were especially popular, as people petitioned the old gods for healing" (Elliott, 2024, p. 112). Statues of Apollo were erected, and sacrificial offerings were made. Charms against plague were devised, such as phrases invoking the protection of Apollo written on amulets and above household doorways (Elliott, 2024).

In medieval Europe, the plague incited some dramatic religious rituals. The Flagellantism movement rose to prominence early in the second plague pandemic. Centered mainly in Germany, Catholic male penitents took to the roads in small troupes, walking from village to village, praying and whipping themselves bloody in imitation of Christ's Passion. By imitating Christ, they hoped to purge their sins and propitiate God's wrath (Gowen, 1907). The idea was that extraordinary acts of penance could end the plague. Crowds gathered to watch this "traveling penitential pageant" (Byrne, 2006, p. 204). Flagellents sang, prayed, and whipped themselves before moving on to the next town for another performance. The Catholic church condemned flagellants as heretical fanatics, and the practice was banned in some cities. In 1349, Pope Clement IV denounced flagellation as a "superstitious invention" (Aberth, 2010, p. 145). Flagellants were sometimes carriers of plague or fleas, inadvertently spreading disease as they trouped from village to village.

In plague outbreaks in England in the 17th century, church attendance swelled, except in those towns depopulated due to death and fleeing (Slack, 1985). When cholera arrived in Marseilles in 1834, a news correspondent reported that the disease outbreak had "quickened the religious zeal of the inhabitants" (Briggs, 1961, p. 81). According to an eyewitness report from

Barbados in the 1854 cholera pandemic, "the churches were more crowded, and the services performed with a deeper feeling of religion during the cholera than before" (Butcher, 1855, p. 40). Religious revivals also occurred in outbreaks of typhus in the 18th century (Slack, 1985). COVID-19 was associated with increased religious observances worldwide (Bentzen, 2021; Wilson et al., 2020). For example, an increase in religious faith was reported by 24% of Americans, and 55% prayed for the pandemic to be over (Gecewicz, 2020; Pew Research Center, 2020).

Heroes and Hero-Worshipping

Hero-worshipping is a form of combined emotion- and problem-focused coping in which one looks to heroes for inspiration, hope, and salvation. Heroes are people who enhance the lives of others, promote morals, and protect people from harm (Kinsella et al., 2015). Healthcare workers (HCWs) were publicly hailed as heroes in COVID-19. Previously, HCWs were rarely called heroes and tended to draw media attention only when they were recipients of workplace violence or accused of professional misconduct (Bellieni, 2020). In past cholera and plague pandemics, doctors and nurses were often viewed with suspicion due to rumors and conspiracy theories that they were profiting from ailments they were supposed to cure (Chapter 12).

COVID-19 differed from past outbreaks in the scope and magnitude of HCW hero-worshipping, facilitated by news and social media. Frontline doctors, nurses, hospital volunteers, vaccine researchers, and other health experts were hailed as heroes in the news media (Daily Mail, 2021; Holmes, 2021). HCWs were portrayed as Good Samaritans, working long hours for little remuneration (Skog & Lundström, 2022). These workers were celebrated in many countries in a ritual evening cheer in which urban residents stood at their apartment windows or balconies at 7 p.m. to applaud HCWs (Allen & Ellicott, 2020; Boulton et al., 2021; Cox, 2020). Cheering became an end in itself, boosting community morale (Mohammed et al., 2021).

The evening cheers for HCWs were not expressions of hero worship in the usual sense. The applauding public showed no signs of identifying with their heroes, and few seemed willing to emulate their deeds. The cheers were instrumental behaviors urging frontline workers to continue toiling to keep communities safe. The cheers turned to complaints and verbal abuse when HCWs failed to meet public expectations (McKay et al., 2021). Many of the people who cheered HCWs during COVID-19 were xenophobic and terrified of getting infected. These cheering but anxious individuals believed HCWs were sources of infection (Taylor, Landry, Rachor, et al., 2020).

Hero-worshipping amid COVID-19 included the purchase of merchandise commemorating public health leaders. Those praised as heroes included public health officers like Dr. Bonnie Henry in Canada. Dr. Henry's coping mantra—"Be kind, be calm, be safe"—was commemorated on decorative towels, necklaces, coffee mugs, t-shirts, and shoes (Glendinning, 2020; Marsh, 2020). Merchandizers in the early months of COVID-19 also produced hero memorabilia for the U.S. health authority, Dr. Anthony Fauci, including t-shirts hailing Dr. Fauci as a hero and commemorative mugs, pillows, and prayer candles (Byck, 2020). Public opinion soured when COVID-19 proved more challenging than initially expected. Dr. Fauci went from hero to anti-hero, especially among political conservatives, with a corresponding rise of "anti-Fauci" t-shirts and other merchandise (Spocchia, 2021).

In dealing with COVID-19, frontline HCWs unquestionably acted as heroes, although many were uncomfortable being labeled as such (Higgins, 2020; Lipworth, 2020; Rimmer, 2021). While the evening cheers may have provided HCWs with encouragement and comfort, practical resources were needed for these workers. HCW burnout and its management are discussed in Chapter 22.

Nostalgia

People commonly turn to nostalgia as a coping strategy when they feel isolated, lonely, or under existential threat (Garrido, 2018). Nostalgia is a bittersweet emotional state in which people experience a wistful or sentimental longing for some past period (Sedikides & Wildschut, 2018). Nostalgia is bittersweet because it involves a sense of loss and longing for the past, but also happiness at recalling positive memories.

Nostalgia-seeking increases when people feel threatened by infectious diseases (Barauskaitė et al., 2022). In the course of COVID-19, the rise of nostalgia-seeking was suggested by (1) social media trends to share old photos, videos, or other reminiscing (e.g., #MeAt20), (2) the rebroadcasting of classic films, sporting events, and concerts, and (3) a resurgence in popularity in old-fashioned board games (Barauskaitė et al., 2022; Gammon & Ramshaw, 2021; Wildschut & Sedikides, 2022).

Nostalgia can serve as an emotional anodyne—a form of emotion-focused coping that temporarily alleviates distress (Wildschut & Sedikides, 2001). Research shows that engaging in nostalgic reminiscence—that is, reliving, in memory, the "good old days"—typically improves one's mood, increases the meaningfulness of one's life by providing a sense of continuity with the past, and heightens one's sense of connection to others (e.g., by sharing of recollections and old photos or videos) (Garrido, 2018; Leunissen et al., 2021).

As COVID-19 spread through communities, researchers found that fear of the coronavirus could be reduced by engaging in short periods of nostalgic reverie (Dennis & Ogden, 2022). However, its beneficial effects tend to be modest (Frankenbach et al., 2020). Nostalgic reverie provides a mild, short-term respite for people in distress. Nostalgic reverie in COVID-19 flourished partly because of social media. It is unclear whether such reverie was used as a coping method in past pandemics or outbreaks.

Not all forms of nostalgia are beneficial. Some resemble bouts of depressed mood, as seen in historical accounts of nostalgia among American Civil War soldiers, consisting of intense sadness and homesickness, involving an intense longing to return to one's family, friends, and home (Weiss & Dube, 2021). For these darker forms of nostalgia, reminiscences are more bitter than sweet. Chronic worriers are more likely to experience these adverse effects (Verplanken, 2012). If people use nostalgic reverie as a coping method, they should be mindful of possible adverse effects.

Coping Fads

A fad is an abruptly arising, widely shared, short-lived enthusiasm. Coping fads occur in disease outbreaks. John of Ephesus (543 AD) documented an especially dramatic example in his account of the Plague of Justinian in Constantinople (Pearse, 2017). A rumor spread that plague would leave the city if people tossed clay water jugs from their upper-story windows, smashing on the streets below. According to John of Ephesus, "the rumour spread from this quarter to another, and over the whole city, and everybody succumbed to this foolishness" (Pearse, 2017, p. 1).

Another coping fad involved the use of sulfur during the Spanish flu. There were reports of people using small amounts of sulfur in their shoes as influenza preventives (Atlanta Constitution, 1918; Pettigrew, 1983). For example, Vancouver resident, George B., a glazier and window washer in frequent contact with the public, "believed he kept himself safe by sprinkling a bit of powdered sulphur into his shoes every morning before leaving the house" (Pettigrew, 1983, p. 114). The choice of sulfur was probably not coincidental, especially in an era when it was mistakenly believed that a bacterium caused the Spanish flu. Sulfur has long been used for its antibacterial properties (Kan et al., 2011).

The use of portable pulse oximeters early in the COVID-19 pandemic is another example of a coping fad. A pulse oximeter is a noninvasive device that clips onto one's finger or earlobe, using a light beam to measure blood oxygen levels. Sensational media reports urged people to buy these devices because of "silent hypoxia" (Halpern, 2021). Media stories recounted how some coronavirus-infected but seemingly healthy people, with no shortness of breath, suddenly collapsed and died from plummeting oxygen levels (Levitan, 2020). The concern turned out to be overblown. Even so, sales of pulse oximeters briefly surged in the opening months of COVID-19 (Kaur, 2020).

In future pandemics, we can expect to see coping fads come and go as frightened people struggle to find ways of feeling safe. Coping fads are mostly harmless efforts to gain control over a disease threat. However, some fads are potentially harmful.

Conclusions

People use various emotion- and problem-focused coping strategies to deal with the stressors associated with disease outbreaks. Ways of coping include seeking support from others, panic buying, turning to religion, assisting others, and relying on traditional remedies. These strategies can focus on solving problems (e.g., turning to folk remedies), managing emotions (e.g., pursuing comforting activities), or both (e.g., seeking practical help and emotional support from others).

The choice of coping strategies in disease outbreaks is influenced by one's past experiences and by observing the behavior of others. People can learn to improve their coping in various ways, such as via cognitive behavior therapy (Chapter 22). News and social media also influence coping, including coping fads. Fads are concerning mainly when the coping method is harmful to oneself—such as consuming toxic "remedies" or panic buying in over-crowded stores—or hazardous to others, such as tossing clay jugs from upper-story windows.

In future pandemics and disease outbreaks, people should be encouraged to pursue coping strategies that don't have adverse consequences for themselves or others. Social support is vital, along with coping strategies to alleviate distress and address practical problems. Nostalgic reverie can provide a mild, transient mood elevation for many people but can worsen mood for others.

Socially affiliative and supportive activities, such as nightly cheers for HCWs, can boost public morale and may offer some comfort to HCWs but do not replace the need for practical resources to alleviate the stress experienced by these workers, as discussed in Chapter 22.

Coping activities foster resilience, help people stay optimistic, and provide a sense of control, real or imagined. However, some coping methods, like relying on unproven remedies, can be harmful. When coping strategies fail or seem likely to fail, people often resort to fleeing—a special form of problem-focused coping discussed in the following chapter.

9
Fleeing
Urban Exodus from Contagion

Introduction

Even before the advent of germ theory, it was widely recognized that the risks of getting sick were greatest in urban settings: villages, towns, and cities. Historically and in modern times, when contagious diseases arise in these places, people commonly flee to places of perceived safety, particularly to the countryside (Cohn, 2018; Slack, 1985; Snowden, 2019). A Latin epigram best expresses the historical advice for staying safe from the plague: *Scilicet cito, longe, et tarde* ("Leave quickly, go far away, and stay away a long time") (Boghurst, 1666). Diarist Miquel Parets, writing during the second plague pandemic, said this:

> There is no better remedy for the plague than to be among the first and farthest to flee and to be among the last to return when the plague has been long forgotten. I say that it is quite right to flee in order not to suffer from this disease, for it is most cruel, but it is just as right to flee in order not to witness the travails and misfortunes and privations that are suffered wherever the plague is found, which are more than any person can stand. (Parets, 1651, pp. 66–67)

Fleeing from infection hotspots causes diseases to spread widely, turning localized epidemics into far-reaching outbreaks. The purpose of this chapter is to review the features, correlates, and consequences of fleeing amid disease outbreaks. Motivators of fleeing are described, and methods for dealing with the problem are discussed. We begin with a case study of the 1994 plague epidemic in India, which illustrates many psychological phenomena associated with fleeing and shows how governments can manage—or mismanage—the problem.

Plague in India, 1994

In August 1994, the Indian village of Mamla experienced an unusually heavy flea infestation associated with large numbers of dead rats in the streets. Shortly thereafter, plague broke out, rapidly spreading to neighboring villages. By September, the plague had reached the city of Surat, over 300 miles (500 km) away, and then spread to other cities. From August to October 1994, over 5,000 cases of suspected plague and 53 deaths were reported in eight states in India (Ramalingaswami, 2001).

Hospitals were flooded with the worried well, who misinterpreted symptoms of minor ailments as signs of plague; "a little runny nose and a cough, you were immediately rushed to the hospital" (Ramalingaswami, 2001, p. 29). People hurriedly manufactured face masks from whatever materials were available. There was panic buying of tetracycline, clinics were looted for medical supplies, and rumors spread that the plague was created as a bioweapon (Ramalingaswami, 2001; Sinha, 2000).

Sensational media reports fueled public anxiety, leading to widespread fleeing (Sinha, 2000). A quarter of Surat's population—an estimated 700,000 people—fled the city (Dutt et al., 2006). In one night alone, an estimated 600,000 fled Surat (Ramalingaswami, 2001). The wealthy fled in private cars (Dutt et al., 2006), while others fled "by whatever means available, including horse carriage, ox car, or even on foot" (Ramalingaswami, 2001, p. 29). Masses of fleeing people, many laden with possessions and some with children or elderly dependents, congested roads, railways, and bus depots. Crowds of frightened people stormed onto trains. Passengers already on the trains tried to block the train doors with suitcases in an unsuccessful attempt to thwart the fleeing crowds from boarding (Burns, 1994b).

Two-thirds of Surat's 400 physicians fled, but most returned when threatened with prosecution (Burns, 1994b). More than 100 patients fled from hospital isolation facilities, "fearing that staying in the wards was a death warrant for anybody who was not already confirmed as having plague" (Burns, 1994b, p. A1). Troops and police were dispatched to prevent further escapes from hospital while police scoured neighborhoods in search of escapees (Burns, 1994d). Senior doctors remaining in Surat appealed to officials to seal off the city with a cordon sanitaire.

In a curiously counterproductive move, the government-run State Transportation Corporation supplied nearly 200 *extra* buses for the fleeing masses, facilitating both the exodus and the spread of infection (Sinha, 2000). The plague followed transportation routes, with outbreaks in Surat followed by outbreaks in several major cities (Burns, 1994c). People hid indoors to avoid infection; "the streets were empty in Bombay, in Delhi, and even in distant places like Calcutta" (Ramalingaswami, 2001, p. 29).

Lasting about two weeks, the plague outbreak created widespread panic and led to short-term bans on travel and exports from India (Dutt et al., 2006; Ramalingaswami, 2001). The economic cost to India was over $US3 billion (Ramalingaswami, 2001). Many of the psychological phenomena seen in pandemics were apparent in this outbreak: Widespread fear, fueled by rumors and conspiracy theories, led to panic buying, looting, and fleeing. Critics blamed the government for mishandling the outbreak (Burns, 1994a). Government responses were inadequate and facilitated the spread of infection by supplying fleeing crowds with transportation.

Descriptive Features of Fleeing

About a decade after the plague in India, a similar episode occurred in Beijing at the onset of the 2003 SARS epidemic. In response to the new infectious threat, thousands of fleeing people mobbed Beijing's West Railway Station. There was panic buying of staples such as rice and vegetables, although sometimes this was impossible because vendors had fled the city, abandoning their market stalls. At the station, people in face masks jostled to buy tickets while scalpers worked the crowd, selling seats at inflated prices to destinations where SARS was scarce (Pomfret, 2003).

Fleeing crowds—often in a sudden, urgent exodus—have been observed in many disease outbreaks, including plague, yellow fever, cholera, SARS, influenza, and COVID-19 (Baltimore Sun, 1918; Barbarossa et al., 2021; Butcher, 1855; Chen et al., 2020; Cohn, 2018; Crampton, 2003; Delaporte, 1986; Fiquepron, 2018; Pomfret, 2003; Rosenberg, 1987; Snowden, 2019).

Flight by only 10% of a community can cause the number of infections to double (Epstein et al., 2008). People flee from both epicenters and surrounding regions. To illustrate, in the early weeks of COVID-19, as a travel ban was about to be implemented for the Wuhan epicenter, a surge of people fled the city, as revealed by cellphone geolocation data (Pang et al., 2022). At the same time, crowds fled from neighboring cities, fearing the arrival of the coronavirus from Wuhan (Pang et al., 2022).

Fleeing turns havens into disease hotspots. In the Antonine plague (165–180 AD), the wealthy fled from crowded urban centers such as Rome to the perceived safety of country villas (Elliott, 2024). Among the fleeing were infected individuals, hoping a trip to the countryside would do them good. Instead, they spread disease. In the Middle Ages, people fleeing the plague commonly sought refuge in monasteries. These havens became hazardous because of the commingling of "the healthy, the ill, and the bearers of infected fleas" (Snowden, 2019, p. 42).

Fleeing occurs even in small towns and villages. In an 1833 outbreak of cholera in the southern United States, "the appearance of cholera in even the smallest hamlet was the signal for a general exodus of the inhabitants, who, in their headlong flight, spread the disease throughout the surrounding countryside" (Rosenberg, 1987, p. 37). When outbreaks reach rural areas, farmers and laborers sometimes also flee, abandoning their crops (Garza, 2008).

Fleeing can occur even when, objectively, there is nowhere safe from infection. People sometimes flee the cities where they live and work, preferring to be in familiar, comforting surroundings with friends and family. Seeking proximity to loved ones is a common reaction in the midst of disasters (Mawson, 2005).

Combined with sickness and death, fleeing leads to temporary societal breakdown because of insufficient workers to perform essential services. When merchants and business owners flee, markets and businesses close, creating unemployment and shortages for those left behind (Anonymous, 1721; Byrne, 2012; Rosenberg, 1987). Historical accounts depict desolate cities during disease outbreaks. When cholera struck New York in 1832, the inhabitants fled to the countryside. Visitors to the city were "struck by the deathly silence of the streets, unaccustomedly clean and strewn with lime" (Rosenberg, 1987, p. 28). Tufts of grass grew in little-used thoroughfares. Even on Broadway, "passers-by were so few that a man on horseback drew curious faces to upper windows" (p. 28).

Fleeing and Conflict

People from all social classes flee amid pandemics. For people in poverty, fleeing can be stressful and risky. Potential hardships include sickness, starvation, assault, and robbery (Cohn, 2018; Kumar et al., 2021; Pearse, 2017). Fleeing is more feasible and less hazardous for people with wealth and resources. But even the wealthy had trouble finding accommodation in rural villages amid plague outbreaks: "Fear of contagion led innkeepers to remove signs, villages to post guards against refugees, and farmers to deny travelers food and roust those sleeping in their barns" (Byrne, 2012, p. 147). In plague outbreaks in the 16th and 17th centuries, villagers met fleeing city-dwellers—"runaways" as they were sometimes called—with suspicion, hostility, and sometimes violence (Byrne, 2012; Cohn, 2018; Dekker, 1625; Slack, 1985; Snowden, 2019; Wear, 1999). On the road, fleeing urbanites were confronted by vigilantes intent on keeping strangers out of their towns or villages. Miquel Parets described official efforts to stem the flow of runaways from plague-infected Barcelona:

> Barcelona was emptied of a great many persons who, terrified by the plague, fled from the city. . . . Those who [fled] suffered great travails and disasters . . . for all Catalonia had been alerted and so many roadblocks had been set up and so many guards were stationed in all the villages and towns and cities that not even a cat could get by. They refused to let anyone get by or even get near. (Parets, 1651, p. 50)

In Sicily in 1887, amid a cholera epidemic, people fled the city of Palermo to the neighboring town of Monreale, 6 miles (10 km) away. Fleeing city-dwellers were confronted by an armed mob: "With guns, the mob forced the refugees to camp in the fields, and stabbed to death and cremated a nine-year-old boy, who approached the town for safety" (Cohn, 2018, p. 247).

COVID-19 was associated with conflicts between locals and fleeing urbanites, but none as dramatic as the Monreale example. During COVID-19, fleeing migrant workers in India faced stigma and hostility on returning to their villages (Patil & Chaukimath, 2020). In the same pandemic in England, Canada, Australia, and America, urbanites fleeing to holiday homes or tourist destinations were met with hostility from locals, who slashed tires and placed notes under windscreens of parked cars, telling the runaways to "go home" (Keogh, 2020; Malatzky et al., 2020; Stanford, 2020; Stewart, 2020). Residents of some American tourist towns tried to block the influx of fleeing urbanites. In Cape Cod, Massachusetts, more than 12,000 residents signed a petition asking authorities to turn away visitors and nonresident homeowners (Barrett, 2020). Similar community-led isolation efforts were initiated in other holiday destinations, including the Florida Keys and North Carolina's Outer Banks (Barrett, 2020; Keogh, 2020).

Motivators and Triggers for Fleeing

Fear Is Contagious

Fleeing illustrates the phenomenon of fear contagion. Humans, being social animals, tend to spontaneously and automatically mimic one another, including facial expressions, body movements, vocal expressions, and emotions (Hatfield et al., 2014; Hatfield et al., 2020). Fear is contagious, spread by observing others behaving fearfully (Bandura, 1986; Debiec & Olsson, 2017;

Gump & Kulik, 1997; Hatfield et al., 1994; Hatfield et al., 2014). Even the smell of sweat from frightened people can evoke fear in others (De Groot et al., 2014). Fear contagion is a building block of human interaction, allowing people to understand one another by "feeling themselves into" the other's emotions (Hatfield et al., 2014). Even someone downplaying a disease threat will likely grow apprehensive when everyone around them is frightened.

Perceived Narrowing of Escape Routes

Fleeing gives frightened people a sense of control—a sense of doing something to deal with an infectious threat (Kumar et al., 2021; Wear, 2015). Fleeing from infected cities is intensified when people fear that travel restrictions will block escape routes (Pang et al., 2022). During COVID-19, fleeing occurred in many urban centers in anticipation of government lockdowns and travel restrictions (Barbarossa et al., 2021; Chen et al., 2020; Kinetz, 2020; Sen & Pandya, 2021). For example, at 2 a.m. on January 23, 2020, in Wuhan, residents were notified that from 10 a.m., all public transport would be suspended, and residents would not be allowed to leave the city without permission. Consequently, more than 300,000 people fled Wuhan by train and other means, spreading the infection to surrounding regions (Barbarossa et al., 2021; Chen et al., 2020; Kinetz, 2020). In India and Italy during COVID-19, the threat of impending lockdowns also triggered fleeing from infection hotspots, with crowds sometimes numbering in the thousands (Barbarossa et al., 2021; Kotoky, 2021; Sen & Pandya, 2021).

Economic Pressures and Mistrust of Government

Fleeing is often driven by economic pressures. Many people flee when faced with lockdown and unemployment, fearing they will not receive government assistance if they remain behind (Kumar et al., 2021). In the words of a fleeing migrant worker during COVID-19, one of the thousands fleeing New Delhi for his home village, "I have just 100 rupees ($1.34) left with me, and I don't know how long this lockdown is going to last ... the government did ask us stay back, but can you trust the government?" (Sen & Pandya, 2021, p. 171)

At the onset of COVID-19, before the first lockdown was imposed in India in March 2020, hundreds of thousands of workers fled the cities to avoid lockdowns that would have rendered them unemployed and without financial support (Sen & Pandya, 2021). Workers and their dependents fled to their hometowns and villages, often hundreds of miles away (Kumar et al., 2021). They gave their main reason for fleeing as financial, although many were also concerned for their safety and that of their family members (Chander et al., 2021; Kumar et al., 2021). The departure was temporary. Workers returned to the cities when restrictions were lifted and their employment resumed. A year later, the cycle was repeated: The threat of a second lockdown triggered another wave of fleeing, with workers returning when the restrictions were lifted (Gettleman et al., 2021).

Social Factors

Peer pressure influences the decision to flee. For migrant workers in India in the time of COVID-19, the decision to flee was influenced by news stories, rumors of fleeing elsewhere, and the opinions of their peers (Kumar et al., 2021). Migrant workers often travel in groups, typically composed of people from the same geographic region. Accordingly, once a group's majority has decided to flee, others feel obliged to conform. These workers and their dependents fled the cities, seeking the familiarity of their home villages and towns (Kumar et al., 2021).

Do Travel Restrictions Work?

For COVID-19, the travel ban from Wuhan, implemented on January 23, 2020, arrived too late to stem the spread of infection. By that time, most Chinese cities had received infected travelers (Chinazzi et al., 2020). According to statistical modeling by Chinazzi and colleagues, the travel ban delayed disease progression by only three to five days in mainland China, but it had a greater impact on the international spread of the disease, at least in the first few weeks of the pandemic.

Systematic research reviews provide mixed support for the efficacy of travel restrictions in controlling disease outbreaks. According to one review, preventing international travel by closing borders is among the most effective ways of pandemic mitigation (Haug et al., 2020). Cordon sanitaire—placing entire towns or cities in quarantine—was rated as moderately effective (Haug et al., 2020). Conclusions from other researchers were less supportive of restrictions. Errett et al. (2020) concluded that there was insufficient research on travel bans to determine their efficacy (Errett et al., 2020). Another group of investigators found "no evidence in favor of international border closures"

(Shiraef et al., 2022, p. 1). Grépin et al. (2023) concluded that there was little evidence for the efficacy of travel restrictions. Border closures were considered helpful in stemming infection "only when coupled with strong domestic public health measures" (Grépin et al., 2023, p. 1). In short, travel restrictions might be helpful depending on how and when they are implemented, but research is lacking.

In some circumstances, travel restrictions are unenforceable, especially when thousands flee en masse. Some experts argue that public education is the key to discouraging fleeing during infectious disease outbreaks (Ramalingaswami, 2001). Others disagree, noting that it's pointless to tell people not to flee if the only other option is to starve; "putting up roadblocks and beating stragglers will only encourage them to find new routes, off the main highways" (Hajari, 2020, p. 1). From this perspective, fleeing can be reduced by bolstering the public's trust in the government to ensure their protection and well-being amid large-scale emergencies, such as by providing financial assistance to unemployed workers while in lockdown.

Historical Advice: Flee Responsibly

Historically, efforts to thwart fleeing involved a combination of travel restrictions, appeals to altruism and morality, and shaming, fines, and arrests (Byrne, 2006; Cohn, 2018; D'Irsay, 1927). A famous tract on fleeing was Martin Luther's sermon *Whether one may flee from a deadly plague* (Luther, 1527). Luther, a Christian theologian, argued that people should avoid needless exposure to disease while maintaining social order and performing one's ethical and civic duties. Luther contended that people in a position of responsibility—such as government officials, providers of essential services, and people caring for dependents—have a moral obligation to remain behind rather than flee.

Luther further argued that people have a moral responsibility for the well-being of their neighbors: "No one should dare leave his neighbor unless there are others who will take care of the sick in their stead and nurse them" (Luther, 1527, p. 120). Ethically, you were permitted to flee so long as there was someone to cover your personal and civic responsibilities. Feeling extremely anxious about a disease outbreak was seen as a legitimate reason for fleeing, so long as you didn't shirk your moral and civic responsibilities (Luther, 1527). Later writers echoed Luther's views: Although the plague was viewed by many as a punishment from God for a community's collective sins, it was acceptable to flee so long as you didn't abandon your dependents or neglect critical responsibilities (Boghurst, 1666; Dekker, 1625; Kephale, 1665).

The arguments raised by Luther and others are relevant today, although there are further considerations. Fleeing causes infectious diseases to spread widely, which is an argument for *not* fleeing infection hotspots while also taking steps to remain safe. To this end, governments play a vital role in providing people with safety and assurances so that fleeing is unnecessary.

Conclusions

Fleeing from infection hotspots has long been recognized as a common, socially disruptive phenomenon that contributes to the spread of infection and leads to transient societal breakdown. Medical and religious writers have discussed fleeing since the earliest plagues, with the consensus that fleeing is acceptable under some circumstances but not others. However, a concern is that fleeing can cause diseases to spread widely, turning localized epidemics into large-scale outbreaks.

Fears of sickness and economic hardship are among the leading causes of fleeing. Government messaging, or the lack thereof, has an impact on fleeing. Governments can address economically induced fleeing by ensuring that community members, especially financially vulnerable individuals, have financial and other support in the course of government-imposed lockdowns. Travel restrictions reduce but do not eliminate fleeing. People are less likely to flee if they feel assured that government interventions will protect them from disease and economic distress. A deeper understanding of the motivations for fleeing can be attained by looking at the psychological processes involved in threat perception and the roles of rumors and conspiracy theories, as discussed in the following chapters.

PART II
PSYCHOLOGICAL PROCESSES AND MECHANISMS

10
Exposure to News and Social Media

Introduction

This chapter examines how the news and social media influence people's appraisals of and responses to disease threats, today and historically. We begin with information exposure—the amount or dose of information a person receives—and how one's cognitive processing style (monitoring vs. blunting) influences information exposure. The effects of news and social media are then discussed. Both types of media can fuel anxiety but also lead to the polarization of attitudes and emotions, affecting how people respond to pandemic threats and mitigation measures. The remainder of the chapter considers the infodemic and fake news, historically and during COVID-19, and discusses contemporary efforts to help people navigate the morass of digitally available health information.

Information Exposure

The type and dose of media information that people receive modulate many pandemic-related phenomena, including the propagation of ideas (e.g., rumors and conspiracy theories) and behaviors (e.g., fleeing). People with little exposure to the news and social media may be unaware of an impending infectious threat and blindsided when disaster arrives. Other people, such as those consuming large doses of media, may be exposed to much threat-related information, including misinformation. Some occupations are associated with more information exposure than others. Journalists covering COVID-19, for example, had high levels of exposure to stories of death and suffering.

A person's cognitive processing style influences the tendency to seek out or avoid health-related information. Some people have a "monitoring" information-seeking style, while others have a "blunting" style (Miller, 1989). People who are monitors seek detailed information about health risks and risk-reduction strategies, whereas blunters avoid health-related information (Kim & Choi, 2017; Miller et al., 2001; Zhuo et al., 2021).

People with a monitoring cognitive style would likely have expressed great interest in the *Lord Have Mercy* broadsheets published in the 1665 Great Plague of London (Sperry, 2018). Named after their title banners, these news publications supplied the public with detailed information about the plague's progress, including local burial statistics. The broadsheets also provided readers with resources such as prayers of repentance and recipes for supposed plague preventives (e.g., garlic mixed with milk). The prayers and recipes encouraged readers to believe they had control over their risk of infection. The broadsheets—filled with plague-related information—would appeal to people with a monitoring coping style, whereas blunters would likely avoid these broadsheets and their morbid contents.

Monitoring and blunting each have shortcomings as self-protective strategies. Although blunting is generally associated with less health-related worry and distress, blunters risk ignoring critical health-related threats, thereby failing to take precautionary measures (Miller, 1996). Compared to blunters, monitors perceive a given health threat as riskier and are more likely to worry about their health in general (Davey et al., 1992; Miller, 1996; Miller et al., 2005). Monitoring was associated with high levels of distress during COVID-19: Among the people in greatest distress were those who repeatedly checked their news and social media feeds for COVID-related information (Taylor et al., 2020).

COVID-19 received intense media attention—on television, the internet, and social media—making the pandemic almost impossible to ignore. When news programs are filled with stories about a disease outbreak, monitors and blunters will be anxious for different reasons. Monitors will become alarmed because of the high volume of threat-related information, and blunters will become anxious because the threatening information is difficult or impossible to avoid. To better manage their anxiety, monitors can learn to focus on positive, reassuring information, such as advice about what one can do to stay safe (Miller, 1996). Blunters may benefit from messages involving logical appeals about protective measures. Such appeals are less likely to trigger avoidance than fear-evoking messages (Kim & Choi, 2017). Public messaging campaigns could consider using different messages to target monitors and blunters.

News Media

COVID-19 arose in an era of global digital interconnectivity and real-time 24-hour news reporting. This led to anticipatory anxiety preceding the arrival of the coronavirus, where people became alarmed about infection even though the disease had yet to reach their community (Taylor et al., 2020). The situation was similar during the 1889 Russian flu, the first pandemic in an era of cheap, mass-circulation newspapers and global communication via telegraph (Honigsbaum, 2010; Kempińska-Mirosławska & Woźniak-Kosek, 2013). So prevalent were fear-evoking newspaper accounts amid the Russian flu that one physician remarked that the fear of flu was "started by telegraph" (Lancet, 1890, p. 88). People became alarmed about the flu even when cases were only in other countries.

The news media has been criticized for exaggerating dangers and creating undue public fear (Brown et al., 2019). The news media can fuel fear and uncertainty with speculative stories about worse-case scenarios of what might happen in a disease outbreak. Modern journalism's adversarial style, where one position or viewpoint is pitted against another, is poorly suited for objectively discussing uncertainty, with the risk of reducing uncertainties to overly simplified either-or arguments (Corner et al., 2012). In attempts to exaggerate controversies to sell stories or in misguided efforts to provide balanced reportage, media stories can give the misleading impression that opposing views on some issue are equally supported, even when the evidence favors one view over discredited views (Corner et al., 2012).

During the SARS outbreak, the media overstated the dangerousness and contagiousness of the virus, leading to widespread but short-lived public anxiety and xenophobia (Muzzatti, 2005). U.S. news coverage of the outbreak "saturated viewers with images of East and Southeast Asians wearing masks and creatively-framed camera angles provided footage of deserted Chinatowns in American urban centers, further fueling the stigma" (Muzzatti, 2005, p. 123). Absent from most media coverage was the fact that SARS was not easily communicable, nor was it fatal in most cases.

The news media was criticized amid the 2004–2007 outbreaks of avian flu for exaggerating the threat by using emotionally toned language, making misleading comparisons between the avian flu and the deadlier Spanish flu, the selective use of statistics, and sensationalized speculations about the death toll and economic costs (Abeysinghe & White, 2010). Experts interviewed by the media can add to the sensationalism. When commenting on the avian flu outbreak, a prominent British virologist was quoted in *The Guardian* as saying, "Forget al-Qaeda, the biggest terrorist threat we face today is Mother Nature" (Nerlich & Halliday, 2007, p. 59).

Analyses of media reports concerning the 2009 swine flu pandemic suggest that the media contributed to heightened risk perceptions primarily through the high volume of coverage and an emphasis on dangers while giving less attention to things people could do to stay safe (Klemm et al., 2016). Responsible reporting need not be devoid of frightening details but should be balanced with information about protective measures (Brown et al., 2019).

Social Media

Traditional news services, such as newspapers, radio programs, and television broadcasts, offer one-way dissemination of information to the receiving public. Social media platforms have changed the way news is spread. These platforms—such as Facebook, Reddit, X (Twitter), Telegram, and YouTube—enable users to selectively share (amplify) some news coverage and create their own stories (Brown et al., 2019). Users who express interest in a particular news story, such as by liking a post on Facebook, signal the value of the story to other social media users (Strekalova, 2017). Stories are most likely to be believed and shared if they evoke strong negative emotions, such as intense fear or moral outrage (Bebbington et al., 2017; Brady et al., 2020; Guadagno et al., 2013; Martel et al., 2020; Rubenking, 2019).

Social media has become a significant source of health information and advice (Adebayo et al., 2017; Devine et al., 2017). As of April 2024, there were 5.1 billion social media users worldwide, representing 63% of the world's population (Datareportal, 2024). The average user spends more than two hours daily on social media, with YouTube, Facebook, and WhatsApp being the most popular platforms (Datareportal, 2024).

Social media provides users with a mix of accurate and misleading information. Surveys of YouTube videos about infectious diseases found that 20% to 30% contained misinformation (Bora et al., 2018; Tang et al., 2018). News stories on Ebola on Reddit were more sensational than those on mainstream news sites (Brown et al., 2019). A survey of Facebook posts amid the Zika pandemic found that 12% of posts about the virus contained misinformation; "the majority of these contained content related to the pandemic as a way to depopulate third-world countries or called Zika virus a hoax intended to cover up chemical teratogens manufactured by major multinational corporations" (Sharma et al., 2017, p. 302). The most widely circulated misleading post was a video titled "10 reasons why Zika virus fear is a fraudulent medical hoax," with over half a million views and about 20,000 shares (Sharma et al., 2017). Misleading posts about the Zika virus were more likely to be shared than posts containing accurate information (Sharma et al., 2017).

People who used social media as a news source were likelier to believe and share COVID-19-related misinformation (Ahmed & Rasul, 2022; Allington et al., 2021). Pro- and anti-vaccination groups were active on social media during COVID-19 (Pilkington & Glenza, 2019; Stuart & Cady, 2023). For both groups, social media provided a vehicle for recruitment and proselytization. Anti-vaccination groups offered tips on how to avoid mandatory COVID-19 vaccination (Thomas, 2021). Pro-vaccination social media groups emphasized the prosocial and personal benefits of vaccines and criticized people holding anti-vaccination attitudes (Stuart & Cady, 2023).

There is no simple relationship between social media use and mental health. On the one hand, social media can provide social support, which should protect mental health. On the other hand, social media is a source of alarming misinformation, inducing needless fear. A meta-analysis found that, overall, there was *no* relationship between social media use and subjective well-being in the course of COVID-19 (Wong et al., 2024). The findings were inconsistent with pre-COVID studies showing that social media use is associated with poorer mental health. Lockdowns may have altered the way social media was used. Overall, any positive and negative effects of social media appear to have canceled each other out during COVID-19 (Wong et al., 2024). Further research is needed to determine how communities and individuals might enjoy the benefits of social media while minimizing its adverse effects.

Media Use and Attitude Polarization

Opinions concerning moral behavior, health, and safety are commonly polarized in pandemics (Garza, 2008; Hirst, 1953; Procopius, 551 AD). Polarized opinions include views concerning the appropriateness of fleeing, whether lockdowns should be used, and whether the disease's severity has been over- or understated. Some people become anxious about the threat of disease, while others dismiss the danger as overstated (Taylor, 2019). People who view news reports as exaggerated are less likely to adopt the health behaviors recommended by health authorities (Rubin et al., 2009).

Polarized attitudes tend to be firmly held and resistant to persuasion (Bienenstock et al., 1990; Brauer et al., 1995). Preexisting attitudes on emotionally charged health-related issues—such as beliefs concerning the safety and necessity of vaccination for one's children—can become entrenched as people take sides and argue their positions. People with extreme attitudes are sometimes willing to risk sickness, death, or unemployment to defend their views. In COVID-19, for example, thousands of healthcare workers lost their jobs for refusing mandatory vaccination (CBC News, 2022; Furey, 2021; Herhalt, 2021; Kirkey, 2023; Lazaruk, 2022; Mitchell, 2021).

Contemporary news and social media enhance attitude polarization because the media enables users to filter information selectively and selectively associate with like-minded individuals (Modgil et al., 2021). People tend to choose media consistent with their attitudes and values (Gvirsman, 2014). Filtering increases the likelihood of exposure to stories that affirm and strengthen one's beliefs. People prefer interactions with like-minded others (McPherson et al., 2001). Accordingly, people holding views on some critical issue (e.g., vaccination) tend to affiliate with like-minded individuals. Such groups provide camaraderie, a shared view, and a common goal on some personally important topic. There is also the "undeniable appeal to joining a group that is fired up with righteous indignation" (Stern, 2016, p. 106).

When like-minded people congregate, such as in social media groups, the repeated expression of their beliefs and hearing others voice similar opinions can strengthen their views, thereby shifting the group to hold more extreme (polarized) attitudes (Brauer et al., 1995). This process can involve strengthening one's ideas by being exposed to novel supporting arguments and refutations of counterarguments. Members may copy others for approval by taking similar or somewhat more extreme positions, which group members may regard as "taking a good idea even further" (Brauer et al., 1995; Forsyth, 2020).

The Infodemic

The term "infodemic" was coined in 2003 by *Washington Post* journalist David J. Rothkopf, writing in the context of SARS. The infodemic consists of "facts, mixed with fear, speculation and rumor, amplified and relayed swiftly worldwide by modern information technologies" (Rothkopf, 2003, p. B01). According to Rothkopf, the infodemic is a complex phenomenon, more than simply a high volume of news combined with an excess of rumors. The infodemic emerges from mainstream news media, websites, and social media. The output from these diverse sources consists of a blend of fact, interpretation, rumor, and propaganda. The information may be difficult to verify for news consumers, and the picture may be shifting and incomplete. Confusion and conflict may arise as news consumers try to make sense of the mass of information.

Early in COVID-19, the WHO warned the public about an infodemic concerning the coronavirus (WHO, 2020). Online misinformation spread faster than the disease itself (Kucharski, 2020; Weiss, 2020). Misinformation about COVID-19 came from various sources, including political leaders of the United Kingdom, America, and Brazil (BBC News, 2021). U.S. President Trump was a prominent source of misinformation about the coronavirus and its treatment (Evanega et al., 2020). The preponderance of vaccine misinformation came from a small number of individuals—dubbed the Disinformation Dozen. An analysis of Facebook and Twitter data indicated that 65% of anti-vaccine content was attributable to the Disinformation Dozen (Center for Countering Digital Hate, 2021).

Infodemics were apparent in past disease outbreaks, albeit not to the extent seen today. Fiquepron (2018) examined newspaper coverage of yellow fever and cholera epidemics in Buenos Aires, Argentina, from 1867 to 1871. Although there were few news outlets compared to today, a small-scale infodemic was evident. Newspapers, barely two pages long, contained facts mixed with opinions and false claims. Included were critiques of how cholera was being managed, scientific reports, advertisements for quack cures appearing alongside articles discussing evidence-based preventives, descriptions of sick rooms, and jokes. People read these newspapers aloud to one another in cafés and elsewhere, facilitating the circulation of opinions and rumors (Fiquepron, 2018).

The Russian flu was the first pandemic in the era of the telegraph and mass-circulation newspapers (Honigsbaum, 2010). Not surprisingly, the Russian flu was associated with an infodemic comprised of a mix of accurate reports on the spread of infection combined with confusing or erroneous accounts of how the disease was caused and how it might be treated. Consider, for example, page 3 of the *London Evening News and Post* on January 7, 1892. In separate articles, that page contained contradictory explanations of the cause of the pandemic. One piece reported that a "Bloomsbury physician has advanced the perfectly feasible theory that influenza is the result of iodine poisoning, the iodine being taken from a surcharged atmosphere." The other article declared that "the influenza bacillus has been discovered almost simultaneously at two institutes entirely independent of each other" (London Evening News and Post, 1892, p. 3). Both articles were mistaken. The pandemic was caused by neither iodine nor bacteria. Instead, it arose from an influenza virus or coronavirus (Chapter 1).

Fake News

Fake news is a pernicious form of misinformation in which stories are deliberately concocted to mislead (Lazer et al., 2018). The stories mimic true ones and typically consist of dramatic, fabricated, or grossly inaccurate claims intended to be spread on social media, often with highly partisan political content to drive reader engagement (Pennycook & Rand, 2019). Fake news can start with a grain of truth (e.g., "COVID-19 began when 5G telecommunications towers were erected in Wuhan"), which is spun into some dramatic claim (e.g., "5G radiation causes COVID-19"). Fake news headlines often evoke fear or moral outrage, which increases the odds that the stories will be shared. People do not always believe what they share. Sometimes, fake news is shared because of inattention to accuracy rather than an intent to circulate falsehoods (Pennycook & Rand, 2021).

Numerous fake news stories, images, and videos were widely circulated during COVID-19. The infamous "bat soup" video showed a smiling Chinese woman holding a cooked bat with chopsticks. After taking a bite, she observed, "The bat tastes very fresh, like chicken meat" (Zhou, 2020, p. 1). The video sparked outrage. Bats are possibly a reservoir for the coronavirus causing COVID-19, and the video could imply that Chinese eating habits—specifically, the consumption of exotic animals from wet markets—could be responsible for COVID-19. However, the video was not taken in China. It was filmed for an online travel program in 2016 in the pacific archipelago of Palau. The clip was originally posted as part of an online travel program where the host sampled local delicacies. In 2020, the clip was reposted by unknown internet users to imply that Chinese eating habits were the source of COVID-19.

People circulated the clip for various reasons, even if they did not believe it was true (Long et al., 2021). However, many people, including news reporters and outspoken politicians, thought the clip was from Wuhan (Ritchie, 2021; Rozsa, 2020; Scheirer, 2020; Shen-Berro, 2020). "China is to blame," declared the U.S. Republican Senator John Cornyn, because they "eat bats and snakes and dogs and things like that" (Shen-Berro, 2020, p. 1). Media outlets circulated the video, and "thousands of Twitter users blamed supposedly 'dirty' Chinese eating habits—in particular the consumption of wildlife—for the outbreak" (Palmer, 2020, p. 1). Chinese officials vigorously denied that people eat bats in their country (Chinese Embassy, 2020).

Distinguishing factual from fake news is increasingly challenging as fakes become more sophisticated, such as "deepfake" videos mimicking real people. Underscoring the difficulty in deciding whether a news story is fake, a study found that healthcare professionals were no better than college students in spotting false stories about COVID-19 (Gruner & Kruger, 2021).

People are more likely to believe fake news if they (1) rely on intuition rather than analytical thinking, (2) overestimate their knowledge about the topic, and (3) tend to ascribe profundity to meaningless statements (Pennycook et al., 2020; Pennycook & Rand, 2020). The source of a news story (e.g., whether it came from a political leader) and the number of social media "likes" also influence the story's perceived veracity (Pennycook & Rand, 2021). People who believe misinformation about one health issue (e.g., statin medications) are likely to accept other sorts of health misinformation (e.g., vaccines) (Scherer et al., 2021). The tendency to believe in health misinformation is correlated with lower educational attainment, distrust in the healthcare system, and positive attitudes toward alternative medicine (Scherer et al., 2021).

Dealing with Misinformation and the Infodemic

Approaches for fighting fake news and other types of misinformation include social media algorithms for censoring or down-weighting problematic content (Pennycook & Rand, 2021). During COVID-19, the social media platform Pinterest altered its search algorithm to make it harder to find vaccine misinformation. Google attempted to dilute the impact of misinformation by preferentially displaying links to reputable health sources when people searched for information about COVID-19 (Kucharski, 2020). Mainstream social media platforms, such as Facebook, Instagram, and YouTube, attempted to regulate their content by removing posts containing misinformation about vaccines and other public health measures. Among the items widely banned by mainstream social media was a slick, misinformation-packed "documentary" called *Plandemic* (Butler, 2021). Among its bogus claims were allegations that mask-wearing "activates" the coronavirus and that vaccines contain tracking microchips.

For better or worse, people usually find ways around censorship (Dorfman, 2022). Material banned on mainstream social media (e.g., Facebook) may appear on alternative social media outlets such as Telegram or Truth Social. Censorship is challenging in an era when almost everyone can use cell phones to record and upload content, including screenshots of censored or deleted internet material. People can be encouraged to self-censor, that is, to be selective in what they share with others on social media.

Tags or warnings attached to fake news stories (e.g., "disputed" or "rated false") can reduce, to some extent, the believability of questionable stories (Clayton et al., 2020). However, one study found that tagging a story as false had little effect on the perceived accuracy and likelihood of sharing the story on social media (Kreps & Kriner, 2022). More effective in reducing misperceptions and sharing were journalistic fact-checks appended to the stories. These are notes stating reasons why a story is false (Kreps & Kriner, 2022).

The ability to distinguish true from fake news can be enhanced by improving one's media and health literacy. Media literacy is the ability to assess the probable accuracy of information from news and social media (Dorr, 2001). Health literacy refers to a person's knowledge, motivation, and competence to access, understand, critically appraise, and apply health information for their healthcare (Sørensen et al., 2012). People with poor media or health literacy are especially likely to have difficulty distinguishing truth from fake news and are liable to fall for conspiracy theories.

Educating people in analytical thinking can reduce belief in fake news (Bago et al., 2020; Bronstein et al., 2019). Checklists of potential red flags can aid people in this regard (e.g., did the story come from a reputable news source?) (Guess et al., 2020). Encouraging people to deliberate on a news story or think about the accuracy of its claims can improve judgments of its accuracy (Ecker et al., 2022). People do not routinely evaluate the credibility of news sources, but when they do, the impact of misinformation can be reduced (Lewandowsky et al., 2020).

Preemptive (pre-bunking) strategies have been developed to inoculate audiences before they encounter misinformation. These strategies involve detailed refutations and alternative explanations (Lewandowsky et al., 2020). Debunking is a related strategy for correcting misconceptions. For example, the WHO published a series of "myth-busting" infographics to debunk misconceptions about COVID-19 (WHO, 2022).

Brief exposure to corrective information tends to have short-lived benefits (Craig & Vijaykumar, 2023; Roozenbeek et al., 2020). Repeatedly presenting accurate COVID-19 information increases its perceived veracity (i.e., the repetition-induced truth effect: Chapter 11). However, experimental research suggests that the benefits are attenuated if the person subsequently encounters misinformation (Craig & Vijaykumar, 2023). If repetition of myth-busting information is used as a debunking method, the effects may be short-lived if followed by misinformation. Booster doses of corrective information may be needed.

A potential problem with myth-busting is that it increases people's exposure to false information (i.e., the myths), which can increase the perceived truthfulness of the myths. These "backfiring" effects are uncommon but can be disruptive when they occur (Ecker et al., 2022). Backfiring was demonstrated in a study of misinformation about COVID-19 vaccines. Repeated exposure to vaccine myths increased the credibility of the misinformation (Lee & Bissell, 2024). Rather than myth-busting (myth plus corrective facts), presenting corrective information (facts only) might be more effective (Lee & Bissell, 2024).

Another approach to myth-busting involves recruiting social media influencers and celebrities to share accurate, health-promoting information (Tang et al., 2018; Yun et al., 2016). This approach is problematic. Most celebrities and influencers are not content experts and might just as easily pass on misleading information, as was the case with the Disinformation Dozen. The public should be encouraged to seek authoritative, reliable information sources.

Conclusions

During disease outbreaks, people differ in their degree of information exposure. Some individuals are exposed to, or seek large amounts of information about the infectious threat, while others try to limit their consumption of frightening disease-related news. There are pros and cons to each of these monitoring and blunting styles. Nevertheless, given the pervasiveness of today's news and social media, it can be difficult to avoid news about large-scale disease outbreaks. The rapid dissemination of news contributes to anticipatory anxiety early in disease outbreaks.

People who use social media as their primary news source are more likely to believe and share misinformation, including unfounded rumors and conspiracy theories. Sensational news and social media stories can have polarizing effects, leading some people to become highly alarmed while others dismiss the reports as overstated. Social media and news media augment attitude polarization, in which divergent opinions on an issue—such as views concerning the efficacy and necessity of vaccination—become increasingly extreme and entrenched.

The vast amount of news and social media data creates an infodemic comprising an uncertain mélange of facts, rumors, speculation, and misinformation. The mix of information creates confusion and hampers efforts to control disease outbreaks. Attempts have been made to regulate social media to stem the spread of misleading information. People can learn to improve their media literacy, although it can be difficult to spot fake news.

11
Heuristics and Biases in Threat Evaluation

Introduction

In the preceding chapter, we discussed the characteristics of disease-related information received from news and social media. The present chapter focuses on how people use or process this information—the cognitive mechanisms in threat perception. People are often inaccurate in their risk estimates, where the degree of concern does not match the objective odds of harm (Frost et al., 1997; Young et al., 2008). Rather than appraising evidence objectively, people are prone to biases and other errors in evaluating and assimilating information, leading people to over- or underestimate risk.

This chapter reviews cognitive mechanisms known as heuristics and biases and discusses how they influence appraisals of disease threats. Heuristics and biases are rapid, efficient cognitive processes that play a pervasive role in human life. When confronted with uncertainty, people use heuristics and biases to guide their decision-making (Ludolph & Schulz, 2017; Tversky & Kahneman, 1974). Among other things, heuristics and biases shape our judgments of the probability (likelihood) and cost ("badness") of potential threats. Heuristics and biases operate non-consciously, analogous to a computer software program running silently in the background. Accordingly, people are usually unaware that heuristics and biases shape their thinking (Pohl, 2017).

Heuristics and biases play an important role in intuitive thinking. Evidence suggests that the human mind is modular, consisting of multiple systems. The distinction can be made between two cognitive systems, one that relies on intuition and another depending more on deliberation (De Neys, 2018; Kahneman, 2011). Intuitive thinking is automatic (non-conscious, involuntary), effortless, and fast. Deliberative thinking is slower, more effortful, and sometimes necessary to correct erroneous intuitions. Both systems, especially the more automatic, intuitive system, involve heuristics and biases (Kahneman et al., 2021; Pohl, 2017).

Heuristics and biases are generally adaptive but lead to systematic (predictable) errors of judgment (Kahneman et al., 2021). Heuristics and biases can lead to distorted risk perceptions and unsafe behaviors during disease outbreaks. In the following sections, we review eight heuristics and biases because of their relevance to pandemics: The anchoring heuristic, confirmation bias, availability heuristic, repetition-induced truth effect, exponential growth bias, affect heuristic, hindsight bias, and temporal discounting.

Anchoring Bias

The anchoring bias occurs when the initial source of information serves as an anchor or basis for subsequent decision-making (Rehana & Huda, 2021; Tversky & Kahneman, 1974). The bias is evident when people cling to initial opinions, failing to update them when new information emerges. Thus, initial, inaccurate information can persistently bias one's views.

The anchoring bias influences how people appraise threats. An initial impression that a disease is not severe ("It's just a cold") may bias subsequent judgments. The anchoring bias can play a role in nonadherence to pandemic mitigation measures. Consider the World Health Organization's (WHO) shifting recommendations on the necessity and efficacy of face masks in public places in 2020. Initially, masks were deemed unnecessary in nonclinical settings, but then, as evidence accrued, mask-wearing was strongly recommended in public places (Chapter 5). An anchoring bias was evident in people who adhered to the initial view, discounting later recommendations on masks (Madison et al., 2021).

The present is a powerful anchor when predicting the future. The anchoring bias is relevant for understanding pessimistic expectations. Amid a pandemic, when people are subject to lockdowns and other restrictions, they may doubt that life will return to the way it was before. People may expect—erroneously—that they will never be able to hug one another, kiss, or shake hands because of the threat of infection (Pendleton, 2020). We imagine the future based on how things appear today. Despite pessimistic expectations in the midst of a pandemic, in the aftermath people routinely return to pre-pandemic ways of living, including the resumption of social rituals such as hugging and shaking hands (Chapter 23).

The anchoring bias is relevant for understanding medical misdiagnosis. In medical settings, the anchoring bias consists of "the focus on a single—often initial—piece of information when making clinical decisions without sufficiently adjusting to later information" (Ly et al., 2023, p. 818). The anchoring bias contributes to medical misdiagnosis because anchoring on an initial diagnosis can lead to the inappropriate exclusion of alternatives (Ly et al., 2023; O'Sullivan & Schofield, 2018; Saposnik et al., 2016).

Pandemics provide conditions conducive to the anchoring bias in emergency room settings, in which there is a high likelihood that patients have the pandemic disease. Such was the case in COVID-19 epicenters, where there was a general expectation that most cases of respiratory infection were due to the coronavirus. Many instances of anchoring-induced misdiagnoses were reported, where clinicians failed to consider alternative diagnoses because they assumed the correct diagnosis was COVID-19 (Abu-Rumaileh et al., 2021; Bhula et al., 2022; Harada et al., 2020; Patel et al., 2021; Zamora et al., 2023). Even if initial tests were negative for COVID-19, "physicians often anchored on the diagnosis of COVID" (Patel et al., 2021, p. 456A). In one case, multiple physicians evaluating a patient were "fixated on COVID-19 pneumonia" as a diagnosis despite evidence to the contrary (Abu-Rumaileh et al., 2021, p. 1).

The anchoring bias is difficult to overcome (Bahnik et al., 2017). Nonetheless, there are several informative guides for understanding and attenuating the effects of anchoring and other heuristics and biases (Croskerry et al., 2013a, 2013b; Daniel et al., 2017; Ecker et al., 2022; Lewandowsky et al., 2020; O'Sullivan & Schofield, 2018). Slowing down to critically reflect on a piece of information is a widely used strategy (O'Sullivan & Schofield, 2018). Other methods for dealing with anchoring and other heuristics and biases include education in meta-cognition—thinking about one's thinking—to help people identify judgment errors. For clinicians, the anchoring bias can be attenuated with structured aids such as checklists of guiding prompts (e.g., "consider alternative diagnoses," "look for disconfirmatory evidence") (Mussweiler et al., 2000; O'Sullivan & Schofield, 2018).

Confirmation Bias

The confirmation bias involves selectively searching for evidence and arguments to support one's views while neglecting or dismissing contrary views (Mercier, 2017). The confirmation bias is a logical consequence of the anchoring bias, in which the person selectively seeks information to confirm their initial (anchored) position. The confirmation bias is so powerful and pervasive that, according to the cognitive scientist Raymond S. Nickerson, "one is led to wonder whether the bias, by itself, might account for a significant fraction of the disputes, altercations, and misunderstandings that occur among individuals, groups, and nations" (Nickerson, 1998, p. 175).

The confirmation bias can perpetuate beliefs in the efficacy of one's coping behaviors. In Chapter 8, we met George B., the glazier and window washer who believed he kept himself safe from the Spanish flu by sprinkling sulfur into his shoes each morning. George regarded the absence of infection as proof of his method—a confirmation bias. Motivated reasoning, such as the wish or desire to be correct in one's judgment, can perpetuate the confirmation bias. If sulfur was George's only coping method, he might be reluctant to scrutinize its efficacy in case it proved ineffectual. People are often unaware that they are engaging in motivated reasoning, erroneously believing that their judgments are unbiased. This lack of awareness is called the "illusion of objectivity" (Pyszczynski & Greenberg, 1987).

The confirmation bias can exacerbate fear. Expecting danger and selectively searching for it can intensify one's sense of threat (Remmerswaal et al., 2014). A person might fear that an episode of diarrhea signals impending COVID-19. The person searches the internet, finding evidence that diarrhea can be a symptom of the disease. A confirmation bias occurs when the person fails to entertain benign reasons for diarrhea, such as stress or minor food intolerances.

Attitude polarization arises from the confirmation bias when people selectively interpret ambiguous information as supporting their views (Benoît & Dubra, 2019). Consider vaccines, for example. People tend to show a confirmation bias when they search for vaccine information, preferring that which supports their beliefs (Malthouse, 2023; Meppelink et al., 2019; Xu et al., 2023). The selective search for evidence against the safety and efficacy of vaccines can strengthen anti-vaccination sentiments. Similarly, a selective search for pro-vaccine evidence can strengthen pro-vaccine beliefs. The result is an increasing polarization of beliefs about vaccines. Thus, the confirmation bias can lead to polarized attitudes about vaccines, with moderate views about vaccines (for or against) becoming more extreme as people search for information to confirm their initial opinions (Li & Jager, 2023). The confirmation bias can be attenuated with training—for example, by instructing people to look for evidence for *and* against some claim or assertion (Daniel et al., 2017).

Availability Heuristic

The availability heuristic has a powerful influence on threat perception. According to this heuristic, people estimate the probability of some outcome by how easily they can recall or imagine similar instances (Tversky & Kahneman, 1973). The availability heuristic is often accurate because the ease of recalling something usually indicates its prevalence or frequency. However, other factors, particularly vividness, influence probability estimates.

Sensational events—such as plane crashes, terrorist bombings, and shark attacks—are more memorable than bland events, thereby inflating people's estimates of the prevalence of dramatic occurrences (Kahneman & Tversky, 1973; Nisbett & Ross, 1980). Sensational media reports of "what might happen" during a disease outbreak can lead people to overestimate the threat by increasing the ease of envisioning frightening scenarios.

When asked to judge the odds of getting infected with a disease, reliance on the availability heuristic leads people to estimate the probability by recalling similar instances of infection in one's social circle (Sherman et al., 2002). If it is easy to recollect examples, the odds of getting infected are judged high. The odds are considered low if few or no examples can be recalled. Thus, the perceived probability of getting COVID-19 was elevated among people whose close others had sickened or died from the disease (Abel et al., 2021; Botzen et al., 2022; Dryhurst et al., 2020). Consuming a lot of news about the coronavirus can also increase the ease of recalling dramatic COVID-19 cases, exacerbating fear (Taylor et al., 2020).

People can be taught to identify the availability heuristic in their thinking, although it is more challenging to counter its effects. The effects can be attenuated when people are encouraged to slow down and deliberate on their decisions (O'Sullivan & Schofield, 2018). For clinicians, diagnostic prompts can also be helpful in medical decision-making, such as reminders to critically examine the objective basis for one's initial diagnosis (Croskerry et al., 2013b; Daniel et al., 2017).

Repetition-Induced Truth Effect

The believability of a news report or posting on social media is greater when the story is familiar, easy to imagine, and easy to understand (Brashier & Marsh, 2020; Ecker et al., 2022; van der Linden, 2022). Fluency—the ease of understanding and imagining—and familiarity increase with repeated exposure. Repetition may seem empty because no new information is conveyed when a message, image, video, or story is repeated. However, repetition facilitates learning and memory (Unkelbach & Koch, 2019). Thus, the repetition-induced truth effect occurs when the repetition of some claim (e.g., "Cholera is a hoax") heightens its fluency and familiarity, thereby increasing its perceived veracity (Dechêne et al., 2010; Renner, 2017).

The repetition-induced truth effect is an automatic cognitive process based on recognition memory. Believing that one has heard the information previously enhances its perceived truthfulness (Renner, 2017). Repetition increases the perceived truthfulness of all kinds of information—accurate information, misinformation, and conspiracy theories—and also increases one's willingness to share such material on social media (Béna et al., 2023; Pillai & Fazio, 2021; Unkelbach & Speckmann, 2021; Vellani et al., 2023).

Repetition increases belief in misinformation even when the false information contradicts prior knowledge (Pillai & Fazio, 2021). Repeated exposure to vaccine myths can increase the credibility of the misinformation (Lee & Bissell, 2024). The persistent repetition of misinformation during COVID-19 likely contributed to the believability of false claims such as "COVID-19 is no worse than seasonal flu" and "Only old people are at risk." Images and videos are especially compelling in persuading people that something is true—seeing is believing (Brashier & Marsh, 2020). Repeated exposure to sensationalized or fake videos and images—such as the infamous "bat soup" video (Chapter 10)—can distort viewers' beliefs about the origins and dangers of diseases.

Advertisers have long used repetition to enhance their products' memorability and perceived efficacy. Consider Bex, an analgesic powder containing phenacetin that was widely advertised as a headache remedy in Australia in the 1960s. Advertisements were extensively broadcasted on TV and radio, such as one relentlessly repeating the message, "Bex is better." Repetition likely contributed to the perceived truthfulness of the claim. In reality, Bex was not better. Bex was banned in the 1970s because it was addictive and caused kidney and liver damage (Casey, 2018). Unfortunately, misinformation can be sticky. Even if corrected later, misinformation can persistently influence one's thinking (Johnson & Seifert, 1994).

The repetition-truthfulness effect can be attenuated when people are encouraged to think critically about the veracity of a claim, such as whether it came from a reputable source and whether the claim is contradicted by other information (Pillai & Fazio, 2021). Countering the effects of repeated misinformation can be challenging because debunking efforts must describe the misinformation being discredited. Several strategies have been offered to improve the impact of debunking under these circumstances (see Chapter 10).

Exponential Growth Bias

R_0 is the basic reproduction number for a given pathogen, defined as the average number of people infected by transmission from a single infected individual in a population that has not previously encountered the pathogen. When $R_0 > 1$, cases increase exponentially—that is, the cases increase in an accelerating manner. People tend to show an exponential growth bias, expecting growth to be linear rather than exponential (Banerjee et al., 2021; Stango & Zinman, 2009).

The exponential growth bias makes people underestimate the speed at which infection spreads. People lacking knowledge of exponential growth tend to assume that the spread of disease will be linear—that is, slow, progressive growth rather than rapid proliferation. These individuals express "particularly strong confidence in their erroneous forecasts" (Lammers et al., 2020, p. 16,264). Failure to understand exponential growth leads people to underestimate the impact of a single infected person on the community—an impact that could be avoided through social distancing (Misuraca et al., 2022). Thus, people who fail to appreciate exponential growth also fail to see the need for social distancing (Lammers et al., 2020).

Although many people struggle to understand exponential growth, training can reduce the bias (Lammers et al., 2020; Misuraca et al., 2022). During COVID-19, public support for social distancing improved when people were taught to understand how infection spreads rapidly via exponential growth—that is, showing people with words or graphs how the "speed" of contagion increases over time, with cases doubling every few days (Lammers et al., 2020).

Affect Heuristic

People evaluate risk by analyzing the situation and attending to their feelings (Slovic & Peters, 2006). Reliance on feelings, known as the "affect heuristic" or "emotional reasoning," involves attending to feelings and gut reactions to make judgments about safety and danger. Good feelings indicate a benign situation, and bad feelings indicate a problem (e.g., "If I feel anxious about entering a crowded store, then it must be unsafe"). Reliance on the affect heuristic, especially when emotions are strong, can lead to the neglect of other sources of information, such as the objective probability of a given risk (Slovic & Peters, 2006). When emotions are strong, reliance on the affect heuristic inflates risk estimates and increases one's tendency to believe sensationalized news reports (Martel et al., 2020).

People prone to high levels of anxiety are most likely to rely on the affect heuristic when inferring danger (Arntz et al., 1995; Özdemir & Kuru, 2023; Paredes-Mealla et al., 2022). The tendency to infer danger based on anxiety may amplify or exacerbate anxiety (Arntz et al., 1995). That is, inferring danger from anxiety ("I am anxious, therefore there must be danger") leads to further anxiety about being in danger. Thus, a positive feedback loop arises, where the affect heuristic amplifies anxiety. People who are highly frightened of anxiety—that is, people scoring high on a trait known as anxiety sensitivity—are most likely to use the affect heuristic to infer danger (Chapter 18). Reliance on the affect heuristic can be reduced when people are trained to base their judgments on objective measures of risks rather than feelings (Lommen et al., 2013). Cognitive behavior therapy targeting anxiety sensitivity also reduces reliance on this heuristic (Taylor, 2000).

Hindsight Bias

The hindsight bias is a "knew-it-all-along" bias involving the tendency to overestimate the extent to which an outcome could have been foreseen. The bias arises when people overestimate what they had known or expected before learning the outcome (Pohl & Erdfelder, 2017). The hindsight bias is evident when people exaggerate, in retrospect, the availability and reliability of early warnings. To illustrate, people may become frightened early in an outbreak of a novel disease, believing the threat to be great. Afterward, if nothing terrible happened, the hindsight bias is suggested by self-assuring statements like "I knew it wouldn't be that bad." Alternatively, if the person suffered significant personal losses during a disease outbreak, the hindsight bias might be expressed by beliefs such as, "Our leaders should have seen it coming!" Beliefs about foreseeability are linked to perceived responsibility and blame (Blank, 2024).

The hindsight bias stems from cognitive processes involved in memory and appraisal (Giroux et al., 2023). Memory distortion may be involved, such as when outcome information affects one's recollection of what was previously known or believed. Beliefs about the foreseeability and inevitability of an event also influence the hindsight bias. Motivational processes may be involved, such as the need to see the world as orderly and predictable or the need to affirm one's preexisting (anchored) views or beliefs.

The hindsight bias reinforces the illusion that one's world is predictable and controllable, at least when viewed retrospectively. The bias is robust and challenging to overcome (Pohl & Erdfelder, 2017). However, several debiasing strategies have been suggested. For example, asking clinicians to explain their diagnostic reasoning can reduce the bias by encouraging them to reflect on their assumptions (O'Sullivan & Schofield, 2018).

Temporal Discounting

Temporal discounting, also known as discounting the future, is a bias to prefer immediate, smaller rewards over larger, delayed ones (Critchfield & Kollins, 2001; Loewenstein & Prelec, 1992). Steep discounting (devaluing) of future rewards is indicative of shortsighted decision-making (Halilova et al., 2022). Here, "reward" is broadly defined to include the absence of aversive outcomes. Temporal discounting is a common cognitive bias, evident in various kinds of decision-making, including decisions made by individuals and governments (Frederick et al., 2002).

Regarding social distancing, temporal discounting is suggested when the gratification of immediate needs (e.g., socializing with friends) takes precedence over more uncertain, longer-term outcomes (e.g., protection from infection). In the case of vaccine hesitancy, temporal discounting is evident when people opt for "smaller, immediate benefits of not getting vaccinated (e.g., avoiding initial side effects) versus the longer-term benefits of vaccination (e.g., immunity to COVID-19, increased social interaction)" (Halilova et al., 2022, p. 5).

Temporal discounting increases when future outcomes are highly uncertain (Frederick et al., 2002). People are more likely to engage in temporal discounting when experiencing negative emotions such as anxiety, depression, anger, or disgust (Calluso et al., 2021; Zhang et al., 2023). Calluso et al. speculated that the increased preference for immediate gratification "serves as a mechanism of self-reward aimed at down-regulating negative feelings" (p. 1).

Several studies examined temporal discounting during COVID-19. Greater temporal discounting—as indicated by performance on a monetary decision-making task (e.g., assessing preferences about hypothetically receiving $5 now vs. $30 after seven days)—was correlated with lower adherence to mask-wearing and social distancing and greater vaccination hesitancy (Byrne et al., 2021; Freitas-Lemos et al., 2023; Halilova et al., 2022; Lloyd et al., 2021).

Historical descriptions provide suggestive evidence of temporal discounting in disease outbreaks, in which people sought to live for the moment, while ignoring the financial, legal, and other consequences. The Plague of Athens (430–426 BC) provides an example. Here, people resolved to "spend quickly and enjoy themselves, regarding their lives and riches as alike things of a day" (Thucydides, 411 BC, p. 252). Desperate pleasure-seeking amid deadly disease outbreaks is further discussed in Chapter 14.

Temporal discounting is not limited to individual decisions—it also occurs when decisions are made in committees and other groups. Research shows that interacting with others leads decision-makers to become more like their collaborative partners over time, including decisions about temporal discounting (Bixter & Luhmann, 2021).

Discounting the future can undermine pandemic preparedness efforts, including failures to maintain long-term disease surveillance systems. In 2019, a few months before the outbreak of COVID-19, the U.S. government decided to discontinue its $200 million Project PREDICT, a pandemic early warning program (Baumgaertner & Rainey, 2020; Milman, 2020). In operation since 2009, the project focused on zoonotic spillover—the spread of viruses from wildlife to humans—which is the primary cause of pandemics (Chapter 24). The goal of the project was "to speed up and organize the previously haphazard hunt for zoonotic diseases" (McNeil, 2019, p. D3). The project had identified "more than 160 different coronaviruses that had the potential to develop into pandemics, including a virus that is considered the closest known relative to COVID-19" (Milman, 2020, p. 1). The reasons for ending the program were never made entirely clear (Schmidt, 2020). Nevertheless, according to Peter Daszak, who played a key role in the project, "cutting a program that could in any way reduce the risk of things like COVID-19 happening again is, by any measure, shortsighted" (Baumgaertner & Rainey, 2020, p. 1).

Conclusions

Threat perception is influenced by several factors, including the type and dose of information that people receive and how they use or process the information. The human mind filters and evaluates data using heuristics and biases. Research indicates that heuristics and biases influence how people appraise and respond to pandemic-related threats. Heuristics and biases are relevant for understanding a range of errors, including misjudgments of the dangerousness of a disease and failures to prepare for future threats.

Heuristics and biases are associated with attitude polarization and can lead to diagnostic errors when these biases sway clinical judgment. People who rely more on intuitive than analytical thinking are more likely to use heuristics and biases in decision-making and are more prone to associated errors. Further research is needed to determine whether reliance on heuristics and biases varies across personality traits. Some heuristics and biases can be overcome with training and practice, while others are more difficult to modify.

As cognitive processes, heuristics and biases shape people's beliefs about the world. Heuristics and biases can strengthen beliefs, as in the confirmation bias. They can also distort beliefs and expectations. Heuristics and biases influence beliefs in rumors and conspiracy theories, which are discussed in the following chapter.

12
Rumors and Conspiracy Theories

Introduction

This chapter reviews the nature, consequences, and management of pandemic-related rumors and conspiracy theories. We begin with rumors, which are forms of improvised news arising when the demand for information on some vital issue exceeds the known supply of facts (DiFonzo & Bordia, 2007). Rumors can help people to make sense of an uncertain, hazardous situation by providing information about what is safe or dangerous and how to avoid harm or escape danger. Rumors are not trivial. Rumors about alleged treatments for feared diseases sometimes lead to deaths, as described later in this chapter.

Conspiracy theories are extreme types of rumors in which significant events (e.g., a pandemic) are attributed to the actions of nefarious individuals or groups. Belief in conspiracy theories is remarkably widespread. This chapter examines the themes, features, and prevalence of pandemic-related conspiracy theories and considers the kinds of people most likely to endorse and share these theories. The chapter concludes by discussing the methods for managing rumors and conspiracy theories in the course of pandemics.

Rumors: Improvised News

Rumors are stories or claims of unknown provenance and uncertain veracity, passed from person to person. Rumors are improvised news, spreading rapidly when the demand for information exceeds the supply (Shibutani, 1966). Rumors may be true, false, or somewhere in between. Historically, rumors were spread by word of mouth and by print media (e.g., newspapers, pamphlets). Today, digital news and social media are common means of rumor dissemination. As rumors pass from person to person, the narrative usually changes; with retelling, rumors tend to become shorter and simpler, with details omitted, as well as sharper, in which some details are accentuated

The New Psychology of Pandemics. Steven Taylor, Oxford University Press. © Oxford University Press (2025).
DOI: 10.1093/9780197811009.003.0012

or distorted, often to fit cultural expectations, biases, or stereotypes (Allport & Postman, 1947; DiFonzo & Bordia, 2007).

Rumors might start as speculations or even fabrications. With retelling, conjectures get spun into facts. Dramatic rumors are sometimes spread for entertainment purposes or to intentionally frighten people. In the early months of COVID-19, for example, a false rumor circulated that smoke from crematoria could be seen from outer space, implying vast numbers of coronavirus casualties (Lytvynenko, 2020).

Lurid rumors commonly arise during pandemics, such as rumors about victims being mistaken for dead and buried alive. Such rumors were described in outbreaks of plague, cholera, and yellow fever (A Physician of New Orleans, 1854; Butcher, 1855; Cohn, 2017; Hecker, 1844; Morens et al., 2008). Rumors proliferated in Europe amid the 1832 cholera pandemic (Benoiston de Châteauneuf et al., 1834; Morens et al., 2008). People were terrified, "believing the wildest fictions," including conspiratorial rumors that "the deaths were all owing to poison, and that there was no such thing as cholera" (Anonymous, 1849, p. 85).

Rumors reduce uncertainty by suggesting treatments or preventives, giving people ideas about ways of protecting themselves and their loved ones. In the SARS outbreak in China in 2003, there were reports of farmers and urban residents consuming "a sugary elixir of boiled mung beans meant to keep the virus away" (Ang, 2003, p. 1). The idea "stemmed from a rumor about a baby who purportedly spoke immediately after birth and said firecrackers and 'green bean soup' could prevent infection, said an official" (Ang, 2003, p. 1). According to the official, "hundreds of thousands of people in the province, including the capital, Hefei, received the rumor via text messages on their cell phones" (p. 1). The rumor led to a spike in sales of mung beans and fireworks (Ang, 2003). Firecrackers have long been used in rituals to drive off malevolent spirits (Wong, 1987).

By suggesting the sources of diseases, rumors encourage people to avoid particular places, things, animals, or activities. Amid SARS, the Spanish flu, plague outbreaks, and COVID-19, there were rumors that dogs and cats were sources of disease, leading frightened people to abandon or destroy these animals (Barry, 2018; CNN, 2022; Roos, 2021; Slack, 1985; Taylor, 2019). Regarding SARS, a false rumor spread about the prevalence of SARS in New York City's Chinatown (Eichelberger, 2007). Even without a single case of SARS, Chinatown was quickly identified as a hotspot of contagion and risk; "the American public, including Chinatown, had become infected with an epidemic of fear, not of disease" (Eichelberger, 2007, p. 1285).

Rumors spread about unsafe foods in the 1849 cholera pandemic in London. People avoided fish and vegetables, believing they contained cholera (Mayhew, 1865). At the same time, in New York City, people avoided eating unripe berries and other fruit for fear of cholera (Rosenberg, 1987). At points in the 1832 and 1849 cholera pandemics in New York, the sale of fresh fruit, vegetables, and fish from open carts was banned for fear that they were sources of disease (Rosenberg, 1987). There was some truth to the rumors. Raw, unwashed produce is a source of cholera, as is produce washed in cholera-contaminated water (Rabbani & Greenough, 1999).

During COVID-19, rumors spread on social media about the beneficial effects of several drugs, including ivermectin, used to treat parasitic worm infections in people and animals, and hydroxychloroquine, used to treat parasitic infections in freshwater aquaria (Schellack et al., 2022). There were several poisonings and deaths from misusing these drugs (Shepherd, 2020).

Rumors can lead to vigilantism and violence. Rumor-fueled mob violence occurred in cholera outbreaks (Chapter 7). In India during COVID-19, when the country was under lockdown, rumors spread in the small town of Telinipara that "hundreds of Muslims" had been infected with the coronavirus and were spreading the disease to the town's Hindu majority. The rumor, fueled by pre-existing tensions between Hindus and Muslims, triggered violence, with Hindu mobs setting fire to 45 Muslim homes and Muslims attacking Hindu houses and shops (Rahman, 2020).

People of certain professions, especially doctors and gravediggers, were commonly subject to rumors amid disease outbreaks (Cohn, 2012). In cholera outbreaks in the 19th century, doctors were rumored to be complicit in murdering people to provide cadavers for medical school dissection (Burrell & Gill, 2005; Cohn & Kutalek, 2016) (see Chapter 7). Gravediggers—who also collected and conveyed the sick and dead to pesthouses and graveyards—were rumored to be manufacturing plague because they supposedly had a vested interest in the disease (Hirst, 1953). In outbreaks of plague, rumors circulated about various sorts of gravedigger misbehavior, such as stealing food and valuables from the homes of disease victims, sexually assaulting the sick, and dumping the bodies instead of following burial procedures (Anonymous, 1721; Carmichael, 1986; Nohl, 1926; Parets, 1651).

There was some truth to the rumors, as some gravediggers did behave badly. In Warsaw in 1625, four gravediggers were hanged for indecorous treatment of plague victims, such as mocking the dead and stealing from their homes (Wyrobisz, 2000). In other cases, gravediggers were wrongly accused and convicted based on false rumors that they were spreading plague for profit (Nohl, 1926; Wyrobisz, 2000). The notion that gravediggers were fearless profiteers was, of course, hyperbole. Gravediggers often refused to handle the dead for fear of getting infected or demanded higher wages for their hazardous work (Barry, 2005; Benoiston de Châteauneuf et al., 1834; Wyrobisz, 2000).

Conspiracy Theories

Conspiracy theories are based on the premise that big events require big explanations (Lewandowsky & Cook, 2020). Conspiracy theories are extreme kinds of rumors in which important events—a pandemic, for example—are explained in terms of secret plots by powerful, often shadowy individuals or organizations. Such theories emerge in marked opposition to mainstream or official accounts of situations and events. Conspiracy theories provide simple, understandable explanations: why something happened, who benefits from it, and who should be blamed (Weigmann, 2018; Wood, 2018). Conspiracy theories resist falsification because they postulate that conspirators use stealth and deception to cover up their actions, implying that people who try to debunk conspiracy theories may be part of the conspiracy (Douglas et al., 2017). The absence of evidence for a conspiracy theory may be taken as evidence of a cover-up.

Conspiracy theorists defend their views in several ways (Wood, 2018). They go to great lengths to cite supposedly authoritative support for their claims. The claims are often vague (e.g., "Research at Harvard has shown that..."). When challenging mainstream views, conspiracy theorists use ploys such as claiming that something "needs more investigation," thereby raising doubts without presenting any factual basis for their claims. Conspiracy theorists frequently use leading questions in a "just asking" style, raising rhetorical questions to challenge mainstream views. For example, "If vaccines are so safe, then how do you explain the increase in disease X in country Y when people received the vaccine Z?"

Disease outbreaks are commonly the subject of conspiracy theories. In the Spanish flu, arising in the final year of World War I, there was a conspiracy theory that the Bayer pharmaceutical company was covertly spreading influenza via their aspirin tablets. As a result, the U.S. Public Health Service was required to investigate whether "Bayer, producing aspirin under what had originally been a German patent, was poisoning its customers with flu germs" (Crosby, 2003, p. 216). Testing revealed that the tablets were uncontaminated.

Not all unusual ideas are conspiracy theories. Consider the following example from the Russian flu: A newspaper article claimed that "instead of being the work of the usual influenza microbe, the Russian influenza is produced by an entirely new microbe that has been developed by the electric light" (New York Herald (European Edition), 1890, p. 2). It was claimed that the Russian flu "raged chiefly in towns where the electric light is in common use, and has penetrated slowly and reluctantly into towns where the electric lamps are unknown" (p. 2). This example is a fanciful claim, not a conspiracy theory. There is no evidence of malicious intent or cover-up. If the article had proposed that the Edison Illumination Company was covertly using its electrical lights to spread disease, that would be a conspiracy theory. Lightbulbs were a relatively new invention, so there were uncertainties about their potential effects. Thomas Edison began mass manufacturing lightbulbs in 1880, only a decade before the Russian flu (Morris, 2020). New technology is commonly the topic of rumors and conspiracy theories.

Themes and Features of Conspiracy Theories

Conspiracy Theories Behave Like Viruses

Conspiracy theories and viruses have much in common. The origins of both are usually difficult to pinpoint, and both require hosts. Like viruses, conspiracy theories cannot survive without hosts (advocates) to disseminate, promote, and defend the theories. Like viruses, which may proliferate only in particular kinds of hosts, conspiracy theories hold credence only for specific individuals.

As with viruses, conspiracy theories mutate over time, forming strains or variants. For example, there are several variants of the 5G conspiracy theory, such as (1) 5G directly transmits the virus causing COVID-19, (2) 5G radiation weakens the immune system, making one more susceptive to the coronavirus, and (3) COVID-19 was deliberately orchestrated to keep people at home while engineers installed 5G towers and related technology as part of some iniquitous plot (Ahmed et al., 2020). Unlike the Edison lightbulb example mentioned earlier, the 5G conspiracy theory proposes a cover-up—the supposedly harmful effects of 5G telecommunication towers are being kept secret for nefarious reasons.

Shadowy Elites

Conspiracy theories tend to be recycled, with old ones modified to "explain" new threats. Conspiracy theories commonly claim that some shadowy organization of elites—such as the Illuminati, Deep State, or New World Order—is intent on depopulating the planet to facilitate the takeover and installation of a one-world government. A prototypic example is the *Protocols of the Elders of Zion*, a tract published to provoke antisemitism by promoting a fabricated Jewish conspiracy theory about world domination (Hassan & Caven-Atack, 2020). Shadowy elites are often the subject of conspiracy theories concerning disease outbreaks. For example, the Zika pandemic and SARS outbreak were said to be part of a plot for world domination by a fictitious New World Order (Jacobs et al., 2016; Lee, 2014).

Xenophobia

Xenophobia is a common feature of conspiracy theories, in which some outgroup is blamed. For example, in the 2010 cholera outbreak in Haiti, the first in many decades, some Haitians believed that malevolent foreigners deliberately spread the disease for political reasons (Grimaud & Legagneur, 2011). Xenophobia may also be directed at foreign aid workers as part of conspiracy theories about healthcare.

Conspiracy Theories About Healthcare

Conspiracy theories that healthcare workers somehow caused an outbreak, or were harming their patients instead of curing them, led to the assault and murder of healthcare workers in epidemics such as Ebola in Africa in 2014, and in cholera outbreaks in 19th-century Europe (Cohn, 2017; Quick, 2018; Rosenberg, 1987). To illustrate, in 2014, a team of eight healthcare workers and journalists arrived in the Guinean village of Wome to teach the villagers how to protect themselves against Ebola. The villagers, believing the workers had come to spread disease, attacked them with clubs and machetes. The bodies were discovered days later, dumped in a village cistern (Quick, 2018).

The pharmaceutical industry has long been a subject of conspiracy theories (Lynas, 2020). Examples include conspiracy theories about the pharmaceutical industry manufacturing the Zika virus for human population control or profit (Ahmed et al., 2020; Klofstad et al., 2019). A COVID-19 conspiracy theory proposed that billionaire philanthropist Bill Gates, in league with Big Pharma, created the coronavirus as part of a plan to institute mandatory global vaccinations that inject microchips into people for tracking and control (Ahmed et al., 2020; Sallam et al., 2021).

There is an element of truth to some conspiracy theories: Medical malfeasance does occur. The Tuskegee Syphilis Study is an infamous example. Conducted by the U.S. Public Health Service from 1932 to 1972 in Alabama, the purpose was to assess the effects of untreated syphilis in 399 infected African American men. Informed consent was not obtained. Investigators "deceived the men into believing they were being treated for 'bad blood,' a colloquialism for several ailments" (Tobin, 2022, p. 1146). Effective treatment was withheld. Instead, participants were given placeboes consisting of vitamins and aspirin. Lumbar punctures to assess neurosyphilis were conducted for research purposes, with no therapeutic value. Participants were led to believe that the lumbar "spinal shot" was a special free therapy. By 1969, "at least 28 and perhaps 100 men had died as a direct result of syphilis; despite this knowledge, the government scientists continued the experiment" (Tobin, 2022, p. 1146). Unethical medical experiments like the Tuskegee study fuel rumors and conspiracy theories about medical misconduct.

Escaped-from-a-Lab Conspiracies

An oft-recycled conspiracy theory is that a pandemic-causing pathogen was clandestinely created in a civilian or military laboratory, from which it escaped, and the escape was hushed up. According to one conspiracy theory, the Zika virus was accidentally created by a biotech company that had been raising genetically modified mosquitoes to combat dengue fever (Jacobs et al., 2016).

As for COVID-19, U.S. President Trump promoted the conspiracy theory that the coronavirus was created in a Chinese lab (Wu, 2021). Former CDC director Robert Redfield also asserted that the coronavirus was a hushed-up escapee from a Wuhan laboratory (Agence France-Presse, 2021). Chinese officials countered by alleging the coronavirus came from an American military lab (Lynas, 2020; Taylor, 2020; Wu, 2021).

There is a grain of truth to the escaped-from-a-lab conspiracy theories; pathogens sometimes *do* escape from labs. Consider the 1977 influenza pandemic. In May 1977, an influenza A (H1N1) virus "genetically and antigenically identical to viruses which had been isolated in the 1950s," re-emerged in China and then spread to Russia, Europe, the United Kingdom, the United States, and Australia (Oxford, 2000, p. 128). Genetic studies suggested that "the 1977 outbreak strain had been preserved since 1950" (Zimmer & Burke, 2009, p. 282). According to Oxford (2000), "It is now thought that the virus re-emerged from a laboratory freezer by error" (Oxford, 2000, p. 128). This conclusion was reiterated in an article in the *New England Journal of Medicine*, where it was stated that the virus causing the 1977 influenza pandemic was "probably an accidental release from a laboratory source" (Zimmer & Burke, 2009, p. 282).

Regarding COVID-19, at the time of writing this book in late 2024, there was suggestive evidence that SARSCOV2 might have escaped from a Wuhan laboratory (Chan, 2024), but no firm proof. Wuhan researchers asserted that the virus samples stored in their laboratory contained no close relatives to SARS-CoV-2 (Mallapaty, 2024).

Bioweapon Conspiracies

For a range of disease outbreaks, a recurring conspiracy theory is that the outbreak is caused by a weaponized pathogen or poison (Cohn, 2017; Taylor, 2022). There are numerous historical examples. When the Plague of Athens erupted in the port town of Piraeus in 430 BC, a rumor spread that it was caused by Spartans poisoning the water supply (Thucydides, 431 BC). The two city-states were at war at the time. The infectious agent, later speculated to be typhus or smallpox, entered Athens through the port, killing a quarter of the city's inhabitants (Cunha, 2004).

When the plague swept across Europe in 1545, the Protestant theologian John Calvin promoted the conspiracy theory that the disease was caused by malefactors smearing poison on door handles (Bonnet, 1858). In the 1665 plague outbreak in England, a rumor spread that the French had brought bottles of plague-infected air to poison the English (Achinstein, 1992). In an 1832 outbreak of cholera in Paris, "rumors of mass poisoning of the water supply led vigilante mobs to roam the streets searching for suspected poisoners, attacking and sometimes killing innocent people" (Morens et al., 2008, p. 715).

During the Spanish flu, arising in the final year of World War I, conspiracy theories circulated in America that influenza was being spread by German infiltrators secretly infecting Americans (Crosby, 2003; New York Times, 1918; Schoch-Spana, 2004). According to an article appearing in the *New York Times*, "outbreaks of Spanish influenza ... may have been started by German agents who were put ashore from a submarine" (New York Times, 1918, p. 11). At the same time in England, a rumor published in *The Times* claimed that the Spanish flu was "directly traceable to the German use of poison gas, the after-effects of which have induced the growth of a new type of streptococcus" (Johnson, 2006, p. 186). There was no evidence that influenza was spread by German agents or poison gas.

At the height of the HIV/AIDS pandemic in the 1980s, there were several bioweapon conspiracy theories (Heller, 2015; Parsons et al., 1999; Turner, 1993). One claimed that the CIA developed HIV/AIDS to kill African Americans and homosexuals (Heller, 2015). Another purported that HIV/AIDS was a bioweapon that had escaped from a lab (Turner, 1993).

In the 1994 plague outbreak in India, described in Chapter 9, the pathogen was a novel strain of *Yersinia pestis* with an unusual infection pattern. It mainly afflicted men aged 20–45 years and reportedly did not spread through households (Kumar, 1995). These features fueled speculation, published in *The Lancet*, that "the organism is being used as a biological warfare agent, most likely by the USA or Pakistan" (Kumar, 1995, p. 443). The allegation was "strongly denied by Col Ernest Takafuji, commander of the US Army Research Institute of Infectious Diseases at Fort Detrick" (p. 443). For conspiracy-minded individuals, the denial was likely seen as a cover-up.

Early in the SARS outbreak, Australian health officials were forced to quell rumors that SARS was a bioweapon released by some malevolent country or agency (Lee, 2014). Regarding the 2009 swine flu pandemic, which originated in Mexico and then spread to the US, a conspiracy theory arose in America that terrorists were using infected Mexican immigrants as "walking germ warfare weapons" (Smallman, 2015, p. 5). We can expect to encounter bioweapon conspiracy theories in future pandemics, fueled by mistrust of government, xenophobia, and fear of infection.

Widespread Belief in Conspiracy Theories

Belief in conspiracy theories is a global phenomenon, having been identified in all cultures studied so far (van Prooijen & van Vugt, 2018). Belief in conspiracy theories is widespread. About 60% of Americans believe President John F. Kennedy was killed in a conspiracy involving the Mafia, CIA, or government (Swift, 2013). According to some surveys, more than a third of Americans believe climate change is a hoax perpetrated by vested interest groups such as climate scientists needing research funds (Douglas et al., 2019). About 11% of people think that 9/11 was an inside job, and 4%

believe that NASA faked the moon landings (Statista, 2019; Waldersee, 2019). Health-related conspiracies are widely believed, such as the following, based on a U.S. community survey (Oliver & Wood, 2014):

- The FDA is deliberately preventing the public from getting natural cures for cancer and other diseases because of pressure from drug companies (37% agreed).
- Doctors and the government still want to vaccinate children even though they know these vaccines cause autism and other disorders (20%).
- Health officials know that cell phones cause cancer but are doing nothing to stop it because large corporations won't let them (20%).

Membership in conspiracy-oriented social media groups swelled with the emergence of COVID-19 (BBC, 2020). Coronavirus conspiracy theories garnered widespread media attention, especially when endorsed by political leaders and other prominent figures. Although the news media typically discredited conspiracy theories, widespread media coverage brought these theories to the attention of people who had not heard of them. A 2020 U.K. survey revealed widespread belief in COVID-19 conspiracy theories, as indicated by the percentage of people agreeing with the following statements (Garry et al., 2022):

- The coronavirus is a bioweapon developed by China to destroy the West (32% agreed).
- The UN and WHO have manufactured the virus to take global control (19%).
- Lockdown is a plot by environmental activists to control the rest of us (17%).
- The coronavirus vaccine will contain microchips to control the people (17%).
- Muslims are spreading the virus as an attack on Western values (13%).
- Jews have created the virus to collapse the economy for financial gain (11%).

A survey of adults from Jordan, Kuwait, and other Arab countries found that 28% believed the conspiracy theory that COVID-19 vaccines contain microchips used to monitor the populace (Sallam et al., 2021). Other research likewise revealed widespread belief in COVID-19 conspiracy theories (Freeman et al., 2022).

Suspicious Minds

What are the psychological characteristics of people who believe in conspiracy theories? People differ in the strength of belief in specific conspiracy theories and their general susceptibility to them (Bruder et al., 2013). People who believe in one conspiracy theory tend to accept others (Chan et al., 2021; Douglas et al., 2019; Freeman et al., 2022; Garry et al., 2022; Lewandowsky et al., 2013). For example, people who think that the Zika virus was deliberately spread by the Monsanto corporation also tend to believe that 9/11 was an inside job and that the government is covering up evidence of extraterrestrial contact.

Conspiracy theorists search for patterns, trying to "connect the dots" to find meaning where none might exist (Douglas et al., 2019). Belief in conspiracy theories is driven by motives that can be characterized as *epistemic* (needing to understand one's environment), *existential* (needing to feel safe and in control of one's environment), and *social* (needing to maintain a positive image of oneself and one's in-group) (Douglas et al., 2017). Once formed, conspiracy beliefs resist change (Jolley & Douglas, 2017). As we saw in Chapter 7, conspiracy theories sometimes contradict one another, such as "COVID-19 is a bioweapon," versus "COVID-19 is a hoax used to control the population." Holding contradictory beliefs is a common feature of conspiratorial thinking (Miller, 2020).

Many studies have investigated the correlates of conspiratorial thinking (e.g., Bruder et al., 2013; Cichocka et al., 2016; Craft et al., 2017; Douglas et al., 2017; Douglas et al., 2019; Duplaga, 2020; Galliford & Furnham, 2017; Georgiou et al., 2020; Imhoff & Lamberty, 2018; Lahrach & Furnham, 2017; Lantian et al., 2017; Marchlewska et al., 2018; Moulding et al., 2016; Swami et al., 2014). People who believe in conspiracy theories tend to have the following characteristics:

- Suspiciousness, magical thinking, and the tendency to believe in the paranormal.
- Narcissism and the need to feel special. Conspiracy theories allow people to feel important, believing they possess vital information about a plot or cover-up.
- Worry about health and mortality—for people who believe in health-related conspiracy theories.
- Gullibility, lower media literacy (i.e., poorer ability to critically analyze the source and contents of news stories), lower intelligence, lower education, and poorer skills in analytical thinking.

- Rejection of conventional scientific findings or theories (e.g., the theory of evolution) in favor of pseudoscience (e.g., the belief that prayer is effective in curing terminal diseases).

Belief in COVID-19 conspiracies was associated with nonadherence and other complications (Allington et al., 2021; Alper et al., 2021; Bertin et al., 2020; Biddlestone et al., 2020; Bierwiaczonek et al., 2020; Earnshaw et al., 2020; Freeman et al., 2022; Kowalski et al., 2020; Romer & Jamieson, 2020; Sallam et al., 2020; Taylor & Asmundson, 2021; Taylor et al., 2020). Belief in conspiracy theories was associated with the following:

- COVID-19 anti-vaccination attitudes and anti-vaccination attitudes in general.
- Lower adherence to COVID-19 health guidelines such as social distancing.
- Use of social media as a primary source of one's news about the coronavirus.
- Lower levels of knowledge about COVID-19.
- Less willingness to be tested for COVID-19.
- A greater chance of testing positive for COVID-19.

Conspiracy theorists who saw COVID-19 as personally threatening were more likely to comply with health guidelines (Marinthe et al., 2020). Consistent with earlier research on conspiracy theories, belief in coronavirus conspiracy theories was associated with suspiciousness, lower education levels, and the tendency to believe in other (non-COVID-19) conspiracies, such as the belief that climate change is a hoax (Freeman et al., 2022; Sallam et al., 2020; van Prooijen et al., 2023). Conservative political ideology in the United States was associated with belief in COVID-19 conspiracy theories, such as beliefs that the virus was created in a Chinese laboratory (Havey, 2020; Romer & Jamieson, 2020; Ruiz & Bell, 2021).

COVID-19 conspiracy theorists represented ideologically diverse groups (Thomas, 2021). Groups included far-right White nationalists, who blamed various ethnic groups for spreading or profiting from the disease (Gallotti et al., 2020). The rise of racist conspiracy theories during COVID-19 was associated with an increase in assaults and hate crimes (Gallotti et al., 2020). Conspiracy theorists who sought to impress their views on nonbelievers were commonly met with disbelief or ridicule (Freeman et al., 2022; van Prooijen et al., 2023).

Who Spreads Conspiracy Theories?

People circulate conspiracy theories for many reasons. Several overlapping groups can be identified: conspiracy theorists, fellow travelers, conspiracy entrepreneurs, political opportunists, and trolls. Conspiracy theorists are true believers, who circulate their views to convince others (Freeman et al., 2022). Fellow travelers are curious about conspiracy theories without necessarily believing or being emotionally invested in them. Fellow travelers might wonder whether there is some truth to conspiracy theory, perhaps encouraged by their social group, without having the suspicious mindset of conspiracy theorists.

Conspiracy entrepreneurs spread conspiracy theories for financial or other gains such as attention and notoriety. Conspiracy entrepreneurs might not believe in the theories they promote but use them for marketing quack products and other merchandise: "These conspiracists depend for their market on getting people to believe that evidence-based (i.e. conventional) medicine doesn't work and is a plot by big pharmaceutical companies to make us ill" (Lynas, 2020, p. 1). Politicians sometimes promote conspiracy theories to deflect blame or draw political support (Ahmed et al., 2020; Lewandowsky & Cook, 2020). Trolls promote conspiracy theories for malicious entertainment and other reasons.

Troubles with Trolls

In the early months of COVID-19, the WHO director general, Dr. Tedros Adhanom Ghebreyesus, declared that "we're not just battling the virus, we're also battling the trolls and conspiracy theories that undermine our response" (BBC, 2020, p. 1). A troll is a person who intentionally antagonizes others by circulating inflammatory or offensive comments, claims, stories, and so forth (Merriam-Webster, 2021).

Trolling has long been around in some form but became especially widespread and disruptive with the advent of the internet. To illustrate, a hoaxer in Hong Kong, amid the SARS epidemic, posted a bogus news item on a faux online news site, claiming that Hong Kong would soon be declared an infected zone and sealed off from the outside world. Rumors of the alleged cordon sanitaire quickly spread throughout the city, triggering panic buying of supplies (Cheng & Cheung, 2005).

In Taiwan, amid COVID-19, authorities accused Chinese internet trolls of "sowing panic over the coronavirus outbreak" by "falsely implying the island has an out of control epidemic" (The Straits Times, 2020, p. 1). Elsewhere in the same pandemic, trolls circulated a photo of empty supermarket shelves, which was said to show the effects of panic buying in Vancouver, Canada. The location was faked. Although the photo wasn't from Vancouver, it still fueled panic buying in that city (Young, 2020). COVID-19 hoaxers also circulated fake text messages, allegedly from health officials, claiming that particular cities would completely shut down (Lytvynenko, 2020). Another malicious rumor came with a fake screenshot warning people not to open their doors to strangers because thieving criminals were pretending to be medical staff testing for COVID-19 (Lytvynenko, 2020). As with many rumors, these contained grains of truth; scams rose in prevalence during COVID-19 (Crist, 2020).

Online anonymity facilitates trolling. Research indicates that trolls, typically men, tend to have the following personality features (Buckels et al., 2014; March, 2019; Sest & March, 2017):

- *Psychopathic personality traits*: People with these traits are callous, manipulative, superficially charming, and lack empathy and remorse for their actions.
- *Sadism*: Trolls enjoy hurting and humiliating people and enjoy watching others inflict hurt and humiliation on others.
- *Negative social potency*: Trolls find it rewarding to cause social mayhem. Creating social disruption provides a sense of power.

Trolls enjoy their malicious activities (Buckels et al., 2014; March, 2019). Trolls on the internet have many features in common with the classic Joker villain: "Trolls operate as agents of chaos on the internet, exploiting 'hot-button issues' to make users appear overly emotional or foolish in some manner" (Buckels et al., 2014, p. 97). If some unfortunate is drawn into their trap, "trolling intensifies for further, merciless amusement" (p. 97). Public appeals to stop trolling are usually counter-productive. Better advice comes from the internet adage "do not feed the trolls." That is, don't reward their behaviors with undue attention.

Managing Rumors and Conspiracy Theories

Rumors and conspiracy theories can be addressed using risk communication strategies (Chapter 4). Internet down-weighting and censorship have been used to limit the spread of conspiracy theories and other misinformation (Chapter 10). During COVID-19, online campaigns were organized to correct misinformation about vaccines, masks, and other mitigation methods. These initiatives may have been helpful for people who lacked information but are unlikely to have influenced conspiracy theorists. The latter do not lack information; they cherry-pick facts to fit their theories.

It is challenging to persuade conspiracy theorists to abandon their conspiratorial ideas. Accordingly, conspiracy theories can be managed by focusing on people who are not invested in theories, such as the merely curious. Techniques to stimulate analytical thinking can reduce the belief in conspiracy theories (Swami et al., 2014). Checklists and other educational materials can teach people to spot conspiracy theories (e.g., Lewandowsky & Cook, 2020; Lewandowsky et al., 2020).

People can be inoculated against specific conspiracy theories by educating them about the theory and showing why it is wrong (Douglas et al., 2019; Jolley & Douglas, 2017). The problem is that the inoculation process broadens the audience, giving the theories needless and potentially counterproductive public attention. However, once some socially disruptive or divisive conspiracy theory has gained widespread circulation, community leaders have little option but to attempt to debunk the theory through education (Ecker et al., 2022). Debunking is discussed further in Chapter 10.

Finally, what happens when a conspiracy theory turns out to be true? Can rumors and conspiracy theories be managed in such circumstances? Consider the COVID-19 escaped-from-a-lab conspiracy theory. If the lab conspiracy were proven true, the following would likely occur:

- Conspiracy theories and conspiratorial thinking would flourish as never before. Conspiracy theorists would feel vindicated and wonder, "What else is being covered up?" and "For what purpose was such a dangerous virus created?"
- Xenophobia and suspiciousness would increase in many countries as people focus blame for COVID-19 on China.
- The revelation would significantly undermine public trust in science, particularly if Wuhan scientists were implicated in the pandemic's origins.
- Evidence for a COVID-19 conspiracy would impact how people react to the next pandemic: There would likely be widespread fear and rumors that a weaponized pathogen caused the outbreak. International cooperation would be jeopardized by blame and counter-blame for its alleged origins.

Conclusions

Rumors are forms of improvised news that are especially likely to flourish when critical uncertainties arise. Rumors become shorter, simpler, and sharper with retelling. There are various motivations for spreading rumors during pandemics, including malign and xenophobic motives in which some group is blamed. Unchecked rumors can incite fear, foment confusion, and undermine pandemic management efforts.

Conspiracy theories are rumors in which some event or situation, such as a severe disease outbreak, is attributed to the sinister work of some individual or shadowy group, usually involving some kind of deception or cover-up. People endorsing one conspiracy theory tend to believe in others and are generally suspicious. Various groups circulate conspiracy theories, including conspiracy theorists (true believers), fellow travelers (the merely curious), and those who spread conspiracy theories for financial or political gain (conspiracy entrepreneurs, political opportunists) or for perverse entertainment (trolls).

Rumors and conspiracy theories contribute to anxiety, nonadherence, and conflict in pandemics. Risk communication methods can address rumors, but when facts are scarce and fear is heightened, rumors are likely to be widespread and difficult to contain. Other methods for managing rumors and conspiracy theories involve regulating the internet (down-weighting or censoring some material), public education, and skills training. Despite these efforts, conspiracy theories are widely believed and likely to be prominent in future outbreaks of emerging infectious diseases.

13
Beliefs About Health and Disease

Introduction

Previous chapters examined how people respond to external stimuli during disease outbreaks, such as rumors and media stories. In the present chapter, we consider how people react to *internal* stimuli—bodily sensations and physical changes—and how beliefs about health and disease influence a person's emotional and behavioral reactions to these stimuli. Central to our discussion is the concept of health anxiety—anxiety about one's health arising from worries about diseases and other health threats.

Dysfunctional beliefs about health and disease, typically expressed in health-related worries, are driving factors in excessive or clinically severe health anxiety, hence the title of this chapter. Beliefs about health and disease influence how people feel and what they do in pandemics. In this chapter, we survey these beliefs and examine how particular behaviors can perpetuate health anxiety. The cognitive behavioral model of health anxiety is reviewed, and treatment options are discussed. Our focus is mainly on people prone to excessively high levels of health anxiety, although problems associated with low levels are also considered. Unless stated otherwise, the examples in this chapter are clinically realistic but hypothetical, used to illustrate various aspects of excessive health anxiety.

The Health Anxiety Spectrum

Health anxiety ranges on a continuum from low to severe. A moderate dose of health anxiety is adaptive. It motivates us to visit a doctor if we notice some bodily change or sensation, such as a new rash or persistent cough. A modicum of health anxiety prompts us to avoid unnecessary risks, such as avoiding physical contact with infectious individuals. Health anxiety is maladaptive when it is out of proportion with the objective degree of medical risk. Low anxiety in the face of high risk, or high anxiety in the face of low risk, can cause problems.

Low levels of health anxiety contribute to the spread of infection. Low levels of health anxiety are associated with a lack of concern about the health risks of infectious diseases, neglect of hand hygiene, and nonadherence to social distancing (Gilles et al., 2011; Goodwin et al., 2009; Jones & Salathé, 2009; Rubin et al., 2009; Taylor et al., 2020; Williams et al., 2015; Wong & Sam, 2011).

High levels of health anxiety are characterized by excessive concern about one's health, where the level of concern is disproportionate to objective indices of physical health. Examples include the tendency to worry about minor, harmless bodily changes (e.g., spots or rashes) or bodily sensations (e.g., muscle twitches). People prone to severe health anxiety tend to become highly anxious amid outbreaks of infectious disease (Chapter 19).

Health-Related Worry

Worry, a core cognitive element of anxiety, consists of "a chain of thoughts and images, negatively affect-laden and relatively uncontrollable; it represents an attempt to engage in mental problem-solving on an issue whose future outcome is uncertain but contains the possibility of one or more negative outcomes" (Borkovec et al., 1983, p. 10). As a problem-solving process, worry is used to resolve critical uncertainties, identify potential threats, and develop contingency plans for dealing with threats. Worry persists if the problem-solving process fails to produce a satisfactory outcome, often because it is impossible to rule out all the essential uncertainties for a given threat.

Health-related worries may be realistic, unrealistic, or somewhere in between. People prone to frequent episodes of health anxiety commonly worry about low-probability, high-impact events; that is, unlikely but dangerous outcomes. The following example illustrates how a "what if" thinking style causes unrealistic concerns to spiral into catastrophic ideas during an episode of severe health anxiety:

> I was at the dentist getting an X-ray, which required me to bite down on a mouthpiece. I started thinking about where the mouthpiece had been—all those mouths. I began worrying that the mouthpiece might not have been cleaned properly—what if it held traces of someone else's saliva or blood? If that happened, I might have swallowed COVID vaccine from someone else's bodily fluids. What if that happened? I heard that the vaccine could give you cancer.

Episodes of health-related worry commonly contain the following: cycles of ruminative thinking (e.g., "Did I come in contact with anyone who might be sick?"), "what-if" chains of catastrophic thinking, thoughts of worst-case scenarios, and urgent thoughts about the need for protective measures. In the following example, the worries were based on realistic concerns, fueled by uncertainty, and focused on looming dangers and possible protective measures:

> I've had a slight cough all day. I'm hoping it's just allergies, but I'm worried it might be swine flu. I've been mentally retracing my steps over the past few days to figure out if I could have gotten infected. I worry that if I get sick, I might infect my husband, who has health issues and could die if he gets infected. I try to stay indoors as often as possible to avoid the virus. I can't get my preferred brand of hand sanitizer because of all the panic buying. I found another brand, but I worry it's not good enough. I also worry about the ingredients in hand sanitizers—what if the one I'm using contains harmful chemicals? I try to do everything possible to stay safe, but it feels like it's not enough.

Features of Excessive Health Anxiety

For people prone to excessive health anxiety, their health-related worries are frequent, time-consuming, distressing, and interfere with daily social and occupational functioning. Excessive health anxiety is a feature of several *Diagnostic and Statistical Manual of Mental Disorders*, Fifth Edition (DSM-5) mental disorders, including illness anxiety disorder, somatic symptom disorder, generalized anxiety disorder, obsessive-compulsive disorder, panic disorder, and some phobias (American Psychiatric Association, 2022).

Approximately 6% of people are prone to bouts of excessive health anxiety (American Psychiatric Association, 2022; Sunderland et al., 2013). This percentage likely rises temporarily during pandemics, especially in the early stages, when uncertainties fuel rumors about the disease's potential dangers.

People prone to recurrent bouts of excessive health anxiety tend to have the following characteristics (Bobevski et al., 2016; Eilenberg et al., 2015; Hedman et al., 2016; Sunderland et al., 2013; Taylor & Asmundson, 2017; Wheaton et al., 2010). They tend to:

- Misinterpret bodily sensations as indicators of poor health or severe disease.

- Overestimate the probability and dangerousness of diseases.
- Believe that good health is associated with few or no bodily sensations.
- Selectively attend to, dwell on, and recall health-related information.
- Draw heavily on the healthcare system by persistently seeking medical reassurance for various shifting health concerns.
- Have better-than-average medical knowledge due to checking, reassurance-seeking, and frequent contact with the healthcare system.
- Have a current or past history of mood or anxiety disorders.

The following case of psychogenic fever further illustrates excessive health anxiety (Imataki & Uemura, 2021). Psychogenic fever, also known as stress-induced hyperthermia, is characterized by persistent low-grade temperature elevations (37 to 38°C) in response to chronic stress (Olivier, 2015). Psychogenic fever arises from noninflammatory mechanisms involved in stress reactions (Nakamura & Morrison, 2022). The following case is summarized from Imataki and Uemura (2021):

> The patient was a 46-year-old Japanese man who worried he was infected with COVID-19 and might infect others. His fears persisted despite reassurance. The patient had a mild fever, ranging from 37.4 to 38.1°C. He reported fatigue and a slight reduction in his sense of smell but no change in taste and no chills, shivering, or sweating. He reportedly had never been in contact with anyone diagnosed with COVID-19. The patient repeatedly tested negative for SARS-CoV-2 but doubted the results' validity, believing they might be false negatives. A thorough medical evaluation revealed no evidence of inflammation, infections, allergic reactions, rheumatoid diseases, endocrine disorders, malignancies, or drug-induced conditions. His fever failed to respond to acetaminophen but was rapidly reduced when his anxiety was treated with the benzodiazepine derivative, loflazepate.

As with this case, people prone to excessive health anxiety should be thoroughly evaluated to rule out general medical conditions such as infections and other pathology. Rather than dismissing the patient's concerns as overblown, a thorough assessment is necessary. Clinicians prone to the anchoring bias run the risk of misdiagnosing their health-anxious patients by dismissing the presenting complaints as mere anxiety. Anchoring on an initial diagnostic hypothesis (e.g., "My patient has excessive health anxiety") can lead clinicians to overlook other potential causes; see Chapter 11.

Two Types of Fears

Health anxiety is associated with two kinds of fears, differing in their behavioral consequences: Fear that one *has* or might have a disease, which is associated with approach behaviors, and fear of *acquiring* a disease, associated with avoidance and escape (Côté et al., 1996).

Fear that one has, or might have, a dreaded disease is associated with medical reassurance seeking, recurrent checking of one's body for feared signs of infection (e.g., frequently palpating one's lymph nodes), seeking reassuring information (e.g., checking medical information on the internet, asking for advice on social media), and trying various kinds of remedies (e.g., quack cures). The above-mentioned case study of psychogenic fever illustrates a patient preoccupied with fear of having COVID-19.

Fear of acquiring a disease is associated with avoidance and escape from disease-related stimuli and situations. People who fear acquiring a disease see clinics and medical staff as sources of sickness rather than healing. These fearful individuals may be reluctant to seek medical care for fear of infection and strive to avoid potentially infected people, objects, and situations:

> The coronavirus is really bad where I live. There aren't any tests, the hospitals are overcrowded, and sick people are everywhere. All this scares me. I stay home a lot to stay safe, but I still worry. I get anxious whenever I touch anything contaminated with the virus, like unwiped groceries. I try to remind myself that the risks are low, but I still feel afraid.

If physical avoidance isn't possible, health-anxious people may engage in cognitive avoidance, such as distracting themselves or using calming imagery, as illustrated by the following example:

> I wear a mask and gloves everywhere I go because I'm afraid I'll get COVID. My friends wanted me to go to the beach with them. I was, like, are you crazy? The beach is probably full of infected people. Sometimes, I'll go into a store but immediately leave if I see someone who looks sick. If I have to ride an elevator with other people, I try to hold my breath so I don't breathe their germs. If I can't hold my breath that long, I imagine myself in a protective bubble, which I find calming.

A person can shift from one fear to the other. People frightened of contracting a disease tend to avoid disease-related stimuli, such as hospitals and healthcare workers. However, they promptly seek out doctors and clinics when they believe they have acquired a disease. Understanding the nature of the person's fears can shed light on why health-anxious people sometimes avoid and sometimes assiduously seek medical care.

Cognitive Behavioral Model of Health Anxiety

Several theories of health anxiety have been proposed over the years, with the most well-developed and empirically supported being the cognitive-behavioral model developed by Paul M. Salkovskis and colleagues, from which an effective treatment has been derived (Salkovskis & Warwick, 2001; Taylor & Asmundson, 2004). The cognitive behavioral model is summarized in Figure 13.1.

According to the model, several cognitive and behavioral factors play a role in excessive health anxiety: misinterpretations of health-related stimuli, dysfunctional or distorted beliefs, selective attention toward health threats, and maladaptive coping behaviors that provide some emotional relief in the short term but perpetuate health anxiety in the longer term. Dysfunctional beliefs are central to excessive health anxiety, maintained and perpetuated by maladaptive coping behaviors that prevent the beliefs from being disconfirmed. As predicted by the model, research shows that health anxiety can be reduced by correcting distorted beliefs and reducing maladaptive coping (Taylor & Asmundson, 2004). The following sections describe, in more detail, the central components of the cognitive-behavioral model.

Misinterpretations: Turning Sensations into Symptoms

Episodes of excessive health anxiety are triggered when bodily changes or sensations are detected and misinterpreted as harbingers of danger (Figure 13.1). A physical sensation is a "symptom" only if it signifies an underlying disease or aberrant physiological state. Most bodily sensations are not symptoms. Humans have noisy bodies due to normal physiological processes. Benign bodily sensations are daily or weekly occurrences, even for healthy people (Pennebaker, 1982). People prone to excessive health anxiety tend to believe that many or all bodily sensations or changes are indications of disease (Taylor & Asmundson, 2017).

People interpret their experiences in light of their beliefs. There is ample room for misinterpreting mild, vague, or diffuse bodily sensations. Weakness, fatigue, nausea, and mild aches and pains are common occurrences

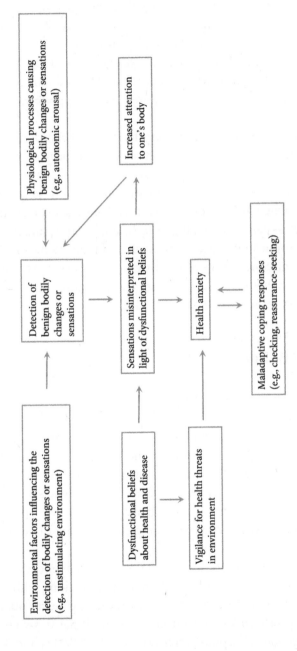

Figure 13.1 Cognitive behavioral model of health anxiety
Source: Taylor, S., & Asmundson, G. J. G. (2004). *Treating health anxiety*. New York: Guilford Press. Reprinted by permission of Guilford Press

that can be interpreted in various ways. People with low levels of health anxiety tend to interpret these reactions as harmless effects of stress, overwork, or physical exertion. People prone to excessive health anxiety become alarmed by bodily reactions, misinterpreting them as signs that their health is in jeopardy (Barsky, 1983). Highly publicized disease outbreaks can lead health-anxious people to misinterpret benign bodily changes and sensations as indications of infection (Wheaton et al., 2012). In the HIV/AIDS pandemic, for example, infection-fearful people misinterpreted fatigue and lack of appetite as indications that they had acquired HIV (Knapp & Vandecreek, 1989).

People prone to excessive health anxiety tend to misinterpret harmless bodily perturbations arising from normal physiological processes, minor diseases, and autonomic arousal (Taylor & Asmundson, 2004). Health-anxious individuals may fail to recognize that their troubling bodily sensations are stress reactions or anxiety responses. That is, sensations associated with autonomic arousal, such as palpitations, fatigue, muscle aches and pains, shortness of breath, and gastrointestinal upset. It is not uncommon for health-anxious people to harbor misconceptions like "anxiety and stress can't cause real body sensations" and thereby misattribute somatic sensations to some severe disease (Taylor & Asmundson, 2004).

Dysfunctional Beliefs

People prone to excessive health anxiety may harbor dysfunctional beliefs about specific physical sensations (e.g., "Coughs are signs of lung cancer") as well as more general beliefs about their health (e.g., "My body is unable to handle physical exertion"). Dysfunctional beliefs fuel anxiety by giving rise to intrusive thoughts and images about the potential horrors of sickness, suffering, and death (Easterling & Leventhal, 1989; James & Wells, 2002; Wells & Hackmann, 1993). For instance, lower back pain may give rise to fears of kidney failure and horrific images of being on agonizing dialysis for the remainder of one's life.

Health-anxious people describe a range of feared consequences of becoming ill. Fears of pain, suffering, and death are common, along with fears of social rejection or inability to care for oneself. Some also worry about getting help from an overburdened healthcare system: "What if my appendix burst and I had to go into a hospital overcrowded with COVID patients?—I'd be exposed to the virus." People highly fearful of death often harbor catastrophic expectations about death and dying (Wells & Hackmann, 1993).

Some believe they will remain aware of their surroundings and body after death (Wells & Hackmann, 1993); "I'll be all alone in the cold earth as my body decomposes." Death-related anxiety is further discussed in Chapter 14.

Health-related experiences can give rise to, or strengthen, dysfunctional beliefs, leading people to mistakenly believe that particular bodily changes or sensations are harbingers of sickness and death (Taylor & Asmundson, 2017). Observational learning—that is, learning from observing the behavior of others—can lead people to misinterpret bodily sensations. Writing in the 17th century, Robert Burton noted in his encyclopedic psychiatric volume, *The Anatomy of Melancholy*, that some people "are afraid that they shall have every fearful disease they see others have, hear of, or read, and dare not therefore hear or read of any such subject ... lest by applying to themselves that which they hear or read, they should aggravate and increase it" (Burton, 1652, p. 294). Observational learning can cause fear to spread widely amid disease outbreaks (Chapter 9).

Misconceptions about disease transmission can lead to undue health anxiety and needless avoidance. For example, if you believed that swine flu was caused by eating pork, you might fear and avoid that meat. In the swine flu pandemic, a substantial proportion of respondents from the United States (9%) and India (41%) believed that eating pork caused swine flu (Kanadiya & Sallar, 2011; Singh et al., 2013), leading to declining sales and bans on pork products (Chapter 4). Surveys of American adults at the height of the HIV/AIDS pandemic in the 1980s found that many believed that HIV could be acquired from a toilet seat (24% yes), eating food handled by someone infected with HIV (19%), or handling money (10%) (Steinbrook, 1985). Such misconceptions lead to needless fear, avoidance, and stigmatization of infected individuals.

The Magnifying Effects of Selective Attention

The perceived threat of infection induces self-focused attention—scanning one's body for sensations or changes—which increases the odds of noticing and misinterpreting benign bodily perturbations (Norris & Marcus, 2014; Witthöft et al., 2016). People with excessive health anxiety tend to be hypervigilant about physical changes and sensations, which increases the chance of detecting and misinterpreting bodily stimuli (Tyrer & Tyrer, 2018). For example, if a health-anxious person was worried about being infected with a respiratory disease (e.g., influenza), then they would tend to focus on respiratory sensations, thereby increasing the odds of detecting and misinterpreting benign sensations (e.g., mild shortness of breath when climbing stairs).

Selective attention to bodily states is influenced not only by internal factors but also by one's surroundings. People are likelier to detect and focus on physical sensations in dull, unstimulating environments containing few or no distractions (Taylor & Asmundson, 2004). Pandemic lockdowns likely amplify health anxiety when people are sequestered alone in their homes for long periods, experiencing boredom mixed with fear of infection. An unstimulating environment in the context of a disease threat provides ideal conditions for focusing on one's body and scanning for "symptoms."

Maladaptive Coping: Solutions That Worsen the Problem

People prone to excessive health anxiety tend to persistently engage in behaviors intended to keep themselves safe, such as repetitive, unnecessary bodily checking (e.g., repeatedly taking one's temperature), checking medical resources (e.g., internet searches), and seeking reassurance from friends, family, and medical professionals (e.g., "Does my face look pale?") (Taylor & Asmundson, 2004; Wheaton et al., 2012). Checking and reassurance-seeking persist because these activities are calming, providing short-term emotional relief (Lucock et al., 1998). In the longer term, checking and reassurance-seeking are counterproductive, perpetuating health anxiety in various ways. Checking can induce bodily sensations, exacerbating rather than assuaging one's anxiety:

> I'm worried that the tickling sensation in my throat is the start of COVID. One of my biggest fears is that my throat will close and I'll be put on a ventilator. I've been checking my throat by swallowing a lot, which has made my throat sore. Now I'm worried I might have damaged my throat.

Health-anxious individuals may go through elaborate decontamination and cleaning rituals to avoid infection, sometimes creating more problems than they solve:

> When I get home, I take off my mask and gloves, remove my clothes and put them in the hamper, shower, and disinfect my phone with wet wipes. I've been using bleach to wipe the virus off groceries and clean my apartment. The other day, after

scrubbing the kitchen, I suddenly felt short of breath and started coughing a lot. I did a Google search. I think I've got chemical pneumonitis from the bleach—or maybe it's COVID.

Repeated internet checking can exacerbate health anxiety. The internet offers health-anxious people an inexhaustible supply of terrifying and often misleading medical information. Instead of being reassured, health-anxious people may be exposed to frightening medical information of uncertain accuracy. Amid COVID-19, people who repeatedly checked the internet for pandemic-related information—a practice colloquially called "doomsurfing" or "doomscrolling"—tended to be highly worried about their health (Anand et al., 2021; Taylor, 2021).

People prone to excessive health anxiety tend to engage in "doctor shopping," where they persistently seek reassurance from numerous clinicians, demanding second and third opinions and repeated medical tests. Doctor shopping burdens the medical system and increases patients' chances of receiving conflicting or confusing medical advice (Taylor & Asmundson, 2004).

Persistent reassurance-seeking and illness preoccupation leads to strained interpersonal relationships with healthcare professionals, friends, and significant others (e.g., "My partner complains that I'm always talking about my health"). Repeated reassurance-seeking by a physically healthy individual has additional self-defeating effects (Salkovskis & Warwick, 2001):

- Reassurance-seeking perpetuates a person's health preoccupation by extending the time they spend discussing their health with others and exposing them to new, potentially frightening medical (mis)information.
- Reassurance-seeking reinforces the person's view that their health is at risk—"My doctor wouldn't be doing all these tests if they didn't think something was wrong."
- It increases the risk of iatrogenic outcomes (e.g., complications due to exploratory surgeries).
- Ultimately, reassurance-seeking fails to reduce uncertainty about one's health because there is always room for doubt. Tests are not entirely accurate, and even a clean bill of health today does not preclude sickness tomorrow ("I was lucky this time; next time could be serious"). Thus, uncertainty persists, prompting further rounds of reassurance-seeking.

Treating Health Anxiety

Cognitive behavior therapy (CBT) conducted by a therapist—in person or by videoconferencing—is a first-line treatment for excessive health anxiety (Taylor & Asmundson, 2017; Tyrer & Tyrer, 2018). CBT targets misinterpretations, dysfunctional beliefs, and maladaptive behaviors, providing the skills necessary to manage or overcome excessive health anxiety. Details of treatment procedures are presented elsewhere (e.g., Abramowitz & Braddock, 2011; Taylor & Asmundson, 2004; Tyrer, 2013).

Self-help materials, such as CBT workbooks and self-directed learning modules on the internet, are promising additional methods for reducing health anxiety (e.g., Asmundson & Taylor, 2005; Cassiday, 2022; Wilson & Veale, 2022). For disease outbreaks in which there is widespread fear, CBT conducted by therapists may be insufficient to meet the demand, hence the need for self-help programs and workbooks (see Chapter 22). Self-help resources are helpful for many health-anxious individuals, although severe cases may require the assistance of a therapist. Certain drugs can also be beneficial in reducing the tendency to experience excessive health anxiety, particularly serotonergic medications such as fluoxetine, fluvoxamine, and paroxetine (Taylor & Asmundson, 2017).

Conclusions

People differ in their tendency to become alarmed by health-related threats. That is, the proneness to experience health anxiety varies on a continuum from low to high. Both extremes are associated with problems. People with low health anxiety rarely worry about their health and may neglect hand hygiene and other recommended health measures because they do not see themselves at risk. In an infectious outbreak, people with very low health anxiety are liable to spread infection due to nonadherence to social distancing and other health guidelines.

At the other end of the spectrum, people prone to severe health anxiety become excessively alarmed during disease outbreaks. These individuals tend to catastrophically misinterpret benign bodily changes or sensations as indications that their health is in jeopardy. Health-anxious people engage in repetitive bodily checking and persistent reassurance-seeking from doctors, burdening an already stressed healthcare system.

Problems arising from low levels of health anxiety are usually addressed via risk communication. Fear-evoking messages are commonly used to motivate people to comply with pandemic-mitigation measures (Chapter 4). The problem is that such messages inflate fears among people already frightened of infection. High levels of health anxiety can be effectively treated with CBT, self-help workbooks, and other educational materials. Such interventions help health-anxious individuals to cope during disease outbreaks and lessen their need for unnecessary medical reassurance.

14
Death Anxiety

Introduction

Anxiety about one's health, discussed in the preceding chapter, concerns the meaning of bodily changes or sensations. These somatic stimuli may be feared because of their possible consequences, such as future pain, suffering, disability, or death. In the present chapter, we focus specifically on death anxiety and related phenomena. The cognitive behavioral model in the preceding chapter is a leading explanation of how bodily changes and sensations are detected and misinterpreted to cause excessive health anxiety. Anxiety specifically about death is further explained by a different model—terror management theory—which is compatible with and complements the cognitive behavioral model. The two theories focus on somewhat different psychological phenomena and mechanisms, as we will see.

Anxiety and fear of death are ubiquitous human experiences (Becker, 1973; Juhl, 2019). To maintain psychological equanimity, psychological mechanisms are needed for dealing with death-related fears and anxieties. Terror management theory describes these mechanisms (Greenberg et al., 1986). The theory proposes that heightened mortality salience—increased awareness that one will eventually die—triggers defensive coping behaviors that enable people to maintain an illusion of immortality: the illusion that one can transcend the fragility and brevity of human existence by construing oneself as a valuable contributor to a meaningful, enduring universe (Pyszczynski et al., 2019).

Terror management theory is a leading account of death anxiety, supported by considerable empirical research (Goldenberg & Arndt, 2008; Greenberg et al., 1986; Greenberg et al., 2008; Pyszczynski et al., 2021). The purpose of this chapter is to review how terror management theory enhances our understanding of how people behave in pandemics. We begin with mortality salience. Next, we discuss the proximal and distal defenses described by terror management theory, and survey four pandemic-related phenomena: infection-related increases in religious nationalism—illustrating distal defenses—and three examples of proximal defenses in disease outbreaks: morbid curiosity, dark humor, and desperate pleasure-seeking.

Mortality Salience

Mortality salience is the awareness of the inevitability of one's demise. Mortality salience increases when people are exposed to reminders of death, such as news stories about fatalities. Research shows that increased mortality salience has a range of effects in addition to triggering death anxiety (Pyszczynski et al., 2021). Mortality salience triggers an increase in the tendency to perceive out-groups (e.g., people from different cultural or religious groups) as dangerous, along with rising hostility toward such groups, which can lead to an escalation in out-group derogation and religious extremism (Shults et al., 2018).

Heightened mortality salience arises from numerous sources in the course of pandemics. In medieval and early modern plague outbreaks, the constant ringing of church bells at funeral services signaled the ever-present threat of death. In some towns, "the funeral bells tolled day and night, as if the living ought to be reminded of their near and inevitable end" (Hecker, 1844, p. 218). Observations recorded in 1665, in the Great Plague of London, depict near-constant mortality salience: "Death stares us continually in the face, in every infected person that passeth by us, in every coffin which is daily and hourly carried along the streets: the bells never cease to put us in mind of our mortality" (Slack, 1985, p. 17).

The practice of tolling church bells was temporarily suspended in many towns in the course of plague outbreaks (Archambeau, 2011; D'Irsay, 1927; Gowen, 1907; Parets, 1651). For example, in medieval Italy, plague regulations included "keeping their citizens in a healthy frame of mind by not tolling the bells to commemorate the dead" (Aberth, 2010, p. 115). Similarly, laws were passed in some European towns forbidding the publication of mortality lists (Gowen, 1907). In Florence, "it was prohibited to publish the numbers of the dead, and to toll the bells at their funerals, in order that the living might not abandon themselves to despair" (Hecker, 1844, p. 40).

In the course of COVID-19, heightened mortality salience arose from a range of sources, including the "ever-increasing death toll statistics, vivid images of the sick and dying in overburdened hospitals, and testimonials of virus survivors, both famous and unknown" (Pyszczynski et al., 2021, p. 176).

Proximal Defenses

Terror management theory distinguishes between two types of psychological mechanisms for dealing with death anxiety: proximal and distal defenses. Proximal defenses are activated when thoughts of death are the current focus of attention and the defenses are logically related to the threat. Proximal defenses are the more obvious reactions to pandemics. For example, when threatened with infection, people typically engage in hygiene behaviors (e.g., handwashing) and avoid sources of contagion. Proximal defenses suppress thoughts of death or enable one to believe that death is not a problem until many years into the distant future. Proximal defenses include the coping behaviors in the preceding chapter for dealing with health anxiety (e.g., checking and reassurance-seeking).

Proximal strategies are attempts to manage conscious death thoughts by relatively direct means, such as denial of one's physical vulnerability to death, avoidance of thoughts about death, and increased efforts to improve one's physical health (e.g., by regularly exercising). During widespread disease outbreaks, distraction and suppression of death-related thoughts become increasingly difficult, especially when there is widespread reporting of the disease in the media and discussion of the infectious threat dominates everyday conversation (Pyszczynski et al., 2021). Proximal defenses are short-term strategies for temporary relief from death anxiety but do not address death's inevitability. For the latter, distal defenses are needed.

Distal Defenses

Distal defenses are activated when death-related thoughts are at the fringes of consciousness—not in focal awareness but still highly accessible. Distal defenses are manifested in the tendency to defend one's worldview (Greenberg et al., 2008). Worldviews are shared beliefs about reality that answer basic questions about life, standards for valued behavior, and the promise of literal or symbolic immortality to those who live up to those standards (Pyszczynski et al., 2021). Worldviews provide people with standards of self-worth (e.g., benchmarks for success), enabling people to believe their lives have meaning and significance (Juhl, 2019). Worldviews involve identification with large, powerful social groups—nationalities, religious organizations, and political groups. Identification with such groups reduces death anxiety because these entities are perceived as more powerful and enduring than mere individuals (Becker, 1973).

Distal defenses can be expressed as legacies or "immortality projects"—things that outlive oneself and foster a sense of symbolic immortality (Becker, 1973). Immortality projects may involve achievements valued by oneself or society, such as creating businesses, accumulating wealth, writing books, composing music, or philanthropic accomplishments. Bearing children is also an immortality project: We live on through our descendants.

Heightened mortality salience strengthens people's commitments to their worldviews, as indicated by increased patriotism, political and ethnic affiliations, and religious observances (Pyszczynski et al., 2021). For example, one study found that asking people to think about pandemic influenza increased their patriotism, involving within-group pride and out-group disparagement (Bélanger et al., 2013).

Political ideologies are central to the worldviews of many people. Some studies show that increased mortality salience leads to a shift toward more conservative political attitudes regardless of political orientation. Other investigations found that increases in mortality salience lead to polarization, with conservatives endorsing increasingly more conservative views and liberals supporting more liberal ones. There is evidence for both phenomena. Research indicates that mortality salience triggers a conservative shift *and* conservative-liberal polarization (Burke et al., 2013). Thus, mortality salience can increase political polarization. Indeed, COVID-19 was politically polarizing in many countries, entailing polarized partisan-based views on the dangerousness of the coronavirus and the necessity for mitigation measures (Chapter 7).

Pandemics can disrupt or interfere with distal coping strategies. Consider funeral rituals. Funerary practices are traditions derived from cultural worldviews concerning the meaning and persistence of existence. Funeral rituals are social responses to death, which, among other things, symbolically conquer death at both a personal and societal level. The deceased lives on in the minds and words of the attendees, along with whatever form of immortality is promised by the person's religion (Bailey & Walter, 2016). Not surprisingly, the bereaved become distressed when these rituals are curtailed or canceled during pandemics.

Religious Nationalism

Religious nationalism is a multifaceted phenomenon. Here, we examine its role as a distal coping strategy and discuss its associated problems. Religious beliefs are calming because they promise immortality if particular rituals or practices are followed. However, nationalistic religious beliefs also increase the odds of infection in pandemics.

In America amid COVID-19, Christian nationalism, not religious commitment per se, was linked to nonadherence to pandemic-mitigation measures (Perry et al., 2020). Blending patriotism with religious fervor, Christian nationalism entails the belief that Christianity defines the American nation and that the government should actively nurture and sustain its Christian heritage (Lee, 2021; Perry et al., 2020). Christian nationalists tend to be authoritarian and xenophobic (Davis & Perry, 2021; Perry et al., 2022). They believed it was acceptable to call COVID-19 "the Chinese virus" and blamed minorities for spreading the disease (Perry et al., 2021).

During COVID-19, some U.S. conservative pastors prophesied God's protection over America. Given a mindset in which it is believed that God will offer special protection over oneself and loved ones, it is unsurprising that Christian nationalism was associated with nonadherence to social distancing, mask-wearing, and hand hygiene (Perry et al., 2020). According to Christian nationalism, the solution to the pandemic lay with religious devotion, appeasement of God's wrath, and moral rectification (Perry et al., 2020).

The rise of Christian nationalism is not just an American issue but a global concern. The rise of Christian nationalism and related ideological groups has been documented in recent years in many places, including Europe, Russia, and Canada (McDonald, 2011; Michel, 2017; Saiya, 2022a, 2022b). Nationalism of other religions, such as Hindu nationalism in India, can similarly lead to problems. In India, a predominantly Hindu nation, xenophobia involved blaming Islamic missionaries and other Muslims for allegedly spreading COVID-19 (Clissold et al., 2020). Religious nationalism is a concern for managing future pandemics, given its association with conflict, xenophobia, and nonadherence to health measures.

Morbid Curiosity

Curiosity is a powerful driver of human behavior. People possess an inherent desire to resolve uncertainty, even if it comes with a price (Hsee & Ruan, 2016). Morbid curiosity is an interest in, or curiosity about, unpleasant things, especially death (Scrivner, 2021). Morbid curiosity leads people to slow their cars to view traffic accidents and to watch disasters unfolding on television. People vary in their degree of morbid curiosity. Some show intense fascination, while others avoid all reminders of death. People with high levels of morbid curiosity agree with statements like "If a head transplant was possible, I would want to watch the procedure" (Scrivner, 2021, p. 4).

Morbid curiosity "manifests as a balance between the costs of exposure to morbid content and the perceived benefits of learning about that content" (Scrivner, 2021, p. 2). Morbid curiosity drives people to learn about threats and how they might be avoided. Morbid curiosity can be regarded as a proximal defense against low or moderate levels of death anxiety. Morbid curiosity is less likely in people who intensely fear death (Scrivner, 2021).

Morbid curiosity is evident in disease outbreaks, where curiosity overrides the fear of infection. In the Great Plague of London, diarist Samuel Pepys (1669) described crowds of people flocking to funeral services: "But Lord! to consider the madness of people of the town, who will (because they are forbid) come in crowds along with the dead corpses to see them buried" (Pepys, 1669, p. 311). In 19th-century New Orleans, amid yellow fever outbreaks, there were reports of "the morbid curiosity of the crowds who gathered about the cemeteries to watch the process of interment, seemingly undisturbed by the ghastly sights and putrid fumes" (Carrigan, 1963, p. 29). Recognizing the commercial value of graveside gawkers, vendors congregated outside cemetery gates selling ice creams and other treats (Carrigan, 1963).

Today, morbid curiosity during disease outbreaks can increase news and social media viewing and other forms of information-seeking, which has a range of effects. On the one hand, curiosity-driven information-seeking can lead people to be better informed and prepared. On the other hand, curiosity can lead people down rabbit holes, exposing them to sensational or fake media stories, rumors, conspiracy theories, and wild claims about disease-related dangers and supposed safety measures.

Dark Humor

Humor involves reappraisal—for example, seeing the light side of a difficult situation (Perchtold et al., 2019). Humor in difficult times can be a salve and shared release (Engle, 2020). Humor is a coping strategy that accentuates positive emotions, psychologically distances oneself from adverse events, and can strengthen social cohesion with friends, acquaintances, and family (Amici, 2020; Fritz et al., 2017; Kuiper, 2012).

Pandemics breed bad jokes. Like other life-threatening hazards, pandemics are associated with a rise in dark humor. Also known as "gallows humor," dark humor involves regarding one's situation with bleak mirth. Dark humor typically juxtaposes morbid and farcical elements involving an illogical or inappropriate response to a desperate situation (Rowe & Regehr, 2010). Dark humor—a proximal defense against death anxiety—was evident in COVID-19, the Spanish flu, swine flu, and HIV/AIDS pandemics, and in outbreaks of plague, cholera, and yellow fever (Alterisio, 2020; Chew & Eysenbach, 2010; Correia, 2018; De Bow's Review, 1853; Dundes, 1987; Engle, 2020; Fiquepron, 2018; King, 1918; Lee, 2014; Munson, 2021; Slack, 1985; Weeks, 1918). The following are some examples.

Dark humor may be expressed as tall tales. According to an anecdote told in New Orleans in 1853, yellow fever "was so bad at the St. Charles Hotel, that as soon as a man arrived and registered his name they immediately took his measure for a coffin, and asked him to note down in which cemetery he desired to be interred" (A Physician of New Orleans, 1854, p. 99). There were witticisms about face masks during the Spanish flu, such as jokes that you are unable to hear long-winded people because of their masks (King, 1918) and jokes about masks providing "the maximum of protection with the maximum of discomfort" (Weeks, 1918, p. 1).

Dark humor was expressed as practical jokes, as illustrated by the following 17th-century English prank, which involved modifying a notice on the door of a plague-infected building (Slack, 1985). The phrase "Lord have mercy upon us" was commonly written on the front doors of infected dwellings as a warning and religious supplication. In one instance, someone modified the door sign of a building in which brass farthings were minted. "Lord have mercy upon us" was changed to "Lord have mercy upon us, for this house is full of tokens." The joke was based on a double entendre. Coins (farthings) and plague lesions (buboes) were both known as tokens.

In 16th- and 17th-century plague outbreaks, pamphleteers published entertaining cautionary tales about disease and death (e.g., Dekker, 1603). Using dark humor, pamphleteers advised readers to avoid extremes, use common sense, and remember their moral obligations (Slack, 1985). The stories denounced city officials who fled and criticized rural folk who shunned the fleeing. Stories denounced foolhardiness, such as the story of the parish official who died after laying on a plague corpse in an attempt to prove that providence would protect him. Readers were encouraged to laugh at absurd precautions, such as avoiding spotted fish, but cautioned about needless risks. This literature "offered ridicule of extremes of behaviour, a defence of charity, and a necessary hard realism which enabled people to come to terms with plague" (Slack, 1985, p. 242).

Dark humor can be adaptive if it keeps people calm and fosters social support. However, using dark humor as a form of coping can be counterproductive when the humor is offensive or alienating (Kuiper, 2012). Despite its widespread use amid disease outbreaks, dark humor may be less effective than other kinds of humor in reducing distress and inducing positive emotions (Perchtold et al., 2019; Samson & Gross, 2012).

Desperate Pleasures

Profligate pleasure-seeking in the face of danger is an extreme form of temporal discounting (Chapter 11) that serves as a proximal defense against death anxiety. Desperate attempts at pleasure-seeking, such as debauched festivities, occurred in outbreaks of plague, cholera, yellow fever, and other diseases (Fiquepron, 2018; Garza, 2008; Gowen, 1907; Procopius, 551 AD; Sorokin, 1942). The debauches were not the partying of people who believed the threat was overstated, as when people flouted restrictions and held illicit parties during COVID-19 (McGee, 2022; Reynolds, 2022). Desperate pleasure-seeking was seen in people who feared they were soon likely to die.

Eyewitnesses to plague outbreaks reported that there was sometimes an "almost carnival spirit of desperate enjoyment that overcame certain sections of the population" (Steel, 1918, p. 95). Amid a plague outbreak in 18th-century Genoa, Italy, people played music, sang, and danced (Gowen, 1907). In plague hospitals, marriages took place; "one day in particular five marriages were performed—four of the bridegrooms being buriers of the dead, dressed in the clothes stripped from the bodies of the deceased" (Gowen, 1907, p. 16).

In the cholera and yellow fever epidemics in Buenos Aires in the period 1867–1871, newspaper reports described a rise in merry-making (Fiquepron, 2018). People gathered in cafes, taverns, and other social venues to sing and dance. People gathered in the streets around bonfires, which were social hubs and means of disinfection—the fires were thought to purify the air against miasma. These diversions provided some respite in a world permeated by death.

The Plague of Athens (430–426 BC), arising in the Peloponnesian War between Athens and Sparta, provides a further example of desperate pleasure-seeking. As the war with Sparta intensified, Athenians retreated into their walled city, where they experienced overcrowding, food shortages, and deteriorating sanitary conditions. When prayers and nostrums proved ineffective in stemming the spread of sickness and death, many Athenians lapsed into dissolute, pleasure-seeking behavior, spending money indiscriminately and defying the law:

> Fear of gods or law of man there was none to restrain them. As for the first, they judged it to be just the same whether they worshipped them or not, as they saw all alike perishing; and for the last, no one expected to live to be brought to trial for his offences, but each felt that a far severer sentence had been already passed upon them all and hung over their heads, and before this fell it was only reasonable to enjoy life a little. (Thucydides, 411 BC, p. 252)

Desperate pleasure-seeking, as an escape from death anxiety, can worsen a person's situation by increasing their exposure to infected others.

Conclusions

The looming threat of death raises issues concerning the meaning, value, and legacy of one's existence. Terror management theory describes mechanisms by which people deal with death anxiety. These include proximal defenses, clearly linked to keeping safe (e.g., hygiene behaviors such as handwashing), and distal defenses, which offer the promise of symbolic or literal immortality, either by personal achievements (legacy projects) or by affiliating with powerful, enduring institutions such as nations, political groups, and organized religions.

Pandemic-related increases in religious activities, political partisanship, and xenophobia exemplify distal defenses against death anxiety. Morbid curiosity, dark humor, and desperate pleasure-seeking can be understood as proximal defenses. The frantic search for desperate pleasures in pandemics highlights how humans, as social creatures, paradoxically seek the company of others during disease outbreaks for solace, support, and diversion, even though socialization increases the risk of what people dread the most—sickness and death.

15
Diseases, Disgust, and Xenophobia

Introduction

Pathogens such as viruses are too small to be directly observed. Therefore, a person's biological immune system is insufficient for detecting and avoiding these agents. It is necessary to rely on perceptible disease cues, such as the sight of people coughing or sneezing, or the smells associated with sickness. The behavioral immune system (BIS) is a theoretical, evolved mechanism for detecting and responding to these cues. Once disease cues are detected, the BIS triggers disgust and fear, which motivate escape from, or avoidance of, disease cues (Ackerman et al., 2018; Schaller & Park, 2011). The BIS complements theoretical accounts of anxiety about health and death (Chapters 13 and 14) by focusing on motivational aspects of disease avoidance. As we will see, the BIS helps us understand the social aspects of disease avoidance, particulary xenophobia and disease-related stigma.

People differ in their degree of BIS sensitivity, as indicated by scores on traits such as the tendency to experience disgust (disgust sensitivity) (Duncan et al., 2009). Individuals with high scores on disgust sensitivity are especially likely to worry about getting infected during disease outbreaks (Taylor, 2019; Taylor et al., 2020). The BIS is biased toward false positives (false alarms). The BIS is sensitive to cues that only superficially resemble signs of infection, which minimizes potentially fatal failures to detect threats but can lead to social problems related to xenophobia. Perceptions of threat, regardless of accuracy, significantly influence the person's emotional and behavioral responses.

In the remainder of this chapter, we will review the BIS and explore its implications for understanding pandemics. We begin with disgust sensitivity and then review how olfactory cues become sources of perceived danger or safety during infectious outbreaks. Outbreak-related xenophobia, discrimination, and racism are then discussed in relation to the BIS and disease avoidance.

Disgust Sensitivity

Disgust is a basic human emotion characterized by aversion, revulsion, and repugnance in response to certain objects, animals, or people. Disgust is central to the BIS. It is probably no coincidence that disgust is also central to the miasma theory of disease, with the latter stating that bad-smelling vapors are sources of contagion. Disgust plays a pervasive but underappreciated role in life.

Disgust-evoking stimuli are related to disease, contamination, and bodily products such as mucus, saliva, and feces (Goetz et al., 2013). Appearance, smell, and taste are common triggers of disgust. Stimuli that people worldwide experience as disgusting include (1) bodily contents and wastes, (2) people who are sick, deformed, or deceased, (3) dirty environments, (4) unfamiliar or spoiled foods, and (5) particular organisms such as worms, rats, and cockroaches (Curtis et al., 2011). People are disgusted not only by things that pose a real risk of infection (e.g., feces) but also by things that superficially resemble real risks (e.g., chocolate fudge sculpted in the shape of feces) (Oaten et al., 2009; Rozin et al., 2008). This is consistent with the idea that the BIS is prone to false alarms as part of a disease-avoidance strategy that errs on the side of caution.

Although disgust appears to be a universal human experience, people differ in their disgust sensitivity. Compared to people scoring low on this trait, high scorers are easily disgusted and experience disgust more strongly (Haidt et al., 1994). People scoring high on disgust sensitivity readily and frequently experience disgust even when exposed to stimuli that are not particularly disgusting, such as the sight of people sneezing from seasonal allergies.

Fear and disgust are closely linked, both serving as motivators of disease avoidance. People with high levels of disgust sensitivity are likely to become particularly disgusted and frightened when threatened with infectious diseases. In the 2009 swine flu pandemic, disgust sensitivity predicted a person's fear of acquiring influenza (Brand et al., 2013; Wheaton et al., 2012). During COVID-19, high levels of disgust sensitivity were associated with intense fear of infection (Díaz & Cova, 2021; Shook et al., 2020; Troisi et al., 2022). Longitudinal COVID-19 research found that pre-pandemic disgust proneness predicted subsequent (peri-pandemic) fear of infection (Cox et al., 2020). People with intense disgust sensitivity tend to be hesitant about vaccination (Yap et al., 2023), which is unsurprising given that vaccination involves injecting pathogen-related material into one's body.

To summarize, disgust is evoked once the BIS detects disease cues, prompting avoidance and escape, even from cues only superficially related to diseases. The degree of disgust sensitivity varies across individuals. Understanding the elements of disgust, such as olfactory cues, provides insights into how people cope with disease threats.

The Smells of Danger and Safety

When threatened with infectious disease, people look for cues to danger and safety, avoiding the former and seeking the latter. Foul odors are potent cues to contagious harm. To evade diseases such as the plague and cholera, medical treatises historically emphasized avoiding "filthy noisome smells" and foul-smelling things (Anonymous, 1721; Burton, 1652; Hodges & Quincy, 1720; Kephale, 1665; Von Pettenkofer, 1873). In the words of a 19th-century physician concerning cholera, "It is a matter of experience, independent of any theory, that we enjoy the better health the purer the air is" (Von Pettenkofer, 1873, p. 332). For centuries, the simple rule "if it smells foul, it could be harmful" has effectively helped people to avoid pathogens.

The BIS is exquisitely attuned to olfactory cues but also responds to learning. People learn to associate some powerful odors with safety, particularly the smells of disinfectants (Tomes, 1999). People even learn to associate noxious smells with safety, such as the putrid smell of asafetida. The latter was a folk remedy in the Spanish flu and other outbreaks (Arnold, 2018; Maclean's, 2009); see Chapter 1.

Powerfully pungent fumigants such as sulfur dioxide have been staples of public sanitation campaigns. In some cases, the smell of sulfurous fumigants was worse than the smell of the dead and dying in their sick rooms (New World, 1840). In an outbreak of yellow fever in New Orleans in 1873, "the large amount of carbolic acid used made the air of a disinfected locality exceedingly irritating to the eyes, and sometimes produced headaches and nausea" (Perry, 1873, p. 190). Strong-smelling fumigants, regardless of efficacy, can be reassuring for infection-fearful people.

There is a long history of using aromatic compounds such as perfumes for their supposed health-promoting properties (King, 2022). In the era of the Antonine plague (165–180 AD), likely caused by smallpox, physicians believed that strong scents could thwart the disease (Elliott, 2024). Dried laurel leaves, with their pleasant fragrance, were placed around infected persons, with the rationale that healthy smells would enter the body and displace diseases trapped therein (Elliott, 2024). It was believed that sweet odors of fragrant oils and perfumes "filled up the sensory passages and kept out the poison in the air; or, if any poison should enter, it would be neutralized by the stronger odors" (Echols, 1961, p. 30). In 17th-century England and Europe, "all manner of sweet-smelling flowers and herbs were supposed to have antiplague properties, and aromatic essences prepared from them were in great demand" (Hirst, 1953, p. 44). Aromatic herbs such as camphor or aloe were burned as plague preventives to "keep the air in a healthful state" (Bradley, 1721, p. 28).

Perfumes, vinegar, sulfur, and chlorine were used by postal services to disinfect the mail against plague in Europe in the 14th century and later (Ellis, 2017). The procedure involved cutting slits or poking holes into sealed letters, exposing the contents to the disinfectant's purportedly purifying fumes. During epidemics of yellow fever in the late 19th century in the southern United States, the mail was similarly fumigated (Ellis, 2017). In the 17th century, coins were rinsed in vinegar as a plague preventive (Inì, 2021; Parets, 1651).

In the 1885 smallpox epidemic in Montreal, a front-page newspaper advertisement for Thymo-Cresol disinfectant exhorted readers to "Beware of odorless disinfectants!!" (Montreal Daily Herald, 1885, p. 1), implying that disinfectant smells were safety cues. However, it has long been recognized that some disinfectants are merely aromatic deodorizers, providing a false sense of security concerning germs (Chapin, 1906; Spirit of The Times, 1848; Sternberg, 1900). In 1900, it was objected that "a large number of the proprietary 'disinfectants' so called, which are in the market, are simply deodorizers," which are "entirely untrustworthy for disinfecting purposes" (Sternberg, 1900, p. 625).

Many of the aromatic purification procedures—including the applications of deodorizers, perfumes, vinegar, acrid smoke, and asafetida—were essentially forms of hygiene theater: conspicuous protective activities that alleviated anxiety by masking smells but offered little or no actual safeguard against infection. A more effective method, of course, is to extirpate the sources of the smells, as per public sanitation. Hygiene theater is discussed in Chapter 17. A meta-analysis of placebo-controlled aromatherapy trials suggests that exposure to pleasant-smelling fragrances is calming (Gong et al., 2020). During disease outbreaks, calming aromatics address the fear of disease rather than the disease itself. Even today, the popularity of deodorizers attests to the widespread practice of hygiene theater.

Regardless of whether a disinfectant is efficacious, any effects are time-limited. Once disinfected, an object or surface may soon become recontaminated. Thus, disinfection is associated with uncertainty, and people commonly resort to rituals or protocols for dealing with uncertainty (see Chapters 16 and 17).

Pathogens and Prejudice

Interpersonal contact is a common way of getting sick, especially when foreign groups intermingle. In this situation, one group introduces a disease the other group has never encountered and has no preexisting immunity (Navarrete & Fessler, 2006). European explorers to the Americas, for example, brought smallpox, influenza, and other diseases, decimating the indigenous inhabitants (Pringle, 2015).

Given that many infections are transmitted through interpersonal interactions, the BIS is said to have evolved to influence social attitudes, including ethnocentrism and negative attitudes toward immigrants and other foreigners (Schaller & Park, 2011). Many studies have shown that when people feel threatened about becoming infected with some pathogen, they tend to become xenophobic, avoiding or stigmatizing out-groups—that is, groups to which a person does not affiliate or identify (Ackerman et al., 2018; Faulkner et al., 2004; Joffe, 1999; Makhanova et al., 2015). Research suggests that xenophobia even extends to disease expectations: People expect seasonal influenza to be more severe if they contact it from a stranger than a friend (Nemeroff, 1995).

Xenophobia during disease outbreaks manifests in various ways, including territoriality, where intruders are confronted and repelled. Banishment of "undesirables" from towns or cities was another common way of dealing with plague outbreaks. Targets included "beggars and vagabonds, and people who are not settled inhabitants, and cannot give a very good account of their business" (Lee, 1869, pp. 429–430). Plague-fearful urban inhabitants fleeing to the countryside were often met with hostility by rural folk (Chapter 9).

Xenophobia is commonly expressed as blame. Throughout history, out-groups have been blamed for causing or spreading diseases because of their supposed lack of hygiene, education, or self-control (Gilles et al., 2013). In outbreaks of plague, for example, the British blamed the Dutch for the disease, whereas the French blamed the British, and Christians blamed Jews (Cohn, 2017; Hirst, 1953; Newitz, 2021).

Fear of infection drives many prejudicial attitudes in the course of disease outbreaks. People most frightened of infection are more likely to avoid foreigners and have negative attitudes toward out-groups (Aarøe et al., 2017; Duncan et al., 2009; Faulkner et al., 2004; Green et al., 2010; Navarrete &

Fessler, 2006; Schaller & Park, 2011; Taylor et al., 2020). The perceived threat of infection is also associated with prejudicial responses against people who display characteristics superficially suggesting poor health, such as physical disability, obesity, and old age (Duncan & Schaller, 2009; Park et al., 2003; Park et al., 2007; White et al., 2014).

Racism

Racism, which conceptually overlaps with xenophobia, refers to "thoughts, attitudes and practices that create hierarchies of superiority and inferiority based on characteristics such as 'race,' ethnicity, and nation . . . and may be expressed through stereotypes, prejudice or discrimination that serve to maintain or exacerbate unfair and avoidable inequalities" (Elias et al., 2021, p. 788). Racism is a complex psychosocial phenomenon in which the BIS plays an important role.

Racism commonly arises when diseases break out in communities. Infection-related racism was a widespread problem in many past outbreaks, including the plague, cholera, swine flu, Russian flu, SARS, and COVID-19 (Alexander, 2009; Ginzburg, 2004; Holmes, 2011; Markel, 2004; McCauley et al., 2013; Nelkin & Gilman, 1988; Todd, 1909; White, 2018). Infection-related racism extends even to nosocomial (hospital-acquired) infections. For example, one study found that the British public tended to blame foreign workers, especially cleaners and nurses, for the spread of methicillin-resistant *Staphylococcus aureus* in hospitals (Joffe et al., 2011).

In the early years of the HIV/AIDS pandemic, Haitians, in addition to gay men, were targets of discrimination (Markel, 2004). During COVID-19, there was a rise in antisemitic hate speech in social media and elsewhere (Institute for Strategic Dialogue, 2021). Amid the Black Death in the years 1347–1351, there was mass violence against Jews, accused, on the basis of unfounded rumors, of poisoning wells and food supplies. Pogroms swept across Europe, with over a thousand Jewish communities affected (Cohn, 2012).

Racism was seemingly less prominent in the Spanish flu. The latter may have moved so swiftly and indiscriminately that it could not easily be blamed on a specific group (Tomes, 2010). However, pandemic-related xenophobia still occurred. For example, some American magazines and newspapers blamed the Germans and Chinese for spreading the infection (Literary Digest, 1918a, 1918b; New York Times, 1918).

Anti-Mexican racism spiked in the United States amid the 2009 swine flu pandemic. Swine flu originated in Mexico and spread to the United States.

There were numerous accounts of racism directed toward Mexicans in the United States, including xenophobic vitriol on the internet and on some American talk shows, alleging that Mexicans were intentionally spreading swine flu across the United States (Alexander, 2009; Holmes, 2011; McCauley et al., 2013).

Anti-Asian racism escalated during SARS, COVID-19, and the Russian flu (Elias et al., 2021; Mussell, 2007; Taylor, 2019; White, 2018). The British media blamed SARS on unhygienic Chinese cultural practices, such as living in close proximity to animals and the habit of spitting in public (Washer, 2004). There were numerous reports of Asian racism in the United States in the course of COVID-19, in which Asian people, including children and seniors, were verbally harassed, coughed and spat upon, and physically assaulted because of the link between China and COVID-19 (Man, 2020; Nick, 2021). Anti-Asian sentiments spread on social media sites like 4chan (Nick, 2021). Racism increased in the context of preexisting global patterns of discrimination and inequality affecting migrants and minority groups (Elias et al., 2021).

Racism is sustained and amplified by rumors and conspiracy theories (Chapter 12). Infection-related prejudice against out-groups may involve beliefs in rumors and conspiracy theories about the role of foreigners in spreading disease (Atlani-Duault et al., 2015; Quick, 2018).

Xenophobia and Beliefs About Immunity

Xenophobia is expressed in beliefs about the health risks posed by fellow citizens versus foreigners. Consider yellow fever, for example. In 19th-century epidemics of yellow fever in New Orleans, it was widely believed that locals were somehow immune because they were "acclimated," either because they had survived past outbreaks of yellow fever or were long-time residents supposedly accustomed to the climate and its diseases (A Physician of New Orleans, 1854; Olivarius, 2019). Inhabitants who saw themselves as acclimated were less likely to flee from New Orleans when yellow fever broke out (Carrigan, 1994).

Before the advent of modern diagnostic testing, immunity was invisible and difficult to verify. Foreigners were viewed with suspicion as potential carriers of disease. Orleanians relied on external cues to judge whether someone was safe or contagious, such as physical appearance, ethnicity, and place of origin. If a person was a newcomer or foreign-born, they were assumed to be unacclimated (Olivarius, 2019). Gaining immunity by surviving yellow fever was a baptism of citizenship in Orleanian society, improving one's opportunities for accommodation, marriage, and employment (Olivarius, 2019). Employers were reluctant to hire and train workers who might succumb to the disease, and landlords were unwilling to house people for the same reason.

The safety of acclimation was illusory for individuals who never acquired yellow fever immunity, such as those who survived diseases misdiagnosed as yellow fever. Even so, beliefs about acclimation provided guidelines for distinguishing safety from danger, allowing disease threats to seem more predictable and controllable by relying on perceptible cues. Beliefs about acclimation led to the development of "fever passes" and other forms of immunity documentation—akin to the vaccine passports used during COVID-19 (see Chapter 5).

Conclusions

Disgust, fear of infection, and xenophobia commonly arise in pandemics as people seek to identify and avoid sources of infection. Pathogens such as viruses are too small to detect with the unaided eye, so detectable cues are needed, such as visual or olfactory signs of disease. The BIS is a hypothetical evolved mechanism for detecting these cues. Once detected, the cues evoke disgust and fear, which motivate escape and avoidance. There are individual differences in the BIS's sensitivity, as indicated by a person's level of disgust sensitivity. When threatened with infection, people scoring highly on this trait readily experience disgust when confronted with disease cues such as the sight of people coughing or sneezing. People learn to associate some cues with danger or safety. Even foul-smelling substances such as asafetida may become learned cues to safety.

The BIS helps us understand societal reactions to infectious threats, such as discrimination against out-groups. Further research is needed to determine how the BIS is conceptually related to the mechanisms for coping with death anxiety, as discussed in the preceding chapter. When the BIS is activated by exposure to disease cues, fear of death may be one of the emotional responses, in which case the proximal and distal defensive strategies would likely be implemented.

Cognitive-behavior therapy can reduce disgust sensitivity (Rast et al., 2023). This treatment could have downstream effects in reducing racism and xenophobia, although this remains to be investigated.

16
Magical Thinking and Superstitious Behavior

Introduction

Magical thinking involves assumptions about causality that don't make sense according to modern science. Examples include beliefs in luck, divination, evil spirits' influential power (e.g., curses, spells), energy transfer (e.g., transferences of good or bad essences between objects), and other paranormal phenomena (Bocci & Gordon, 2007; Eckblad & Chapman, 1983). Magical thinking plays an influential role in how people deal with pathogens. Superstitious rituals are based on magical thinking. Even superstitions acquired by observational learning—watching and imitating others—are based on the assumption of supernatural causes.

The purpose of this chapter is to review the nature of magical thinking and how it relates to superstitious behaviors seen in disease outbreaks. Magical thinking may be part of a mental disorder, such as obsessive-compulsive disorder or schizotypal personal disorder. However, magical thinking is also widespread in the general population, which is our focus here.

This chapter begins with a review of magical thinking in the general population, including its nature and prevalence. The laws of sympathetic magic—that is, the laws of contagion and similarity—are discussed. These laws describe common kinds of magical thinking. Magical thinking leads to various types of superstitious behaviors. Several superstitions related to disease outbreaks are reviewed, including the reliance on talismans, avoidance of tempting fate, and seeking omens. Superstitious rituals based on observational learning are illustrated with a case study of the 1832 religious panic in Ireland, which arose in response to the threat of cholera.

Magical Thinking Is Widespread

Over a quarter of Americans (27%) say "bless you" when someone sneezes, 26% "knock on wood" for luck, 24% carry a lucky charm, and 20% cross their fingers for some hoped-for event (Nguyen, 2018; Orth, 2022). Worldwide, many buildings, including apartment towers and hospitals, lack floors with "unlucky" numbers, such as the number 4 in Asian cultures and 13 in Western and other cultures (Huang & Teng, 2009; Vyse, 2019). For hotels and apartment buildings with a 13th floor, surveys show that many people try to avoid that floor, preferring other floors (Antipov & Pokryshevskaya, 2015; Burakov, 2018; Carroll, 2007). For example, a U.S. survey found that 13% of Americans would be bothered if assigned a hotel room on the 13th floor, and 9% would ask for a room on a different floor (Carroll, 2007).

Very few people display a complete lack of magical thinking (Caspi et al., 2024). Some may be unwilling to admit they are superstitious and yet say "bless you" after someone sneezes, precautiously "touch wood" after discussing some hoped-for future event, or refrain from mentioning the event altogether for fear of tempting fate (Rudski & Edwards, 2007; Subbotsky, 2007). Magical thinking is built into the English language, as illustrated by everyday expressions like "fortunately" and "luckily" to describe personally pleasing outcomes and "fingers crossed" for hoped-for events.

Despite cultural variations, magical thinking is universal, representing a fundamental characteristic of the human mind (Nemeroff & Rozin, 2000). Magical thinking is evident in all spheres of life, persisting throughout human history despite the rise of modern science. Regardless of education level, most adults engage in magical thinking at some point, although some people more than others (Rozin et al., 1992).

Magical thinking develops in childhood and typically persists in attenuated form into adulthood (Brashier & Multhaup, 2017; Rosengren & French, 2013). The tendency to engage in magical thinking arises from a combination of genetic and environmental factors, including learning experiences (Brambilla et al., 2014; Karcher et al., 2014).

Magical thinking may be a by-product of adaptive cognitive processes (Nemeroff & Rozin, 2000; Risen, 2016). Magical thinking coexists with logical, science-based reasoning. People may simultaneously hold contradictory (compartmentalized) beliefs, such as scientific beliefs (e.g., belief in germ theory) and magical beliefs (e.g., belief that an illness can be prevented by wearing a lucky charm). Endorsing supernatural explanations for a disease is not necessarily due to a lack of knowledge of scientific explanations, and learning those explanations does not necessarily reduce belief in supernatural causes (Lobato & Zimmerman, 2018).

People turn to magical thinking in unpredictable, uncontrollable, high-stakes situations (Malinowski, 1955; Markle, 2010; Risen, 2016). In outbreaks of lethal disease, magical thinking enables people to believe that their actions—such as searching for omens (good or bad signs), wearing talismans (amulets or good luck charms), or performing superstitious behaviors (rituals) invoking a deity, fate, or luck—will preserve the health and happiness of themselves and loved ones.

Magical thinking is especially likely in people with high levels of anxiety about health and death, intolerance of uncertainty, and suggestibility (James & Wells, 2002; Keinan, 2003; Subbotsky, 2007; Wong, 2012). During COVID-19, people who intensely feared the disease were likelier to perform superstitious rituals to bring good fortune (Hoffmann et al., 2022).

Sympathetic Magic

Law of Similarity

There are several forms of magical thinking. Each is a style of thinking and behavior that follows a predictable pattern or law. Among the most relevant to pandemics are the sympathetic magical laws of similarity and contagion. People commonly think and behave according to these laws, even without realizing they are doing so (Fraser, 1894; Rozin & Nemeroff, 2002).

The law of similarity has two sub-laws: (1) causes resemble effects, and (2) appearance equals reality (Rozin & Nemeroff, 2002). The first states that "like causes like." For example, strong (foul-tasting) medicines are needed to combat formidable diseases. Indeed, cough syrups elicit a stronger placebo response when they have an unpleasant taste (Eccles, 2020). The assumption that causes resemble effects can lead people to overestimate how difficult it is to destroy or neutralize a virus on contaminated surfaces. Consider HIV, for example. Research findings indicate that "in current lay thought, it is believed by many that because AIDS is lethal and extremely resistant to attempts at cure, the infectious agent (HIV) should have the same potent and indestructible qualities" (Rozin & Nemeroff, 2002, p. 204).

The second sub-law of similarity proposes that appearance (e.g., an image or representation) equals reality. The use of voodoo dolls is based on the belief that harming the doll harms the person the doll represents (Risen, 2016). Conversely, quack cures such as patent medicines may look more appealing to consumers and elicit more powerful placebo responses when the bottles or packaging resembles those of bona fide prescription medicines.

Law of Contagion

According to the law of contagion, when two objects come in contact, they exchange properties, including the permanent transfer of essences, good and bad. There are several sub-laws to the law of contagion (Rozin et al., 1992):

- *Dose insensitivity*: Contamination of the part contaminates the whole—for example, the belief that a drop of urine is sufficient to contaminate an entire barrel of water.
- *Permanence of contamination*: Once contaminated, always contaminated.
- *Negativity bias*: Adverse effects are stronger and more likely to be transmitted than beneficial ones.

The law of contagion resembles but is far broader than germ theory in that all kinds of properties—physical, moral, and spiritual—are believed to be passed from one object to another when they come in contact. Fans may covet a sweater formerly owned by a celebrity because of the law of contagion—the implicit belief that some celebrity essence resides in the clothing. Conversely, items owned by Adolf Hitler may be assiduously avoided for fear of acquiring some evil essence (Rozin & Nemeroff, 2002). People sometimes behave as if foods carry the essence of those who prepared them. For example, office workers might be wary of cupcakes supplied by a co-worker who had recently recovered from a feared infection (Rozin et al., 1992).

Shunned: Once Infected, Always Infected

The sympathetic magical law of contagion is illustrated by the shunning of infected but recovered people. In outbreaks of severe infectious disease, healthy people often shunned these individuals for fear of infection. Such phenomena were documented in outbreaks of MERS, SARS, COVID-19, influenza, cholera, plague, Ebola virus disease, and other diseases (Almutairi et al., 2018; Bax, 2014; CDC, 2007; Henry, 2020; Nursing Standard, 2004; Perry, 2014; Phiri, 2016).

To illustrate, a survivor of Ebola virus disease, a 24-year-old teacher in the West African country of Guinea, was fired from her job—even though she had recovered—for fear she could infect others. "People looked at me like I'd come back from the dead, like I was a zombie," she recalled after being released from 12 days in an isolation ward, "nobody except my relatives wanted anything to do with me anymore" (Bax, 2014, p. 1).

Early in the COVID-19 pandemic, when infected individuals were relatively rare in many communities, people who had been infected and recovered were shunned by others. "It was like I was radioactive," recalled one physician about the shunning he received, even though he had recovered from COVID-19 weeks earlier. Another survivor, Texas resident Sheri Colbert, had been recovered for over a month but was unable to convince her parents that she was safe to be near. When she tried to give her mother a gift for Mother's Day, her mother recoiled. "She told me to leave the gift in the garage so they could wait for the virus to die off of it before they would see it" (Henry, 2020, p. 1). Two months later, the gift was still in the garage.

Talismans

A talisman—a lucky charm or amulet—is an object believed to be endowed with special powers to protect oneself from bad luck or to bring good fortune. The lucky essence of the talisman is supposedly transferred to the wearer according to the sympathetic magical law of contagion.

The use of talismans for disease protection dates back to classical Rome or probably earlier, where they were used to ward off the plague (Jones, 2016). Since then, amulets and charms have been popular protectives against plague, cholera, and other diseases (Byrne, 2006; Jones, 2016; Life Magazine, 1908; Reiner, 1960; Slack, 1985). The following are some examples.

In the 17th century, it was common for people to use talismans to ward off diseases, worn around the neck or fixed to the wrists or armpits. Even among doctors, the practice "enjoyed a surprising vogue and respectability" (Baldwin, 1993, p. 227). Such was the widespread use of talismans that the German physician Jacob Wolff published a 400-page treatise on diseases supposedly treatable by charms and amulets (Wolff, 1692).

During a cholera outbreak in St. Petersburg in 1908, reliance on talismans was hazardous when people relied on them instead of avoiding contaminated water. Popular charms included "belts made of old copper coins rusted green," which were regarded as especially efficacious and commanded a high price (Life Magazine, 1908, p. 1). Authorities were frustrated and bewildered by the widespread reliance on superstition and distributed hot tea to discourage people from drinking contaminated water (Life Magazine, 1908). People may be reluctant to abandon their superstitions, taking the absence of a bad outcome as evidence for the efficacy of their talisman or superstitious ritual. Under these circumstances, people are reluctant to test the ritual by abandoning it or trying something new (Risen, 2016).

The use of talismans is not merely a quaint practice from a bygone era. Throughout COVID-19, there were reports from around the world—Thailand, India, Japan, Mexico, and elsewhere—of people using talismans to protect themselves from the coronavirus (Aaj Bikel News, 2022; O'Neil, 2020; South China Morning Post, 2021; Tanakasempipat, 2022; Thomason, 2022).

Talismans were sold on Amazon.com, such as the Japanese "Omamori charm for goodbye COVID-19" (Amazon, 2023). Jewelers marketed amulets as COVID-19 protectives. One maker claimed their jewelry would "guard the wearer from danger, disease and hardship or serve as a good luck token" (Mobilia Gallery, 2021, p. 1). A microbiologist at the University of Pittsburgh published an article—since debunked and retracted—claiming that jade amulets offered protection against COVID-19 (Bility et al., 2020).

In a 2020 press conference, Mexican President Andres López Obrador proudly displayed two religious amulets from his wallet, asserting they formed a personal "protective shield" against COVID-19 (O'Neil, 2020; Sherman, 2021). The protection was illusory. The president later became ill with COVID-19, for which he received conventional medical care.

Tempting Fate

The laws of sympathetic magic influence luck-related beliefs and behaviors. The number 19, as in COVID-19, became unlucky for gamblers during the coronavirus pandemic (Roger et al., 2023). Even talking about outcomes can be perceived to be lucky or unlucky. An example is the belief that it is bad luck to "tempt fate." Here, the person considers an unwanted outcome (e.g., a miserable vacation) to be more likely when they perform an action that "tempts" a bad outcome (e.g., announcing the trip beforehand) (Risen & Gilovich, 2008).

Superstitious beliefs about tempting fate are common. For example, some travelers believe they are more likely to experience a mishap if they have not purchased travel insurance (van Wolferen et al., 2013). Some people refuse to make a legal will for fear of tempting fate, believing that talking about one's demise increases the odds of dying (Brabant, 2020; Gorvins, 2016).

Health-anxious individuals may fear tempting fate if they tell themselves they're healthy (Taylor & Asmundson, 2004). Joking about COVID-19 was regarded as tempting fate by some people (Levy, 2020; Mackenzie, 2022). Fear of tempting fate can also lead some individuals to refuse vaccination. Some people perceived COVID-19 vaccination as an exercise in tempting fate, increasing the odds of infection (Ichino, 2022).

Omens: Perceived Cues to Danger and Safety

When facing an uncertain threat, people search for signs of danger and safety. Safety signals are potent inhibitors of fear and distress (Christianson et al., 2012), even when the cues offer only illusory signs of safety. Signs of danger and safety are colloquially known as omens—portents or predictors of what will come. Omens can be danger signals (bad omens) or safety signals (good omens). Omens can be true or false in their predictive accuracy. Omen-seeking is influenced by religious and other beliefs, advice from others, and observational learning.

People look for omens in disease outbreaks to attain a sense of prediction and control. Writing in 1527 in Florence during an outbreak of plague, the diplomat and author Niccolo Machiavelli reported that he would not venture outdoors until "the hour when the sun disperses the exhalations which rise from the earth" (Nohl, 1926, p. 217). The absence of exhalations—in other words, the absence of miasma—was Machiavelli's safety signal, indicating that he could venture outdoors.

Some omens in historical pandemics represented legitimate risk factors. To illustrate, John of Ephesus, a Byzantine historian and witness to the Plague of Justinian in 541 AD, documented several omens portending plague (Pearse, 2017). Omens thought to signal impending death included having the youngest member of a household fall ill with plague—a bad omen, for sure. Living with a sick, contagious family member increases the risk of infection for the rest of the household.

There were numerous examples of omen-seeking in the course of COVID-19, in which people sought to make their world more predictable and controllable. Some turned to astrology in search of portents (Piskorz, 2021). Online fortune telling and divination grew in popularity (Tanakasempipat, 2022). In Naples, the failure of a prayed-for miracle was taken as a bad omen concerning COVID-19. In the city's cathedral, a sealed vial containing dried blood of the 4th-century martyr San Gennaro is displayed several times a year. Based on the idea that the saint dispenses favors when he bleeds, the faithful pray for the Miracle of San Gennaro, which is said to occur when the saint's blood liquefies (Dauverd, 2020). According to witnesses, the blood does liquify. The phenomenon can be replicated using a small amount of melted beeswax in olive oil, colored with red pigment. The mixture is solid when cool and liquefies when warmed by body heat or candles (Nickell, 2009). The miracle failed to occur in 2020, despite rounds of praying, which was interpreted as a bad omen concerning COVID-19 (Reuters, 2020).

Religious Panic in Ireland, 1832

Superstitious rituals can be community-wide affairs, fueled by rumors and encouraged by the behaviors of others. This is illustrated by the religious panic in Ireland, which arose in 1832 in response to the looming threat of cholera, a widely feared disease at the time. Over six days, the panic spread across three-quarters of Ireland's counties. The religious panic shows how rumors—in the form of directives—can lead to superstitious rituals. The following account is based on Connolly's (1983) detailed archival investigation.

The panic began on Saturday, June 9, in County Cork, with the widespread rumor that the Virgin Mary had appeared on the altar in the chapel at Charleville. According to a widely circulated story, the Virgin had left a pile of ashes with a warning that the ashes, combined with prayers, were the only protection against cholera and should be collected into small packages and distributed to neighboring homes. The person receiving the ashes was instructed to collect ashes from their chimney, distribute them to four other houses, and so on. The message spread rapidly across 40 miles of Irish counties between midnight and 4 a.m. on June 10. Observers reported messengers running about "as if they were mad," fulfilling the Virgin's orders (Connolly, 1983, p. 216).

The Virgin's message morphed over time, much like a game of telephone, where a message conveyed from person to person becomes distorted with retelling. As the message spread across the country, the instruction to distribute ashes was replaced with messages to distribute turf or straw. Messengers, sometimes in the hundreds, ran in all directions through the towns and villages carrying protective tokens for distribution, such as ashes, straw, turf, or stones. Messengers also brought with them sensational but false rumors of cholera death tolls in neighboring towns or villages.

The religious panic was a largely prosocial event in which people urgently sought to thwart the spread of cholera by distributing tokens and prayers to friends, neighbors, and strangers. But not everyone participated. Messengers arriving at some households were met with disbelief, ridicule, or indifference. Skeptics believed the religious panic was instigated by a practical joker. Messengers reported that they were acting on directives from the clergy. Church authorities denied any involvement.

The religious panic occurred before the advent of germ theory. At the time, cholera and other infectious diseases were frightening and poorly understood. Participants in the religious panic were primarily Catholic, uneducated, and poor, with "a strong and very literal belief in direct supernatural intervention in human affairs" (Connolly, 1983, p. 230). Better education might have dampened the religious fervor but is unlikely to have extinguished it altogether because of preexisting beliefs in religious supernatural events. Doing something—even distributing tokens in a superstitious ritual—furnished an illusion of control over the looming cholera threat.

Superstitious Coping Versus Helpless Resignation

When placed in threatening, seemingly uncontrollable situations, some people struggle to assert control while others become passive, helpless, and resigned to their fate (Rudski, 2004). Whether a person reacts with helplessness or superstitious rituals in uncontrollable situations depends on various factors, including their learning history and beliefs about the causes and controllability of aversive events (Abramson et al., 1989; Alloy et al., 2018). People who believe they have little or no control over their lives are likely to respond to threatening diseases with helplessness. Conversely, people with a strong sense of control may be especially likely to persist in superstitious behaviors (Rudski, 2004). The illusion of control is discussed in Chapter 17.

In the past and today, some people view pandemics as a form of divine punishment. In such cases, we expect to see a variety of reactions. Some individuals may feel helpless, believing their fate is inevitable and they have no control over the outcome. Others might resort to superstitious rituals to change the situation, such as making offerings or supplications to deities. Whether people persist in a superstitious ritual depends, in part, on its perceived efficacy. When persistent pleas to supernatural agents go unanswered, some people lapse into helplessness, resignation, and despair.

Religious practices may become polarized during pandemics. Most religious people increase the frequency of their spiritual practices amid pandemics (Chapter 5). Others lose faith: "From the Plague of Athens onwards, people either sought solace in religious practices or fled from gods which had failed them" (Slack, 1985, p. 4). Increases in both religious rituals and hopeless resignation were observed in the Plague of Athens. While some people petitioned the gods with prayers and offerings, others lapsed into hopelessness and helplessness (Thucydides, 411 BC).

Conclusions

Magical thinking and superstitious behavior are common even in modern society. People behave according to two laws of sympathetic magic: the law of similarity (e.g., "like causes like") and the law of contagion (transfer of properties). Although pathogens spread via physical contact, these laws go beyond germ theory by positing magical (nonscientific) causes and cures for diseases.

When threatened with diseases that seem difficult or impossible to control, people turn to superstitions—rituals, talismans, and omen-seeking—to gain a sense of prediction and control. The superstitious behaviors observed in COVID-19 were remarkably similar to those in historical disease outbreaks. Performing certain rituals or seeking omens can alleviate anxiety and provide a claming but largely false sense of security.

During disease outbreaks, superstitions often involve avoiding or escaping disgusting objects or situations. Further research is needed to understand the relationship between magical thinking, superstitious behaviors, and the behavioral immune system. The latter is a theoretical system for detecting disease cues, such as olfactory and visual cues (Chapter 15). Once these cues are detected, they evoke fear and disgust, thereby motivating escape and avoidance. When avoidance or escape is impossible, people may resort to superstitious rituals to cope with the infectious threat. Thus, the behavioral immune system may be connected to the psychological mechanisms involved in magical thinking and superstitious behavior.

Rumors can lead to the widespread use of superstitious rituals, as was evident in the 1832 religious panic in Ireland. The relationship between magical thinking, superstitions, and conspiracy theories requires further study. People who believe in conspiracy theories tend to engage in magical thinking (Chapter 12), but little is known about the relationship between belief in conspiracy theories and superstitious behaviors.

Magical thinking is a major source of superstitious rituals, but the latter are influenced by additional factors. As noted in this chapter, beliefs about control are important determinants of behavior. The illusion of control and related self-serving biases are discussed in the following chapter.

17
The Illusion of Control and Other Self-Serving Biases

Introduction

People prefer their environments to be predictable and controllable (Rodin, 1986). Having perceived control over one's environment may be essential for psychological well-being and survival. The preference for control is evident even in infants, such as their insistence on feeding themselves. The preference for personal agency appears to be innate—we are "born to choose" (Leotti et al., 2010, p. 457). Perceived personal control, even if illusory, buffers the emotional impacts of stressful events (Alloy & Clements, 1992; Thompson, 2017).

During infectious outbreaks, people seek control in many ways. Individuals may persist in behaviors providing only an illusion of control, making them calmer but not necessarily safer. This chapter discusses these biases and illusions. Although magical thinking can lead to illusory protective behaviors, as discussed in the preceding chapter, the illusions and self-serving biases discussed in the present chapter do not require the types of magical thinking addressed in Chapter 16.

This chapter reviews several interrelated biases and illusions, including the optimism bias, the illusion of control, illusory correlations, and the denial of disease. As illustrated throughout the chapter, many self-serving biases, particularly the illusion of control, are evident in everyday hygiene practices today and in the past, as seen in the practices known as "hygiene theater."

The Optimism Bias

The optimism bias is characterized by persistent, unrealistically positive beliefs about one's future—that is, the tendency to believe that compared to others, one is more likely to experience good things and less likely to experience adversity (Taylor & Brown, 1988; Weinstein, 1980). People with a strong optimism bias tend to undervalue dangers such as diseases, whose existence they acknowledge but do not believe will affect them personally (Makridakis & Moleskis, 2015). The optimism bias is positively correlated with stress-buffering traits such as resilience and hardiness, and negatively correlated with health anxiety and distress-vulnerability traits (Taylor et al., 2021); see Chapter 18.

The optimism bias has been observed in numerous disease outbreaks, including SARS, Swine flu, and COVID-19 (Ji et al., 2004; Kim & Niederdeppe, 2013; Shukla et al., 2021). Research in the course of COVID-19 found that people scoring higher on trait optimism reported lower levels of pandemic-related distress (Shiloh et al., 2023; Taylor et al., 2021). The optimism bias helps people remain calm but can have harmful effects, such as leading people to neglect hand hygiene and vaccination (Kim & Niederdeppe, 2013).

The tendency to be optimistically biased arises from genetic factors and environmental influences such as learning experiences (de Vries et al., 2022; Wootton et al., 2017). Genes and learning experiences likely influence the optimism bias by shaping processes involved in cognition and emotion. The unrealistic optimism bias is resistant to change in the face of disconfirming information (Jefferson et al., 2017; Sharot et al., 2011).

Illusions of Invulnerability and Control

Several self-serving biases are correlated with the optimism bias, including the illusion of unique invulnerability. The latter occurs when people believe they are less likely to be the victims of dangers or misfortunes that befall others (Perloff & Fetzer, 1986). People under the illusion of unique invulnerability are less anxious in response to stressful life events, more likely to drink and drive, more likely to engage in unprotected sex, and less likely to seek vaccination even in pandemics (Chan et al., 2010; Gerrard & Warner, 1994; Hill et al., 2012; Kleiman et al., 2017; Morrell et al., 2016; Ravert et al., 2009; Taha et al., 2013).

Another illusion related to the optimism bias—the illusion of control—occurs when people overestimate their influence over outcomes (Langer, 1975). Most people succumb to the illusion of control, but some more than others. The illusion can be demonstrated with computer-generated tasks, such as when participants try to switch on a light via button pressing. The illusion of control is evident when respondents believe they can control the light when, in fact, the button is disconnected. Using this design, a recent study found that 66% of people experienced an illusion of control, thinking they had some degree of control when, in fact, they had none (Simões et al., 2020).

The illusion of control is shaped by several factors, including (1) the desire or need for a specific outcome (motivated reasoning), (2) perceived but illusory correlations (discussed below), and (3) contextual factors, such as whether one is led to believe a given situation is controllable (Thompson, 2017). In objectively uncontrollable situations, people are more likely to experience the illusion of control when they can choose their actions (Langer, 1975). For example, people are more likely to succumb to the illusion of control over a lottery outcome when the person can select their ticket rather than having it randomly assigned. Hygiene theater is another activity involving the illusion of control, discussed later in this chapter.

The illusion of control typically stays within modest bounds. Illusions that are too extreme will be corrected by environmental feedback (Taylor, 2011). In cases where there is no feedback, the illusion persists. When people are encouraged to assess the situation logically, the illusion of control is attenuated or even eliminated (Thompson, 2017).

Illusory Correlations

Self-serving biases are supported or reinforced by illusory correlations. People look for environmental patterns or regularities to make their world more predictable and thereby more controllable. Illusory correlations are products of this predictive process. An illusory correlation occurs when an observer perceives an association between two variables when, in fact, there is none (Hamilton & Lickel, 2000).

Illusory correlations arise from several factors, including (1) expectations based on beliefs or stereotypes (e.g., believing that people from country A are carriers of disease B), (2) the confirmation bias (Chapter 11), (3) motivational factors, and (4) reliance on small or unrepresentative samples (Fiedler, 2017; Nickerson, 1998). Expectations and illusory correlations can be mutually reinforcing. Expecting two things co-occur can lead you to look for supporting evidence, strengthening the belief that the two are linked.

In addition to playing a role in many of the biases discussed in this chapter, illusory correlations influence people's choice of folk remedies in disease outbreaks. Consider smoking, which has long been a folk remedy for respiratory ailments—even though smoking offers no protection and, in fact, can worsen these conditions (Chapter 8). The "evidence" for smoking's protective powers was based on casual observations, leading to illusory correlations supporting beliefs that smoking was associated with the absence of a feared disease.

Illusory correlations concerning smoking are suggested in assertions made concerning plague and cholera in the 17th to 19th centuries. For example, there were claims that tobacconists rarely caught or died from these diseases (Kell, 1965). In Denver, Colorado, during the Spanish flu, the deputy health commissioner declared that "smokers are not in much danger of influenza, and I have the concrete proof" (Rocky Mountain News, 1918, p. 6). The commissioner's proof consisted of a short list of acquaintances who either smoked and were spared from the flu or didn't smoke and succumbed. Thus, flawed medical advice arose from a perceived but illusory correlation between smoking and the absence of influenza. The use of smoking as a coping strategy is further discussed in Chapter 8.

Illusory correlations can also maintain the superstitious behaviors discussed in the preceding chapter, where the person attributes the absence of an outcome (e.g., infection) to some putatively preventive behavior (e.g., wearing a talisman). Once formed, illusory correlations are resistant to change, affecting subsequent judgments and decision-making (Fiedler, 2017; Hamilton & Lickel, 2000). It can be challenging to eliminate the illusory correlation through training (Fiedler, 2017). Being aware that you are prone to illusory correlations is typically insufficient for overcoming the bias.

Hygiene Rituals and the Illusion of Control

Modern conceptions of personal and household hygiene, dating back to the early 20th century, provide people with guidelines about the behaviors needed to remain safe from infection (Tomes, 1997, 1999). With the advent of germ theory, kitchens, bathrooms, and high-traffic surfaces became targets for disinfecting, scrubbing, and fumigating. Contemporary hygiene involves a range of practices, including those that objectively reduce the odds of infection and those that are calming for infection-fearful people but largely illusory in protective powers.

Hygiene protocols involve ritualized behaviors, such as procedures for sneezing into a tissue and carefully folding and discarding it in a proper receptacle. There is also the familiar three-second rule we teach children: Dropped food is safe to eat if it has been on the ground for less than three seconds. This simple rule—and its more liberal counterpart, the five-second rule—helps distinguish safety from danger, but safety is illusory. A food item becomes contaminated as soon as it touches a pathogen-coated surface. Three or five seconds makes no difference. Nevertheless, with the rise of the modern hygiene movement, cleaning rituals became established procedures for fending off microbial threats, offering people a sense of safety and control—real and illusory—over the threat of infection.

Handwashing with soap and water is a vital hygiene behavior, but there is more to handwashing than disease prevention. Although excessive handwashing is associated with obsessive-compulsive disorder, handwashing rituals are commonly seen in the general population, even in people without mental health problems. Handwashing has become a multipurpose purity ritual in Western society—an all-purpose way of "washing away" all kinds of unpleasant things. Research shows that in addition to removing germs and dirt, handwashing can (1) alleviate guilt or shame after immoral behavior, (2) give people the sense that they are removing bad luck, and (3) make people feel more optimistic after failure (Kaspar, 2013; Khan & Grisham, 2018; Lee et al., 2024; Xu et al., 2012; Zhong & Liljenquist, 2006).

Handwashing has become a prominent self-protective tool for avoiding infection. Ritualized handwashing might involve scrubbing one's hands a set number of times, for a set duration, with specific ways of cleaning one's fingers, using specific cleansing agents (e.g., hand sanitizer). During COVID-19, elaborate posters began appearing in public restrooms, consisting of multipanel pictograms offering guidelines for washing one's hands. It is unclear whether elaborate handwashing rituals were more effective than a brief rinse with plain soap and water. Nevertheless, amid disease outbreaks in an era of germ theory, people gain multiple benefits from handwashing rituals, including relief from distress and a sense of control over microbial threats. Some control is real, such as frequent handwashing with soap and water. More elaborate forms of handwashing, such as those using elaborate washing protocols, might offer additional advantages primarily because of their calming effects.

Hygiene Theater

In the early months of the COVID-19 pandemic, health authorities emphasized the importance of cleaning and disinfecting surfaces and objects that might be contaminated with the coronavirus. In later months, as research accumulated, it became apparent that contaminated surfaces and objects were not as important as once thought and that infection was spread primarily through droplets or aerosols (i.e., coughing and sneezing) (Goldman, 2020). There is limited evidence that SARS-CoV-2 is transmitted via contaminated surfaces (Lewis, 2021). Indeed, disinfecting surfaces is one of the least effective methods for preventing the spread of COVID-19 (Haug et al., 2020). Yet, vigorous cleaning and disinfecting persisted: Trains, buses, and public spaces were vigorously sanitized, and restaurant tables were scrubbed, along with door handles, railings, and other high-contact objects in public places. Some people even cleaned their groceries—for example, using disinfecting towelettes to wipe soup cans and milk containers—in the mistaken belief it reduced their risk of acquiring COVID-19 (Choi, 2020; Koelle et al., 2022).

The excessive cleaning of public places was dubbed "hygiene theatre" (Thompson, 2020). Hygiene theater, a logical consequence of the modern hygiene movement, is a form of coping that provides a largely illusory sense of mastery over the threat of infection. Public displays of cleaning and disinfecting provided comforting but false assurances that these activities keep people safe from infection.

Activities suggestive of hygiene theater occurred in the past, even before the advent of germ theory. Based on the idea that diseases were spread by miasma, especially at night, there were numerous attempts over the centuries to disperse the supposedly unhealthy night air with bonfires and cannon fire. In several New Orleans epidemics of yellow fever in the 1850s, for example, efforts were made to "purify the atmosphere and drive away the pestilence" (Carrigan, 1959, p. 348). The New Orleans Board of Health ordered the daily firing of cannons and burning of barrels of tar in the streets and cemeteries. In plague and cholera outbreaks in the 19th century and earlier, large bonfires were lit in public squares and other public places, as they were thought to drive off pestilence (Clapp, 1857; D'Irsay, 1927; Gallaher et al., 1855; Harper's Weekly, 1865; Harvey, 1892; Smith, 2016; Staiano, 2008; Wear, 2015). In the 2003 SARS outbreak in China, some believed that gunpower "could kill the virus and disinfect the air" (Ang, 2003, p. 1).

Hygiene theater is evident in the use of disinfectants. Over a century ago, concerns were raised that disinfectants largely provided a false sense of security. A pioneer in U.S. public health, Dr. Charles V. Chapin, speaking at the 1906 annual meeting of the American Medical Association, criticized the widespread use of disinfection as a public health measure. Referring to it as "the fetish of disinfection," Chapin argued that "we do not disinfect because the utility of the process has been demonstrated, but because of precedent and authority" (Chapin, 1906, p. 574). In other words, we disinfect because others do it.

Hygiene practices are analogous to medications regarding expectancy (placebo) responses. All medicines are prone to placebo effects in addition to their intended pharmacologic actions. Some drugs elicit stronger placebo reactions than others—for example, a big, brightly colored capsule embossed with a brand name elicits a greater placebo response than a small, plain pill (Benedetti, 2021; Meissner & Linde, 2018). Something analogous may apply to hygiene practices. Regardless of their antimicrobial benefits, some hygiene activities may be more calming than others. Highly public sanitation initiatives, such as scrubbing trains during COVID-19 or strewing lime on the streets during cholera outbreaks, may be especially calming. Much remains to be learned about the placebo effects of current hygiene practices.

How can we tell, ahead of time, whether a cleansing or disinfecting activity is hygiene theater? Stoking bonfires to drive off miasma might have seemed sensible in the 19th century. Today, it would be considered hygiene theater. Some of today's practices—such as using alcohol-based hand sanitizer instead of plain soap and water—might be substantially illusory in their protective advantages. Further research is needed to resolve this issue.

Benefits and Risks of Illusion-Based Coping

The illusion of control can have several consequences, positive and negative. In terms of benefits, increasing one's sense of agency is calming even when control is illusory (Barlow, 2004). The illusion of control is correlated with good mental health (happiness, contentment, resilience), lower depression, and lower levels of distress in response to stressors (Bogdan et al., 2012; Taylor, 2011; Taylor & Brown, 1988, 1994). Perceiving that one's actions can influence outcomes may motivate coping behaviors and offer a buffer against hopelessness and despair (Alloy et al., 2018). Thus, the illusion of control and other self-serving illusions can be beneficial under some circumstances.

A false sense of security is not necessarily bad so long as the illusory protective activity is (1) not inherently harmful, (2) not the sole way of remaining safe, and (3) does not give rise to risk compensation. The latter occurs when the introduction of one protective behavior (e.g., disinfecting surfaces) causes a decrease in other protective behaviors (e.g., social distancing). Research conducted before COVID-19 suggested, across a wide range of health behaviors, that risk compensation does not usually happen (Mantzari et al., 2020). For example, taking preexposure prophylaxis medication decreases the risk of HIV/AIDS but typically does not lead to a reduction in other protective behaviors such as condom use (O Murchu et al., 2022).

There were mixed findings regarding risk compensation during COVID-19. The research—focusing on masks, vaccines, and social distancing—investigated whether adopting one protective measure was associated with reduced use of other measures. Some studies reported that mask-wearing was linked to decreased adherence to social distancing (Aranguren, 2022; Aranguren et al., 2023; Luckman et al., 2021; Wadud et al., 2022; Yan et al., 2021), while other studies found little or no evidence of this relationship (Guenther et al., 2021; Hall et al., 2023; Jørgensen et al., 2021; Liebst et al., 2022; Seres et al., 2021). A systematic review found no consistent evidence that mask-wearing leads to risk compensation (Millest et al., 2024).

Vaccination against COVID-19 did not lead to risk compensation in several studies (Desrichard et al., 2022; Sun et al., 2022; Thorpe et al., 2022). One study found some evidence for growing risk compensation over time. Vaccinated individuals became less likely to avoid social gatherings and less likely to wear masks (McColl et al., 2024). Other research found the opposite of risk compensation: Vaccinated people generally pursued other safety behaviors, such as mask-wearing and handwashing (Sun et al., 2022; Yang et al., 2023).

To summarize, the available research suggests that risk compensation usually does not occur. The findings indicate that pursuing activities providing an illusion of control (e.g., unnecessary cleansing) is unlikely to dissuade people from pursuing empirically supported protective measures such as vaccination.

Denial of Disease

Another self-serving bias—denial—is the refusal to acknowledge facts that threaten one's self-esteem, self-view, or worldview (Baumeister et al., 1998; Cramer, 2015; Freud, 1966). Denial is an observable phenomenon, distinguishable from its theoretical mechanisms (Wallerstein, 1967). In this book, we consider two types of denial: (1) disavowal of infectious cases by government authorities—that is, the concealment and under-reporting for socioeconomic and political reasons, as discussed in Chapter 7, and (2) the denial of personal disease—for example, the refusal to accept test results indicating that one has a feared disease—as discussed in the present chapter.

Denial of disease by patients—and sometimes by their caregivers—is indicated when the patient has been provided with an adequate explanation of their diagnosed medical condition but persistently denies the presence or severity of the condition (Patierno et al., 2023). Denial of physical illness has been documented for a range of medical conditions, including cardiovascular disease, diabetes, cancer, rheumatoid arthritis, and infectious diseases. The reported prevalence of disease denial varies widely, with estimates ranging from 2% to 74%, depending on the type of disease, medical setting, and method used to assess denial (Patierno et al., 2023).

Denial of disease is evident in the way people interpret medical test results. A negative biopsy might be accepted without question, whereas a positive finding, indicative of pathology, may be met with disbelief and insistence on a second opinion (Baumeister et al., 1998). During COVID-19, there were numerous reports of "deathbed denials," in which critically ill patients refused to accept that they were infected with the coronavirus (Hoye, 2021; Miranda, 2021; Salcedo, 2021; Villegas, 2020). Many of these patients—and their family members—were unvaccinated, believed COVID-19 was a hoax, and insisted they were suffering from some other disease. The prevalence of COVID-19 deathbed denials is unclear. Not all healthcare workers reported seeing such cases (Zweig, 2020).

According to terror management theory (Chapter 14) and psychodynamic theories, denial is an unconscious defense mechanism to protect the ego from anxiety. Lack of awareness is a key assumption—we are supposedly unaware of deceiving ourselves (Baumeister et al., 1998; Cramer, 2015). It can be difficult or impossible to determine whether a given instance of denial is unconsciously motivated. In many cases, denial may arise from some mix of conscious and non-conscious cognitive processes. The latter include processes of perception, learning, memory, and thinking that operate below the level of awareness (Kihlstrom, 1987). Denial may share cognitive processes with some heuristics and biases (Chapter 11). For example, the processes underlying the confirmation bias may also play a role in some forms of denial (Bardon, 2019). Denial may also be part of a "blunting" coping strategy (Chapter 10).

Denial of disease is adaptive under some circumstances, such as cases of terminal cancer where, in the initial stages, denial can quell distress, serving as a form of emotion-focused coping. However, denial of illness can also lead to treatment refusal, delayed treatment-seeking, and lack of compliance if treatment is undertaken. For example, denial of HIV infection is associated with delayed initiation of medical management and increased risk of infecting others (Kalichman, 2018; Kiyingi et al., 2023). Thus, denial can hamper community efforts to control the spread of disease.

Little is known about the management of denial. Children are thought to outgrow the tendency to engage in denial once they recognize it as a form of self-deception (Cramer, 2015). Adults may persist in denial, especially when their self-esteem, self-view, or worldview is threatened. Much remains to be learned about disease-related denial, including so-called deathbed denials.

Conclusions

People commonly harbor self-serving biases and illusions, including the optimism bias and the illusion of control. Illusions and self-serving biases, like many psychological phenomena, appear to arise from various factors, including genes, learning experiences (e.g., observing others), and cognitive mechanisms such as the confirmation bias. Self-serving biases and illusions are evident in contemporary hygiene practices, such as cleansing activities collectively known as hygiene theater. These calming activities provide a sense of agency and will likely be seen in future pandemics. Despite their distorting effects on perception and decision-making, self-serving biases and illusions can alleviate distress and enhance a person's well-being, at least temporarily. Sometimes, however, biases and illusions can have harmful consequences. Some cognitive processes, such as those involved in denial, can interfere with the ability to acknowledge and address pandemic-related threats.

18
Personality and Pandemics

Introduction

One of the remarkable things about pandemics is the range of responses that people display. Some react with alarm; others are less concerned. Some have difficulty tolerating the uncertainties associated with disease threats, while others cope well. Some people cannot handle the boredom of lockdown, while others readily adapt. No single theory or research domain explains the many different psychological phenomena that arise in pandemics. Instead, there are various relevant fields. This chapter focuses on personality traits, which are enduring patterns of feeling, thinking, and behaving.

Personality traits are shaped by genetic and environmental factors (Kendler & Prescott, 2006). Personality is relatively stable across the life span but malleable to some degree. Personality traits are measured by validated questionnaires, in which higher scores correspond to the strength of a trait (Watson & O'Hara, 2017). For example, a high score on a measure of trait anxiety indicates that the person frequently becomes anxious in response to stressors.

Research into personality and pandemics is a relatively modern endeavor, with most pandemic-related personality research conducted in the past two decades. Three types of traits are reviewed in this chapter: (1) distress vulnerability traits, (2) stress-buffering traits, and (3) traits related to nonadherence to pandemic mitigation measures.

Distress Vulnerability Traits

Negative Emotionality

Negative emotionality is a broad trait conferring vulnerability to many kinds of mental health problems, including mood and anxiety disorders (Brandes et al., 2019). Negative emotionality, also known as neuroticism, is the tendency to become easily upset or distressed. People scoring high on this trait frequently experience negative emotions—anxiety, depression, anger, irritability, loneliness, shame, and guilt—in response to stressors or other events (Costa & McCrae, 1987).

Compared to low scorers, people scoring high on negative emotionality tend to overestimate the probability of adverse events and underestimate the likelihood of positive ones (Booth & Sharma, 2021). People with high levels of negative emotionality tend to misinterpret bodily sensations as indications of severe disease (Ferguson, 2000). The severity of a person's negative emotionality predicts their likelihood of becoming distressed when their health is threatened, such as by infectious diseases (Asmundson et al., 2001; Boelen & Carleton, 2012; Fergus et al., 2015; Smith et al., 2009; Taylor, Fong, et al., 2021; Taylor, Paluszek, et al., 2021; van Dijk et al., 2016).

High levels of negative emotionality were associated with severe distress in pandemics and other outbreaks. In the SARS epidemic, negative emotionality predicted high levels of distress among medical staff caring for patients with suspected SARS (Lu et al., 2006). In the course of COVID-19, higher levels of negative emotionality predicted more frequent worry about COVID-19 and health in general (Taylor, Fong, et al., 2021). Compared to low scorers, people scoring high on negative emotionality tended to have the following characteristics (Baker & Merkley, 2023; Götz et al., 2020; Horwood et al., 2023). High scorers during COVID-19, compared to low scorers:

- Perceived the coronavirus as more dangerous.
- Reported greater adherence to social distancing.
- Experienced more household conflicts in the pandemic.
- Reported greater hesitancy about getting vaccinated.
- Were more pessimistic about how fast society would recover from the outbreak.

Negative emotionality is composed of several narrower, overlapping traits (Brandes et al., 2019; Fournier et al., 2019; Subica et al., 2016). These include trait anxiety, harm avoidance, overestimation of threat, worry proneness, intolerance of uncertainty, and anxiety sensitivity. Studying these component traits, as described in the following sections, yields further insights about the relationship between personality and pandemic-related psychological phenomena.

Trait Anxiety and Harm Avoidance

Trait anxiety and harm avoidance are conceptually overlapping traits. Trait anxiety is the proneness to experience anxiety. People scoring high on trait anxiety tend to view the world as dangerous and threatening and frequently experience anxiety (Spielberger, 1979). Harm avoidance is the tendency to avoid potentially risky or threatening situations. People with high levels of harm avoidance tend to be fearful and worry excessively (Cloninger, 1994).

Harm avoidance and trait anxiety are both correlated with anxiety and mood disorders and with excessive worry about one's health (Taylor, 2019b). Amid SARS and COVID-19, high levels of trait anxiety were associated with intense fear of infection (Brosch et al., 2022; Cheng & Cheung, 2005; De Landsheer & Walburg, 2022; Nürnberger et al., 2022). Harm avoidance predicted greater adherence to COVID-19 lockdowns (Lo Presti et al., 2022).

Overestimation of Threat

People scoring high on the overestimation of threat tend to have inflated expectations about the probability and cost ("badness") of aversive events (Frost & Steketee, 2002). High scorers tend to agree with statements such as "The world is a dangerous place" and "Bad things are more likely to happen to me than to other people." As these examples suggest, the overestimation of threat is negatively correlated with the optimism bias (Chapter 17).

High scores on the overestimation of threat are associated with anxiety disorders and the tendency to worry about one's health (Arnáez et al., 2021; Green & Teachman, 2013; Obsessive-Compulsive Cognitions Working Group, 2005). People scoring highly on the overestimation of threat tend to be anxious amid disease outbreaks. This finding has been described in numerous outbreaks, including SARS, Ebola, swine flu, avian flu, and COVID-19 (Bish & Michie, 2010; Blakey & Deacon, 2015; Jessup et al., 2022; Lau et al., 2008; Wheaton et al., 2012; Xie et al., 2011).

Worry Proneness

Chapter 13 discussed health-focused worry. Here, we consider worry more broadly. People differ in their general tendency to worry. People scoring high on trait worry—chronic worriers—tend to worry about all sorts of things, with their concerns touching on multiple areas of life, including health, finances, world events, and the opinions of others. Chronic worriers tend to be indecisive, have low confidence in their problem-solving abilities, and repeatedly seek reassurance to allay their fears (Llera & Newman, 2020; Schut et al., 2001). Not surprisingly, chronic worriers tend to suffer from insomnia (McGowan et al., 2016).

Chronic worriers generally believe that worry keeps them safe from danger (Llera & Newman, 2020). They may deliberately initiate episodes of worry about some issue (e.g., start worrying about running out of hand sanitizer), then find themselves unable to control their worrying. The concerns may broaden and intensify via chains of "what if?" thinking (e.g., "What if we run out of food in addition to hand sanitizer? What if shortages lead to looting and rioting?").

People prone to chronic worry tended to be highly distressed during COVID-19 (Duplaga & Grysztar, 2021). As people worry more about one issue, they tend to neglect others (Weber, 2015). At a community level, this was seen in COVID-19, where a study of nearly 19 million tweets found that as the number of tweets about the pandemic rose, the number of tweets about climate change declined (Smirnov & Hsieh, 2022). As the threat of COVID-19 subsided, chronic worriers likely shifted their focus to other issues or concerns.

Intolerance of Uncertainty

People generally dislike uncertainty; some dislike it a lot (Keren & Gerritsen, 1999). The intolerance of uncertainty is a personality trait characterizing the extent to which a person is anxious about the uncertainties in daily life. People scoring high on this trait have a strong desire for predictability. They agree with statements such as "You should always look ahead to avoid surprises." When faced with uncertainty, they are indecisive and tend to procrastinate (Birrell et al., 2011).

People who are intolerant of uncertainty also tend to score high on trait worry. They are prone to episodes of anxiety and depression (Fergus, 2015; Gentes & Ruscio, 2011; O'Bryan & McLeish, 2017; Rosser, 2018; Shihata et al., 2016; Thibodeau et al., 2015). When confronted with threats, they commonly engage in repetitive checking and reassurance-seeking (Dugas & Robichaud, 2007; Shihata et al., 2016). When faced with health-related uncertainties, people scoring high on the intolerance of uncertainty tend to check and recheck the internet for medical information and persistently seek reassurance from doctors (Bottesi et al., 2017; Fergus, 2015; Lauriola et al., 2018; Norr et al., 2015).

During pandemics, people who are unable or unwilling to accept uncertainty are likely to experience considerable distress, especially if they perceive themselves as having limited control over the threat (Taha et al., 2014). In the 2009 swine flu pandemic, people scoring high on the intolerance of uncertainty, compared to low scorers, were most likely to become anxious about contracting the virus (Taha et al., 2014). High scorers endorsed statements such as "Even though there is a one in a million chance of me dying from the flu, so long as there is a chance, no matter how small, I'm worried that it could happen." In COVID-19, high levels of intolerance of uncertainty were associated with worry about the coronavirus, high levels of distress (anxiety, depression), panic buying, and vaccination hesitancy (Brun et al., 2022; Gillman et al., 2023; Karataş & Tagay, 2021; Rettie & Daniels, 2020; Taylor, Fong, et al., 2021; Taylor et al., 2020).

Intolerance of uncertainty can be expressed as ambiguity aversion, which is the tendency to choose an option with a known rather than unknown risk (Azarpanah et al., 2021; Fox & Tversky, 1995). Ambiguity aversion can contribute to vaccination hesitancy, especially when the vaccine lacks an established track record. People intolerant of uncertainty are more likely to select an option with a known risk (e.g., the odds of getting COVID-19) than one with an unknown risk (e.g., the odds of having an adverse reaction to a novel vaccine). These ambiguity-aversive individuals are more likely to choose the disease instead of vaccination because more is known about the risks of the former than the latter. In future pandemics, widely publicized doubts about vaccine safety will lead to worry and procrastination, especially among people who have difficulty tolerating uncertainty.

Need for Cognitive Closure

Uncertainty and lack of information do not prevent people from forming firm opinions. People intolerant of uncertainty tend to have a strong need for cognitive closure. The latter is a personality trait defined by the need for definitive answers to personally relevant issues (Kruglanski, 1989). People with a strong need for cognitive closure are distressed by ambiguity and strongly motivated to seek predictability, order, and structure (Webster & Kruglanski, 1994). People with a strong need for closure tend to "seize and freeze" on conclusions, which are rapidly reached, firmly held, and resistant to persuasion (Kruglanski & Fishman, 2009). Compared to low scorers, people scoring high on the need for cognitive closure (1) seek less information before reaching a decision, (2) express greater confidence in their hasty judgments, (3) avoid or dismiss information that challenges or questions their conclusions (i.e., are reluctant to return to a state of uncertainty), (4) have difficulty taking the perspectives of others, (5) tend to pressure others to accept their views, and (6) prefer in-groups that are homogenous and similar to themselves (Kruglanski & Fishman, 2009).

As a mechanism for reducing uncertainty, striving for cognitive closure can lead to polarization, where different groups "seize and freeze" on different answers to a given problem (Acar-Burkay et al., 2014). Conspiracy theories and simple explanations based on stereotypes appeal to people with a strong need for cognitive closure (Baldner et al., 2019; Marchlewska et al., 2018). Such explanations are especially appealing when authorities fail to answer important questions such as "Where did the outbreak start?" and "Who is to blame?" When the plague broke out in San Francisco at the turn of the 20th century, some blamed Chinese residents simply because the disease originated in China (Todd, 1909). This view provided the predominantly White residents of San Francisco with a simple explanation and an illusion of control; they could stay safe from the plague—so they believed—if they stayed away from Chinatown and its inhabitants (Todd, 1909).

Anxiety Sensitivity

People differ in their tendency to be frightened of anxiety. Anxiety sensitivity is the fear of arousal- or anxiety-related bodily sensations, arising from beliefs that the sensations have harmful consequences (Taylor, 2019a). People with high levels of anxiety sensitivity tend to have misconceptions about anxiety, believing that intense anxiety leads to death, insanity, or loss of control. Highly anxiety-sensitive people strongly agree with statements such as "Whenever I get short of breath, I worry I might suffocate," "Whenever my heart beats rapidly, I worry I might have a heart attack," and "Too much anxiety can kill a person." People with elevated anxiety sensitivity tend to rely on the affect heuristic described in Chapter 11: "If I feel anxious, there must be danger" (Muris et al., 2003).

Anxiety sensitivity is an amplification factor that intensifies anxiety and fear (Taylor, 2019a). When highly anxiety-sensitive individuals experience anxiety, they become alarmed about being anxious, which worsens their anxiety. In disease outbreaks in which there is widespread fear of infection, people with heightened anxiety sensitivity are likely to be notably anxious. Compared to people scoring low on anxiety sensitivity, high scorers reported greater fear of infection in the COVID-19, swine flu, and Zika pandemics

(Blakey & Abramowitz, 2017; Ojalehto et al., 2021; Saulnier et al., 2022; Wheaton et al., 2012; Yunus et al., 2022).

Stress-Buffering Traits

Resilience

Resilience is the ability to endure and overcome adversities (Bonanno & Diminich, 2013). If resilient people become depressed or anxious during stressful periods, they quickly recover once adversity passes. Greater resilience is associated with higher levels of happiness, life satisfaction, and mental health (Fan et al., 2022; Färber & Rosendahl, 2020; Hu et al., 2015). In COVID-19, people with high levels of resilience, compared to less resilient individuals, reported lower levels of distress (Fernández et al., 2020; Kavčič et al., 2021).

Several factors contribute to resilience, including hardiness (discussed below), social support, and psychological flexibility (Kashdan & Rottenberg, 2010; Kunicki & Harlow, 2020; Maddi, 2013). The latter involves the ability to manage shifting environmental demands effectively. A meta-analysis of COVID-19 studies found that high levels of psychological flexibility were associated with low levels of anxiety and depression (Yao et al., 2024).

Resilience is substantially heritable, just like other personality traits. Research using identical and fraternal twins shows that 40% of the variance in resilience scores is due to genetic factors, with the remainder due to environmental influences (Waaktaar & Torgersen, 2012). Substantial heritability does not mean that resilience is immutable. Like other traits, resilience is generally stable but can be modified (Köhne et al., 2022; Linnemann et al., 2020). Although chronic stress can erode resilience, the latter can be strengthened through "toughening up" exercises used in stress management training (Maddi, 2013; Taylor, 2017). The latter include stressful or challenging exercises (e.g., physical exercise programs) that provide a sense of mastery.

Hardiness

Hardiness is the cognitive core of resilience. Hardiness buffers the harmful effects of stress on physical and mental health and facilitates functioning in daily living (Kobasa, 1979; Maddi, 2013). Hardiness consists of mindsets (perspectives, attitudes) and learned skills that help people confront, adapt, and grow from adversity. Hardy attitudes motivate people to engage in the following:

- Problem-solving coping instead of denial or avoidance.
- Reappraisal coping, such as reframing the meaning of a stressor to reduce its emotional impact (Chapter 22).
- Socially-supportive interactions.
- Beneficial self-care (e.g., stress management).

Three mindsets characterize high levels of hardiness: commitment, control, and challenge (Kobasa, 1979; Maddi, 2013). Commitment is the tendency to involve oneself in activities and have a genuine interest in, and curiosity about, one's environment. Commitment entails believing that no matter how bad things get, it is vital to remain involved with whatever is happening rather than sink into detachment, hopelessness, and alienation. The control mindset entails believing one can influence the stressors in one's life, which is the opposite of powerlessness and passivity. The challenge mindset entails believing that change, rather than stability, is the norm. Stressful circumstances are seen as opportunities for growth rather than security threats.

Hardiness is correlated with optimism, but the two differ in several ways. Hardiness is characterized by specific mindsets leading to active coping, whereas optimism can involve passivity or complacency, where people hope good things will happen without doing anything (Maddi, 2013).

Low hardiness is associated with intolerance of uncertainty, nihilism, and fear of stressors (Maddi, 2013; Oral & Karakurt, 2022). Compared to high scorers, people scoring low on hardiness had more severe anxiety and depression during COVID-19 (Bartone et al., 2022; Epishin et al., 2020). Low hardiness was also associated with burnout among healthcare workers (Vagni et al., 2022).

Other Traits

It has been speculated that introversion may be protective during lockdown because introverted people, compared to extroverts, may be better able to endure the isolation of lockdown because introverts do not require a high degree of social interaction. Research does not support this view. Some COVID-19 studies found little difference between introverts and extraverts in lockdown-related distress (Taylor, Paluszek, et al., 2021), while other investigations found that introverts reported *more* distress than extraverts (Horwood et al., 2023; Schmit et al., 2024; Smrdu et al., 2023). Research is needed to understand the reasons why introverts might fare worse in lockdown, as compared to extraverts. The differences might be due to social support. Extraverts, compared to introverts, tend to have larger social networks (Swickert et al., 2002). The larger networks likely provided a greater degree of social support even during lockdown, in which social media and other means of indirect social interaction were available.

Personality and Nonadherence to Mitigation Measures

Authoritarianism

Authoritarianism is a trait characterized by a cluster of attitudes concerning (1) the need for strict adherence to conventional values, (2) deference to authority figures, (3) insistence on subservience from people regarded as lower in status, and (4) animosity toward those who depart from traditional norms (Altemeyer, 2009). Authoritarianism can be right-wing (conservative) or left-wing (liberal) (Altemeyer, 2009; Costello et al., 2022; Manson, 2020; Peng, 2022). Both are characterized by dogmatism, punitive attitudes toward dissenters, fear of out-groups (xenophobia), and obedience and respect for authority (Altemeyer, 1996; Manson, 2020).

People with authoritarian attitudes see the world as dangerous (Altemeyer, 1996; Costello et al., 2022). They tend to be highly sensitive to threats, particularly threats to the integrity and cohesion of their in-group (e.g., threats to one's culture or country). Authoritarians cope with threats by obeying strong leaders, conforming to societal norms, and aggressing against norm-violators (Deason & Dunn, 2022; Passini, 2022).

Despite their tendency to see the world as dangerous, authoritarians do not necessarily adhere to pandemic mitigation measures. They follow the advice of their leaders. COVID-19 vaccine acceptance was higher among left-wing than right-wing authoritarians, in line with the views of their respective political leaders (Peng, 2022). Right-wing authoritarians in America were more likely to have negative attitudes about wearing masks, which was also in keeping with the attitudes expressed by their political leaders (Prichard & Turner, 2023).

Like other personality traits, authoritarianism is somewhat malleable, increasing or decreasing in response to environmental contingencies. In community-wide emergencies, people look to their leaders to keep them safe. The strength of authoritarian attitudes increases, at least temporarily, amid crises such as economic crashes, terrorist attacks, and pandemics (Bilewicz et al., 2023; Golec de Zavala et al., 2021; Hartman et al., 2021; Karwowski et al., 2020; Maher et al., 2022; Pazhoohi & Kingstone, 2021; Tybur et al., 2016). In the course of COVID-19 in America, scores on authoritarian traits rose as infections increased (Pazhoohi & Kingstone, 2021). In other words, as infection grew more widespread, people increasingly exhibited a "preference for an authoritarian socially conservative value system, as a protection against possible contamination from outgroup members" (Pazhoohi & Kingstone, 2021, p. 3).

Psychological Reactance

Pandemic mitigation requires that people agree to forfeit some of their freedoms, at least for the short term. People must agree to curtail their travel and social activities, wear masks, and receive vaccinations. If people understand the importance of such measures, most are willing to comply (Taylor & Asmundson, 2021). However, a minority vigorously object to such restrictions. The objections arise for various reasons, for example, questioning the safety and efficacy of vaccines or challenging the government's legitimacy to impose restrictions on mobility. A theme commonly running through these objections involves psychological reactance, which plays a role in many kinds of pandemic nonadherence behaviors, including nonadherence to masks, vaccines, and social distancing (Taylor, 2019b; Taylor & Asmundson, 2021).

People scoring high on the trait of psychological reactance strongly value their autonomy and resist rules, regulations, and other impingements on their freedom (Brehm, 1966; Rosenberg & Siegel, 2018). For these high-scorers, perceived threats to freedom motivate them to assert their independence by rejecting attempts at persuasion, often with anger and counter-arguments (Brehm, 1966; Brehm & Brehm, 1981; Rains, 2013). Psychological reactance is correlated with antisocial and narcissistic personality traits and political conservatism (Frank et al., 1998; Irmak et al., 2020; Lewing & Caraway, 2019; Ma et al., 2019). The latter is not surprising, given that conservative ideology favors limiting government involvement in the private lives of citizens (Crawford et al., 2017).

People scoring high on psychological reactance were less likely to adhere to mitigation measures such as mask-wearing, adherence to social distance, and vaccine uptake during COVID-19 (Ball & Wozniak, 2022; Díaz & Cova, 2021; Soveri et al., 2024; Taylor & Asmundson, 2021).

Boredom Proneness

Lockdown and quarantine are conducive to boredom. Boredom is an unpleasant state of being weary and restless—where time drags, and nothing maintains one's interest or focus of attention. Boredom motivates people to seek new experiences, even if those experiences have adverse consequences (Bench & Lench, 2019). Boredom is not simply an unpleasant psychological state. Boredom can be a health issue. Hospital patients notice more symptoms and consume more analgesic medication when their hospital rooms are dull and unstimulating, compared to rooms containing posters, decorations, windows, and so forth (Taylor & Asmundson, 2004).

Boredom proneness is characterized by the tendency to become bored in many situations (Farmer & Sundberg, 1986). In COVID-19, boredom proneness was correlated with (1) the tendency to experience negative emotions such as depression, anxiety, loneliness, and irritability, (2) substance-use disorders and related conditions such as problem gambling and internet addiction, (3) difficulty adjusting to stay-at-home orders and closures, (4) the tendency to disregard social-distancing guidelines, and (5) increased risk of getting infected with the coronavirus (Boylan et al., 2021; Brosowsky et al., 2021; Drody et al., 2022; Liang et al., 2022; Weiss et al., 2022; Yang et al., 2020). These findings suggest that "high boredom proneness is an important vulnerability factor for poor psychological health and risky behaviors" (Weiss et al., 2022, p. 1).

Narcissism and Psychological Entitlement

Narcissism and psychological entitlement are related but distinguishable constructs. Psychological entitlement refers to the tendency to claim excessive and unearned rewards and resources and to demand undeserved special treatment (Campbell et al., 2004; Neville et al., 2024). Narcissism is a broader construct involving self-absorption, grandiosity, arrogance, and entitlement (Rose & Anastasio, 2014). Thus, entitlement can be a component of narcissism, but high levels of entitlement can also occur in the absence of narcissism. A person can feel entitled to special treatment without necessarily having an inflated sense of self-worth. A sense of relative deprivation is one way a person might feel entitled without necessarily being grandiose—for example, "I was deprived of my grad party last year because of lockdown, so I deserve to be out having fun with my friends this year."

Narcissism and psychological entitlement are associated with pandemic fatigue (Taylor et al., 2022) (see Chapter 6). During COVID-19, when people were urged to refrain from nonessential social activities, individuals scoring high on narcissism and psychological entitlement were likelier to flout social-distancing guidelines (Vint et al., 2024; Zitek & Schlund, 2021). They were more likely to visit restaurants, spas, salons, nightclubs, and casinos (Neville et al., 2024). People with high levels of narcissism and entitlement were less likely to wear masks and less likely to seek vaccination (Giancola et al., 2023; Hatemi & Fazekas, 2023; Prichard & Turner, 2023; Vint et al., 2024). But if they wore masks, they tended to tell others to wear one (Hatemi & Fazekas, 2023). People scoring high on narcissism and psychological entitlement are more likely to endorse conspiracy theories, including conspiratorial beliefs about COVID-19 and vaccines (Neville et al., 2024).

Conscientiousness

People scoring high on the conscientiousness personality trait are responsible, efficient, organized, self-disciplined, and diligent (Costa & McCrae, 2005). People scoring low on this trait tend to be laid-back, spontaneous, and disorganized, disliking rules, schedules, and regulations. Not surprisingly, compared to high scorers, people scoring low on conscientiousness were less adherent to COVID-19 social distancing and hygiene behaviors (e.g., hand-washing) (Götz et al., 2020; Khosravi et al., 2022; Telaku et al., 2022; Turk et al., 2023; Zuffianò et al., 2023).

There were mixed findings regarding the relationship between conscientiousness and vaccination hesitancy in COVID-19. Some, but not all, studies found that low conscientiousness was associated with greater vaccination hesitancy (Baker & Merkley, 2023; Ngo et al., 2023; Reagu et al., 2023; Sabatini et al., 2023). Baker et al. (2023) found that differences in vaccination hesitancy diminished over time between people scoring high and low on conscientiousness (Baker & Merkley, 2023). Any effects of low conscientiousness on vaccination hesitancy were apparently overridden by other factors shaping vaccine uptake, such as nudges and mandates (Chapter 5).

Modifying Personality Traits

Although personality traits tend to be stable over time, they can be modified. Cognitive behavior therapy (CBT) can reduce the severity of distress vulnerability traits, including negative emotionality, trait anxiety, harm avoidance, the overestimation of threat, intolerance of uncertainty, worry proneness, and anxiety sensitivity (Frost & Steketee, 2002; Molton et al., 2019; Querstret & Cropley, 2013; Robichaud, 2013; Sauer-Zavala et al., 2021; Talkovsky & Norton, 2016; Taylor, 2019a; Torbit & Laposa, 2016; Wilson et al., 2023). CBT can also strengthen stress-buffering traits such as hardiness (Maddi, 2013).

Several cognitive behavioral methods are used to achieve these ends, including cognitive restructuring, problem-solving training, and stress-management techniques. Transdiagnostic CBT targeting multiple traits is especially promising. Here, a single treatment protocol can treat a range of emotional problems (Barlow et al., 2017; Payne et al., 2021). In addition to reducing distress, these treatments can increase positive emotions (Boettcher et al., 2019). Internet-based transdiagnostic CBT can lower distress vulnerability traits and improve resilience (Timulak et al., 2022).

CBT and other psychotherapies can effectively treat people suffering from narcissistic personality disorder (Cukrowicz et al., 2011). However, people scoring high on narcissism may not see their personality as something needing modification. Little is known about modifying other traits, such as boredom proneness, entitlement, psychological reactance, and authoritarianism. Boredom proneness is negatively correlated with mindfulness (Regan et al., 2020), which raises the question of whether mindfulness training might reduce boredom proneness.

Conclusions

Personality traits arise from genetic and environmental influences. These traits are measured with questionnaires whose scores indicate the severity or "dose" of a given trait. Some people acquire, via a combination of genes and the environment, doses of traits that can create problems for themselves and society.

Distress vulnerability traits include negative emotionality and its component traits such as trait anxiety, overestimation of threat, and intolerance of uncertainty. Other traits are linked to low distress and better adjustment in the course of pandemics. These include resilience, trait optimism, and hardiness. A third set of personality traits is associated with nonadherence to pandemic mitigation methods. These traits include psychological reactance, boredom proneness, and psychological entitlement.

Authoritarianism increases in community-wide crises such as pandemics. Authoritarian personality traits are associated with xenophobia and punitive attitudes toward rule violators. Although authoritarians tend to see the world as dangerous, they do not necessarily adhere to pandemic mitigation measures. Instead, they follow the examples set by their leaders. Authoritarianism is associated with nonadherence when authoritarian leaders express negative attitudes toward pandemic mitigation measures.

Personality traits tend to be stable but have some malleability. Cognitive behavioral interventions can reduce distress-related traits and strengthen stress-buffering traits. Less is known about modifying other personality characteristics associated with nonadherence, such as psychological reactance and entitlement. Instead of changing these traits, nudges or mandates are used to improve adherence.

PART III
MENTAL HEALTH

19
Pandemics and Mental Health

Introduction

Mental disorders can be understood as arising from diatheses-stress interactions. That is, psychological problems are most likely to occur when stressors impinge on people possessing particular biopsychosocial vulnerability characteristics, such as specific genetic polymorphisms, personality traits, or other factors. If a person is highly vulnerable to psychopathology (e.g., has very high scores on distress-vulnerability traits; Chapter 18), then even minor stressors could trigger mental health problems. If stressors are sufficiently severe and prolonged, mental disorders are likely to arise even in people with few vulnerability factors.

Pandemic-related stressors can trigger or exacerbate a range of mental health problems. This chapter presents a broad survey of mental health problems arising in pandemics. We begin by reviewing general pandemic-related distress (i.e., anxiety and depression). Seven types of pandemic-related mental health issues are then reviewed: fears and phobias, post-traumatic stress disorder, prolonged grief disorder, obsessive-compulsive disorder, addictive behaviors, interpersonal violence, and suicide. Vignettes and other examples are included to illustrate clinical phenomena that might not be familiar to all readers.

Anxiety and Depression

COVID-19

Several hundred studies have been published concerning the impact of COVID-19 on anxiety and depression. Participants in these studies, drawn mainly from the community rather than clinics or hospitals, were mostly uninfected with the coronavirus. The results of subsets of these studies were combined, analyzed, and summarized in dozens of meta-analyses (Arora et al., 2020; Bello et al., 2022; Blasco-Belled et al., 2022; Bueno-Notivol et al., 2021; Cénat et al., 2021; Chen et al., 2021; Chen et al., 2022; COVID-19 Mental Disorders Collaborators, 2021; Daniali et al., 2023; Duc et al., 2022; Fang et al., 2022; Geoffroy et al., 2024; Huang et al., 2024; Luo et al., 2020; Metin et al., 2022; Miao et al., 2023; Necho et al., 2021; Nochaiwong et al., 2021; Pappa et al., 2020; Prati & Mancini, 2021; Racine et al., 2021; Ren et al., 2020; Robinson et al., 2022; Salanti et al., 2022; Salari et al., 2020; Sokouti et al., 2023; Sun et al., 2023; Wu et al., 2021).

Before reviewing the meta-analytic findings, we must consider the methodologies used in the studies included in those meta-analyses. For each study, researchers used one of three designs—either a cross-sectional design or one of two longitudinal ones. The design used in most studies was cross-sectional. Here, anxiety and depression were assessed at some point in the pandemic and compared to preexisting data on pre-pandemic levels. For example, one might administer an anxiety or depression questionnaire early in the disease outbreak and compare the findings to previously published, pre-pandemic scores on the same measure.

Two alternative designs were longitudinal, typically involving two assessment points. In one design, investigators sought out people who happened to have pre-pandemic scores on some questionnaire (e.g., an anxiety scale). The researchers then obtained a score on the same measure from the same participant in the pandemic. In the other design, participants were longitudinally assessed at two (or sometimes more) points during the pandemic.

All three designs have strengths and limitations. Longitudinal studies are subject to attrition biases: People who drop out before completing the Time 2 assessment may be psychologically different from those who complete the study. Cross-sectional studies require accurate estimates of pre-pandemic anxiety or depression. The accuracy of these estimates is sometimes doubtful. All three designs fail to characterize the dynamic nature of pandemics. The fluctuating patterns of anxiety and depression are not accurately portrayed in cross-sectional or two-wave longitudinal designs.

Despite these limitations, several noteworthy findings emerged. For studies using cross-sectional designs, most meta-analyses reported increases in anxiety and depression in COVID-19, especially in the first wave—that is, the first six months of the pandemic (Bello et al., 2022; Blasco-Belled et al., 2022; Bueno-Notivol et al., 2021; Cénat et al., 2021; Chen et al., 2022; COVID-19 Mental Disorders Collaborators, 2021; Daniali et al., 2023; Duc et al., 2022;

Fang et al., 2022; Luo et al., 2020; Necho et al., 2021; Nochaiwong et al., 2021; Pappa et al., 2020; Prati & Mancini, 2021; Racine et al., 2021; Salari et al., 2020; Wu et al., 2021).

For studies using longitudinal designs, most meta-analyses also reported increases in anxiety and depression, particularly in the opening months of COVID-19 (Cénat et al., 2021; Huang et al., 2024; Miao et al., 2023), followed in later months by decreased, stable, or other symptom trajectories (Robinson et al., 2022; Salanti et al., 2022). One longitudinal meta-analysis reported minimal increases in anxiety and depression in COVID-19 (Sun et al., 2023), while another concluded that there were insufficient data to draw firm conclusions (Geoffroy et al., 2024).

Emotional and other reactions commonly associated with anxiety and depression were also examined in several meta-analyses and other investigations. Results indicated that COVID-19 led to increases in irritability, agitation, and insomnia (Cénat et al., 2021; Cost et al., 2021; Daniali et al., 2023; Ravens-Sieberer et al., 2021; Wu et al., 2021). Nightmares also increased, with themes of sadness, anger, contamination, and cleanliness (Davis et al., 2020; Mota et al., 2020).

After communities emerged from lockdown, anxiety and depression improved on average, even when restrictions on social gatherings were still in place and vaccines had not yet become available (Richter et al., 2021; Zhou et al., 2020).

Although anxiety, depression, and related phenomena tended to increase early in COVID-19, there is uncertainty about the magnitude of these effects. Some researchers suggested that the increases were significant but modest (e.g., Penninx et al., 2022). Other investigators drew darker conclusions. A review and meta-analysis appearing in *The Lancet* estimated that the prevalence of major depressive disorder and anxiety disorders increased globally amid COVID-19—with estimated increases of 28% and 26%, respectively—corresponding to 53 million cases of major depressive disorder and 76 million cases of anxiety disorders (COVID-19 Mental Disorders Collaborators, 2021). The true picture likely lies somewhere between the extremes described by Penninx et al. and the COVID-19 Mental Disorders Collaborators.

To summarize, hundreds of studies of depression and anxiety during COVID-19 have been aggregated in dozens of meta-analyses. Design limitations prevent these analyses from identifying patterns of fluctuation, but they provide information about overall levels of distress in the first two years of COVID-19. Results generally indicate that anxiety, depression, and associated reactions, such as irritability, insomnia, and nightmares, tended to increase. The severity of anxiety tended to peak early in the pandemic. Anticipatory anxiety—anxiety ahead of the arrival in one's community (Chapter 1)—is part of the early peak in anxiety. Less is known about the trajectories of other reactions, such as depression, irritability, and insomnia. These reactions may persist when social restrictions are prolonged and pandemic fatigue sets in (Chapter 6).

Moderating Variables

There was a great deal of heterogeneity of findings among the studies included in the meta-analyses, suggesting exceptions to the trends described above. Moderator analyses were reported in several meta-analyses to investigate whether COVID-related changes in anxiety and depression differed across demographic groups and geographic regions.

Severe anxiety and depression were likely to be reported by people with preexisting emotional disorders or previous exposure to trauma (Lahav, 2020; Robillard et al., 2021; Taylor, 2022). Compared to the general population, some groups—particularly women, youth, and healthcare workers (HCWs)—reported higher levels of anxiety and depression. There was some evidence that anxiety was especially prevalent among inexperienced frontline nurses (Chutiyami et al., 2022). Hospitalization for COVID-19 was also associated with heightened anxiety and depression (Xie et al., 2022).

Ethnic and gender minorities were at heightened risk for anxiety and depression (Batra et al., 2023; Fruehwirth et al., 2021; Kidd et al., 2021; Moore et al., 2021). The disproportionate impact of COVID-19 on minority groups may be related to the stressful inequalities and healthcare obstacles encountered by these groups. The female gender findings are consistent with previous data showing that women tend to report higher levels of anxiety than men for various biopsychosocial reasons (reviewed in Craske, 2003).

The meta-analyses revealed substantial geographical variation in the prevalence of anxiety and depression but few firm trends. Increases in anxious and depressive symptoms tended to be greatest in communities with high infection rates and tight restrictions on mobility (e.g., lockdown) (COVID-19 Mental Disorders Collaborators, 2021; Every-Palmer et al., 2020; Giuntella et al., 2021; McDowell et al., 2021; Prati & Mancini, 2021; Zheng et al., 2021).

Comparisons to Other Outbreaks

As with COVID-19, the Russian flu, Spanish flu, swine flu, plague, and SARS were associated with community-wide increases in emotional distress (Bristow, 2012; Chau et al., 2021; Honigsbaum, 2013; Moote & Moote, 2004; Smith, 1995; Taylor, 2019). In the years following both Russian and Spanish flu pandemics, there was also evidence of increases in first-time admissions to psychiatric hospitals (Mamelund, 2010).

Compared to these outbreaks, the 1957 and 1968 influenza pandemics were unusual because they were associated with little apparent distress (Honigsbaum, 2020; Wilson et al., 2009). These pandemics were relatively mild, attracted little media attention, and social restrictions such as lockdown were not used (Chapter 1). The pandemics of 1957 and 1968 are instructive because they show that widespread distress is not an inevitable concomitant of pandemics.

Fears and Phobias

Fear of Infection

The difference between fears and phobias is a matter of degree. Phobias are severe, persistent, and excessive fears that tend to interfere with social or occupational functioning (American Psychiatric Association, 2022). Most of the research into pandemics has not distinguished between fears and phobias. In the following discussion, we use "fear" as an umbrella term encompassing both fears and phobias.

Historical descriptions contain numerous references to infection-related fears, with examples including "flu-phobia" in the Spanish flu, references to "coronaphobia" in COVID-19, and fear reactions described in outbreaks of plague, Zika virus, and swine flu (Blakey & Abramowitz, 2017; Blakey et al., 2015; Evening Express, 1918; Spokesman Review, 1918; Taylor, 2021; Wheaton et al., 2012).

There are numerous examples of infection fears in the historical record. A survivor of the Spanish flu recalled feeling constantly afraid because of the widespread death; "people were afraid to kiss one another, people were afraid to eat with one another, they were afraid to have anything that made contact because that's how you got the flu" (Barry, 2018, p. 346). The diarist Miquel Parets described widespread fears in the second plague pandemic in

Barcelona: "People fled and shunned not only the sick but also the well, as no one dared to get near anyone else for fear that they might carry plague stuck in their clothes" (Parets, 1651, p. 59). Some healthy but highly fearful people hid in their homes to avoid exposure to the plague (Byrne, 2006).

Fear Syndromes

There is more to pandemic-related fears than simply the fear of infection. Research on past outbreaks (e.g., Zika, swine flu, SARS) suggested that fear of infection is commonly associated with obsessive-compulsive contamination symptoms (health-related checking and reassurance seeking) and traumatic stress symptoms (pandemic-related nightmares and intrusive thoughts) (Taylor, 2021). Research early in COVID-19 found evidence of a COVID stress syndrome characterized by five features, with fear of infection being the central (most important) element (Taylor et al., 2020b):

- Fears of becoming infected, including fear of contact with potentially infected objects or surfaces.
- COVID-19-related xenophobia: fear of coming into contact with foreigners for fear that they might be infected.
- Fear of socioeconomic hardships arising from the pandemic (e.g., job loss, financial problems).
- Repetitive checking and reassurance-seeking about pandemic-related threats (e.g., repetitively checking the news and social media for pandemic-related information or repeatedly checking one's temperature for signs of infection).
- Traumatic stress symptoms about the pandemic (e.g., nightmares and unwanted intrusive thoughts about the pandemic).

In terms of the *Diagnostic and Statistical Manual of Mental Disorders*, Fifth Edition (DSM-5), the COVID stress syndrome is an adjustment disorder (Taylor, 2021). Adjustment disorders often remit once the precipitating stressor has passed, although they can become chronic (Bachem & Casey, 2018; O'Donnell et al., 2016). People with severe forms of COVID stress syndrome were more likely to have preexisting risk factors for mental health problems, such as high scores on traits such as negative emotionality and the intolerance of uncertainty (Taylor et al., 2020a, 2020b). Further research is needed to investigate the COVID stress syndrome's long-term course and to determine whether similar syndromes can be identified in future pandemics.

Fear of Sexually Transmitted Diseases

Sexually transmitted diseases might seem quite different from respiratory ailments like influenza and COVID-19. However, there are many similarities in terms of reactions, particularly xenophobia, fear of infection, and reassurance-seeking. Clinical descriptions of syphilis phobia in the 19th century highlighted the intense fear experienced by some people (Knapp & Vandecreek, 1989). Syphilis "aroused fear, stigmatisation and moralistic responses, as well as a desperate scramble to find an effective means of control" (Darby, 2015, p. 573). In the 1980s, the HIV/AIDS pandemic evoked similar reactions.

HIV/AIDS—transmitted via sexual intercourse, intravenous drug use, and contaminated blood products—was not subject to lockdown, social distancing, or border closures. Yet, the HIV/AIDS pandemic was similar to other pandemics in that there was widespread fear and xenophobia. The disease was widely feared even among people at no risk of infection (Bouton et al., 1987). Fear of HIV/AIDS peaked in the mid-to-late 1980s, declining thereafter with the advent of retroviral therapies and pre-exposure prophylactic drugs (Bayramoğlu, 2021; Moskowitz et al., 2009).

The term "AIDS phobia" was coined in the late 1980s to describe people who were intensely frightened that they had, or might acquire, HIV (Jäger et al., 1988). People with AIDS phobia presented in great distress to doctors. Repeatedly negative antibody tests failed to reassure these anxious individuals (Jäger-Collet, 1988). They went from doctor to doctor to obtain reassurance, but relief was short-lived; they were "satisfied for two or three days, but then again experienced great anxiety" (Sander, 1988, p. 8). They avoided people, places, and activities perceived as risky for acquiring HIV, including objectively low-risk activities such as sitting on toilet seats (Logsdail et al., 1991; Wright et al., 2007). The following is a clinical description of a heterosexual man suffering from AIDS phobia, summarized from Sander (1988):

> After 14 years of faithful marriage, the patient had sex with a prostitute. He then became highly alarmed upon learning that sex workers can transmit HIV. Frightened that he might be infected, he began recurrently taking his temperature, inspecting his mouth in the mirror, checking his body for rashes, and palpating his lymph nodes for signs of swelling. His sleep became restless and he would awake bathed in sweat. He worried that if he was infected, he might infect his family. He no longer slept with his wife, avoided intimate and social contacts, and lost interest in his job, believing he might not live much longer. He was tested for HIV six times.

The result was negative each time, but reassurance was short-lived, and his fears returned.

People with AIDS phobia commonly have a history of obsessive-compulsive symptoms, health anxiety, and anxiety-proneness in general (Harrell & Wright, 1998; Jacob et al., 1989; Sander, 1988). Much stigma was attached to HIV/AIDS. Fear of stigma, along with fear of the disease itself, dissuaded people from getting tested. Infected people were also reluctant to reveal their HIV-positive status for fear of discrimination (Evangeli & Wroe, 2017). Preexisting homophobia likely fueled the widespread fear of HIV/AIDS (O'Donnell et al., 1987).

Post-Traumatic Stress Disorder

PTSD in Contemporary Disease Outbreaks

Post-traumatic stress disorder (PTSD) arises when a person experiences a traumatic event that triggers four sets of symptoms, which persist for a month or more: (1) intrusive thoughts or recollections of the trauma (e.g., nightmares and flashbacks), (2) persistent avoidance of trauma reminders (e.g., avoiding people, places, and things that trigger trauma recollections), (3) negative changes in mood and cognition (e.g., negative emotions such as fear, anger, guilt, or shame, and negative beliefs about oneself and the world), and (4) marked alterations in arousal and reactivity (e.g., hypervigilance and exaggerated startle) (American Psychiatric Association, 2022).

The worldwide lifetime prevalence of PTSD arising from any trauma—such as natural disasters, combat exposure, or sexual assault—is about 4% (American Psychiatric Association, 2022). PTSD can be triggered by traumatic pandemic-related stressors such as exposure to widespread death, the death of loved ones, and personally life-threatening infections (Chapter 2). PTSD or symptoms of the disorder were reported in studies of SARS, MERS, HIV/AIDS, avian flu, and COVID-19 (Asmundson & Taylor, 2021; Martin & Kagee, 2011; Rogers et al., 2020; Tang et al., 2016).

A meta-analysis of SARS-related PTSD reported a prevalence of 32% (Rogers et al., 2020). For PTSD arising from COVID-19, meta-analytic estimates ranged from 5% to 50% (Arora et al., 2020; Cénat et al., 2021; Nagarajan et al., 2022; Xiong et al., 2020; Yuan et al., 2021). Most estimates were based on self-report measures of PTSD symptoms. Very few studies assessed PTSD using structured clinical interviews, which form the gold standard for diagnosing the disorder. An exception was an Italian study of 381 COVID-19 patients evaluated with a diagnostic interview (Carfì et al., 2020; Janiri et al., 2021). Most patients were severely ill because of COVID-19, and most were hospitalized. The prevalence of PTSD due to COVID-19 was 30%.

Risk factors for COVID-related PTSD were female gender, history of psychiatric disorders, delirium or agitation in the acute phase of COVID-19 infection, and persistent COVID-19 symptoms, most commonly fatigue and dyspnea (Carfì et al., 2020; Janiri et al., 2021). Female gender, delirium, and history of psychopathology are previously established risk factors for PTSD in general (Taylor, 2017).

A life-threatening illness requiring inpatient treatment can be terrifying. For patients admitted to intensive care units (ICUs) for any life-threatening condition, more than 9% die and, of the survivors, about a quarter develop PTSD symptoms in the weeks and months following discharge (Demass et al., 2023; Gonçalves-Pereira et al., 2023; Parker et al., 2015). The following is an example of PTSD arising from hospital experiences due to a life-threatening COVID-19 infection (summarized from Skilbeck & Byrne, 2022):

> A 46-year-old Asian British man with no history of mental health problems was referred to a psychology clinic for treatment of PTSD and panic attacks after developing severe COVID-19. He also had Long COVID, managed by a separate clinic. His episode of COVID-19 began with severe breathlessness, requiring admission to an intensive care unit for six weeks, which included four weeks in an induced coma. Family members were not permitted to visit. In lucid moments, the patient felt helpless and alone and feared he was going to die. After discharge from the hospital, his problems persisted. He felt weak and vulnerable, with an ever-present sense of danger ("It's going to happen again"). Reexperiencing phenomena were his main PTSD symptoms. Although his memories of the hospital experience were sparse and fragmented due to coma and delirium, there was sufficient recollection for him to have recurrent nightmares and flashbacks related to his hospital stay. He described recurrent, intrusive, vivid memories of being unable to move and flashbacks of hallucinatory experiences in the ICU, where he believed medical staff were trying to kill him. He tried to avoid reminders that triggered intrusive recollections. Triggers included hospitals, ambulances, HCWs, media stories about the coronavirus, and the smell of hospital disinfectant. PTSD and panic attacks were successfully treated with 16 weekly sessions of CBT via videoconferencing.

Research is needed to understand the long-term course of PTSD arising from pandemics and other disease outbreaks. A 12-year longitudinal Taiwanese study, based on information from hospital records, found that SARS survivors, compared to matched controls, were more likely to experience a range of psychiatric problems, including PTSD symptoms, in the years after recovering from acute infection (Tzeng et al., 2020). In the coming years, we can expect similar studies on the long-term psychological effects of COVID-19.

PTSD in the Historical Record

PTSD was formally introduced into the diagnostic nomenclature only in 1980 (American Psychiatric Association, 1980) and, therefore, was not investigated in disease outbreaks before that time. An issue of debate is whether PTSD is a timeless, universal disorder or a modern idiom of distress—that is, a socially and culturally determined way of expressing emotional suffering (McNally, 2003). Despite this issue, descriptions from the Spanish flu and other outbreaks suggest PTSD-like symptoms. Persistent, death-related intrusive recollections were reported by the bereaved, HCWs, and others (Bristow, 2012; Honigsbaum, 2009; Taylor, 2019). A 96-year-old survivor of the Spanish flu reported being haunted by intrusive childhood recollections—"like a film in my head"—of the funeral of her parents and brother, who perished decades earlier in the Spanish flu. She vividly recalled the hearse and other details—"the black horses with the plumes made from ostrich feathers," "the gun carriage with my dad's coffin covered with the union flag," her mother's coffin in "a big glass hearse," with her brother's coffin under the driver's seat (Honigsbaum, 2009, p. 104).

Trauma-related recollections and dreams are emotionally charged and often compelling in their realism. When experiencing flashbacks or nightmares, the person is not simply recalling the trauma; they feel like they are back in the traumatic situation. Reverend Theodore Clapp reported being haunted by recurrent nightmares and recollections of his experiences 35 years earlier while ministering to the sick and dying in several New Orleans epidemics of cholera and yellow fever. In his nightmares, he was tormented by recurrent images of distorted, sickly faces, convulsing and groaning in pain. The nightmares had a vivid, compelling quality; "they come up before my mind's eye like positive, absolute realities" (Clapp, 1857, p. 189). Of course, there is more to PTSD than intrusive recollections and nightmares. Archival research and other investigations are needed to determine whether there is evidence of other PTSD symptoms among survivors of historical pandemics, such as hyperarousal and emotional numbing.

Prolonged Grief Disorder

Bereavement is widespread in pandemics, as dramatically demonstrated by COVID-19 research. On average, each COVID-19 death in the United States caused five immediate family members to be bereaved—parents, siblings, spouses, and children (Verdery et al., 2020). As of 2024 in the United States, there had been 1.2 million COVID-19 fatalities (CDC, 2024), leading to an estimated 6 million people bereaved of immediate family members (Verdery et al., 2020). The prevalence of bereavement was likely higher in countries with greater fatality rates.

A consequence of widespread bereavement is an increase in prolonged grief disorder, also known as persistent complex bereavement disorder (American Psychiatric Association, 2022; WHO, 2019b). This severe, chronic grief reaction is characterized by persistent yearning and preoccupation with the deceased and intense emotional distress about the loss (e.g., sadness, guilt, anger, and blame) (Shear & Gribbin, 2016).

According to a meta-analysis, 46% of people bereaved in COVID-19 experienced intense short- or long-term grief, although the prevalence of prolonged grief disorder remains unclear (Kustanti et al., 2023). Research before COVID-19 suggests that prolonged grief disorder afflicts 10% of the bereaved (Lundorff et al., 2017). Assuming a 10% prevalence of prolonged grief disorder and an estimated 6 million Americans bereaved of immediate family members, there may be 600,000 U.S. cases of prolonged grief disorder due to COVID-19. The actual number may be higher because mitigation measures (social restrictions) thwarted the usual grieving process. Culturally prescribed mourning rituals were prevented, and final farewells were not possible for patients in isolation. Even funerals were held virtually (Petry et al., 2021). Studies are needed to determine the global prevalence and impact of pandemics on prolonged grief disorder.

Obsessive-Compulsive Disorder

Severe, debilitating obsessions and compulsions define obsessive-compulsive disorder (OCD) (American Psychiatric Association, 2022). There are several types of obsessions and compulsions. Among the most common are contamination-related obsessions (e.g., preoccupations about contact with germs), which typically lead to persistent, time-consuming washing and cleaning compulsions. People with OCD may devote hours daily to handwashing and household cleaning. Milder (subclinical) obsessions and compulsions, insufficient in severity or debility for a diagnosis of OCD, are prevalent in the general population (Muris et al., 1997; Rachman & de Silva, 1978; Salkovskis & Harrison, 1984).

Infectious disease threats exacerbate contamination obsessions and washing/cleaning compulsions. Preexisting contamination-related obsessions and compulsions tended to worsen amid COVID-19 (AlDandan et al., 2023; Rosa-Alcázar et al., 2023; Taylor et al., 2020a). The following case illustrates obsessions and compulsions in OCD during COVID-19, as summarized from Wiese et al., 2022:

> AR, a 33-year-old male, presented for treatment of OCD and major depression. His OCD, which predated COVID-19, involved obsessive fears of becoming sick or contaminated, with compulsive washing and avoidance. He avoided "contaminated" items, avoided driving because of fear of striking pedestrians, and avoided people when possible. After the onset of COVID-19, AR became preoccupied with contracting COVID-19. In addition to his preexisting compulsions, AR developed new ones focused on COVID-19. Compulsive rituals involved the following: Wearing latex gloves in public, bathing on returning home, avoiding doorknobs in the home, excessive use of hand sanitizer (not limited to hands), "quarantining" mail and packages for days at a time, and wiping down groceries even though health authorities deemed this unnecessary. His obsessions and compulsions about COVID-19 persisted even after he received two doses of coronavirus vaccine. Indeed, he reported obsessional doubts about the effects of the vaccine.

In the first year of COVID-19, there was an increase in subclinical obsessions and compulsions in the general population, especially contamination obsessions and compulsive handwashing (Malas & Tolsá, 2022). These symptoms, likely influenced by handwashing advisories, rose and fell in concert with the rise and fall of COVID-19 infections (Pugi et al., 2023). For many people, the symptoms were temporary phenomena, abating once the pandemic had passed. For others, the symptoms were more enduring.

Pandemics are of special relevance to the treatment of OCD. Evidence-based treatments include cognitive behavior therapy (CBT) and serotonergic pharmacotherapies (e.g., fluvoxamine, fluoxetine, and clomipramine) (Nathan & Gorman, 2015). COVID-19 interfered with the treatment of OCD, with a more significant impact on CBT than pharmacotherapy (Sharma et al., 2021; Storch et al., 2021). The effects of CBT were attenuated for several reasons. The treatment involves exercises where patients are asked to touch objects or surfaces (i.e., exposure) and refrain from washing, checking, and reassurance-seeking (response prevention). In COVID-19, people with OCD were understandably reluctant to perform these exercises. Indeed, refraining from washing or cleaning was counter to WHO and CDC guidelines. Suggestions for modifying CBT were offered (Shafran et al., 2020). Nevertheless, many clinicians considered pharmacotherapy to be more feasible for OCD during COVID-19 (Fineberg et al., 2020). The same will likely apply to future pandemics where health authorities strongly encourage handwashing and other hygiene measures.

Addictive Behaviors

Alcohol and recreational drugs are commonly used as forms of emotion-focused coping (Chapter 8). Alcohol consumption increased in some countries amid COVID-19 (e.g., the United States, the United Kingdom, and Canada) and decreased in others (e.g., Sweden) (Acuff et al., 2022; Kilian et al., 2022). Consumption was limited by availability. In some countries, alcohol was considered an essential item (e.g., the United States, Canada, and the United Kingdom), while in other countries it was considered nonessential and restricted in availability (e.g., India, South Africa, and Greenland).

A meta-analysis of alcohol consumption in 58 countries in the early months of COVID-19 found no overall increase. A substantial proportion of people increased their alcohol intake (23%), while an equally substantial proportion (23%) decreased their consumption (Acuff et al., 2022). The authors concluded that "the pandemic differentially affected drinking based on multiple individual and contextual variables" (p. 1). The problem with Acuff et al.'s conclusion is the lack of a non-pandemic control condition. What percentage of people increase or decrease their alcohol intake in non-pandemic times? For example, what percentage of people increased or decreased their consumption over the course of 2019, and were these values different from the 23% reported during COVID-19?

Although it is unclear whether COVID-19 led to changes in patterns of alcohol consumption, heavy drinking was a problem for many people. Risk factors for increased alcohol consumption in COVID-19 included (1) working from home rather than in-person, (2) socioeconomic hardship (e.g., job loss), (3) being an essential worker, (4) age 25–45 years, (5) concurrent depression or other mental health problems, and (6) a history of heavy drinking (Acuff et al., 2022). There were no consistent gender differences in pandemic-related changes in alcohol consumption (Acuff et al., 2022).

Compared to alcohol, less research was devoted to illicit or recreational substance use during COVID-19. Studies of adults reported various patterns of substance use, including decreases, increases, and no change. Some studies found that substance use tended to decline while people were in lockdown, rising after that (Remesan et al., 2023). Other research found increases in lockdown-related substance use (Taylor et al., 2021). The picture concerning pandemic-related substance use in adults remains to be clarified. When looking at changes in substance use, one needs to consider the confounding effects of changes in substance availability. A pandemic may be associated with increases in substance seeking but decreases in availability due to supply chain restrictions and business closures. Increases in substance seeking may be canceled out by reductions in substance availability, producing no net increase in substance abuse.

The picture is clearer concerning youth. In the decade before COVID-19, alcohol and substance use among youth were generally declining (Hoots et al., 2023). Surveys of youth amid COVID-19 found that alcohol and substance use typically declined or remained unchanged despite worsening anxiety and depression (Hoots et al., 2023; Zolopa et al., 2022). Declining use was reported for various substances, including cannabis and tobacco products (Layman et al., 2022). In contrast, there was an increase in gaming disorder among adolescents during COVID-19, likely reflecting attempts to cope with the stress and boredom of stay-at-home restrictions (Teng et al., 2021). Gaming disorder is a pattern of online, digital, or video gaming characterized by a preoccupation with gaming to the neglect of other activities, impaired control over gaming (e.g., inability to cut down), and persistent or increased gaming despite harmful social, educational, or occupational consequences (WHO, 2019a).

Regarding gambling problems in adults, there was an overall reduction in gambling in COVID-19 but marked increases in some groups, particularly young adults and people with pre-existing gambling problems (Quinn et al., 2022). When casinos closed due to COVID-19 restrictions, people with gambling problems responded in various ways. Some heavy gamblers moved to online gambling, while others shifted from gambling to substance abuse (Xuereb et al., 2021).

Not much is known about addictive behaviors in pandemics before COVID-19. Historical records suggest increases in alcohol abuse in outbreaks of plague, cholera, yellow fever, and other diseases (Fiquepron, 2018; Garza, 2008; Gowen, 1907; Procopius, 551 AD; Sorokin, 1942). There is little information on the prevalence of alcohol abuse in the Russian and Spanish flu pandemics. In both pandemics, small quantities of liquor were commonly used as tonics or palliatives for influenza, which increased liquor demand

(Saunders-Hastings & Krewski, 2016). However, it is unknown whether this resulted in an increase in alcohol abuse. At the time of the Spanish flu, the temperance movement was gaining momentum in America, which may have impacted the prevalence of alcohol misuse.

Interpersonal Violence

Violence—particularly domestic or intimate partner violence—is often associated with mental health problems of the perpetrators (e.g., substance-use disorders) and can lead to mental health problems in the victims (e.g., anxiety and related disorders). Perpetrators of intimate partner violence are typically men, and their victims are usually women. Intimate partner violence includes physical aggression, sexual coercion, verbal abuse, and controlling behaviors. It is unknown whether past pandemics or outbreaks were associated with increases in interpersonal violence. A great deal of research shows an increase in interpersonal violence during COVID-19.

Irritability and anger increased widely in COVID-19 (Suthaharan et al., 2021). Intimate partner violence increased globally by 8% during COVID-19, as compared to previous years (Piquero et al., 2021). Such violence was most frequent in low-income countries (Kifle et al., 2024). Heavy alcohol use, lack of social support, and unemployment were risk factors (Krishnakumar & Verma, 2021; Lee et al., 2021).

Firearm purchases and firearm violence increased substantially in the United States amid COVID-19 (Donnelly et al., 2021; Kim & Phillips, 2021; Schleimer et al., 2021; Sun et al., 2022; Yeates et al., 2021). A comprehensive U.S. nationwide survey found increases in firearm-related incidents (15% increase), nonfatal injuries (34%), and deaths (28%) (Sun et al., 2022). The increase in firearm mortality primarily arose in urban settings (Lundstrom et al., 2023).

Lockdown was associated with an increase in intimate partner violence (Piquero et al., 2021). Lockdown may increase the risk of violence by confining victims with abusive partners, reducing opportunities for assistance or escape, and exacerbating risk factors for violence, such as financial distress and alcohol consumption (Costa et al., 2024; Piquero et al., 2021).

Globally, the prevalence of child abuse increased in COVID-19, compared to previous years, especially in low-income countries (Lee & Kim, 2023). The global prevalence of child maltreatment in the pandemic was estimated at 39% for psychological abuse (i.e., emotional or verbal abuse) and 18% for physical abuse (Lee & Kim, 2023). High rates of parental stress from financial and other pressures and lack of child care increase the risk of child abuse (Lee & Kim, 2023; Sethuraman et al., 2021).

Workplace violence against HCWs was prevalent in COVID-19. According to two meta-analyses, 9% to 11% of these workers reported being physically assaulted, and 46% to 48% were verbally abused (Hadavi et al., 2023; Zhang et al., 2023). These remarkably high figures were *not* higher than the rates of HCW violence before COVID-19. Workplace violence against healthcare professionals is a longstanding, widespread problem that substantially and needlessly increases the stress experienced by these workers.

Suicide

Does Suicide Increase During Disease Outbreaks?

The Russian flu coincided with a marked rise in the suicide rate (Honigsbaum, 2010; Smith, 1995). For example, in Paris, suicides increased by 25% (Leichtenstern, 1905). Regarding the Spanish flu, an analysis of U.S. Census data from 1910 to 1920 revealed that suicide rates increased in the Spanish flu, even after controlling for the effects of World War I, which overlapped with the first nine months of the pandemic (Wasserman, 1992). An analysis of U.S. Spanish flu data found that social distancing—such as closures of schools, businesses, and places of worship—was associated with an increased suicide rate (Stack & Rockett, 2021). Such closures created financial hardship and social isolation.

The HIV/AIDS pandemic was associated with increased suicide among infected individuals (Aro et al., 1995; Rafiei et al., 2023). The risk of completed suicide for people living with HIV/AIDS (10.2 suicides per 1,000 people) was 100 times higher than that of the general population (0.11 per 1,000) (Pelton et al., 2021). Brief suicide-prevention programs show promise for people newly diagnosed with HIV (Govender et al., 2014).

In Hong Kong during the SARS outbreak, the suicide rate among seniors (>65 years) tripled from previous years to 38 deaths per 100,000 (Chan et al., 2006; Yip et al., 2010). The spike in suicides coincided with the peak of SARS infection. SARS was also associated with increased suicide in Taiwan (Tzeng et al., 2020), but this was not found in the United States, where SARS was far less prevalent (Okusaga et al., 2011).

Meta-analyses found that suicidal ideation and suicide attempts increased over the course of COVID-19 (Dubé et al., 2021; Farooq et al., 2021; Madigan et al., 2023; Yan et al., 2023). Risk factors for suicidal ideation in COVID-19 were much the same as those in non-pandemic periods. Risk factors included female gender, younger age, poorer physical and mental health, social isolation, and low social support (Dubé et al., 2021; Farooq et al., 2021).

Regarding completed suicide, there were more than 850,000 suicides in the first 15 months of COVID-19, according to research from 33 medium- and high-income countries (Pirkis et al., 2022). Overall, the research revealed no change in completed suicide from previous years (da Cunha Varella et al., 2024; Pirkis et al., 2022; Yan et al., 2023). There was no evidence that COVID-19 altered suicide rates for most countries and no evidence that COVID-19 differentially impacted any age or gender group in terms of suicide rate (Pirkis et al., 2022). The study obtained limited data from low- and lower-middle-income countries. Pirkis and colleagues observed that the omission was concerning because "there appeared to be concerning uplifts in suicides in the areas of India and Iran for which we had data" (Pirkis et al., 2022, p. 15). In any given year, about 77% of suicides occur in low- and middle-income countries (WHO, 2023). Many of these countries were severely impacted by COVID-19, including economic and mental health impacts. Research from these countries is needed to understand the impact of pandemics on suicide rates.

In summary, previous pandemics were associated with increases in suicide. As for COVID-19, there is little information for low-income countries, where suicides tend to be most prevalent. For high- and middle-income countries, the suicide rate remained stable compared to previous trends despite increases in suicidal ideation and suicide attempts, rising depression, and other mental health problems. The pattern of findings can be understood by considering the pathway from suicidal ideation to completed suicide. The path can be blocked at any point. Emerging mental health problems in the course of COVID-19 were met with increases in mental health resources in many countries (Chapter 22). When suicidal people seek mental health support, suicidal ideation is targeted to prevent suicidal ideation from translating into suicidal action. Plausibly, for COVID-19, the increase in mental health services countered the effects of rising suicidal ideation, such that the suicide rate did not increase.

Motives and Risk Factors

Although COVID-19 was not associated with an increase in suicide—at least in middle- and high-income countries—it is essential to understand the motives for pandemic-related suicides for the purpose of suicide prevention.

Several factors have been linked to heightened suicide risk during infectious outbreaks (Bhuiyan et al., 2020; Dsouza et al., 2020; Goyal et al., 2020; Iob et al., 2020; Jahan et al., 2021; Mamun & Griffiths, 2020):

- Fear of infection and its consequences (e.g., infecting loved ones).
- Desire to escape the pain and suffering from a disease.
- The emotional pain of losing loved ones.
- Social isolation (e.g., due to quarantine or lockdown).
- Job loss and economic hardship, including the inability to feed and care for one's family.
- Rejection or shunning because of suspected infection.

Fear of infection is a significant risk factor for suicide in severe disease outbreaks. People frightened of infection during COVID-19 were more likely to have thoughts of self-harm (Killgore et al., 2020). In a study of 69 COVID-19 suicides in India, common motives were fear of being infected or infecting others (30%) and financial crisis (28%) (Dsouza et al., 2020). Regardless of whether one was infected, fear of disease was sufficient to precipitate suicide (Goyal et al., 2020).

Fear of becoming infected appears to have triggered some suicides in the Russian flu and Spanish flu pandemics (London Standard, 1890; Rice, 2005; Woolley, 1963). During SARS, suicides among seniors were associated with low social support (social isolation), fear of infection, and concerns about burdening one's family by becoming ill (Cheung et al., 2008; Yip et al., 2010).

Healthcare Worker Suicide

Research is lacking concerning the question of whether HCW suicide increases in pandemics. Nevertheless, HCW suicide is a pressing problem. Physicians tend to have higher suicide rates than the general population, even in non-pandemic times (Dutheil et al., 2019). Physicians are often reluctant to seek mental health services out of career concerns, work culture, or a predisposition toward self-reliance (Duarte et al., 2020). Regarding COVID-19 and the Spanish flu, there were numerous reports of physicians, nurses, paramedics, and other HCWs attempting or committing suicide (Berger, 2020; Jahan et al., 2021; Knoll et al., 2020; Mortier et al., 2021). Some took their lives because they felt unable to provide adequate care for their patients (Moutier et al., 2021).

Risk factors for suicidal ideation or attempts in HCWs include (1) female gender, (2) specific medical specialties (anesthesiology, psychiatry, general practice, and surgery), (3) being infected with a serious disease and fear of passing it to loved ones and others, (4) being a frontline worker, (5) having a preexisting mental disorder, (6) having relationship or career difficulties, and (7) work-related stress and burnout (e.g., overwork and feeling that one was ineffective at one's job) (Duarte et al., 2020; Dutheil et al., 2019; Jahan et al., 2021; Mortier et al., 2021; Shi et al., 2021).

Suicide Mitigation

Contemporary suicide-mitigation methods include public education, government assistance to offset economic stressors, e-health resources (e.g., internet-based crisis counseling), telephone hotlines, and preemptive approaches targeting at-risk populations (e.g., resiliency training for HCWs, and outreach programs for socially isolated seniors) (Gunnell et al., 2020; John et al., 2020; Karamouzian et al., 2020; McIntyre & Lee, 2020; Moutier et al., 2021; Reger et al., 2020). These and other interventions for mental health problems are discussed in Chapter 22.

Conclusions

Various psychological problems can arise or worsen in pandemics. Although people tend to be resilient to stress, pandemics are often associated with increases in anxiety, depression, and other mental health problems. Distress fluctuated over the COVID-19 pandemic, tending to be greatest in the early stages and then fluctuating over time in response to infection rates and stressors. Research on other outbreaks, such as SARS and the Spanish flu, although not as extensive as the corpus of COVID-19 investigations, paints a similar picture of rising mental health problems. Some demographically defined groups are more affected than others, particularly women, youth, HCWs, and ethnic and gender minorities. Social restrictions such as lockdowns worsen anxiety and depression.

In many cases, anxiety, depression, and other mental health problems diminish once an outbreak has passed. Some mental health problems may become chronic if untreated. Much remains to be learned about the long-term mental health effects of pandemics. For pandemics such as COVID-19, in which extensive restrictions were in place, long-term psychological effects could arise from disruptions to education and socialization opportunities for children and economic and other hardships for adults. For children and adults, long-term consequences could include persistent grief and the lingering effects of infection, such as post-viral syndromes. The latter are discussed in the following chapter.

20
Infection-Induced Psychopathology

Introduction

In the preceding chapter, we considered pandemic-related mental health in general terms. Mental health problems commonly arise from, or worsened by, the effects of pandemic stressors such as the illness or death of loved ones, economic hardships, and the stressful effects of mitigation measures. To attain a comprehensive understanding of the mental health impacts of pandemics, it is essential to explore how the infection itself can lead to psychopathology.

This chapter examines five infection-induced syndromes: sickness behavior, delirium, encephalitis lethargica, post-intensive care syndrome, and postviral reactions. These phenomena differ in several ways, including severity and time course. This chapter discusses what is known about the etiology of these syndromes and reviews their management. We begin with sickness behavior, which is thought to arise mainly from inflammatory processes.

Sickness Behavior

People acutely infected by viral or bacterial agents may develop a syndrome called sickness behavior (Dantzer et al., 2008). This is a nonspecific, immune-mediated reaction, not linked to any particular disease. Signs and symptoms include nausea, fatigue, lethargy, loss of appetite, sleep disturbance, depression, irritability, reduced sociability, and mild cognitive impairment. The latter consists of problems colloquially called "brain fog," consisting of difficulties in word-finding, decision-making, memory, and attention (Andreasson et al., 2018; Dantzer et al., 2008; McFarland et al., 2021).

Sickness behavior is triggered by proinflammatory cytokines such as tumor necrosis factor-α, interleukin-6, and interleukin-1β (Shattuck & Muehlenbein, 2016). Sickness behavior is not simply a reaction to the discomfort of fever. Sickness behavior and fever are distinguishable reactions to infection. One can occur without the other, and treatments for fever (e.g., paracetamol, ibuprofen) may not affect sickness behavior (Corrard et al., 2017). Sickness behavior has been observed in animals—indicated by reductions in appetite, activity, and social interaction—suggesting that sickness behavior might be a vestigial response to infection involving energy conservation (Hart, 1988; McFarland et al., 2021).

There are individual differences in sickness behavior. One person suffering from a cold may be miserable and bedridden, while someone else—suffering from the same cold—might experience only minor discomfort (Lasselin, 2021). People predisposed to emotional disorders may be particularly prone to sickness behavior (Dantzer, 2009). Sickness behavior is correlated with the personality trait of negative emotionality and with preexisting (pre-sickness) levels of stress and anxiety (Lasselin, 2021). There have been mixed findings regarding the association between sickness behavior, age, and gender. Recent studies found no correlation between sickness behavior and these demographic variables (McFarland et al., 2021; Shattuck et al., 2020). Expectations may influence sickness behavior, analogous to nocebo reactions (Chapter 21), where people expect to have symptoms and then notice those reactions.

Treatments for anxiety and depression—including cognitive behavior therapy and drugs like selective serotonin reuptake inhibitors—might be effective in managing sickness behavior (Dantzer, 2009). However, given that sickness behavior is a relatively mild, short-lived reaction, treatment for sickness behavior per se is usually unnecessary.

What are the practical implications of sickness behavior during pandemics? When infection is rampant, sickness behavior will be widespread, including widespread but transient depression, irritability, and foggy thinking. Some people experiencing these reactions—especially people prone to excessive health anxiety (Chapter 13)—may become unduly alarmed, mistakenly believing the symptoms to be the precursors of more serious problems. Public education may help prevent these misinterpretations.

Neuroinvasive Pathogens

Sickness behavior arises regardless of whether a pathogen infiltrates the nervous system. Additional syndromes may arise when pathogens invade the central nervous system. Neuroinvasive infections can lead to neuroinflammation, increased intracranial pressure, and immune-mediated complications such as Guillain-Barré syndrome (Pezzini & Padovani, 2020). Neurotropic infections can produce a range of signs and symptoms, including fever, headache, nausea, vomiting, seizures, acute paralysis, dizziness, confusion, disorientation, and impairment in taste and smell (Chen et al., 2021; Collantes et al., 2021; Favas et al., 2020; Leibovitch & Jacobson, 2016; Ortelli et al., 2021).

Many pathogens are neurotrophic. Examples include the viruses causing influenza, HIV/AIDS, COVID-19, yellow fever, Zika, measles, and dengue fever (Halani et al., 2021; Harapan & Yoo, 2021; Hogan & Wilkins, 2011; Leibovitch & Jacobson, 2016; Tomori, 2004; Zhou et al., 2020). It has been conjectured that the Russian flu was caused by the OC43 coronavirus (Antia & Halloran, 2021; King, 2020). OC43 and the virus causing SARS—SARS-CoV-1—are potentially neuro-invasive (Pezzini & Padovani, 2020).

Delirium

Neuroinvasive infections causing critical illness can lead to a range of syndromes, including delirium. Delirium is an acute, usually short-term impairment of consciousness characterized by disturbed attention, reduced awareness of one's surroundings, and other cognitive impairments. Hallucinations and delusions may occur. Sometimes, delirious patients become highly agitated, expressing great fear or anger (American Psychiatric Association, 2022).

Delirium during severe illness is common. According to a meta-analysis of mostly older (>65 years) COVID-19 patients, 53% of those admitted to an intensive care unit (ICU) developed delirium, and almost half (45%) of these patients died (Shao et al., 2021). Risk factors for delirium among hospitalized COVID-19 patients included pre-infection cognitive impairment (e.g., dementia) and ICU admission requiring mechanical ventilation (Guo et al., 2023).

Delirium can be a terrifying experience. Consider, for example, the following description offered by a physician who developed acute delirium as a result of COVID-19 (Arumi et al., 2021). In the course of his stay in an ICU, he experienced intensely realistic, terrifying hallucinations of being drowned in a pool by nursing staff. Although he was in a dream-like state and never fully aware of his surroundings, he also had "tremendously clear memories ... as if they were reality" (p. 2). Then, "little by little, I became aware that I was coming out of a delirium" (p. 2).

In the bright, noisy environment of the ICU, patients experience pain, discomfort, sleep disruption, sedation, and partial consciousness, and may be unable to communicate or move. Staff wearing masks may look terrifying to delirious patients (Murray et al., 2020). Social support is limited because visitors are usually not allowed, and patients commonly fear they will die. When these factors are combined with intensely realistic and frightening hallucinations, it is not surprising that delirium can lead to mental health problems such as post-traumatic stress disorder (Chapter 19).

Historical descriptions suggestive of infection-related delirium can be found in accounts of plague, influenza, and other outbreaks (Kraepelin, 1912; Parets, 1651; Pearse, 2017; Procopius, 551 AD). Diarist Miquel Parets (1651) provided the following eyewitness account of what appears to be plague-related agitated delirium:

> From time to time one saw some of the plague-stricken who had gone mad run through the city, for there were many who went crazy from this disease. If they could escape from bed or from those nursing them, they went out into the streets completely naked or however they were dressed at the time and no one dared stop them. Instead, everyone fled them unless they could find some grave diggers or the nurse in charge of them, who made them return home. But often they were so strong that it was not easy to hold them down, and no one could help them, instead everyone ran away. It was a pity to see how some who, if they could get to the window, suddenly threw themselves to the street and died. Unlike the other sick, ... the frantic were so strong that they could not be kept down, and in this way many of them died. Few survived among those who went mad. And some who went insane and were taken to Jesus [the plague hospital at the Jesus Monastery] had to be tied to the stretchers for the dead or else they would escape. And they screamed all the way there. (Parets, 1651, pp. 66–67)

Agitated delirium can be associated with hyperthermia. Febrile, plague-stricken people often developed an inner burning heat and insatiable thirst (Chicoyneau, 1721; Creighton, 1891; De Mertens, 1799; Hodges & Quincy, 1720; Kephale, 1665). Some died from drinking too much water in an attempt to quench their thirst (Boghurst, 1666). Others immersed themselves in cold water. Thucydides (431 BC) provided the following description of hyperthermic cases during the Plague of Athens:

> Internally it burned so that the patient could not bear to have on him clothing or linen even of the very lightest description; or indeed to be otherwise than stark naked. What they would have liked best would have been to throw themselves into cold water; as indeed was done by some of the neglected sick, who plunged into the rain-tanks in their agonies of unquenchable thirst; though it made no difference whether they drank little or much. (Thucydides, 411 BC, p. 246)

To uninfected bystanders, it must have been deeply disturbing to watch agitated, plague-stricken people immersing themselves in tanks supplying the city's drinking water.

Post-Intensive Care Syndrome

Modern medical care increases the odds of surviving life-threatening infections. Still, problems may persist in the form of post-intensive care syndrome (PICS). The latter consists of new or newly worsened impairments in physical or mental health arising from any illness requiring intensive care and persisting after hospital discharge (Inoue et al., 2019). PICS resembles Long COVID (discussed below), with symptoms including muscle weakness and fatigue, foggy thinking, and psychiatric symptoms (e.g., depression and anxiety) (Berger & Braude, 2021; Inoue et al., 2019; Ohbe et al., 2022).

About 50% of ICU patients develop PICS, which can last for months or years (Berger & Braude, 2021). The pathophysiology of PICS is multifactorial, with possible causes including sepsis, organ failure, hypoxia, neuroinflammatory processes, and the effects of anesthetics (Ramnarain et al., 2021). PICS risk factors include prolonged mechanical ventilation and immobility (Inoue et al., 2019). Protracted mechanical ventilation increases the risk of lung injury, pneumonia, and diaphragmatic myotrauma (Berger & Braude, 2021). Although older age is a risk factor for PICS, it can occur even in young people.

PICS is managed with the ABCDEF bundle, consisting of (A) assessing and managing pain, (B) breathing exercises as part of ventilator weaning, (C) sedatives and analgesics as needed, (D) delirium assessment and management, (E) early mobility and exercise, and (F) family engagement (Pun et al., 2019). The ABCDEF bundle, focusing on symptom relief, can be used with any patient regardless of their ventilation status and reason for needing intensive care (Ramnarain et al., 2021).

Post-Viral Syndromes

The lingering effects of infection are not limited to people requiring intensive care. Even relatively milder illnesses can have persistent symptoms. Postinfectious cough, for example, is common, affecting 11% to 25% of adults after a respiratory infection, lasting three to eight weeks, and typically abating without treatment (Liang et al., 2024). Other symptoms can be more severe and enduring. For many infectious diseases—the Russian flu, Spanish flu, SARS, MERS, and COVID-19—there were reports of people experiencing chronic (months or longer) post-viral problems, with common symptoms being chronic fatigue, neuralgia (aches and pains), shortness of breath, anxiety, depression, and concentration difficulties (Ahmed et al., 2020; Honigsbaum, 2013; Jelliffe, 1918; Kraepelin, 1912; Kwek et al., 2006; Moldofsky & Patcai, 2011; Rozen, 2020; Smith, 1995; The Hospital, 1897, 1900).

Commenting on patients seen in the Russian flu pandemic, one physician observed that "many patients recovering from a case of influenza which had run a normal unchecked course frequently suffered for six or nine months, or even a year, from pronounced symptoms such as depression, neurasthenia, neuritis, and other ills which we could only describe as 'nervous'" (Turner, 1919, p. 77). The psychopathologist Emil Kraepelin (1912) made similar observations about the lingering effects of influenza. He observed that some patients failed to recover their former vitality after recovering from acute infection; they had low energy and were very susceptible to fatigue. The patients had difficulty thinking clearly but were not disoriented or hallucinating. Emotionally, they were "sad and troubled, sometimes irritable, and occasionally at night they suddenly develop a state of great anxiety" (Kraepelin, 1912, p. 131).

Long COVID

About 20% to 50% of COVID-19 patients report symptoms persisting for weeks or months after recovering from their initial infection (Chen et al., 2022; Fernandez-de-Las-Peñas et al., 2024; Navis, 2023; Stone et al., 2023; Woodrow et al., 2023; Zeng et al., 2023; Zheng et al., 2023). People suffering from the long-term effects of COVID-19 coined the term "Long COVID" to draw attention to this poorly understood post-viral condition (Callard & Perego, 2021). Long COVID is also known by other labels such as "post-Acute COVID-19 syndrome" (National Institute for Clinical Excellence, 2020).

Symptoms of Long COVID have been reported from every major organ system (Stone et al., 2023). Symptoms in children are similar to those of adults (Ludvigsson, 2021). Common symptoms of Long COVID—fatigue, weakness, dyspnea, myalgia, sleep problems, foggy thinking, anxiety, and depression—overlap with PICS (Alkodaymi et al., 2022; Baldwin & Anesi, 2022; Chen et al., 2022). In some cases, breathing difficulties ascribed to

Long COVID are due to having been on a ventilator. However, Long COVID can arise even in patients not hospitalized or ventilated (Baldwin & Anesi, 2022). Even patients who initially experienced mild symptoms may develop Long COVID (Nature Medicine, 2020). There may be periods of remission and relapse, along with the emergence of new symptoms (Altmann & Boyton, 2021; LaVergne, 2021; National Institute for Clinical Excellence, 2020). It can be challenging to determine whether newly arising symptoms are features of Long COVID or coincidental, arising for some other reason.

Risk factors for Long COVID include preexisting medical or psychiatric conditions, severe acute COVID-19 requiring hospitalization, obesity, and older age (Chen et al., 2022; Rayner et al., 2024; Sudre et al., 2021; Zakia et al., 2023; Zeng et al., 2023). The pathophysiology of Long COVID is unclear. Long COVID is likely to be etiologically heterogeneous. Several hypotheses have been proposed, including those implicating immune dysregulation, autoimmunity, persistent viral reservoirs, and microvascular dysfunction (Navis, 2023).

Studies of Long COVID have focused mainly on the direct physiological effects of viral infection. The role of expectations remains to be investigated. In some cases, a form of nocebo effect may be at work. Fearful expectations of persistent symptoms can lead a person to misattribute bodily aches, pains, and other bodily sensations to Long COVID. Physical deconditioning due to inactivity may also play a role because it dramatically increases the likelihood of exertion-related fatigue (Taylor & Asmundson, 2004).

Uncertainty about the course of Long COVID can be distressing for patients and loved ones. Long COVID has been likened to chronic fatigue syndrome, also known as myalgic encephalomyelitis. Although Long COVID could be a post-viral form of chronic fatigue syndrome, it is hazardous to label it simply as "chronic fatigue" because that could dissuade medical practitioners from adequately investigating the causes of the symptoms (Atherton et al., 2021).

Rehabilitation programs using physical exercise show promise in reducing symptoms of Long COVID-19, particularly dyspnea, fatigue, and depression (Zheng et al., 2024). It is unclear whether cognitive behavior therapy effectively treats Long COVID-19, given concerns about whether this therapy can ameliorate chronic fatigue (Vink & Vink-Niese, 2020). Vaccination against COVID-19 decreases the risk of developing Long COVID-19 (Ceban et al., 2023; Watanabe et al., 2023). Once a person develops Long COVID, getting vaccinated does not alter the course of the condition.

Encephalitis Lethargica: An Anomalous Pandemic

A complete understanding of the psychology of pandemics requires a consideration of those outbreaks eliciting comparatively little public concern. The encephalitis lethargica (EL) pandemic is an example. EL was the world's first neuropsychiatric pandemic, lasting from 1915 to 1927 and disappearing after that (Hoffman & Vilensky, 2017; Shorter, 2021).

EL, colloquially known as "sleeping sickness," afflicted over a million people worldwide, primarily children and young adults (Hoffman & Vilensky, 2017; Ravenholt & Foege, 1982). EL had a complex clinical presentation and multiple forms. It typically began with flu-like symptoms followed by stupor, persistent somnolence, ocular motility disturbances, and movement disorders (Giordano et al., 2020). People surviving the acute phase recovered to varying degrees. Then, one to five years later, many survivors developed chronic neurological disorders, typically Parkinsonism, although there is debate about whether Parkinsonism was etiologically linked to EL (Hoffman & Vilensky, 2017).

The pathophysiology of EL remains unclear. The EL pandemic overlapped with the Spanish flu, but evidence is lacking for a causal connection between the two (Shorter, 2021). Several other sources of pathogenesis have been proposed, such as EL being caused by an enterovirus, by some environmental toxin, or arising as a post-infectious autoimmune disorder (Bond et al., 2021; Hoffman & Vilensky, 2017).

EL was widely presumed to be caused by some infectious agent, but there is scant evidence of its contagiousness. Some documented cases suggested that EL was contagious, but these were exceptions (Hoffman & Vilensky, 2017). Unlike influenza, where entire families succumbed, it was common for only one case of EL to appear in a given household.

The EL pandemic was remarkable in that the disease was widespread, sometimes lethal, debilitating for those who survived, unknown in terms of etiology and mode of transmission, and lacking in treatment. EL was unpredictable and uncontrollable. Yet there is no record of widespread, community-wide fear of EL. Numerous newspaper reports of sleeping sickness occurred during the EL pandemic. But unlike the gruesome descriptions of Spanish flu victims, news stories of EL were often humorous or wonderous in their descriptions of what it was like to experience EL (e.g., Charlevoix County Herald, 1919; New Britain Herald, 1920; Washington Evening Star, 1925).

To illustrate, one survivor recounted being in a persistent dreamlike state where he "could hear the ringing of what seemed a million cathedral chimes" and reported visions, primarily beach scenes with hundreds of bathers: "No matter what I saw, I could always hear the sound of the surf as it broke against the shore, and sooner or later I found myself on the beach again" (Charlevoix County Herald, 1919, p. 2).

EL occurred in an era when infectious diseases were among the leading causes of death, especially for children. EL was one of many severe diseases, including influenza, tuberculosis, diphtheria, and poliomyelitis. Although EL had a high fatality rate, medical authorities understated its seriousness (Copeland, 1923; Lima Daily News, 1919; Philadelphia Inquirer, 1923). One U.S. health officer, for example, assured the public that "it is only another form of influenza," which "can be combated by the same practical methods as used before, and put out of business" (Lima Daily News, 1919, p. 11).

The news media at the time largely ignored the EL pandemic, focusing on the Spanish flu and the events of World War I. There were no government restrictions due to EL—no lockdowns, quarantines, mandated masks, or business closures—because there was no good evidence that EL was contagious. Accordingly, EL did not have the disruptiveness and socioeconomic impact of the Spanish flu and did not evoke widespread distress. As discussed in Chapter 1, disease outbreaks are more likely to be feared if the symptoms are disgusting, the disease is portrayed as dangerous by the media, and governments impose onerous restrictions to stem the spread of infection. EL was associated with none of these.

Conclusions

Infectious diseases, including those causing pandemics, can have neurological consequences. This chapter examined several syndromes, including a relatively mild and typically short-lived reaction (sickness behavior), a severe acute condition (delirium), post-acute syndromes (post-intensive care syndrome and post-viral syndromes), and the enigmatic EL. Acute infections and post-acute syndromes may be associated with cognitive impairment (e.g., foggy thinking) and psychiatric symptoms (e.g., anxiety, depression). Delirium can be terrifying for sufferers, sometimes leading to mental health problems such as PTSD.

Various etiological factors are involved in infection-related psychopathology, including brain inflammatory (immunological) reactions. Expectations about the nature and persistence of symptoms may influence the odds of experiencing symptoms (nocebo reactions), although further research is needed to investigate this issue. Uncertainties about the lingering (e.g., post-viral) effects of infection are a source of distress for patients and loved ones.

Sickness behavior can be managed by reassuring patients that the symptoms are likely to be short-lived. Severe acute conditions (e.g., delirium) require inpatient medical management. Protocols are available for treating post-intensive care syndrome. Treatment for EL involved supportive medical management. People with Long COVID may benefit from rehabilitation programs involving physical exercise. Long COVID can be prevented by vaccination against COVID-19. Vaccination, however, sometimes comes with problems, as discussed in the following chapter on vaccination stress reactions.

21
Immunization Stress Reactions

Introduction

Vaccination—also known as immunization or inoculation (CDC, 2021)—is a process involving psychosocial elements such as lining up with other people, watching others getting vaccinated, receiving the vaccine—via injection, oral administration, or intranasal spray—and sitting with others in the recovery area. For most people, vaccination is a low-stress procedure with few or no adverse effects. However, some people experience intense adverse reactions.

There are two kinds of adverse reactions to vaccines: those attributable to the vaccine's ingredients and those arising from the vaccination process. Immunization stress-related reactions (WHO, 2019) are caused by the vaccination process, not the vaccine's components. This chapter describes these stress responses, discusses how they arise, and reviews their management and implications for vaccination hesitancy.

Varieties of Immunization Stress Reactions

Immunization stress-related reactions have been documented worldwide (Loharikar et al., 2018; WHO, 2019). These reactions may arise before, during, or after vaccination. These stress-related reactions tend to occur when new vaccines are introduced or when there are changes to an established vaccination program, such as offering the vaccine to a new (e.g., younger) age group or changing the vaccination setting (Buttery et al., 2008; Loharikar et al., 2018).

There are four overlapping types of stress reactions arising from the immunization process: (1) acute anxiety and stress responses, (2) vasovagal reactions, (3) mass psychogenic illness, and (4) functional neurological disorders (Loharikar et al., 2018; WHO, 2019).

Regarding the distinction between anxiety and stress reactions, the two phenomena overlap substantially. However, there are differences, mainly concerning worry (a defining feature of anxiety) and irritability (a characteristic stress response). Stress reactions are characterized by difficulty relaxing, agitation, nervousness, irritability, and a tendency to be easily upset. Anxiety is characterized by apprehension, worry, vigilance for future danger, increased muscle tension, and avoidance and escape behaviors (American Psychiatric Association, 2022).

In the following sections, we discuss immunization stress reactions in more detail, with an emphasis on the most severe, disruptive reactions—mass psychogenic illness and functional neurological disorders.

Acute Anxiety and Stress Responses

Vaccination-related acute anxiety or stress reactions include palpitations, headache, dizziness, faintness, and sometimes hyperventilation (WHO, 2019). These reactions typically occur when vaccines are administered in schools or other closed, cohesive social settings where it is possible to observe others being vaccinated (line-of-sight transmission). As discussed in Chapter 9, fear is contagious, spread by observing others behaving fearfully. Observing one or two people having adverse reactions (e.g., fainting, collapsing, or crying) can spread fear to others awaiting vaccination.

Acute anxiety- or stress-related adverse effects have occurred for many kinds of vaccines, including those for tetanus, hepatitis B, cholera, human papillomavirus, and influenza. In all cases, the affected people, typically children and young adolescents, recovered quickly. More significantly, however, the stress reactions disrupted vaccine administration and eroded public trust in vaccine safety (Loharikar et al., 2018).

Vasovagal Reactions

Some people experience vasovagal reactions when they receive injections. These reactions begin with increased heart rate, followed by bradycardia, faintness, and sometimes syncope (fainting). If the person faints, it typically happens soon after receiving an injection. Virtually all (98%) episodes of immunization-triggered syncope occur within 30 minutes after vaccination (WHO, 2019). Vasovagal reactions can occur in isolated form or as a part of blood-injury-injection phobia (American Psychiatric Association, 2022).

Observational learning influences the odds of vasovagal reactions. Blood donors, for example, are more likely to report feeling faint or lightheaded during a blood draw if they observe other donors having the same responses (Mennitto et al., 2022). Blood donors scoring high on emotional empathy—the ability to "feel" another's emotions—are most likely to report vasovagal reactions triggered by observing these reactions in others (Mennitto et al., 2022).

Cognitive-behavior therapy involving a technique called applied tension can effectively reduce vasovagal reactions and injection fears (McMurtry et al., 2015; Öst & Sterner, 1987). Alternatively, vasovagal reactions can be circumvented if injections are replaced with other inoculation methods, such as syrups, drops, or intranasal sprays.

Mass Psychogenic Illness

Mass psychogenic illness (MPI)—colloquially known as "mass hysteria"—is the collective occurrence of a constellation of bodily reactions suggestive of a neurological affliction but without an identified pathophysiological cause (Clements, 2003). Common reactions include headache, dizziness, weakness, nausea, trembling, and fainting, and sometimes functional neurological symptoms—that is, reactions mimicking neurological disorders—such as difficulty walking, speech problems, and pseudoseizures (Buttery et al., 2008; Clements, 2003). Pseudoseizures consist of tonic-clonic movements resembling epileptic seizures without other seizure features such as tongue-biting, urinary incontinence, cyanosis, or neurological abnormalities.

Vaccine-related MPI is like other forms of MPI in terms of symptoms, line-of-sight transmission (e.g., seeing others have adverse reactions to vaccination), and demographics, with children and young adolescents most affected (Clements, 2003). MPI typically occurs in closed, cohesive social settings, such as schools. MPI tends to have an acute onset and rapid spread, with symptoms resolving within hours or days after the sufferers—and their parents in the case of children and adolescents—have been reassured. MPI can be exacerbated by media coverage, such as televised images of afflicted school children being rushed to hospital by ambulance.

There have been many episodes of vaccine-triggered MPI throughout the world, including those triggered by vaccinations for influenza, cholera, tetanus, diphtheria, helminths (parasitic worms), papillomavirus, and Japanese encephalitis (Buttery et al., 2008; Clements, 2003; D'Argenio et al., 1996; Dodoo et al., 2007; Dreger, 1992; Huang et al., 2010; Kharabsheh et al., 2001; Khiem et al., 2003; Marchetti et al., 2020; Peiró et al., 1996; Peñas et al., 2018; Simas et al., 2019; Yasamy et al., 1999).

The odds of an MPI outbreak increase when there is community distrust about the safety and necessity of vaccination (Kharabsheh et al., 2001). Rumors and misinformation can aggravate outbreaks of MPI. To illustrate, MPI broke out during a 2007 mass deworming program in Ghana, in which school children were treated with oral mebendazole (Dodoo et al., 2007). Within hours of the children taking the tablets, local radio stations began circulating stories of deaths and severe side effects. There was widespread public alarm. Schools were shuttered, and there were reports of teachers being attacked by irate parents (Dodoo et al., 2007). In fact, there were no deaths and only scattered reports of mild gastrointestinal upset, a known side effect of mebendazole. Over 350 children were hospitalized for evaluation. As with other outbreaks of MPI, there was no evidence that the vaccine had harmed the children. They and their parents were reassured and sent home.

Mass vaccination for COVID-19 was unprecedented in scope. Over 12.7 billion vaccine doses were administered worldwide (Bloomberg, 2022). MPI was rare in the deployment of COVID-19 vaccines. An episode of COVID-19 vaccine-related MPI was reported in Portugal in 2021 (Reis Carneiro & Araújo, 2023). The outbreak occurred at a vaccination center in Mafra, near Lisbon, when a group of young people were vaccinated. Within minutes, 21 of them, all under 30 years old, fainted. Investigators found no evidence of defective vaccines.

The rarity of MPI during COVID-19 was remarkable given the widely held expectation that COVID-19 vaccines have adverse effects, such as pain at the injection site and intense but transient flu-like symptoms. The vaccination procedures likely reduced the risk of MPI because the most vulnerable groups for MPI—children and adolescents—were usually not vaccinated in isolation from other groups. Vaccination was a community affair rather than limited to a single school or clinic. Moreover, children and adolescents were vaccinated *after* adults had received their shots. During the vaccine rollout, the media depicted politicians, health authorities, and healthcare workers getting vaccinated without adverse effects. Evidence of safe vaccination in adults likely assuaged vaccine concerns among children and adolescents. Similar procedures could be considered in future pandemics to limit the odds of MPI.

Functional Neurological Disorders

While vaccine-related MPI was rare during COVID-19 vaccine deployment, several hundred cases of functional neurological disorders (FNDs) were reported (Albu et al., 2023; Alonso-Canovas et al., 2023; Apiwattanakul et al.,

2022; Butler, Coebergh, et al., 2021; De Souza et al., 2023; Demartini et al., 2023; Ercoli et al., 2021; Fasano & Daniele, 2022; Fung et al., 2023; Sanjeev et al., 2022; Takahashi et al., 2022; Zhu & Burke, 2022).

Previously known as conversion disorders, FNDs are mental disorders characterized by one or more motor or sensory reactions resembling neurological symptoms but incompatible with known neurologic diseases (American Psychiatric Association, 2022). FNDs are commonly characterized by weakness, paralysis, movement disorders, speech impairment, and pseudoseizures.

Rather than being a diagnosis of exclusion, FND is diagnosed by identifying positive signs of the condition, such as tremors that abate when the person is distracted (Espay et al., 2018). Detailed discussions of methods for assessing FNDs (e.g., Hoover's sign) can be found elsewhere (Espay et al., 2018; Perez et al., 2021; Scamvougeras & Howard, 2018; Stone & Sharpe, 2001).

FNDs can be transient, lasting a few days, or chronic, persisting for months or longer. FND and MPI can overlap, as in cases of outbreak of pseudoseizures in school settings. However, MPI is more likely to be fleeting, mainly affecting groups of young people, especially children. FND affects mainly adolescents and adults rather than children, tends to arise sporadically in single individuals rather than affecting groups of people, and can be chronic if untreated (Espay et al., 2018).

Acute physiological reactions to immunization, such as localized pain at the injection site, vasovagal responses, and flu-like symptoms, can evolve into FNDs (Butler, Coebergh, et al., 2021). FNDs have been triggered by influenza vaccinations, including those for seasonal and swine flu (Lin et al., 2011; Reismann & Singh, 1978; Ryu & Baik, 2010; Yang et al., 2017).

FNDs arising after vaccination for COVID-19 are illustrated by research from Thailand, consisting of a retrospective chart review from March to July 2021 of reported adverse reactions to the COVID-19 vaccines (Apiwattanakul et al., 2022). More than 200 patients were identified with transient stroke-like symptoms following vaccination (e.g., temporary left-sided weakness), which in most cases (75%) were on the same side as the injection site. All had unremarkable neuroimaging results (CT, MRI). Most were women (84%) in their thirties or forties. Adverse reactions occurred within an hour after vaccination, and the time from injection to recovery was typically two days.

The following case further illustrates vaccination-related FND (Butler, Coebergh, et al., 2021). The patient—a 38-year-old healthy British woman—received the first dose of the COVID-19 Pfizer-BioNTech vaccine in her left arm. Twenty minutes later, she developed a feeling of "weakness" around her left ear, which rapidly spread to her mouth and left arm and leg, persisting for the remainder of the day. On waking the next morning and for the next two days, the patient experienced weakness and difficulty moving her left arm and leg. Two months after vaccination, a clinical examination revealed mild weakness in the lower left leg but no evidence of neurological deficits. An MRI brain scan was normal.

Vaccine-related FNDs attract a great deal of publicity and fuel vaccination hesitancy. Several videos circulated on social media sites (e.g., YouTube), some garnering millions of views, purportedly showing the neurological adverse effects of COVID-19 vaccines (Kim et al., 2021). In several instances, neurologists reviewing the videos found evidence that the adverse reactions were FNDs (Kim et al., 2021).

Heightened body-focused attention, anxious arousal, and other factors play a role in the pathophysiology of FND (Kim et al., 2021). Research shows that FNDs are associated with heightened suggestibility, involving increased responsiveness to direct verbal suggestions (Wieder et al., 2021). Some vaccine-related FNDs may be nocebo reactions, that is, being led to expect dramatic adverse side effects and then experiencing them (discussed below).

Treatment of FND involves education about the disorder, physical rehabilitation, and cognitive behavior therapy (Gutkin et al., 2021; Kim et al., 2021; Scamvougeras & Howard, 2018). Patients are informed that the symptoms are real but caused by an aberration in brain circuitry rather than structural lesions. For a detailed discussion of the management of FNDs, see Scamvougeras and Howard (2018).

The Nocebo Effect

The nocebo effect occurs when negative expectations about a medical intervention—such as taking a drug or receiving an injection—cause the person to experience adverse side effects (Kennedy, 1961). Nocebo effects can involve nausea, headache, muscle pain, numbness, tingling, and motor impairment (e.g., unsteadiness, twitching, tics, and speech impairment) (Bagarić et al., 2022; Feldhaus et al., 2021; Horváth et al., 2021). Negative expectations can lead people to misinterpret immunization stress reactions as vaccine side effects.

In clinical drug trials comparing medication to pill placebo, a quarter of patients receiving a placebo discontinue because of side effects—that is, nocebo reactions (Colloca & Barsky, 2020). COVID-19 vaccines were primed to produce nocebo reactions because people were told to expect intense side effects (e.g., flu-like symptoms) from these new vaccines.

A meta-analysis of 12 double-blind placebo-controlled trials of two-dose COVID-19 vaccines revealed a substantial nocebo effect in terms of systemic adverse reactions—that is, reactions not limited to the injection site. The placebos were inert substances (e.g., saline), having no pharmacologic effects. For people taking placebos in these trials, systemic adverse effects, most commonly headache or fatigue, were reported by 35% of recipients after the first dose of placebo and 32% after the second, indicating a substantial nocebo response (Haas et al., 2022). For patients receiving the vaccine, Haas and colleagues estimated that nocebo reactions occurred in 76% of patients after the first dose and 52% after the second.

Nocebo reactions are more likely for painful injections and unpleasant-tasting oral vaccines (Colloca & Barsky, 2020; Khiem et al., 2003). The odds of nocebo reactions are also increased for people possessing the following characteristics (Bagarić et al., 2022; Petrie et al., 2004):

- High scores on negative emotionality and other distress vulnerability traits.
- Somatic preoccupation—the tendency to focus on one's body for indications of illness.
- The tendency to misinterpret benign bodily sensations as signs of danger.

These are also the characteristics of people prone to excessive health anxiety (Chapter 13). People experiencing strong nocebo reactions tend to have a history of anxiety disorders, mood disorders, and medically unexplained physical symptoms (Amanzio et al., 2021; Feldhaus et al., 2021; Kern et al., 2020).

Negative expectations about vaccinations can be acquired in many ways, including (1) explicit warnings about side effects from vaccine providers, (2) exposure to news or social media stories about adverse reactions, (3) previous experiences with vaccines, and (4) observing other people having adverse reactions (Bagarić et al., 2022; Colloca & Barsky, 2020; Petrie & Rief, 2019).

Implications for Vaccination Hesitancy

Public health authorities should plan to prevent or manage immunization stress reactions, beginning with public education about how unpleasant reactions such as fatigue, lightheadedness, and headache can be harmless vaccination-related stress responses. Simply warning about nocebo effects can reduce the odds of these reactions (Pan et al., 2019). Positive framing is also effective in eliminating nocebo reactions. Instead of informing patients that "a minority of patients experience side effects," the message could be reframed as "the majority of people don't experience side effects" (Mao et al., 2021). The odds of immunization stress reactions can be further reduced by administering the vaccine in a room or cubicle that shields the patient from the view of others, thereby eliminating line-of-sight transmission of stress reactions.

Prompt management of immunization stress reactions is essential because reports of these adverse effects can spread rapidly in the news and social media, exacerbating vaccination hesitancy. Ideally, the healthcare workers administering vaccines would be trained to recognize immunization stress reactions and assure patients when necessary.

If there is an outbreak of MPI, health authorities need to conduct a thorough assessment rather than dismissing the outbreak as "hysteria"; vaccine recipients and the public need to be reassured that due diligence has been followed to rule out the possibility that the adverse reactions were due to a "bad batch" of vaccine. Further details on assessing and managing immunization stress reactions can be found elsewhere (Butler, Tamborska, et al., 2021; Espay et al., 2018; Loharikar et al., 2018; WHO, 2019).

Conclusions

Immunization stress-related reactions are caused by the vaccination process, not the vaccine components. Mild stress reactions to vaccination are common, especially for individuals with preexisting vaccination fears. People's expectations influence the odds of adverse reactions—the nocebo effect. Severe stress reactions, such as MPI and FND, are rare, but due to their dramatic nature, they garner much media attention and fuel vaccination fear and hesitancy. While there were few episodes of MPI amid COVID-19, there were numerous cases of FND reported in the media.

When immunization stress-related reactions occur, people often assume the vaccines are flawed or contaminated. Accordingly, the integrity of the vaccine batch must be tested, and the results communicated to the public. The odds of immunization stress reactions can be reduced by educating people about these reactions and organizing vaccination clinics to reduce line-of-sight transmission of stress reactions. These reactions may abate untreated or respond to reassurance and psychotherapeutic interventions. However, FND can be chronic, requiring specialized treatment.

22
Managing Mental Health During Pandemics

Introduction

This chapter considers contemporary treatments for pandemic-related mental health problems, focusing on empirically supported therapies and how they can be adapted to best serve communities in pandemics and other outbreaks of severe infectious diseases. The discussion focuses primarily on cognitive behavior therapy (CBT), a first-line psychotherapy for many mental health conditions, and the subject of extensive research before and throughout COVID-19.

The chapter begins with an overview of CBT, followed by a discussion of e-health, which enabled CBT and other therapies to be available throughout COVID-19. The chapter then reviews the comprehensive mental health program deployed in Chengdu, China, in the early months of COVID-19. This innovative, rapidly implemented program offered valuable mental health support for people in lockdown. The chapter then reviews methods for overcoming pandemic fatigue and improving personal resilience. Also discussed are mental health resources for healthcare workers (HCWs), including strategies for dealing with burnout and moral injury.

Cognitive Behavior Therapy

CBT is a first-line treatment for several clinical conditions, including mood and anxiety disorders, post-traumatic stress disorder, obsessive-compulsive disorder, and substance-use disorders (Nathan & Gorman, 2015). CBT can also effectively treat infection-related phobias such as AIDS phobia (Jäger, 1988; Logsdail et al., 1991; Taylor & Asmundson, 2004). CBT and interpersonal psychotherapy show promise in treating prolonged grief reactions (Bryant et al., 2014; Iglewicz et al., 2020).

CBT teaches people to identify and counter maladaptive patterns of thinking and behaving, as well as teaching stress management and other skills. Although CBT is a modern invention, emerging in the late 1950s, simple cognitive behavioral methods were used historically. In past outbreaks, including plague, yellow fever, and the Spanish flu, simple cognitive strategies were recommended for anxious people, involving distraction and avoidance of negative thinking (e.g., "think of something else," "focus only on the moment"), along with positive thinking and reappraisal strategies—for example, warning people about misinterpreting cold symptoms as indications of dangerous infection (Boghurst, 1666; Fiquepron, 2018; Literary Digest, 1918).

Detailed descriptions of modern CBT protocols are available from several sources (e.g., Barlow, 2021; Barlow et al., 2017; Beck, 2020; Clark, 2019; Resick et al., 2024; Segal et al., 2018).

Community-Wide Interventions: The Rise of E-Health

Telephone Hotlines

Pandemics increase the need for mental health services but also impact the delivery of those services when lockdowns and other social restrictions are used. Face-to-face psychological consultations may not be possible due to lockdown and related restrictions, and the magnitude of people requiring such services may exceed the availability of suitably trained clinicians. Accordingly, there is a need for inexpensive, widely available, and remotely accessible mental health services during and after a pandemic. CBT skills can be taught via self-help books and other instructional materials. However, at least initially, consultation with a live mental health professional may be necessary concerning diagnosis and treatment advice.

Telephone hotlines involving CBT or other interventions are promising ways of managing mental health problems, including those arising in pandemics (Coughtrey & Pistrang, 2018; Gates & Albertella, 2016; Malakouti et al., 2020; Mathieu et al., 2021). An advantage of telephone hotlines, compared to face-to-face or online (internet-based) services, is that they require little technology or technological expertise and can be run as "pop-up" services, mobilized when needed. Lay counselors supervised by mental health professionals can be trained to administer these interventions and to provide emotional support.

Globally, there was an increase in mental health services amid COVID-19, mainly telephone hotline services, phone apps, and internet-based programs

(Berdullas Saunders et al., 2020; Ransing et al., 2020; Strudwick et al., 2021; Wang et al., 2020; Zgueb et al., 2020). To illustrate, in China, there were 63 crisis hotlines before COVID-19, which swelled to 625 hotlines during the pandemic (Wang et al., 2020). Telephone-administered counseling in COVID-19, provided by lay counselors under supervision, reduced loneliness, depression, and anxiety in housebound adults (Kahlon et al., 2021). If hotline services cannot address a given mental health issue, patients can be referred to a mental health professional for a face-to-face or online consultation.

Online Programs

Online interventions such as videoconferencing and internet-based programs are promising for reducing pandemic-related distress in children, adolescents, and adults (Amanvermez et al., 2023; Fischer-Grote et al., 2024; Jasti et al., 2020). A meta-analysis of controlled trials of online interventions used in COVID-19 suggested that CBT and related methods helped to reduce distress, especially anxiety (Hao et al., 2023).

Regarding the treatment of specific clinical conditions, videoconferencing using CBT can reduce symptoms of post-traumatic stress disorder (Fina et al., 2020; Hagerty et al., 2020; Held et al., 2021). Brief online, self-guided CBT reduces excessive worry (Wahlund et al., 2020). Mindfulness training—an intervention often used in CBT—can be delivered online to improve resilience to pandemic-related stress (Yuan, 2021). Brief CBT delivered online or as a phone application can treat insomnia (Cheng et al., 2020). Online stress management interventions—involving relaxation exercises, exercise and diet guidance, and simple cognitive restructuring exercises—were also found helpful in reducing COVID-19-related distress (Amanvermez et al., 2023; Batastini et al., 2021; Jasti et al., 2020).

Recent research underscores the value of simple, online cognitive behavioral reappraisal exercises for reducing pandemic-related distress (Wang et al., 2021). Reappraisal exercises are simple, adaptable, efficient, and among the most effective cognitive interventions for changing emotional responses (Webb et al., 2012). Two related types of reappraisal were found to be especially effective in reducing distress during COVID-19: reconstrual and repurposing (Wang et al., 2021). The former focuses on changing negative interpretations of stressful situations, while the latter focuses on what benefits can be derived.

Reconstrual involves changing how a situation is interpreted or understood. That is, reconstrual involves reframing one's situation. For example, instead of saying to oneself, "I will never get through this pandemic," one could say, "I know from world history that keeping calm and carrying on gets us through tough times." Repurposing is a related strategy that focuses on potentially positive outcomes of an aversive situation. For example, instead of saying to oneself, "Lockdown is horrible," one could say, "Lockdown helps me realize the importance of cultivating a good social network." Reconstrual and repurposing are simple reappraisal strategies. If used consistently, they can help people cope with daily stressors by reducing distress and by encouraging people to search for possible benefits during difficult times. Benefit-finding is associated with personal growth during crises, as discussed in Chapter 23.

Stepped Care

Overall, therapy delivered by telephone or video appears to be as effective as consultations with a live therapist, at least for reducing anxiety (Krzyzaniak et al., 2024). However, some patients require more intensive interventions. The concept of triage is well-developed in general medicine, in which the severity and urgency of cases determine treatment methods and priorities. Similarly, stepped care can be used to treat pandemic-related mental health problems, in which cases are screened to determine the type and intensity (dose) of intervention. Mild or moderately severe cases can be treated with online materials or consultations via video or telephone. Severe or complex cases may require more intensive interventions, such as face-to-face consultation. Inpatient psychiatric treatment may be needed if patients are severely depressed or suicidal. Further discussion of pandemic-related screen-and-treat methods can be found elsewhere (Taylor, 2019).

Comprehensive Mental Health Management

The approach to mental health services during the COVID-19 pandemic was largely piecemeal and reactive rather than proactive; mental health services arose in response to widespread increases in mental health problems. The treatment program developed and implemented in Chengdu, China (He et al., 2020) is an example of a proactive approach to pandemic-related mental health needs. This wide-reaching, multicomponent program was rapidly deployed in the early months of the pandemic. The program, delivered by a multidisciplinary team of mental health professionals, was designed to reach people in the community and at-risk groups. The program had four components:

- TV and radio programs were broadcasted nightly, discussing COVID-19-related psychological problems and offering information and advice. These were supplemented and promoted through Chinese social media platforms (WeChat, Weibo, and TikTok), drawing millions of viewers.
- Twenty-four-hour hotline consultations provided free advice through six dedicated hotlines.
- In cases where telephone consultation was insufficient, online video consultation sessions were offered, in which psychological interventions were implemented or pharmacotherapy was prescribed.
- On-site (hospital or clinic) crisis interventions were offered to frontline HCWs and patients hospitalized or quarantined for COVID-19.

The Chengdu program was well-received according to service utilization data collected in the first two months of COVID-19 (He et al., 2020). There were 4,236 hotline consultations. Most callers (60%) requested assistance with mental health problems, 28% needed help with practical difficulties, and 13% requested advice for sleep problems. A total of 233 patients received psychological treatment via videoconferencing. Most (85%) were referred from telephone hotlines, while the remainder were from COVID-19-designated hospitals and testing sites. Thirty-nine inpatients diagnosed with COVID-19 received psychological assistance, and numerous frontline HCWs received training in cognitive behavioral methods.

The Chengdu program is a promising model for delivering evidence-based mental health services amid pandemics. It was rapidly deployed, comprehensive, widely available to people in lockdown, and well-received. Further research is needed to evaluate such programs and determine who will most likely benefit.

Overcoming Pandemic Fatigue

Counseling and therapist consultations, by telephone or videoconferencing, are commonly sought by people in crisis. Pandemic fatigue is a more insidious mental health problem requiring a somewhat different approach.

During pandemics, lockdowns and other social-distancing restrictions may be unavoidable. Lockdowns, closures, and social distancing are effective in stemming the spread of infection but adversely affect mental health and thwart the natural inclination of people to socialize. To better manage the adverse effects of lockdown and other restrictions, it is necessary to address the problem of pandemic fatigue. Pandemic fatigue is a burnout-related amotivational syndrome that emerges with prolonged pandemic-related restrictions on socialization. Pandemic fatigue is associated with emotional exhaustion and growing nonadherence to social distancing (Chapter 6).

Reinvigorating people to follow social distancing and other guidelines requires input from all levels of society—individual, community, and government. The WHO (2020) outlined four principles for managing pandemic fatigue:

- Understand the needs of people to develop targeted, tailored policies, interventions, and communications.
- Engage people and communities as part of the solution.
- Allow people to live their lives—ease restrictions as much as possible while maintaining safety.
- Acknowledge and address the hardship that people experience and the profound impact that the pandemic and pandemic restrictions have on their lives.

At a government level, leaders must serve as role models—refraining from flouting travel restrictions—and their risk communication messages should be clear and consistent. As pandemic fatigue sets in, previously effective public health messages become less effective (WHO, 2020). People may increasingly tune out oft-repeated messages from health authorities about the need for social distancing. Something similar arises during flu season when people increasingly tune out messages to get the seasonal influenza vaccine (Taylor, 2019).

To counter pandemic fatigue, health authorities and other community leaders must periodically revise messages and messaging strategies to reengage and reinvigorate the public. Messages should be pilot-tested because they can backfire. Messaging may be improved when governments actively involve communities in crafting messages (i.e., enhancing stakeholder involvement), including particular demographic groups (e.g., encouraging young people to develop public health announcements targeting their demographic group).

Coping strategies at an individual level involve general stress management (e.g., physical exercise, healthy lifestyle) and self-motivation to stay the course, as one would in a physical exercise program. Self-motivation might involve (1) reminding oneself of the importance of adherence to health guidelines for bringing the pandemic to an end, (2) finding ways of staying positive (e.g., trying cognitive behavioral reappraisal exercises), and (3) reminding yourself that if you've come this far, you can see it through. Other coping strategies involve community support, such as seeking encouragement from like-minded people (e.g., friends motivating one another) and looking for new opportunities to socialize safely within the limits of pandemic restrictions.

Strengthening Personal Resilience

Resilience is the capacity to withstand or quickly recover ("bounce back") from adversity. Resilience can be improved by training in cognitive behavioral coping skills, such as those described above. Resilience can be enhanced by the following (Bilsker & Gilbert, 2020; Joyce et al., 2018):

- Finding a sense of purpose, such as finding meaning in work or other activities.
- Improving self-acceptance and reducing self-criticism.
- Obtaining social support—having the practical and emotional support of friends or family in difficult times.
- Attaining a work-personal life balance—for example, understanding how imbalances arise, taking breaks from one's job, finding ways to relax during or after the workday, staying engaged in hobbies, and taking time for family life.
- Engaging in physical self-care, such as pursuing an exercise program.

Targeting particular personality factors, particularly distress vulnerability traits such as the intolerance of uncertainty, can improve resilience. People who are highly intolerant of uncertainty are likely to have particular difficulty coping with stressors that involve a high degree of uncertainty, such as pandemics. Cognitive behavioral interventions that improve one's tolerance for uncertainty can improve personal resilience (Dugas & Robichaud, 2007). Targeting other traits, such as anxiety sensitivity and worry proneness, can also enhance resilience (Chapter 18).

Burnout and Moral Injury Among Healthcare Workers

Burnout

Workplace-related burnout, as defined in the 11th edition of the International Classification of Diseases (WHO, 2019), is a syndrome arising from chronic workplace stress, characterized by the following:

- Feeling depleted of energy and exhausted.
- Having diminished job commitment or cynical attitudes toward one's job.
- Experiencing a sense of ineffectiveness and lack of accomplishment.

Workplace-related burnout among HCWs is a longstanding problem that worsens in disease outbreaks, especially for workers directly involved in patient care (Bai et al., 2004; Chor et al., 2020; Crosby, 2003; Fiest et al., 2021; Lee et al., 2018; Paton, 2020; Ward, 2021; Xiao et al., 2020). According to a meta-analysis, physicians and nurses had high levels of COVID-19-related burnout (Macaron et al., 2023). Based on 45 observational studies, the meta-analysis found that 55% of HCWs experienced burnout, with frontline workers reporting the highest levels. Doctors and nurses were equally affected.

Several work-related factors are linked to high levels of burnout among HCWs. These include heavy workload and high job demands, working in unsafe settings (e.g., lacking adequate personal protective equipment), inexperience and lack of training, limited opportunities for downtime (i.e., limited sleep, recreation, time with friends or family), and lack of support from peers and management (D'Ettorre et al., 2021; Morgantini et al., 2020). HCWs may be fearful of infecting others, especially family members (Ho et al., 2005; Taylor, 2019). The children of HCWs may worry about their parents becoming infected. Some HCWs may choose to protect their families by living apart in a disease outbreak despite the emotional toll of separation (Mollica et al., 2021).

Moral Injury

Moral injury, also known as moral stress, is a burnout-related phenomenon. It involves events or actions that violate one's moral code or values (Litz et al., 2009). Moral stressors are unavoidable in clinical practice when there are numerous patients and limited resources. Moral stress can involve, for example, deciding which patients receive life-saving resources in short supply, such as ventilators.

Emotions associated with moral injury include shame, guilt, anger, disgust, sadness, anxiety, self-condemnation, and demoralization. People experiencing moral injury may (1) lose faith in their profession, workplace, or leaders and (2) experience existential or spiritual crises—for example, losing faith in previously held religious beliefs or loss of belief in a just world (Phoenix Australia, 2020). Moral injury is part of a broad constellation of work-related stressors encountered by HCWs, including stigma against HCWs for fear that they are sources of infection (Duffy et al., 2020; Elhadi et al., 2020; Taylor et al., 2020).

Adverse Effects on Healthcare Workers and Healthcare

Burnout and moral injury are risk factors for job turnover, absenteeism, and mental health problems, including post-traumatic stress disorder, anxiety disorders, mood disorders, and substance-use disorders (Phoenix Australia, 2020; Varner, 2021; Ward, 2021). Burnout has also been implicated in HCW suicide, including suicides during COVID-19 by exhausted physicians or nurses who felt powerless to deal with the surge of infected cases (Jahan et al., 2021; Knoll et al., 2020; Moutier et al., 2021). Burnout is also a safety issue as it may undermine the ability of HCWs to provide optimal patient care (Hartzband & Groopman, 2020; Ward, 2021).

HCW burnout and moral injury are longstanding problems that worsen in widespread disease outbreaks. Efforts to address burnout and moral injury have been criticized as inadequate and ineffectual. As observed by Mollica et al. (2021), "The medical system's anemic pre-pandemic response to burnout, such as dinners for doctors and relaxation classes, while helpful, were not sufficient to aid health practitioners in dealing with the intense exhaustion and pain caused by the large scale human suffering of the COVID-19 pandemic" (Mollica et al., 2021, p. 3).

Enhancing Healthcare Worker Resilience

Managing and preventing burnout and moral injury requires structural resources (e.g., a safe, adequately supplied work environment), organizational support (e.g., the availability of supportive, responsive team leaders who address the work-related concerns of their members), social support (e.g., peer support), and individual-focused interventions (Wu et al., 2020). The latter includes essential self-care (e.g., adequate sleep, rest, and diet) and stress management (Borges, 2019; Farnsworth et al., 2017; Gray et al., 2012; Haller et al., 2020; Mollica et al., 2020).

Self-assessment questionnaires can improve staff awareness of whether they are developing problems such as burnout and whether they should seek help (Wei et al., 2020). Organizational changes can reduce burnout, such as reducing administrative burdens (Borges et al., 2020; Dean et al., 2019; Ward, 2021). Clear communication and guidelines about safety protocols are needed but without onerous administrative procedures or constantly changing instructions (Duffy et al., 2020).

Military organizations, such as the U.S. Department of Defense, have developed training programs to enhance the resilience of personnel working in combat zones. Recently, these procedures have been adapted to improve resiliency in HCWs (Albott et al., 2020; Wei et al., 2020). Methods include educational webinars, skills training, and structural changes to workplace operations. Education about the nature and risk factors for workplace-related burnout and emotional disorders is provided. Stress reactions are framed as reactions one should expect and plan to address. Skills training involves education about simple, practical coping strategies (e.g., reaching out to colleagues, positive self-talk, limiting exposure to disturbing news media, maintaining a healthy lifestyle, and other stress-reducing activities such as yoga or meditation) (Albott et al., 2020; Wei et al., 2020).

Buddy systems can strengthen HCW resilience. The Battle Buddies program (Albott et al., 2020) involves HCWs pairing up such that pairs are similar in demographics, occupational roles, and seniority. Buddies are matched as far as possible on these variables because the nature of occupational stressors can differ considerably across demographics, roles, and seniority (e.g., people in managerial positions face different stressors than people in junior positions). Members of each pair debrief one another each day, brainstorm potential solutions to problems, and provide mutual support. In daily check-ins, buddies share their reactions to stressors (e.g., "I'm afraid I'm going to bring the virus home"), validate each other's experiences (rather than debating or arguing), offer their perspectives and discuss possible solutions, and encourage the seeking of additional help if stressors or anxieties escalate (Albott et al., 2020). Ideally, buddies are not close friends, confidantes, or spouses because sometimes difficult conversations are needed, without fear of jeopardizing close relationships.

Research is needed to evaluate the Battle Buddies program for reducing HCW burnout. Studies are also required to investigate whether this or similar programs can reduce burnout in other groups, such as essential service workers and others exposed to high levels of occupational stress. Journalists, for example, may be exposed to high doses of disturbing media content in pandemics and other collective crises. Burnout among journalists reportedly increased amid COVID-19, leading to calls for increased support for these workers (Morell, 2020; Relly & Waisbord, 2022).

Conclusions

When communities are threatened with a severe, highly transmissible infection, governments need to be proactive in addressing likely mental health needs. The treatment program developed in Chengdu, China, implemented early in the COVID-19 pandemic, serves as a model of how mental health needs in the community can be rapidly and widely addressed. Research is needed to refine and evaluate programs like that used in Chengdu.

Research is also needed to determine how the mental health needs of communities differ with different types of infectious diseases. The Chengdu program looks promising for addressing the mental health needs of pandemics arising from respiratory infections, such as influenza and coronavirus diseases, and perhaps insect-borne infections, such as Zika virus disease. It is unclear whether a Chengdu-style mental health program would be optimal or sufficient for managing the mental health needs arising from sexually transmitted diseases—such as a pandemic arising from variants of mpox, HIV, or syphilis. These diseases are stigmatizing and elicit moral condemnation and xenophobia (Chapter 2).

COVID-19 highlighted the substantial burden that pandemics place on HCWs. Various methods for alleviating HCW burnout have been devised, including stress management and structural changes that provide more resources and reduce unnecessary burdens. These methods could be applied to other occupational groups, such as journalists and essential service workers.

COVID-19 accelerated the societal trend toward using digital technologies to provide mental health services. Numerous mental health phone apps and Internet programs were deployed during the pandemic, and telephone mental health hotlines increased to meet the rising demand. Although these methods have limitations, they permit unprecedentedly large numbers of people to receive mental health assistance. Such programs will likely be required in future pandemics.

Research is needed to further refine and evaluate treatments for pandemic-related mental health problems. Given the existential threat posed by pandemics, existential issues will likely be prominent concerns for many people—for example, issues concerning the meaning and fragility of life. Several variants of CBT help people find purpose and meaning in life, such as Acceptance and Commitment Therapy (ACT; Hayes et al., 2016). This treatment is efficacious in treating a range of emotional and other problems, including death anxiety (Binder et al., 2024; Ferreira et al., 2022; Nasirnia Samakoush & Yousefi, 2022; Nejad-Ebrahim Soumee et al., 2024; Rowe-Johnson et al., 2024). There was encouraging preliminary evidence for ACT's usefulness in helping people cope with COVID-19 (Otared et al., 2021; Shepherd et al., 2022; Wallace-Boyd et al., 2023).

PART IV
AFTERMATH AND FUTURE

23
Life in the Aftermath

Introduction

Previous chapters explored what happens during pandemics. We now consider how pandemics end and what happens in the aftermath, including mental health outcomes, alterations in hygiene behavior, and broader societal changes. The "end" of a pandemic is "as much a process of social and political negotiation as it is biomedical" (Charters & Heitman, 2021, p. 210). The chapter begins with a discussion of these endings and what happens when they are prematurely announced. The chapter also reviews hygiene practices in the aftermath and how pandemics can catalyze personal growth and societal shifts. Pandemics can lead to chronic mental health problems, which may persist after the outbreak has ended. Accordingly, pandemic-related mental health services are needed in the post-pandemic period. Although some individuals develop persistent mental health issues as a result of a severe disease outbreak, many people report positive personal growth as a result of surviving the ordeal.

How Do Pandemics End?

We can distinguish between two types of pandemic endings—social and physical—with the former arising before the latter. The social ending is defined by the mindset that the pandemic is essentially over, accompanied by the resumption of pre-pandemic social and commercial activities, even though infection is still prevalent in communities.

The physical ending of a pandemic—defined in terms of morbidity and mortality—occurs when any of the following occur: (1) Humans adapt to the pathogen, with or without the aid of vaccines, (2) pathogens mutate to become less virulent, (3) vectors of disease transmission are disrupted (e.g., mosquito eradication), or (4) the pathogen runs out of human hosts by wiping out a large portion of the population.

The physical ending of a pandemic may be evident only in retrospect because of uncertainty about whether there will be subsequent waves of infection. Sometimes, pandemics or other outbreaks end because the microbe seemingly disappears or is entirely eradicated by vaccination. The SARS epidemic ended as abruptly as it arrived before a vaccine became available (Davis, 2021).

The pathogens causing pandemics may never entirely disappear; they may circulate in low frequency (endemic) among humans or in host animals (pathogen reservoirs), sometimes mutated into a less-virulent form (CDC, 2012). Endemic diseases persist in specific geographic regions, punctuated by spikes of infection corresponding, for example, with seasonality (e.g., increased prevalence in the winter months as people gather indoors) (Antia & Halloran, 2021).

Some past pandemics ended in endemicity, such as the Russian flu, Zika virus, swine flu, Spanish flu, COVID-19, and cholera pandemics (Aborode et al., 2021; Antia & Halloran, 2021; Bernhard et al., 2023; Brüssow, 2022; Kayembe et al., 2022; Van Reeth et al., 2012). Some infectious diseases become endemic only in animals. The plague bacterium *Yersinia pestis* is endemic in rodents, not humans (Mahmoudi et al., 2021). Plague is endemic in diminished virulence in rodents in semi-arid areas worldwide, such as regions of the western United States (Barbieri et al., 2020; CDC, 2024). Research suggests climate change could increase the prevalence of *Y. pestis* in rodents, increasing the risk of spillover to humans (Carlson et al., 2022).

False and Uncertain Endings

Public trust can be eroded when health authorities prematurely declare the physical ending of an outbreak. In 2015–2016, the World Health Organization (WHO) erred twice in announcing the end of an outbreak of Ebola virus disease in West Africa (WHO, 2015a, 2015b, 2016). The WHO erroneously declared on two occasions that the outbreak was over because there were seemingly no more cases. The WHO changed its criteria on the third occasion, stating that the outbreak was over except for sporadic flare-ups.

In other outbreaks, the WHO was more cautious in what it meant when declaring an outbreak over. For the 2009 swine flu pandemic, the WHO didn't claim an ending but instead announced the onset of a "post-pandemic period" characterized by continued outbreaks of swine flu that were expected to follow the seasonal pattern of influenza (WHO, 2010). For COVID-19, the WHO declared in 2023 that the ongoing outbreak was no longer qualified as a global emergency even though the coronavirus still circulated in communities (WHO, 2023).

Uncertainty is unavoidably inherent in these declarations. People who have difficulty tolerating uncertainty will likely worry that the declarations offer premature assurance, especially when there are still active cases of infection. Brief surges or spikes of infection are a further source of anxiety. When restrictions are eased and people start congregating again, respiratory infections may spike due to common pathogens causing cold- or flu-like symptoms (e.g., rhinoviruses, respiratory syncytial virus), especially among children. A brief surge of such infections arose in China and other countries when COVID-19 restrictions were lifted (Davidson, 2023). Such surges are fear-provoking, especially for health-anxious individuals who worry that the threat is not over.

Rise and Fall of Personal Hygiene

Hand Hygiene

The concept of cleaning hands with an antiseptic agent emerged in the early 19th century, gradually gaining importance in clinical settings and later by the public (Boyce & Pittet, 2002). Handwashing in the community became an essential part of the hygiene movement in the 20th century (Tomes, 1999).

The prevalence of handwashing and other hygiene behaviors rises and falls with infectious outbreaks. As an example, consider the 2009 swine flu pandemic. The frequency of handwashing and other forms of hand hygiene increased during the pandemic, declining afterward (Garcia-Continente et al., 2013; Manning et al., 2010). Hand sanitizer became "the new bottled water," so widespread was its use: "It's the new, expensive version of something we used to get for free, namely soap and water" (Albom, 2009, p. 35). Hand sanitizer sales rose dramatically in 2009 compared to the previous year, declining thereafter (Forrester, 2012; Mass Market Retailers, 2009).

As with swine flu, hand sanitizer was also hotly coveted in sprees of panic buying as COVID-19 spread worldwide in 2020. Hand sanitizer sales increased by 600% (Terlep, 2021). But that was short-lived. Sales dropped precipitously in 2021 (Kang, 2021).

Face Masks

In Western countries amid the Spanish flu, the use of masks increased dramatically from 1918 to 1920, and then the practice mostly disappeared outside of hospital settings. In San Francisco in 1918, the end of mandatory mask-wearing was a cause for celebration (San Francisco Examiner, 1918).

Even in countries where mask-wearing is a common practice to prevent colds and flu, mask-wearing declines as pandemics abate. Regarding the swine flu pandemic, mask-wearing increased amid the outbreak and declined afterward in both Western and Asian countries (Garcia-Continente et al., 2013; Shu-Ru & Jiun-Hau, 2012). The rise and fall of mask-wearing also occurred in COVID-19 (Floyd et al., 2022; MacIntyre et al., 2021; Wollast et al., 2023).

Kissing, Hugging, and Shaking Hands

In the Spanish flu, Dr. Royal S. Copeland, health commissioner of New York, advised parents to avoid kissing their children to prevent infection (Robins, 2005). Meanwhile, in Chicago, there was an attempt to replace handshakes with salutes to prevent passing disease on to others (Ruth, 1990). In Prescott, Arizona, it briefly became illegal to shake hands (Fincher, 1989). But once the Spanish flu had passed, people returned to the old social habits of hugging, kissing, and shaking hands.

In the first year of COVID-19, there was speculation about whether handshaking and hugging would endure (Bower, 2020). People temporarily became alarmed about shaking hands. White House health advisor Dr. Anthony Fauci declared, "I don't think we should ever shake hands ever again" (Scipioni, 2020, p. 1). Despite temporary reductions in the frequency of kissing, hugging, and shaking hands during COVID-19, these social customs returned when infection levels dropped. The social and emotional value of human physical contact can take precidence over concerns about infection.

Emerging from Lockdown

People are generally resilient. After being released from lockdown after the first wave of the Spanish flu in 1918, crowds thronged Boston's theater district, breaking attendance records: "Long before the time for the start of the performances, standing room was at a premium in practically every show house that was opened" (Boston Post, 1918, p. 4).

A similar situation emerged over a century later in Wuhan, China, the epicenter of the COVID-19 pandemic. After Wuhan inhabitants emerged from lockdown in late 2020, many remained anxious, avoided going out, wore masks when they did go out, and worried that COVID-19 could return. Some grieved the loss of loved ones or felt anger about deaths perceived to be avoidable. Yet, the subways were crowded with commuters, and restaurants, karaoke bars, and music clubs were filled with revelers (Sabrie et al., 2021).

Not everyone bounces back. In the aftermath of COVID-19, there was an increase in hikikomori, a syndrome that superficially resembles agoraphobia in which people become recluses, reluctant to leave their living quarters. Hikikomori, defined as severe social withdrawal lasting six months or longer (Teo, 2010), was once regarded as a syndrome limited to Japan but has become increasingly recognized in other countries (Bowker et al., 2019).

According to a 2022 Japanese government survey, an estimated 1.5 million working-age people, representing 2% of people aged 15–64, were classified as having hikikomori, with 21% of cases attributed to stressors associated with COVID-19 (Asia Pacific Foundation of Canada, 2023; McCurry, 2023). Japan did not enforce lockdowns, but people were asked to avoid unnecessary outings. Bars and restaurants closed early, and working or studying from home was encouraged.

Advances in technology make it increasingly simpler and easier for people to withdraw into their homes. Hikikomori may have been facilitated by societal trends accelerated by COVID-19, such as trends toward a home-centric lifestyle, where people live, work, and shop from home. Phenomena like hikikomori were rarely reported in previous disease outbreaks. For future disease outbreaks in which lockdowns or shelter-in-place orders are used, the prevalence of hikikomori won't be known until after these orders have been lifted and people are free to leave—or not leave—their homes.

More generally, many kinds of mental health problems arising or worsening in a pandemic may become chronic, persisting into the post-pandemic period. These problems—discussed in Chapters 19 to 21—include mood and anxiety disorders, post-traumatic stress disorder, and post-viral syndromes. The need for mental health services for pandemic-related problems does not end with the end of a pandemic. Post-pandemic mental health is a neglected but vital concern.

Personal Growth

Some people grow as human beings after enduring a pandemic without needing to consult a therapist. Personal growth refers to positive psychological changes from undergoing some major stressful event. Changes include a deeper appreciation for friends and family, improved resilience, enhanced spirituality, greater confidence in one's ability to handle adverse events, a greater appreciation for life, and recognition of new possibilities or paths in life (Tedeschi & Calhoun, 2004).

Stress-related personal growth has been documented worldwide (Taku et al., 2021). Over half (53%) of survey respondents report personal growth after some stressful life event (Wu et al., 2019). During SARS, some people developed a greater appreciation of friends and family, while some healthcare workers reported a strengthening sense of professional identity and perceived importance of their jobs (Heung et al., 2005; Lau et al., 2006). In COVID-19, most people (39% to 98%) reported some degree of personal growth (Asmundson et al., 2021; Chen et al., 2021; Pietrzak et al., 2021). Personal growth included a greater appreciation for life, improved social relationships, and greater resilience (Asmundson et al., 2021; Pietrzak et al., 2021). Personal growth was associated with active coping rather than passivity, higher education level, attempts to make sense of the pandemic, openness to experience, hope, and the availability of social support (Huecker et al., 2020).

Personal growth can be real or illusory (Asmundson et al., 2021; Frazier et al., 2009). For some people reporting personal growth, this appears to be part of a self-deceptive strategy (Boerner et al., 2020; Engelhard et al., 2015; McFarland & Alvaro, 2000). For example, an anxious person might try to assure themselves that they're becoming more resilient to stress, even though their anxiety persists or grows. A series of studies by McFarland and Alvaro (2000) led to the conclusion that "perceptions of personal improvement reflect, at least in part, motivated illusions that are designed to help people cope with threatening experiences" (p. 327). Illusory growth is not necessarily harmful. Positive illusions about personal development may lead to positive changes (Calhoun & Tedeschi, 2006). However, genuine personal growth, including an actual increase in resilience, is more likely to aid the person in dealing with stressors.

Cognitive behavior therapy and other psychotherapeutic methods can enhance personal growth (Liu et al., 2020; Roepke, 2015; Xu et al., 2016). Personal growth can be facilitated by using adaptive coping styles such as positive reframing—that is, looking for benefits in stressful times—and by seeking advice and encouragement from supportive others (Aliche et al.,

2019; Mangelsdorf & Eid, 2015; Peters et al., 2021). Detailed protocols for facilitating personal growth have been developed by Richard Tedeschi and colleagues (Tedeschi & Moore, 2016; Tedeschi et al., 2018).

Pandemics and Societal Change

There is a reciprocal interplay between pandemics and society. Pandemics can alter society, and societal factors can affect how pandemics unfold. Prepandemic societal factors, such as preexisting poverty and a fragile healthcare system, can influence morbidity, mortality, and mental health during pandemics. These problems are likely greater when the healthcare system cannot handle the influx of patients. Preexisting poverty means people have fewer resources to cope with pandemics and mitigation measures, such as fewer resources to survive unemployment due to lockdowns.

Pandemics sometimes serve as catalysts, accelerating pre-existing societal changes. The plague pandemic in the 14th century and the associated decimation of the labor force led to improved working conditions for low-income people as the demand for workers soared (Ziegler, 2016). Farm rents steeply declined, and wages increased, at least initially (Cantor, 2001; Herlihy, 1997; Kenny, 2021).

The cholera pandemics in the 19th century were an impetus for improving public sanitation (Rosenberg, 1987). Regarding the Spanish flu, one historian concluded that it "did not spur great changes in the structure and procedures of governments, armies, corporations, or universities" (Crosby, 2003, p. 309). However, the Spanish flu did lead to some innovations, particularly public health improvements, such as centralized, publicly funded healthcare and early warning (surveillance) systems to detect disease outbreaks (Spinney, 2017). Public health also rose in political importance due to the Spanish flu.

COVID-19 accelerated societal changes that were previously underway. Trends before COVID-19, amplified by the pandemic, included tendencies for people to increasingly work from home, to watch movies at home instead of going to the cinema, to shop online instead of going to stores, to use home delivery food services instead of going to restaurants, and to attend classes or business meetings online rather than in person (David, 2021; Karp, 2020; Plaugic, 2018; PR Newswire, 2020; Singh, 2019; Tilley, 2020; U.S. Census Bureau, 2013, 2014). COVID-19 may have facilitated the transition from hard currency to electronic transactions, as contamination-conscious individuals viewed paper money and coins with growing aversion.

COVID-19 accelerated trends for the digital delivery of health services via videoconferencing, internet platforms, and phone apps. Mental health professionals rapidly adapted to the restrictions imposed by COVID-19 by moving their clinical practices to online or telephone formats when face-to-face consultations became impractical because of lockdown and related restrictions.

Conclusions

The physical endings of pandemics are slow and uneven, with gradual declines in infection interspersed with sporadic outbreaks. Pathogens causing pandemics may never entirely disappear. They may become endemic, circulating in low levels in human populations or residing in animal reservoirs. There is usually much uncertainty about whether a pandemic is over. Even health authorities may mistakenly declare the physical ending to an outbreak.

The social ending of a pandemic precedes its physical ending. The social ending is when people decide the risk of infection has declined sufficiently to resume life as before the pandemic. Hygiene measures—such as handwashing, hand sanitizer, and mask-wearing—rise and fall in prevalence during disease outbreaks, increasing with growing disease threat and declining as the threat diminishes. Pandemics and society reciprocally influence one another. Societal factors, such as the robustness of the healthcare system, affect the course of pandemics. Pandemics, in turn, can serve as agents of change, accelerating pre-pandemic societal trends.

Although pandemics can be terrifying events that increase the odds of mental health problems, many people report personal growth, in which they describe positive changes as a result of living through the ordeal. However, as we saw in previous chapters, a substantial minority of individuals develop new or worsened mental health problems, which can become chronic if untreated. Mental health services initiated in response to a pandemic should be continued in the aftermath to address persistent problems.

24
Future Pandemics

Introduction

Pandemics are unlikely to be preventable, primarily because of human activities and population growth. As our highly mobile population expands, diseases spread increasingly rapidly and widely. Human encroachment on wildlands increases the odds of exposure to novel pathogens. The odds of outbreaks are also influenced by climatic changes causing shifts in pathogen habitat. The next pandemic might not be preventable, but its effects can be ameliorated.

Obstacles to pandemic preparation include mindsets, such as forgetting the past and discounting the future (Chapter 11). In this final chapter, we review factors that influence the odds of pandemics and summarize the complex process of preparing for future pandemics, including the formulation of predictions and scenarios. The chapter concludes by summarizing the main findings of this book, organized according to the overarching themes of uncertainty, fear, control, and conflict.

Forgetting the Past

More than a century ago, the French psychologist and polymath Gustave Le Bon observed that the Russian flu, which claimed thousands of lives in Paris, soon faded from public consciousness once the outbreak was over (Le Bon, 1895). After the SARS outbreak, pandemic emergency plans were drafted by various agencies (e.g., CDC, 2007; WHO, 2005). However, "as the emergency receded and fear subsided, citizens and governments reverted to business as usual" (Cohn, 2018, p. 103). Funds for emergency response programs were cut and agencies disbanded.

The historian Frank M. Snowden observed that pandemics are characterized by "a recurring pattern of societal amnesia," where "each microbial challenge has been followed by a period of frenetic activity at every level, internationally and nationally, but has concluded with a lapse into forgetfulness" (Snowden, 2019, p. 92).

Forgetting or failing to consider the past may have undermined our ability to deal with COVID-19. The psychological phenomena observed in COVID-19—such as panic buying, racism, vaccine hesitancy, mask nonadherence, and lockdown protests—took community leaders by surprise. Panic buying in 2020 is one example. Bewildered and exasperated community leaders exhorted shoppers to "stop panicking," but such pleas were ineffective or likely backfired. It is well-known that panic buying occurs in pandemics, so it was surprising that there was seemingly little or no preparation to address the problem. Racism and other pandemic-related societal issues should have been anticipated and prepared for because they commonly occurred in past pandemics and other outbreaks. The hindsight bias, of course, makes all these problems seem obvious in retrospect. Even so, failure to learn from the past will likely be a problem in preparing for future pandemics.

Pandemics Are Not "Once-in-a-Lifetime" Events

The false belief that pandemics are rare can leave communities unprepared for emerging infectious diseases. Seven pandemics have arisen in the past six decades (Chapter 1). Outbreaks of emerging infectious diseases are inevitabilities of human existence. With the expanding global population, increased population mobility due to mass transportation networks, and the potential change in disease dynamics due to climate change, infectious outbreaks are likely to become more prevalent (Daszak, 2021).

Climate change is a significant driver of emerging infectious diseases (Marani et al., 2021). Data from past epidemics and pandemics, combined with the estimated effects of climate change on disease prevalence, suggest a 38% or greater chance of a pandemic of similar impact to COVID-19 occurring in one's lifetime. This percentage "may double in the coming decades" due to climate change and other factors (Marani et al., 2021, p. 1).

Zoonotic Spillover

Zoonotic spillover—the transmission of pathogens from animals to humans—is the predominant source of pandemics (One Health High Level Expert Panel, 2023). Three-quarters of all emerging infectious diseases in humans have some connection to wildlife (WHO, 2021b). Zoonotic spillover is caused by human activity. Wet markets—markets selling raw meat, fish, live animals, and animal products—and human-induced land changes near dense, animal-rich forests are significant drivers of emerging infectious diseases (Allen et al., 2017; Shah et al., 2018). Land changes include deforestation to accommodate population growth and agriculture. These changes bring pathogens and pathogen carriers (vectors) into increasingly more frequent contact with humans.

The odds of zoonotic spillover are increased by the trade and transport of wildlife and exotic animals used for personal consumption (e.g., African bushmeat) or prepared for folk medicines (Castillo-Chavez et al., 2015). Such products are sold in wet markets in China, Southeast Asia, and Africa. In these markets, live animals and animal products are typically stored and sold in open-air environments, with few or no health safety measures (Nuwer, 2020). Stressed animals in crowded cages are susceptible to infection and, if infected, are likely to shed viruses.

Wet markets and bushmeat consumption are culturally sanctioned practices in many countries. There have been calls to ban wet markets, typically made by American or European commentators urging the closure of Asian or African markets (Aguirre et al., 2020). During SARS and COVID-19 in China, wet markets were closed, but only temporarily (Nuwer, 2020).

If wet markets are an integral part of a country's culture, then calls for closures will likely go unheeded (Zhu & Zhu, 2020). Improved sanitary standards in these markets may be a partial solution. Programs have been proposed and piloted in Africa to reduce bushmeat consumption. These include education programs and programs to reduce dependency on bushmeat through alternative farming approaches (Castillo-Chavez et al., 2015). Research is needed to evaluate the acceptability and efficacy of these approaches.

Older, Sicker, Hotter, More Crowded

Evidence suggests that the world's population will become older and sicker as our planet becomes hotter and more crowded. With these changes comes an increasing risk of pandemics. According to the United Nation's 2024 report on world population, the current population—8.2 billion in 2024—is expected to increase in the next 50 to 60 years, peaking at 10.3 billion by the mid-2080s and then declining somewhat to 10.2 billion by the end of the 21st century (United Nations Department of Economic and Social Affairs 2024). Population growth will partly arise from increased life expectancy despite the predicted global reduction in birth rate, resulting in an expanding, aging population. By 2080, people aged 65 or older will outnumber those under 18 (United Nations Department of Economic and Social Affairs 2024). Infection-related morbidity and mortality will likely increase as the population contains increasingly more medically vulnerable (older) individuals.

Much of the anticipated population growth is expected in Africa, India, and Pakistan. Africa will play "a central role in shaping the size and distribution of the world's population over the coming decades" (United Nations, 2022, p. 1). Hotspots for emerging infectious diseases are regions with high population densities and excessive poverty, located near dense forests where human-led land changes are underway. Numerous African regions meet these criteria (Shah et al., 2018). Human population expansion in disease hotspots will increase the risk of zoonotic spillover.

Climate change will cause many species to migrate in search of suitable habitat. Disease vectors, such as particular species of bats and mosquitoes, will migrate, carrying pathogens. Even a 1-degree increase in global temperature will significantly increase the risk of zoonotic spillover, creating opportunities for countless viruses to find new hosts (Carlson et al., 2022). Thus, people will be more frequently infected with diseases they have not previously encountered. Forced human migration due to climate change will likely increase the prevalence and severity of localized outbreaks of water-borne diseases such as cholera, especially in places where sanitation is poor and access to clean drinking water is limited.

The perception of environmental change is relative to one's observational standpoint (Welzer, 2017). A hotter, more crowded world may be stressful for the current generation, but likely less distressing for future generations, born into a world where crowding, sickness, and extreme weather events are the norm. People will be more resilient simply because they have grown up experiencing and dealing with stressors associated with climate change, such as wildfires, droughts, and hurricanes. But there are limits to resilience and adaptation.

Variations over Time, Culture, and Context

The psychological phenomena discussed in this book show remarkable consistency across pandemics despite differences in diseases, historical epochs, and cultures. Examples include fleeing, panic buying, conspiracy theories, and xenophobia, which have been features of many past pandemics and other outbreaks, past and present. Cultural and technological developments, such as the rise of digital technology and social media, appear to have amplified or accelerated previously identified psychological phenomena—such as panic buying, protests, and conspiratorial thinking—rather than introducing hitherto unobserved phenomena.

Future outbreaks of emerging infectious diseases will likely be associated with psychological phenomena similar to past outbreaks. However, temporal context modulates the psychological response to pandemics. Temporal context includes, among other things, where a pandemic falls relative to other disease outbreaks. For example, does it come on the heels of some other widespread disease, or is it the first severe emerging disease in many decades? What are the relevant recent memories or experiences of affected communities? A pandemic might arise amid longstanding government mistrust, undermining compliance with mitigation measures. If a past pandemic is recent, people's behaviors will be influenced by their recollections of what happened last time. Among other things, this may lead to earlier onset panic buying, as people try to anticipate the behaviors of others.

The effects of temporal context can be further examined by considering the following hypothetical scenario: What if COVID-19 had arisen in 2011 instead of 2019? COVID-11, as we will call it, would have come on the heels of the 2009 swine flu pandemic, which officially ended on August 10, 2010 (CDC, 2019). Swine flu was feared but mild, and health authorities were criticized for overreacting (Klemm et al., 2016). Given this backdrop, there would likely be widespread under-reaction to COVID-11. "It's probably another false alarm" would be a view expressed by many. There would be a widespread initial under-reaction, followed by heightened anxiety once people realized the unexpected seriousness of COVID-11. Thus, COVID-11 and COVID-19 would likely differ in their patterns of fear, at least initially.

Vaccine technologies in 2011 were less advanced than in 2019, meaning that vaccine availability for COVID-11 would likely have taken much longer than for COVID-19. As a result, the COVID-11 pandemic might have lasted longer, with greater reliance on lockdowns, thereby having a more significant impact on mental health. There are additional differences between 2011 and 2019, such as the greater prominence of social media and other digital technologies in 2019 and different political leaders. Accounting for temporal context is a challenge in planning for future pandemics.

Possible Futures: Predictions and Scenarios

Predictions and scenarios are used to anticipate and prepare for future pandemics. Predictions about outcomes or events are building blocks to develop scenarios. The latter are evidence-based narratives of what the future could hold, depending on an interplay of critical factors (Brom et al., 2022; WHO, 2022b).

Scenarios help decision-makers to anticipate and plan for various possibilities, such as best-case, worst-case, and most-likely scenarios. Scenarios can be tied to a specific time frame (e.g., within the next five years) or not. Planning for wildcards is essential. Wildcards are low-probability, high-impact events, either positive or negative. An example of a wildcard event would be the occurrence of two overlapping pandemics, compounding problems and complicating methods for containing the diseases.

The World Health Organization (WHO) organized a pandemic scenario-building exercise during COVID-19. Experts from various disciplines, including the present author, participated in a series of consultations and panel discussions (WHO, 2021a, 2022a, 2022b). The goal was to identify and explore plausible scenarios for the future of COVID-19. The scenarios were developed as a pandemic planning exercise rather than to produce a list of actionable recommendations.

The process began with experts identifying key trends and factors that would likely shape the future of COVID-19. Then, four plausible scenarios were developed for the next three to five years, and their implications were explored. Four detailed, realistic scenarios—titled after popular songs—were created with three key factors in mind: (1) pathogen and host characteristics, (2) public health and social measures, and (3) contextual factors. The scenarios and their defining contingencies are summarized in Table 24.1.

In Scenario 1, "A Little Happiness," the pandemic is essentially over. COVID-19 is under control, and most people have vaccine-acquired or natural immunity. COVID-19 has become endemic but mild. Mitigation efforts lead to a greener, fairer, better-prepared world. The infodemic is managed, and countries use the lessons learned to prevent new pandemics. Climate change slows; people respect science-based decisions, and humanity works together. This scenario, developed in 2021, accurately predicted the decline of the pandemic but was overly optimistic about economic hardships, mental health impacts, the infodemic, and climate change.

The remaining scenarios paint darker portraits. Scenarios 2 and 3 represent "futures dichotomized by amplified disparities and variants of continuous emergence of COVID-19" (WHO, 2022b, p. 58). In Scenario 2 ("I Love You, I Hate You"), SARS-CoV-2 continues to evolve, leading to a catch-up process where vaccines must be continually modified to deal with the latest coronavirus variant. Additional viruses emerge with pandemic potential. Strict mitigation measures are implemented, including lockdowns. Healthcare systems struggle with the surge of cases, economies suffer, trust in government

Table 24.1 Elements of Four COVID-19 Future Scenarios, as Conceived in 2021

Contingency	Scenario			
	1. "A Little Happiness"	2. "I Love You, I Hate You"	3. "Heart-Break Hotel"	4. "Here Comes Trouble"
Virus becomes milder.	Y	N	N	N
Global cooperation.	Y	N	N	N
Climate targets are met.	Y	N	N	N
Infodemic is fixed.	Y	N	N	N
Transmissibility increases.	N	N	Y	N
Vaccines prove inadequate.	N	Y	Y	Y
Strict mitigation measures.	N	Y	Y	Y
Rising lockdown protests.	N	Y	Y	Y
Global disparities increase.	N	Y	Y	Y
Stress on healthcare system.	N	Y	Y	Y
Economic hardship.	N	Y	Y	Y
Pandemic fatigue.	N	Y	Y	Y
Widespread fear of infection.	N	Y	Y	Y

Note: Data in this table were extracted and summarized from the WHO (2022a).

plummets in many countries, extreme weather events become more frequent, and the protracted stress of a pandemic amid climate change wears people down. Demonstrations and civil unrest are constant phenomena. Ecosystem degradation and diminishing biodiversity contribute to the emergence of new pandemics.

In Scenario 3 ("Heartbreak Hotel"), SARS-CoV-2 has become more virulent. Vaccine-resistant strains emerge, most infected people develop Long COVID, healthcare systems struggle to keep up, economies suffer, misinformation is widespread, and the fight against climate change fails to yield results. Vaccine nationalism emerges—that is, reduced international cooperation for sharing vaccines and vaccine technology. A "two-speed world" emerges, characterized by increasing socioeconomic, technological, environmental, and political disparities between high- and low-income countries. People become increasingly fearful of the virus, hesitant about vaccines, and increasingly avoid in-person social contact. Mental health problems escalate as people struggle to manage COVID-19 in addition to other hardships, including other health risks, economic stressors, and the rapidly growing impacts of climate change.

Scenario 4 ("Here Comes Trouble") describes a double pandemic in which a Zika-like arbovirus emerges during COVID-19. Healthcare systems and societies are overwhelmed, economies struggle or collapse, cooperation between countries deteriorates, vaccines are unavailable or inefficacious, protests and civil unrest become increasingly frequent, and extreme weather events become more prevalent. Countries relatively unaffected by the coronavirus attract waves of migration, placing pressure on their healthcare systems and infrastructure and catalyzing conflict. Species go extinct, while some surviving animals—for example, rats and bats—host potentially harmful pathogens.

Roundtable discussions of these scenarios highlighted the importance of sustainable development, trust in government, equity of resources (e.g., vaccine equity across nations), and community solidarity in dealing with pandemics (WHO, 2022a). In addition to these general conclusions, the scenario process highlighted the complexity of pandemic preparation, with multiple contingency variables.

The WHO scenarios included a best-case scenario and three realistic worst-case scenarios. The scenarios were devised for COVID-19 as a planning exercise. The same or similar scenarios could be developed for other pathogens. For example, scenarios for an influenza pandemic could be based on scenarios 1–4, with minor modifications.

Challenges for this scenario-based approach concern the selection of scenarios and the scenario development process. Protocols are needed to ensure the process is objective, transparent, and reproducible. Many pandemic scenarios could be developed from permutations of contingencies, including, but not limited to, those in Table 24.1. How might one prepare for pandemics with a potentially limitless number of scenarios, including several worst-case scenarios? More work is needed to establish the practical value of scenario-based methods and determine whether they fundamentally change how pandemics are managed. The utility of scenarios can be compared with alternative approaches. An alternative is to focus on potential or likely problems rather than specific scenarios. Plans or guidelines could be developed for dealing with common pandemic-related issues, such as those described throughout this volume—fleeing, panic buying, xenophobia, vaccination hesitancy, and so forth.

Worst-Case Scenarios

Worst-case scenarios can be useful for government agencies to prepare for disasters, but how helpful are these scenarios for the public? In an editorial in the leading journal *Nature*, risk-communication consultant Peter M. Sandman argued that the government must help people to envision worst-case scenarios to prepare themselves (Sandman, 2009). Regarding the 2009 swine flu pandemic, Sandman asserted that "the CDC's biggest failure [was] in not doing enough to help people visualize what a bad pandemic might be like so they can understand and start preparing for the worst" (p. 322).

Sandman argued that people need to be educated as to how they can protect themselves rather than being treated as passive victims: "Officials need to ask themselves whether they see the public as potential victims to be protected and reassured, like young children, or as pandemic fighters—grown-ups—who can play an active part in the crisis that might be ahead" (p. 323). Sandman argued that giving people things to do increases their sense of control and that "urging people to prepare can calm those whose concern is excessive and rouse those whose concern is insufficient" (p. 323).

Research is needed to evaluate the benefits and risks of presenting the public with worst-case scenarios and to determine whether these scenarios have the benefits claimed by Sandman. The risks may exceed any benefits. Worst-case scenarios, long used in sensational media reports, can induce undue fear among some people while leading others to dismiss the threat as overblown. A further problem is that there is no single worst-case scenario; there are many, as exemplified by the scenarios in Table 24.1.

False Alarms

Pandemic preparation involves considering the possibility of false alarms and their consequences. The 1976 swine flu scare provides an example of a pandemic false alarm and its impact. Not to be confused with the 2009 swine flu pandemic, the 1976 event arose when a recruit at Fort Dix, New Jersey, died, and another 500 were infected from a novel form of influenza dubbed swine flu (Neustadt & Fineberg, 1983). Fort Dix recruits were the only ones infected, and there was only one death. Nevertheless, disease experts raised the alarm about a possible pandemic. Some pundits speculated that the virus could kill a million Americans (Fumento, 2005). Vaccines were rushed into production with unprecedented speed. More than 40 million Americans were vaccinated in 10 weeks. The rushed vaccine proved more hazardous than the disease itself (Fisher, 2020). The program was abruptly terminated due to the unusually high prevalence of Guillain-Barré Syndrome triggered by the vaccine (Neustadt & Fineberg, 1983). Approximately 450 vaccinated people developed the neurological syndrome (Eschner, 2017).

Disease-surveillance systems are never perfect, and it is better to err on the side of caution. We can expect future pandemic-related false alarms—predicted outbreaks that fail to materialize. Pandemic-related false alarms have occurred before and can create undue anxiety, create economic hardships (e.g., preemptive closures of businesses), and undermine public confidence in health authorities. When planning for future pandemics, it is essential to consider how false alarms might be minimized and their effects mitigated without sacrificing the ability of a surveillance system to detect true alarms.

Conclusions: Lessons Learned

Pandemics are complex, multifaceted events in which psychology plays a central role. Human behavior drives all significant aspects of pandemics, ranging from the emergence of pathogens (e.g., zoonotic spillover) to the management of infection (vaccines, masks, and social distancing). No single theory can explain all the psychological phenomena associated with pandemics. Instead, several psychological theories offer valuable frameworks from the fields of personality, social, and cognitive psychology.

Over the centuries, humans have changed very little in their reactions to disease outbreaks. Despite modern developments such as germ theory, the psychological phenomena observed during COVID-19 were essentially the same as those observed historically. Pandemics are associated with three major classes of psychological phenomena:

- Nonadherence to health guidelines (e.g., disregard for social distancing, vaccination hesitancy, mask refusal).
- Societally disruptive phenomena (e.g., panic buying, fleeing, protests).
- Worsening or new-onset mental health problems (e.g., mood and anxiety disorders), but also personal growth in many people.

Common themes across these phenomena concern uncertainty, fear (and anxiety), control, and conflict. The evidence examined in this book leads to the conclusions outlined in the following subsections.

Uncertainty

- Uncertainty pervades all aspects of pandemics, from their zoonotic (or other) origins to their social and physical endings. Uncertainties complicate decision-making processes for individuals and governments. People generally dislike uncertainty, preferring their environments to be predictable and controllable. People scoring highly on some personality traits (e.g., the intolerance of uncertainty) tend to become highly anxious when confronted with uncertainties associated with pandemics.
- Rumors and conspiracy theories are circulated to reduce uncertainty by providing "answers" to essential questions about an outbreak's causes, consequences, and control. However, given their uncertain and questionable veracity, rumors and conspiracy theories add to the infodemic of disease-related information, fueling uncertainty about what is true and what advice to follow. The infodemic will likely be a feature of future pandemics.
- When individuals and governments make judgments or decisions in uncertain circumstances, they often fall prey to systematic errors in threat evaluation. These errors, driven by cognitive mechanisms such as heuristics and biases, can lead to problems. For individuals, this can result in excessive fear and nonadherence to pandemic mitigation guidelines. For governments, biases such as the tendency to discount the future can hinder efforts to prepare for future outbreaks of emerging infectious diseases. Recognizing these biases is crucial but typically insufficient. De-biasing strategies are necessary to counter their effects.

Fear (and Anxiety)

- Pandemics commonly evoke fear and anxiety. The two emotions overlap conceptually and phenomenologically. Fear and anxiety rise early in a pandemic, and they generally decline over time as people adapt to the infectious threat. Some people may experience new or worsened anxiety disorders and other emotional problems. However, resilience is a more common response, in which distress abates once the pandemic has passed.

- Fear is influenced by news and social media coverage, rumors, conspiracy theories, and the actions or inactions of government leaders. Even the name given to a disease influences its fearfulness.
- Extremes of fear arise in pandemics, with some people becoming highly fearful while others dismiss the threat as overblown. Low levels of fear are associated with nonadherence to pandemic mitigation measures, while high levels of fear are associated with panic buying and fleeing.
- Panic buying occurs when lockdowns are anticipated or shortages are rumored. Medicines and food are the most common targets, although items with little or no protective value (e.g., toilet paper) may also become targets. Panic buying can be managed preemptively by imposing limits on purchases.
- Fleeing from infection hotspots is a frequent response that causes diseases to spread widely. Fleeing is likely to occur when there are rumors or announcements of an impending cordon sanitaire or border closure. Fearful people flee even when there is no haven from infection, such as when they flee from cities to their hometowns to be with family.
- Xenophobia—fear of strangers—can be widespread in pandemics. Xenophobia is thought to arise, in part, from psychological mechanisms for detecting and avoiding pathogens. When people feel threatened with infection, there is a rise in racism (e.g., directed at the people from countries where the pandemic supposedly arose) and stigmatization (e.g., shunning people associated with infection, such as healthcare workers or recovered patients). People scoring high on disgust sensitivity tend to become especially frightened, disgusted, and xenophobic when threatened with infection. Political leaders exacerbate xenophobia by blaming some nation or ethnic group for the outbreak.

Control

- People endure pandemics with problem-focused coping (searching for ways of staying safe) and emotion-focused coping (engaging in calming activities). Magical thinking and superstitious rituals are evident during pandemics as people try to exert control over invisible infectious threats. Some coping behaviors provide an illusion of control, making people calmer but not safer.
- People tend to become more authoritarian during widespread calamities such as pandemics, demanding that leaders take charge. Authoritarianism is associated with xenophobia and harsh attitudes toward rule breakers.

- Public confidence in health authorities and government leaders is essential for ensuring adherence to pandemic mitigation measures.
- Governments try to control pandemics by restricting social mobility and encouraging people to follow particular guidelines (e.g., hand hygiene). Various methods increase public adherence, including fear-evoking messages, nudges, and mandates. Interventions to control one problem may worsen others. Lockdown, for example, is moderately effective in mitigating pandemics but can harm mental health. Alternatives to lockdown are test-trace-isolate approaches using digital surveillance. Although promising, the alternatives come with problems.
- Risk communication and community involvement are essential for ensuring adherence to pandemic mitigation measures. Risk communication needs to be carefully crafted and pilot-tested to be optimally effective and avoid unintended consequences such as triggering outbreaks of panic buying.
- Vaccination hesitancy is as old as vaccination itself and will almost certainly be a feature of the next pandemic. Nevertheless, the vaccination efforts during COVID-19 showed that it was possible to vaccinate nearly three-quarters (72%) of the world's population. Education, vaccine safety assurances, nudges, and mandates enhance vaccine uptake.
- Nudges are benign, low-effort, and effective ways of improving adherence to health behaviors such as mask-wearing, vaccination, and adherence to social distancing. If nudges prove insufficient, mandates may be implemented.
- Healthcare worker burnout is a significant, longstanding problem that hampers pandemic preparedness and control. Resources are needed to ensure that essential workers—particularly frontline healthcare workers—can perform their duties in public health emergencies such as pandemics.
- To address mental health problems in pandemics, large-scale, remotely accessible community mental health resources, such as internet-based treatment programs are needed. Persistent mental health problems and post-infection syndromes may emerge, requiring treatment.

Conflict

- Efforts at controlling community-wide outbreaks can elicit conflicts over the necessity, efficacy, and fairness of mitigation measures. Attitudes may be polarized in pandemics, leading to conflict. People may adopt strong

views for or against vaccines, masks, and social distancing. Social and cognitive processes contribute to attitude polarization.
- Irritability, anger, suspiciousness, and interpersonal conflict increase when people feel threatened by dangerous contagious diseases. Blaming particular groups (scapegoating) can make a pandemic seem more predictable and controllable but exacerbates societal discord.
- The study of personality traits sheds light on conflicts over mask-wearing, vaccination, and social distancing. Some people would sooner die of infection than be told what to do. People scoring high on a trait known as psychological reactance tend to resist government-mandated measures, valuing personal freedom above all else.
- Societal tensions may be exacerbated in the course of pandemics, such as tensions between governments and marginalized groups (e.g., people in poverty). This is an important consideration when planning mitigation measures that might impact one group more than others.
- Protests, such as those against masks, vaccines, and social restrictions, periodically arise amid pandemics. People participate in protest rallies for various reasons. Protests can lead to rioting when restrictions are perceived as unfair or frustrating, such as when lockdowns are rescinded and reimposed (recurrent lockdowns) and new limits are added to existing ones (e.g., imposing a curfew in addition to existing restrictions on personal mobility). Protests, although disruptive and sources of superspreading, can provide valuable feedback to health authorities about problematic mitigation measures.

Psychological factors will almost certainly play vital roles in the next pandemic, with issues including vaccination hesitancy, conspiratorial thinking, and nonadherence to mask-wearing and social distancing. Preparing for the next pandemic requires long-term planning, which is undermined when people focus exclusively on immediate concerns. Allocating resources to far-off potential problems can be problematic when communities and countries face immediate challenges, such as geopolitical conflicts, pressing social inequalities, and the threat of extreme weather events associated with climate change. Nevertheless, pandemic preparation is vital because there will be more pandemics and other outbreaks in the years and decades ahead.

References

Chapter 1

Agamben, G. (2005). *State of exception*. University of Chicago Press.

Aguirre, A. A., Catherina, R., Frye, H., & Shelley, L. (2020). Illicit wildlife trade, wet markets, and COVID19: Preventing future pandemics. *World Medical & Health Policy, 12*(3), 256–265. https://doi.org/10.1002/wmh3.348

Ahmad, F. B., & Anderson, R. N. (2021). The leading causes of death in the US for 2020. *JAMA, 325*(18), 1829–1830. https://doi.org/10.1001/jama.2021.5469

Almagro-Moreno, S. (2022). How bacterial pathogens emerge. *American Scientist, 110*, 162–169.

Alsharif, M., & Almasy, S. (2020, October 22). Nearly 50 people contracted coronavirus after fellowship event at a small church in Maine. *CNN*. https://www.cnn.com/2020/10/22/us/maine-church-covid-19-outbreak/index.html

Altemeyer, B. (2009). *The authoritarians*. Cherry Hill Publishing.

Angus Reid Institute. (2020). COVID-19: Canadian concern over falling ill on the rise again. http://angusreid.org/covid-concern-rising/

Arnold, C. (2018). *Pandemic 1918: Eyewitness accounts from the greatest medical holocaust in modern history*. St. Martin's Press.

Aschwanden, C. (2020). How "superspreading" events drive most COVID-19 spread. *Scientific American*. https://www.scientificamerican.com/article/how-superspreading-events-drive-most-covid-19-spread1/

Asmundson, G. J. G., & Taylor, S. (2020). Coronaphobia revisited: A state-of-the-art on pandemic-related fear, anxiety, and stress. *Journal of Anxiety Disorders, 76*, article 102326. https://doi.org/10.1016/j.janxdis.2020.102326

Associated Press. (2021). India's crematoriums overwhelmed as COVID-19 patients scramble for medical help. *Associated Press*. https://www.cbc.ca/news/world/india-covid19-patients-creamatorium-1.6001536

Barry, J. M. (2018). *The great influenza*. Penguin Random House.

Becker, K. M. (2020). More than 200 COVID-19 cases linked to Fitchburg church. *NBC News*. https://www.nbcboston.com/news/local/more-than-200-covid-19-cases-linked-to-fitchburg-church/2225433/?amp

Berche, P. (2022). The enigma of the 1889 Russian flu pandemic: A coronavirus? *Presse Meédicale, 51*(3), article 104111. https://doi.org/10.1016/j.lpm.2022.104111

Bernheim, B. D., Freitas-Groff, Z., Buchmann, N., & Otero, S. (2020). *The effects of large group meetings on the spread of COVID-19: The case of Trump rallies*. Stanford Institute for Economic Policy Research, https://drive.google.com/file/d/1VfgazJSEAg3m0QZOOSauSwNLhbTrYovr/view

Brittany, S., Knowles, H., & Keating, D. (2021, November 24). Sturgis motorcycle rally linked to more than 100 coronavirus infections amid delta surge. *Washington Post*. https://www.washingtonpost.com/health/2021/08/26/sturgis-motorcycle-rally-covid-cases/

Brooks, J. (1996). The sad and tragic life of Typhoid Mary. *Canadian Medical Association Journal, 154*, 915–916.

Burrell, S., & Gill, G. (2005). The Liverpool cholera epidemic of 1832 and anatomical dissection: Medical mistrust and civil unrest. *Journal of the History of Medicine and Allied Sciences*, 60(4), 478–498. https://doi.org/10.1093/jhmas/jri061

Butler, T. (2023). Plague gives surprises in the second decade of the twenty-first century. *American Journal of Tropical Medicine and Hygiene*, 109(5), 985–988. https://doi.org/10.4269/ajtmh.23-0331

Byrne, J. P. (2006). *Daily life during the Black Death*. Greenwood.

Cagnassola, M. E. (2021, May 5). Narendra Modi, India's Prime Minister, called a COVID "super-spreader" by medical official. *Newsweek*. https://www.newsweek.com/narendra-modi-indias-prime-minister-called-covid-super-spreader-medical-official-1588876

Caley, P., Philp, D. J., & McCracken, K. (2008). Quantifying social distancing arising from pandemic influenza. *Journal of the Royal Society Interface*, 5, 631–639.

Cauchemez, S., Ferguson, N., Wachtel, C., Tegnell, A., Saour, G., Duncan, B., et al. (2009). Closure of schools during an influenza pandemic. *Lancet Infectious Diseases*, 9, 473–481. https://doi.org/10.1186/1471-2334-14-207

CDC. (2007). *Interim pre-pandemic planning guidance: Community strategy for pandemic influenza mitigation in the United States*. Author.

CDC. (2024). Ebola outbreak history. https://www.cdc.gov/ebola/outbreaks/

Cha, S. (2021). A little-known cult is South Korea's latest COVID-19 outbreak. *CTV News*. https://www.ctvnews.ca/health/coronavirus/a-little-known-cult-is-south-korea-s-latest-covid-19-outbreak-1.5678947

Chan-Yeung, M., & Xu, R. H. (2003). SARS: Epidemiology. *Respirology*, 8(Suppl 1), S9–S14. https://doi.org/10.1046/j.1440-1843.2003.00518.x

Chen, P. Z., Koopmans, M., Fisman, D. N., & Gu, F. X. (2021). Understanding why superspreading drives the COVID-19 pandemic but not the H1N1 pandemic. *Lancet Infectious Diseases*, 21(9), 1203–1204.

Clapp, T. (1857). *Autobiographical sketches and recollections, during a thirty-five years residence in New Orleans*. Phillips, Sampson & Co.

Collinson, S., Khan, K., & Heffernan, J. M. (2015). The effects of media reports on disease spread and important public health measurements. *PLOS ONE*, 10, e0141423. https://doi.org/10.1371/journal.pone.0141423

Daly, M., Jones, A., & Robinson, E. (2021). Public trust and willingness to vaccinate against COVID-19 in the US from October 14, 2020, to March 29, 2021. *JAMA*, 325(23), 2397–2399. https://doi.org/10.1001/jama.2021.8246

Daly, M., & Robinson, E. (2021). Willingness to vaccinate against COVID-19 in the US: Longitudinal evidence from a nationally representative sample of adults from April-October 2020. *American Journal of Preventive Medicine*, 60, 766–773. https://doi.org/10.1101/2020.11.27.20239970

Davis, K. C. (2018, September 21). Philadelphia threw a WWI parade that gave thousands of onlookers the flu. *Smithsonian Magazine*. https://www.smithsonianmag.com/history/philadelphia-threw-wwi-parade-gave-thousands-onlookers-flu-180970372/

Dawood, F. S., Iuliano, A. D., Reed, C., Meltzer, M. I., Shay, D. K., Cheng, P.-Y., et al. (2012). Estimated global mortality associated with the first 12 months of 2009 pandemic influenza A H1N1 virus circulation: A modelling study. *Lancet Infectious Diseases*, 12(9), 687–695. https://doi.org/10.1016/S1473-3099(12)70121-4

DeFranza, D., Lindow, M., Harrison, K., Mishra, A., & Mishra, H. (2021). Religion and reactance to COVID-19 mitigation guidelines. *American Psychologist*, 76(5), 744–754. https://doi.org/10.1037/amp0000717

Dixon, M. G., & Schafer, I. J. (2014). Ebola viral disease outbreak—West Africa, 2014. *Morbidity and Mortality Weekly Report*, 63(25), 548–551.

Economist. (1969, January 18). Feverish. *The Economist*, 230, 40–41.
Eisenberg, M., & Mordechai, L. (2019). The Justinianic Plague: An interdisciplinary review. *Byzantine & Modern Greek Studies*, 43(2), 156–180. https://doi.org/10.1017/byz.2019.10
Elliott, C. (2024). *Pox Romana: The plague that shook the Roman world*. Princeton University Press.
Fenner, F., Henderson, D. A., Arita, I., Jezek, Z., & Ladnyi, I. D. (1988). *Smallpox and its eradication*. WHO.
Fiquepron, M. R. (2018). Places, attitudes and moments during the epidemics: Representations of yellow fever and cholera in the city of Buenos Aires, 1867–1871. *História, Ciências, Saúde*, 25(2), 1–16. https://doi.org/10.1590/S0104-59702018000200003
Fung, T. K. F., Namkoong, K., & Brossard, D. (2011). Media, social proximity, and risk: A comparative analysis of newspaper coverage of avian flu in Hong Kong and in the United States. *Journal of Health Communication*, 16(8), 889–907. https://doi.org/10.1080/10810730.2011.561913
Galvani, A. P., & May, R. M. (2005). Dimensions of superspreading. *Nature*, 438, 293–295.
Garfin, D. R., Silver, R. C., & Holman, E. A. (2020). The novel coronavirus (COVID-2019) outbreak: Amplification of public health consequences by media exposure. *Health Psychology*, 39(5), 355–357. https://doi.org/10.1037/hea0000875
Garza, R. P. (2008). *Understanding plague: The medical and imaginative texts of medieval Spain*. Peter Lang.
Gestefeld, M., Lorenz, J., Henschel, N. T., & Boehnke, K. (2022). Decomposing attitude distributions to characterize attitude polarization in Europe. *SN Social Sciences*, 2(7), article 110. https://doi.org/10.1007/s43545-022-00342-7
Glatter, K. A., & Finkelman, P. (2021). History of the plague: An ancient pandemic for the age of COVID-19. *American Journal of Medicine*, 134(2), 176–181. https://doi.org/10.1016/j.amjmed.2020.08.019
Gowen, B. S. (1907). Some aspects of pestilences and other epidemics. *American Journal of Psychology*, 18(1), 1–60. https://doi.org/10.2307/1412171
Green, T. (2020, October 10). What are we so afraid of? *Washington Post*. https://www.washingtonpost.com/nation/2020/10/10/coronavirus-denier-sick-spreader/?arc404=true
Halani, S., Tombindo, P. E., O'Reilly, R., Miranda, R. N., Erdman, L. K., Whitehead, C., et al. (2021). Clinical manifestations and health outcomes associated with Zika virus infections in adults: A systematic review. *PLOS Neglected Tropical Diseases*, 15(7), article e0009516. https://doi.org/10.1371/journal.pntd.0009516
Herrera-Valdez, M. A., Cruz-Aponte, M., & Castillo-Chavez, C. (2011). Multiple outbreaks for the same pandemic: Local transportation and social distancing explain the different "waves" of A-H1N1pdm cases observed in México during 2009. *Mathematical Biosciences and Engineering*, 8, 21–48. https://doi.org/10.3934/mbe.2011.8.21
Hirst, L. F. (1953). *The conquest of plague*. Clarendon.
Hoffman, L. A., & Vilensky, J. A. (2017). Encephalitis lethargica: 100 years after the epidemic. *Brain*, 140(8), 2246–2251. https://doi.org/10.1093/brain/awx177
Honigsbaum, M. (2010). The great dread: Cultural and psychological impacts and responses to the "Russian" influenza in the United Kingdom, 1889–1893. *Social History of Medicine*, 23(2), 299–319. https://doi.org/10.1093/shm/hkq011
Honigsbaum, M. (2020a, October 18). How do pandemics end? In different ways, but it's never quick and never neat. *The Guardian*. https://www.theguardian.com/commentisfree/2020/oct/18/how-do-pandemics-end-in-different-ways-but-its-never-quick-and-never-neat
Honigsbaum, M. (2020b). Revisiting the 1957 and 1968 influenza pandemics. *Lancet*, 395, 1824–1826. https://doi.org/10.1016/S0140-6736(20)31201-0

Humphreys, M. (2002). No safe place: Disease and panic in American history. *American Literary History*, *14*(4), 845–857. https://doi.org/10.1093/alh/14.4.845

Iezzoni, L. (1999). *Influenza 1918: The worst epidemic in American history*. TV Books.

Kanungo, S., Azman, A. S., Ramamurthy, T., Deen, J., & Dutta, S. (2022). Cholera. *Lancet*, *399*(10333), 1429–1440. https://doi.org/10.1016/S0140-6736(22)00330-0

Kelly, H., Peck, H. A., Laurie, K. L., Wu, P., Nishiura, H., & Cowling, B. J. (2011). The age-specific cumulative incidence of infection with pandemic influenza H1N1 2009 was similar in various countries prior to vaccination. *PLOS ONE*, *6*(8), e21828. https://doi.org/10.1371/journal.pone.0021828

LaGrassa, J. (2020, October 30). Blenheim church an example of a "quintessential super spreader event." *CBC News*. https://www.cbc.ca/news/canada/windsor/covid-19-church-spreader-event-1.5783090

Lammers, J., Crusius, J., & Gast, A. (2020). Correcting misperceptions of exponential coronavirus growth increases support for social distancing. *PNAS*, *117*(28), 16264–16266. https://doi.org/10.1073/pnas.2006048117

LeHardy, J. C. (1888). The yellow fever panic. *Atlanta Medical and Surgical Journal*, *5*(10), 605–616.

Lewis, D. (2021). Superspreading drives the COVID pandemic—and could help to tame it. *Nature*. https://www.nature.com/articles/d41586-021-00460-x

Littman, R. J. (2009). The plague of Athens: Epidemiology and paleopathology. *Mt Sinai Journal of Medicine*, *76*(5), 456–467. https://doi.org/10.1002/msj.20137

Lloyd-Smith, J., Schreiber, S., Kopp, P., & Getz, W. (2005). Superspreading and the effect of individual variation on disease emergence. *Nature*, *438*(7066), 355–359.

London St. James Gazette. (1890, January 11, 19). The influenza: The epidemic abating in London. *London St. James Gazette*.

Lycett, S. J., Duchatel, F., & Digard, P. (2019). A brief history of bird flu. *Philosophical Transactions of the Royal Society of London. Series B, Biological Sciences*, *374*(1775), article 20180257. https://doi.org/10.1098/rstb.2018.0257

MacCarthy, F. D. (1969). Hong Kong Flu. *BMJ*, *1*, 182. https://doi.org/10.1136/bmj.1.5637.182-b

Majra, D., Benson, J., Pitts, J., & Stebbing, J. (2021). SARS-CoV-2 (COVID-19) superspreader events. *Journal of Infection*, *82*(1), 36–40. https://doi.org/10.1016/j.jinf.2020.11.021

Mathieu, E., Ritchie, H., Rodés-Guirao, L., Appel, C., Giattino, C., Hasell, J., et al. (2024). Coronavirus pandemic (COVID-19). *Our World in Data*. https://ourworldindata.org/coronavirus

McCoy, J., Rahman, T., & Somer, M. (2018). Polarization and the global crisis of democracy: Common patterns, dynamics, and pernicious consequences for democratic polities. *American Behavioral Scientist*, *62*(1), 16–42. https://doi.org/10.1177/0002764218759576

McDonnell, W. M., Nelson, D. S., & Schunk, J. E. (2012). Should we fear "flu fear" itself? Effects of H1N1 influenza fear on ED use. *American Journal of Emergency Medicine*, *30*, 275–282. https://doi.org/10.1016/j.ajem.2010.11.027

McEvoy, J. (2021, September 2). Covid surges nearly 700% in South Dakota after Sturgis motorcycle rally—an even higher rate than last year. *Forbes*. https://www.forbes.com/sites/jemimamcevoy/2021/09/02/covid-surges-nearly-700-in-south-dakota-after-sturgis-motorcycle-rally-an-even-higher-rate-than-last-year/?sh=760f1cbe74c6

McGee, L. (2022, January 12). Boris Johnson apologizes for attending Downing Street "bring your own booze" party during lockdown. *CNN*. https://www.cnn.com/2022/01/12/uk/boris-johnson-pmqs-downing-street-party-intl-gbr/index.html

Michaelis, M., Doerr, H. W., & Cinatl, J. (2009). Novel swine-origin influenza A virus in humans: another pandemic knocking at the door. *Medical Microbiology and Immunology*, *198*(3), 175–183. https://doi.org/10.1007/s00430-009-0118-5

Mohindra, R., Ghai, A., Brar, R., Khandelwal, N., Biswal, M., Suri, V., et al. (2021). Superspreaders: A lurking danger in the community. *Journal of Primary Care & Community Health, 12*, 1–4. https://doi.org/10.1177/2150132720987432

Mordechai, L., Eisenberg, M., Newfield, T. P., Izdebski, A., Kay, J. E., & Poinar, H. (2019). The Justinianic Plague: An inconsequential pandemic? *PNAS, 116*(51), 25546–25554. https://doi.org/10.1073/pnas.1903797116

Morens, D. M., Folkers, G. K., & Fauci, A. S. (2008). Emerging infections: A perpetual challenge. *Lancet Infectious Diseases, 8*, 710–719. https://doi.org/10.1016/S1473-3099(08)70256-1

National Collaborating Centre for Infectious Diseases. (2024). H5N1 highly pathogenic avian influenza A virus (bird flu). https://nccid.ca/debrief/avian-influenza-h5n1/

Parets, M. (1651). *A journal of the plague year: The diary of the Barcelona tanner Miquel Parets 1651 (J. S. Amelang, trans. & ed., 1991)*. Oxford University Press.

Paules, C. I., Eisinger, R. W., Marston, H. D., & Fauci, A. S. (2017). What recent history has taught us about responding to emerging infectious disease threats. *Annals of Internal Medicine, 167*(11), 805–811. https://doi.org/10.7326/M17-2496

Peckham, R. (2020). Viral surveillance and the 1968 Hong Kong flu pandemic. *Journal of Global History, 15*(3), 444–458. https://doi.org/10.1017/S1740022820000224

Penninx, B. W. J. H., Benros, M. E., Klein, R. S., & Vinkers, C. H. (2022). How COVID-19 shaped mental health: From infection to pandemic effects. *Nature Medicine, 28*(10), 2027–2037. https://doi.org/10.1038/s41591-022-02028-2

Primrose, S. B. (2022). *Microbiology of infectious disease: Integrating genomics with natural history*. Oxford University Press. https://doi.org/10.1093/oso/9780192863843.003.0003

Procopius. (551 AD). *History of the wars: Book II (H. B. Dewing, trans, 1914)*. Heinemann.

Ramamurthy, T., & Ghosh, A. (2021). A re-look at Cholera pandemics from early times to now in the current era of epidemiology. *Journal of Disaster Research, 16*(1), 110–117. https://doi.org/10.20965/jdr.2021.p0110

Reynolds, C. (2022). Transport Canada fines passengers on Sunwing party flight. *Globe and Mail*. https://www.theglobeandmail.com/business/article-transport-canada-fines-passengers-on-sunwing-party-flight-2/

Robinson, E., & Daly, M. (2021). Explaining the rise and fall of psychological distress during the Covid-19 crisis in the United States: Longitudinal evidence from the Understanding America Study. *British Journal of Health Psychology, 26*(2), 570–587. https://doi.org/10.1111/bjhp.12493

Shin, Y., Berkowitz, B., & Kim, M. J. (2020). How a South Korean church helped fuel the spread of the coronavirus. *Washington Post*. https://www.washingtonpost.com/graphics/2020/world/coronavirus-south-korea-church/

Shryock, R. H. (1960). *Medicine and society in America, 1660–1860*. New York University Press.

Snowden, F. M. (2019). *Epidemics and society: From the Black Death to the present*. Yale University Press.

Soper, G. A. (1939). The curious career of Typhoid Mary. *Bulletin of the New York Academy of Medicine, 15*, 698–712.

Spinney, L. (2017). *Pale rider: The Spanish flu of 1918 and how it changed the world*. Vintage.

Spinney, L. (2020, March 11). Closed borders and "black weddings": What the 1918 flu teaches us about coronavirus. *The Guardian*. https://www.theguardian.com/world/2020/mar/11/closed-borders-and-black-weddings-what-the-1918-flu-teaches-us-about-coronavirus#:~:text=Zamora%20went%20on%20to%20record,of%20the%20highest%20in%20Europe.&text=He%20died%20of%20flu%20a,is%20vastly%20different%20from%201918

Spokane Daily Chronicle. (1918, October 29). Wholesome fear of influenza is needed by city. *Spokane Daily Chronicle*, 1.

Stango, V., & Zinman, J. (2009). Exponential growth bias and household finance. *Journal of Finance, 64*(6), 2807–2849. https://doi.org/10.1111/j.1540-6261.2009.01518.x

Steel, D. (1918). Plague writing: From Boccaccio to Camus. *Journal of European Studies, 11*, 88–110.

Stein, R. A. (2010). Super-spreaders in infectious disease. *International Journal of Infectious Disease, 15*, e510. https://doi.org/10.1016/j.ijid.2010.06.020

Swenson, R. M. (1988). Plagues, history, and AIDS. *American Scholar, 57*(2), 183–200.

Taylor, S. (2021). Understanding and managing pandemic-related panic buying. *Journal of Anxiety Disorders, 78*, article 102364. https://doi.org/10.1016/j.janxdis.2021.102364

Taylor, S. (2022). The psychology of pandemics. *Annual Review of Clinical Psychology, 18*, 581–609. https://doi.org/10.1146/annurev-clinpsy-072720-020131

Taylor, S., Landry, C. A., Paluszek, M. M., Fergus, T. A., McKay, D., & Asmundson, G. J. G. (2020). Covid stress syndrome: Concept, structure, and correlates. *Depression and Anxiety, 37*, 706–714. https://doi.org/10.1002/da.23071

Temime, L., Opatowski, L., Pannet, Y., Brun-Buisson, C., Boëlle, P. Y., & Guillemot, D. (2009). Peripatetic health-care workers as potential superspreaders. *PNAS, 106*, 18420–18425. https://doi.org/10.1073/pnas.0900974106

Thucydides. (431 BC). *The history of the Peloponnesian War* (R. Crawley, Trans., 2009). Project Gutenberg. www.gutenberg.org

Tomori, O. (2004). Yellow fever: The recurring plague. *Critical Reviews in Clinical Laboratory Sciences, 41*(4), 391–427. https://doi.org/10.1080/10408360490497474

Tzeng, N., Chung, C., Chang, C., Chang, H., Kao, Y., Chang, S., et al. (2020). What could we learn from SARS when facing the mental health issues related to the COVID-19 outbreak? A nationwide cohort study in Taiwan. *Translational Psychiatry, 10*(1), article 339. https://doi.org/10.1038/s41398-020-01021-y

Verdery, A. M., Smith-Greenaway, E., Margolis, R., & Daw, J. (2020). Tracking the reach of COVID-19 kin loss with a bereavement multiplier applied to the United States. *PNAS, 117*, 17695–17701. https://doi.org/10.1073/pnas.2007476117

Walker, P. (2021, August 20). 9,000 Covid cases linked to Euro 2020 games in mass events scheme. *The Guardian*. https://www.theguardian.com/world/2021/aug/20/9000-covid-cases-linked-to-euro-2020-games-in-mass-events-scheme

WHO. (2021). Preventing the next pandemic. *Bulletin of the World Health Organization, 99*(5), 326–327. https://doi.org/10.2471/BLT.21.020521

WHO. (2023a). Cholera. https://www.who.int/news-room/fact-sheets/detail/cholera

WHO. (2023b). Statement on the fifteenth meeting of the IHR (2005) Emergency Committee on the COVID-19 pandemic. https://www.who.int/news/item/05-05-2023-statement-on-the-fifteenth-meeting-of-the-international-health-regulations-(2005)-emergency-committee-regarding-the-coronavirus-disease-(covid-19)-pandemic

WHO. (2024a). HIV. https://www.who.int/data/gho/data/themes/hiv-aids#:~:text=Global%20situation%20and%20trends%3A,people%20have%20died%20of%20HIV

WHO. (2024b). MERS situation update. https://www.emro.who.int/health-topics/mers-cov/mers-outbreaks.html

Wilson, J. M., Iannarone, M., & Wang, C. (2009). Media reporting of the emergence of the 1968 influenza pandemic in Hong Kong: Implications for modern-day situational awareness. *Disaster Medicine & Public Health Preparedness, 3*(Suppl 2), S148–S153. https://doi.org/10.1097/DMP.0b013e3181abd603

Wnuk, A., Oleksy, T., & Maison, D. (2020). The acceptance of Covid-19 tracking technologies: The role of perceived threat, lack of control, and ideological beliefs. *PLOS ONE, 15*(9), article e0238973. https://doi.org/10.1371/journal.pone.0238973

Wu, J. S.-T., Hauert, C., Kremen, C., & Zhao, J. (2022). A framework on polarization, cognitive inflexibility, and rigid cognitive specialization. *Frontiers in Psychology, 13*. https://doi.org/10.3389/fpsyg.2022.776891

Zinn, J. O. (2020). "A monstrous threat": How a state of exception turns into a "new normal." *Journal of Risk Research, 23*(7–8), 1083–1091. https://doi.org/10.1080/13669877.2020.1758194

Chapter 2

American Psychiatric Association. (2022). *Diagnostic and statistical manual of mental disorders* (5th ed., text rev.). Author.

Anonymous. (1849). Fear a cause of epidemics. *New England Botanic, Medical & Surgical Journal, 3*(5), 84–86.

Associated Press. (2021). India's crematoriums overwhelmed as COVID-19 patients scramble for medical help. *Associated Press*. https://www.cbc.ca/news/world/india-covid19-patients-creamatorium-1.6001536

Bai, Y., Lin, C.-C., Lin, C.-Y., Chen, J.-Y., Chue, C.-M., & Chou, P. (2004). Survey of stress reactions among health care workers involved with the SARS outbreak. *Psychiatric Services, 55*, 1055–1057. https://doi.org/10.1176/appi.ps.55.9.1055

Barrett, R., & Brown, P. J. (2008). Stigma in the time of influenza: Social and institutional responses to pandemic emergencies. *Journal of Infectious Diseases, 197*(Suppl 1), S34–S37. https://doi.org/10.1086/524986

Barry, J. M. (2018). *The great influenza*. Penguin Random House.

Bhuiyan, A., Sakib, N., Pakpour, A., Griffiths, M., & Mamun, M. (2020). COVID-19-related suicides in Bangladesh due to lockdown and economic factors: Case study evidence from media reports. *International Journal of Mental Health and Addiction, 19*, 2110–2115. https://doi.org/10.1007/s11469-020-00307-y

Bishop, G. D., Alva, A. L., Cantu, L., & Rittiman, T. K. (1991). Responses to persons with AIDS: Fear of contagion or stigma? *Journal of Applied Social Psychology, 21*(23), 1877–1888. https://doi.org/10.1111/j.1559-1816.1991.tb00511.x

Bower, J. E., & Kuhlman, K. R. (2023). Psychoneuroimmunology: An introduction to immune-to-brain communication and its implications for clinical psychology. *Annual Review of Clinical Psychology, 19*, 331–359. https://doi.org/10.1146/annurev-clinpsy-080621-045153

Bower, J. E., Radin, A., & Kuhlman, K. R. (2022). Psychoneuroimmunology in the time of COVID-19: Why neuro-immune interactions matter for mental and physical health. *Behaviour Research and Therapy, 154*, article 104104. https://doi.org/10.1016/j.brat.2022.104104

Butcher, T. (1855). *"Mordichim": Recollections of cholera in the Barbados, during the middle of the year 1854*. Partidge, Oakey, & Co.

Cabrini, L., Grasselli, G., & Cecconi, M. (2020). Yesterday heroes, today plague doctors: The dark side of celebration. *Intensive Care Medicine, 46*, 1790–1791. https://doi.org/10.1007/s00134-020-06166-4

Cameron, A. (1996). *Procopius and the sixth century*. Routledge.

Cameron, E. (2014). Internalized stigma. In S. O. Okpaku (Ed.), *Essentials of global mental health*. (pp. 72–77). Cambridge University Press. https://doi.org/10.1017/CBO9781139136341.010

Chan, B. T., & Tsai, A. C. (2017). Personal contact with HIV-positive persons is associated with reduced HIV-related stigma: Cross-sectional analysis of general population surveys from 26 countries in sub-Saharan Africa. *Journal of the International AIDS Society, 20*(1), article 21395. https://doi.org/10.7448/IAS.20.1.21395

Chang, A., Schulz, P. J., Tu, S., & Liu, M. T. (2020). Communicative blame in online communication of the COVID-19 pandemic: Computational approach of stigmatizing cues and negative sentiment gauged with automated analytic techniques. *Journal of Medical Internet Research, 22*(11), article e21504. https://doi.org/10.2196/21504

Chen, Y., Qin, G., Chen, J., Xu, J., Feng, D., Wu, X., et al. (2020). Comparison of face-touching behaviors before and during the coronavirus disease 2019 pandemic. *JAMA Network Open, 3*, article e2016924. https://doi.org/10.1001/jamanetworkopen.2020.16924

Cheng, C. (2004). To be paranoid is the standard? Panic responses to SARS out-break in the Hong Kong Special Administrative Region. *Asian Perspective, 28*, 67–98. https://doi.org/10.1353/apr.2004.0034

Chenneville, T., Gabbidon, K., Drake, H., & Rodriguez, L. (2019). Preliminary findings from the HIV SEERs project: A community-based participatory research program to reduce HIV stigma among youth in Kenya. *Journal of the Association of Nurses in AIDS Care, 30*(4), 462–473. https://doi.org/10.1097/JNC.0000000000000019

Clapp, T. (1857). *Autobiographical sketches and recollections, during a thirty-five years residence in New Orleans.* Phillips, Sampson & Co.

Cohn, S. K. (2012). Pandemics: Waves of disease, waves of hate from the Plague of Athens to A.I.D.S. *Historical Research, 85*(230), 535–555. https://doi.org/10.1111/j.1468-2281.2012.00603.x

Cohn, S. K. (2018). *Epidemics: Hate and compassion from the plague of Athens to AIDS.* Oxford University Press.

Crocker, J., Major, B., & Steele, C. (1998). Social stigma. In D. Gilbert, S. T. Fiske, & G. Lindzey (Eds.), *Handbook of social psychology* (4th ed.) (pp. 504–553). McGraw-Hill.

D'Irsay, S. (1927). Defense reactions during the Black Death, 1348–1349. *Annals of Medical History, 9*, 169–179.

Frye, V., Paige, M. Q., Gordon, S., Matthews, D., Musgrave, G., Kornegay, M., et al. (2017). Developing a community-level anti-HIV/AIDS stigma and homophobia intervention in New York City: The project CHHANGE model. *Evaluation and Program Planning, 63*, 45–53. https://doi.org/10.1016/j.evalprogplan.2017.03.004

Glaser, R., & Kiecolt-Glaser, J. K. (2005). Stress-induced immune dysfunction: Implications for health. *Nature Reviews Immunology, 5*, 243–251. https://doi.org/10.1038/nri1571

Goffman, E. (1963). *Stigma: Notes on the management of spoiled identity.* Simon and Schuster.

Gowen, B. S. (1907). Some aspects of pestilences and other epidemics. *American Journal of Psychology, 18*(1), 1–60. https://doi.org/10.2307/1412171

Graves, C. (1969). *Invasion by virus: Can it happen again?* Icon Books.

Gronholm, P. C., Nosé, M., van Brakel, W. H., Eaton, J., Ebenso, B., Fiekert, K., et al. (2021). Reducing stigma and discrimination associated with COVID-19: Early stage pandemic rapid review and practical recommendations. *Epidemiology and Psychiatric Sciences, 30*, article e15. https://doi.org/10.1017/S2045796021000056

Herek, G. M., & Capitanio, J. P. (1993). Public reactions to AIDS in the United States: A second decade of stigma. *American Journal of Public Health, 83*, 574–577. https://doi.org/10.2105/ajph.83.4.574

Irwin, M. R., & Slavich, G. M. (2017). Psychoneuroimmunology. In J. T. Cacioppo, L. G. Tassinary, & G. G. Berntson (Eds.), *Handbook of psychophysiology* (4th ed., pp. 377–397). Cambridge University Press.

Jäger, H. (1988). AIDS—psychosocial aspects. In H. Jäger, Welch, J., & Francis, J. L. (Eds.), *AIDS phobia: Disease pattern and possibilities of treatment* (pp. 35–46). Halstead.

Jäger, H., Welch, J., & Francis, J. L. (1988). *AIDS phobia: Disease pattern and possibilities of treatment*. Halsted.

Jefferson, T., Dooley, L., Ferroni, E., Al-Ansary, L. A., van Driel, M. L., Bawazeer, G. A., et al. (2023). Physical interventions to interrupt or reduce the spread of respiratory viruses. *Cochrane Database of Systematic Reviews*, CD006207. https://doi.org/10.1002/14651858.CD006207.pub6

Johnson, N. (2006). *Britain and the 1918–19 influenza pandemic*. Routledge.

Keren, G., & Gerritsen, L. E. M. (1999). On the robustness and possible accounts of ambiguity aversion. *Acta Psychologica*, 103(1–2), 149–172. https://doi.org/10.1016/S0001-6918(99)00034-7

Khare, V. (2021). The India Covid patients whose lonely death went viral. *BBC News*. https://www.bbc.com/news/world-asia-india-57098625

Kiecolt-Glaser, J. K. (2009). Psychoneuroimmunology: Psychology's gateway to the biomedical future. *Perspectives on Psychological Science*, 4, 367–369. https://doi.org/10.1111/j.1745-6924.2009.01139.x

Koh, D., Lim, M., Chia, S., Ko, S., Qian, F., Ng, V., et al. (2005). Risk perception and impact of severe acute respiratory syndrome (SARS) on work and personal lives of healthcare workers in Singapore: What can we learn? *Medical Care*, 43, 676–682. https://doi.org/10.1097/01.mlr.0000167181.36730.cc

Kumar, P. R. K. (2013). The role of social rituals in well-being. In A. Morandi & A. N. Narayanan Nambi (Eds.), *An integrated view of health and well-being: Bridging Indian and Western knowledge* (Vol. 5, pp. 83–98). Springer. https://doi.org/10.1007/978-94-007-6689-1_6

Lee, W. (1869). *Daniel Defoe: His life, and recently discovered writings* (Vol. 2). Hotten.

Lin, A. L., Vittinghoff, E., Olgin, J. E., Pletcher, M. J., & Marcus, G. M. (2021). Body weight changes during pandemic-related shelter-in-place in a longitudinal cohort study. *JAMA Network Open*, 4(3), article e212536. https://doi.org/10.1001/jamanetworkopen.2021.2536

Lohiniva, A.-L., Benkirane, M., Numair, T., Mahdy, A., Saleh, H., Zahran, A., et al. (2016). HIV stigma intervention in a low-HIV prevalence setting: A pilot study in an Egyptian healthcare facility. *AIDS Care*, 28(5), 644–652. https://doi.org/10.1080/09540121.2015.1124974

Lyon, I. P., Tenney, C. F., & Szerlip, L. (1919). Some clinical observations on the influenza epidemic at Camp Upton. *JAMA*, 72(24), 1726–1731. https://doi.org/10.1001/jama.1919.02610240014004

Markel, H. (2004). *When germs travel: Six major epidemics that have invaded America since 1900 and the fears they have unleashed*. Pantheon.

Moote, A. L., & Moote, D. C. (2004). *The great plague: The story of London's most deadly year*. Johns Hopkins University Press.

Moraes, L. J., Miranda, M. B., Loures, L. F., Mainieri, A. G., & Mármora, C. H. C. (2017). A systematic review of psychoneuroimmunology-based interventions. *Psychology, Health & Medicine*, 23, 635–652. https://doi.org/10.1080/13548506.2017.1417607

Morens, D. M. (2011). Remembering Daumier's Blue Period. *EcoHealth*, 8(4), 527–530. https://doi.org/10.1007/s10393-012-0745-y

Morens, D. M., Folkers, G. K., & Fauci, A. S. (2008). Emerging infections: A perpetual challenge. *Lancet Infectious Diseases*, 8, 710–719. https://doi.org/10.1016/S1473-3099(08)70256-1

Nardi, P. M., & Bolton, R. (1991). Gay-bashing: Violence and aggression against gay men and lesbians. In R. Baenninger (Ed.), *Targets of violence and aggression*. (pp. 349–400). North-Holland. https://doi.org/10.1016/S0166-4115(08)61062-6

Nohl, J. (1926). *The Black Death: A chronical of the plague*. Allen & Unwin.

Olson, G. (2002). Plague on the prairie: The cholera epidemic of 1833 and its impact on one Illinois town. *Illinois Heritage*, 5(1), 6–9.

Parets, M. (1651). *A journal of the plague year: The diary of the Barcelona tanner Miquel Parets 1651* (J. S. Amelang, trans. & ed., 1991). Oxford University Press.
Pearse, R. (2017). John of Ephesus describes the Justinianic plague. https://www.roger-pearse.com/weblog/2017/05/10/john-of-ephesus-describes-the-justinianic-plague
Pettigrew, E. (1983). *The silent enemy: Canada and the deadly flu of 1918*. Western Producer Prairie Books.
Phillips, A. C., Carroll, D., Burns, V. E., & Drayson, M. (2005). Neuroticism, cortisol reactivity, and antibody response to vaccination. *Psychophysiology, 42*, 232–238. https://doi.org/10.1111/j.1469-8986.2005.00281.x
Prasad, S. K., Karahda, A., Singh, P., & Gupta, R. (2020). Role of mental health professionals in dealing with the stigma attached to COVID-19. *General Psychiatry, 33*(5), article e100298. https://doi.org/10.1136/gpsych-2020-100298
Procopius. (551 AD). *History of the wars: Book II* (H. B. Dewing, trans, 1914). Heinemann.
Rosenberg, C. E. (1987). *The cholera years: The United States in 1832, 1849, and 1866*. University of Chicago Press.
Sander, U. (1988). The delusion of being infected. In H. Jäger, Welch, J., & Francis, J. L. (Ed.), *AIDS phobia: Disease pattern and possibilities of treatment* (pp. 7–10). Halstead.
Sandhu, P., Shah, A. B., Ahmad, F. B., Kerr, J., Demeke, H. B., Graeden, E., et al. (2022). Emergency department and intensive care unit overcrowding and ventilator shortages in US hospitals during the COVID-19 pandemic, 2020–2021. *Public Health Reports, 137*(4), 796–802. https://doi.org/10.1177/00333549221091781
Schibalski, J. V., Müller, M., Ajdacic-Gross, V., Vetter, S., Rodgers, S., Oexle, N., et al. (2017). Stigma-related stress, shame and avoidant coping reactions among members of the general population with elevated symptom levels. *Comprehensive Psychiatry, 74*, 224–230. https://doi.org/10.1016/j.comppsych.2017.02.001
Schoch-Spana, M. (2004). Lessons from the 1918 pandemic influenza: Psychosocial consequences of a catastrophic outbreak of disease. In R. J. Ursano, A. E. Norwood, & C. S. Fullerton (Eds.), *Bioterrorism: Psychological and public health interventions* (pp. 38–55). Cambridge University Press.
Shryock, R. H. (1960). *Medicine and society in America, 1660–1860*. New York University Press.
Slack, P. (1985). *The impact of plague in Tudor and Stuart England*. Routledge.
Taylor, S. (2017). *Clinician's guide to PTSD* (2nd ed.). Guilford.
Taylor, S. (2022). The psychology of pandemics. *Annual Review of Clinical Psychology, 18*, 581–609. https://doi.org/10.1146/annurev-clinpsy-072720-020131
Taylor, S., Landry, C. A., Rachor, G. S., Paluszek, M. M., & Asmundson, G. J. G. (2020). Fear and avoidance of healthcare workers: An important, under-recognized form of stigmatization during the COVID-19 pandemic. *Journal of Anxiety Disorders, 75*, article 102289. https://doi.org/10.1016/j.janxdis.2020.102289
Taylor, S., Paluszek, M., Rachor, G. S., McKay, D., & Asmundson, G. J. G. (2021). Substance use and abuse, COVID-19-related distress, and disregard for social distancing: A network analysis. *Addictive Behaviors, 114*, article 106754. https://doi.org/10.1016/j.addbeh.2020.106754
Thucydides. (431 BC). *The history of the Peloponnesian War* (R. Crawley, Trans., 2009). Project Gutenberg. www.gutenberg.org
Tomes, N. (1999). *The gospel of germs: Men, women, and the microbe in American life*. Harvard University Press.
Vega, M. Y. (2016). Combating stigma and fear: Applying psychosocial lessons learned from the HIV epidemic and SARS to the current Ebola crisis. In J. Kuriansky (Ed.), *The psychosocial aspects of a deadly epidemic: What Ebola has taught us about holistic healing*, (pp. 271–286). Praeger.

White, R., & Cunningham, A. M. (1991). *Ryan White, my own story*. Dial.

WHO. (2020a). *Advice on the use of masks the community, during home care and in health care settings in the context of the novel coronavirus (2019-nCoV) outbreak*. WHO.

WHO. (2020b). *Mask use in the context of COVID-19*. WHO.

Xu, J., Sun, G., Cao, W., Fan, W., Pan, Z., Yao, Z., et al. (2021). Stigma, discrimination, and hate crimes in Chinese-speaking world amid Covid-19 pandemic. *Asian Journal of Criminology, 16*(1), 51–74. https://doi.org/10.1007/s11417-020-09339-8

Yuan, K., Huang, X., Yan, W., Zhang, Y., Gong, Y., Su, S., et al. (2022). A systematic review and meta-analysis on the prevalence of stigma in infectious diseases, including COVID-19: A call to action. *Molecular Psychiatry, 27*(1), 19–33. https://doi.org/10.1038/s41380-021-01295-8

Chapter 3

Aiello, A., Coulborn, R., Aragon, T., Baker, M., Burrus, B., Cowling, B., et al. (2010). Research findings from nonpharmaceutical intervention studies for pandemic influenza and current gaps in the research. *American Journal of Infection Control, 38*, 251–258. https://doi.org/10.1016/j.ajic.2009.12.007

Baldwin, P. C. (2003). How night air became GOOD AIR, 1776–1930. *Environmental History, 8*(3), 412–429. https://doi.org/10.2307/3986202

Bloomberg. (2022a). The best and worst places to be as world enters next Covid phase. https://www.bloomberg.com/graphics/covid-resilience-ranking/#xj4y7vzkg?leadSource=uverify%20wall?leadSource=uverify%20wall

Bloomberg. (2022b). Methodology: Inside Bloomberg's Covid Resiliency Ranking. https://www.bnnbloomberg.ca/inside-bloomberg-s-covid-resilience-ranking-1.1526943

Byrne, J. P. (2006). *Daily life during the Black Death*. Greenwood.

CDC. (2020). Considerations for wearing masks, https://www.cdc.gov/coronavirus/2019-ncov/prevent-getting-sick/cloth-face-cover-guidance.html

CDC. (2024). Aerial spraying. https://www.cdc.gov/mosquitoes/mosquito-control/aerial-spraying.html#:~:text=Aerial%20spraying%20is%20used%20to,from%20a%20mosquito%2Dborne%20disease

Charles River Editors. (2020). *The 1889–1890 flu pandemic: The history of the 19th century's last major global outbreak*. Author.

Chicago Herald and Examiner. (1918, October 4). Police given order to war on influenza. *Chicago Herald and Examiner*. http://hdl.handle.net/2027/spo.1480flu.0001.841

Cohn, S. K. (2008). Epidemiology of the Black Death and successive waves of plague. *Medical History Supplement, 27*, 74–100.

Cohn, S. K. (2018). *Epidemics: Hate and compassion from the plague of Athens to AIDS*. Oxford University Press.

Elliott, C. (2024). *Pox Romana: The plague that shook the Roman world*. Princeton Universtiy Press.

Erasmus, V., Daha, T. J., Brug, H., Richardus, J. H., Behrendt, M. D., Vos, M. C., et al. (2010). Systematic review of studies on compliance with hand hygiene guidelines in hospital care. *Infection Control & Hospital Epidemiology, 31*, 283–294. https://doi.org/10.1086/650451

Gilles, I., Bangerter, A., Clémence, A., Green, E., Krings, F., Staerklé, C., et al. (2011). Trust in medical organizations predicts pandemic (H1N1) 2009 vaccination behavior and perceived efficacy of protection measures in the Swiss public. *European Journal of Epidemiology, 26*, 203–210. https://doi.org/10.1007/s10654-011-9577-2

Haug, N., Geyrhofer, L., Londei, A., Dervic, E., Desvars-Larrive, A., Loreto, V., et al. (2020). Ranking the effectiveness of worldwide COVID-19 government interventions. *Nature Human Behaviour, 4*(12), 1303–1312. https://doi.org/10.1038/s41562-020-01009-0

Hoffmann, T., Bakhit, M., Krzyzaniak, N., Del Mar, C., Scott, A. M., & Glasziou, P. (2021). Soap versus sanitiser for preventing the transmission of acute respiratory infections in the community: A systematic review with meta-analysis and dose-response analysis. *BMJ Open, 11*(8), article e046175. https://doi.org/10.1136/bmjopen-2020-046175

Jefferson, T., Dooley, L., Ferroni, E., Al-Ansary, L. A., van Driel, M. L., Bawazeer, G. A., et al. (2023). Physical interventions to interrupt or reduce the spread of respiratory viruses. *Cochrane Database of Systematic Reviews*, CD006207. https://doi.org/10.1002/14651858.CD006207.pub6

Judah, G., Donachie, P., Cobb, E., Schmidt, W., Holland, M., & Curtis, V. (2010). Dirty hands: Bacteria of faecal origin on commuters' hands. *Epidemiology and Infection, 138*, 409–414. https://doi.org/10.1017/S0950268809990641

Karamanou, M., Panayiotakopoulos, G., Tsoucalas, G., Kousoulis, A. A., & Androutsos, G. (2012). From miasmas to germs: A historical approach to theories of infectious disease transmission. *Le Infezioni in Medicina, 20*(1), 58–62.

Lazarus, J., Romero, D., Kopka, C., Karim, S., Abu-Raddad, L., Almeida, G., et al. (2022). A multinational Delphi consensus to end the COVID-19 public health threat. *Nature, 611*(7935), 332–345. https://doi.org/10.1038/s41586-022-05398-2

Mead, R. (1744). *A discourse on the plague* (9th ed.). Millar.

New York Times. (1918, November 17). Epidemic lessons against next time. *New York Times*, 42.

Pfattheicher, S., Strauch, C., Diefenbacher, S., & Schnuerch, R. (2018). A field study on watching eyes and hand hygiene compliance in a public restroom. *Journal of Applied Social Psychology, 48*, 188–194. https://doi.org/10.1111/jasp.12501

Robins, N. (2005). *Copeland's cure: Homeopathy and the war between conventional and alternative medicine*. Knopf.

Slack, P. (1985). *The impact of plague in Tudor and Stuart England*. Routledge.

Spokane Daily Chronicle. (1918, October 29). Wholesome fear of influenza is needed by city. *Spokane Daily Chronicle*, 1.

Taylor, S., Paluszek, M., Landry, C., Rachor, G. S., & Asmundson, G. J. G. (2020). Worry, avoidance, and coping during the COVID-19 pandemic: A comprehensive network analysis. *Journal of Anxiety Disorders, 76*, article 102327. https://doi.org/10.1016/j.janxdis.2020.102327

Tomes, N. (1999). *The gospel of germs: Men, women, and the microbe in American life*. Harvard University Press.

Tomes, N. (2010). "Destroyer and teacher": Managing the masses during the 1918–1919 influenza pandemic. *Public Health Reports, 125 (Suppl. 3)*, 48–62. https://doi.org/10.1177/00333549101250S308

WHO. (2008). *WHO outbreak communication planning guide*. Author.

WHO. (2012). Vaccines against influenza WHO position paper. *Weekly Epidemiological Record, 87*, 461–476.

WHO. (2021a). Coronavirus disease (COVID-19) advice for the public. https://www.who.int/emergencies/diseases/novel-coronavirus-2019/advice-for-public

WHO. (2021b). Preventing the next pandemic. *Bulletin of the World Health Organization, 99*(5), 326–327. https://doi.org/10.2471/BLT.21.020521

WHO Writing Group. (2006). Nonpharmaceutical interventions for pandemic influenza, national and community measures. *Emerging Infectious Diseases, 12*, 88–94.

Wolfe, M. K., Gallandat, K., Daniels, K., Desmarais, A. M., Scheinman, P., & Lantagne, D. (2017). Handwashing and Ebola virus disease outbreaks: A randomized comparison of soap, hand sanitizer, and 0.05% chlorine solutions on the inactivation and removal of model organisms Phi6 and E. coli from hands and persistence in rinse water. *PLOS ONE, 12*(2), article e0172734. https://doi.org/10.1371/journal.pone.0172734

Chapter 4

Abel, E. L. (2018). Syphilis: The history of an eponym. *Names: A Journal of Onomastics, 66*(2), 96–102. https://doi.org/10.1080/00277738.2017.1415522

Altman, L. K. (1982, May 11). New homosexual disorder worries health officials. *New York Times*, C1. https://www.nytimes.com/1982/05/11/science/new-homosexual-disorder-worries-health-officials.html

Brennan, R. O., & Durack, D. T. (1981). Gay compromise syndrome. *Lancet, 2*(8259), 1338–1339. https://doi.org/10.1016/s0140-6736(81)91352-0

Business North Carolina. (2010). Pork producers aren't living high on the hog. *Business North Carolina, 30*(1), 18.

Copeland, R. S. (1923, April 24). What sleeping sickness is and what is known about it. *Logansport Pharos Tribune*, 6.

Dodsworth, L. (2021). *A state of fear: How the UK government weaponised fear during the COVID-19 pandemic*. Pinter & Martin.

Evans, H., & Bartholomew, R. E. (2009). *Outbreak! The encyclopedia of extraordinary social behavior*. Anomalist Books.

Giordano, A., Schwarz, G., Cacciaguerra, L., Esposito, F., & Filippi, M. (2020). COVID-19: Can we learn from encephalitis lethargica? *Lancet Neurology, 19*(7), p. 570. https://doi.org/10.1016/S1474-4422(20)30189-7

Goldenberg, J. L., & Arndt, J. (2008). The implications of death for health: A terror management health model for behavioral health promotion. *Psychological Review, 115*, 1032–1053. https://doi.org/10.1037/a0013326

Kanadiya, M. K., & Sallar, A. M. (2011). Preventive behaviors, beliefs, and anxieties in relation to the swine flu outbreak among college students aged 18–24 years. *Journal of Public Health, 19*, 139–145. https://doi.org/10.1007/s10389-010-0373-3

Kaur, H., Sidhu, T. K., & Coonar, P. S. (2015). Knowledge, attitude and practices regarding swine flu among adult population. *Indian Journal of Community Health, 27*(3), 402–410.

Kupferschmidt, K. (2015). Rules of the name. *Science, 348*(6236), p. 745. https://doi.org/10.1126/science.348.6236.745

MacArthur, K., & Thompson, S. (2005). KFC preps bird-flu fear plan. *Advertising Age, 76*(45), 1–2.

National Chicken Council. (2021). Questions and answers on avian influenza ("bird flu"), https://www.nationalchickencouncil.org/bird-flu-its-not-in-your-food/questions-and-answers-on-avian-influenza/

Nerlich, B., & Halliday, C. (2007). Avian flu: The creation of expectations in the interplay between science and the media. *Sociology of Health & Illness, 29*, 46–65. https://doi.org/10.1111/j.1467-9566.2007.00517.x

Nick, I. M. (2021). In the name of hate: An editorial note on the role geographically marked names for COVID-19 have played in the pandemic of anti-Asian violence. *Names: A Journal of Onomastics, 69*(2), 1–10. https://doi.org/10.5195/names.2021.2276

Peters, G.-J. Y., Ruiter, R. A. C., & Kok, G. (2013). Threatening communication: A critical re-analysis and a revised meta-analytic test of fear appeal theory. *Health Psychology Review, 7* (Suppl. 1), S8–S31. https://doi.org/10.1080/17437199.2012.703527

Pilkington, E. (2009, April 28). What's in a name? Governments debate "Swine Flu" versus "Mexican Flu." *The Guardian*. http://www.theguardian.com/world/2009/apr/28/mexican-swine-flu-pork-name

Singh, S., Kaur, P., & Singh, G. (2013). Study to assess the awareness, perception and myths regarding swine flu among educated common public in Patiala district. *International Journal of Research & Development of Health, 1*(2), 54–60.

Taylor, S. (2019). *The psychology of pandemics: Preparing for the next global outbreak of infectious disease*. Cambridge Scholars Publishing.

Taylor, S. (2022). The psychology of pandemics. *Annual Review of Clinical Psychology, 18*, 581–609. https://doi.org/10.1146/annurev-clinpsy-072720-020131

Tomes, N. (2010). "Destroyer and teacher": Managing the masses during the 1918–1919 influenza pandemic. *Public Health Reports, 125 (Suppl. 3)*, 48–62. https://doi.org/10.1177/00333549101250S308

Toppenberg-Pejcic, D., Noyes, J., Allen, T., Alexander, N., Vanderford, M., & Gamhewage, G. (2019). Emergency risk communication: Lessons learned from a rapid review of recent gray literature on Ebola, Zika, and yellow fever. *Health Communication, 34*(4), 437–455. https://doi.org/10.1080/10410236.2017.1405488

Viveki, R. G., Halappanavar, A. B., Patil, M. S., Joshi, A. V., Gunagi, P., & Halki, S. B. (2012). Swine flu (H1N1 influenza): Awareness profile of visitors of swine flu screening booths in Belgaum city, Karnataka. *Journal of the Indian Medical Association, 110*(6), 358–361.

White, A. E., Johnson, K. A., & Kwan, V. S. Y. (2014). Four ways to infect me: Spatial, temporal, social, and probability distance influence evaluations of disease threat. *Social Cognition, 32*, 239–255. https://doi.org/10.1521/soco.2014.32.3.239

WHO. (2005). *WHO checklist for influenza pandemic preparedness planning*. Author.

WHO. (2008). *WHO outbreak communication planning guide*. Author.

WHO. (2015). World Health Organization best pratices for the naming of new human infectious diseases. https://apps.who.int/iris/bitstream/handle/10665/163636/WHO_HSE_FOS_15.1_eng.pdf

WHO. (2022). WHO recommends new name for monkeypox disease. https://www.who.int/news/item/28-11-2022-who-recommends-new-name-for-monkeypox-disease

Wilson, M. (2009, October). "Swine" flu destroying pork market. *Irish Farmers Monthly*, 20.

Chapter 5

Alcalde-Cabero, E., Almazán-Isla, J., López, F., Ara-Callizo, J., Avellanal, F., Casasnovas, C., et al. (2016). Guillain-Barré syndrome following the 2009 pandemic monovalent and seasonal trivalent influenza vaccination campaigns in Spain from 2009 to 2011: Outcomes from active surveillance by a neurologist network, and records from a country-wide hospital discharge database. *BMC Neurology, 16*, article 75. https://doi.org/10.1186/s12883-016-0598-z

Antommaria, A. H., & Prows, C. A. (2018). Content analysis of requests for religious exemptions from a mandatory influenza vaccination program for healthcare personnel. *Journal of Medical Ethics, 44*, 389–391. https://doi.org/10.1136/medethics-2017-104271

Babcock, H. M., Jernigan, J. A., & Relman, D. A. (2014). The importance of influenza vaccination. *JAMA Internal Medicine, 174*, 644–645. https://doi.org/10.1001/jamainternmed.2013.11174

Bamji, A. (2019). Health passes, print and public health in early modern Europe. *Social History of Medicine, 32*(3), 441–464. https://doi.org/10.1093/shm/hkx104

Bangerter, A., Krings, F., Mouton, A., Gilles, I., Green, E. G. T., & Clémence, A. (2012). Longitudinal investigation of public trust in institutions relative to the 2009 H1N1 pandemic in Switzerland. *PLOS ONE, 7*, article e49806. https://doi.org/10.1371/journal.pone.0049806

Beard, K. R., Brendish, N. J., & Clark, T. W. (2018). Treatment of influenza with neuraminidase inhibitors. *Current Opinion in Infectious Diseases, 31*, 514–519. https://doi.org/10.1097/QCO.0000000000000496

Behrman, A., & Offley, W. (2013). Should influenza vaccination be mandatory for healthcare workers? *BMJ (Clinical Research Ed.), 347*, article f6705. https://doi.org/10.1136/bmj.f6705

Berman, J. M. (2021). When antivaccine sentiment turned violent: The Montréal Vaccine Riot of 1885. *Canadian Medical Association Journal, 193*(14), E490–E492. https://doi.org/10.1503/cmaj.202820

Bliss, M. (1991). *Plague: A story of smallpox in Montreal.* HarperCollins.

Bloomberg. (2022). More than 12.7 billion shots given: Covid-19 tracker. https://www.bloomberg.com/graphics/covid-vaccine-tracker-global-distribution/

Born, K., Ikura, S., & Laupacis, A. (2015). The evidence, ethics and politics of mandatory health care worker vaccination. *Journal of Health Services Research & Policy, 20*, 1–3. https://doi.org/10.1177/1355819614546960

CDC. (2018). Influenza vaccination recommendations, 2017–2018. https://www.cdc.gov/vaccines/ed/flu-recs/

CDC. (2023a). Influenza vaccination coverage for persons 6 months and older. https://www.cdc.gov/flu/fluvaxview/interactive-general-population.htm

CDC. (2023b). Safety of COVID-19 vaccines. https://www.cdc.gov/coronavirus/2019-ncov/vaccines/safety/safety-of-vaccines.html#print

Chen, C., Liu, X., Yan, D., Zhou, Y., Ding, C., Chen, L., et al. (2022). Global influenza vaccination rates and factors associated with influenza vaccination. *International Journal of Infectious Diseases, 125*, 153–163. https://doi.org/10.1016/j.ijid.2022.10.038

Clements, C. J. (2003). Mass psychogenic illness after vaccination. *Drug Safety, 26*(9), 599–604. https://doi.org/10.2165/00002018-200326090-00001

Dolan, B. (2020). Unmasking history: Who was behind the anti-mask league protests during the 1918 influenza epidemic in San Francisco? *Perspectives in Medical Humanities.* https://doi.org/10.34947/M7QP4M

Du, S.-Y., Dai, Y.-X., Li, P.-W., Zhao, N., Li, S., & Zheng, Y. (2022). Vaccinated or not? Survey on attitude toward "approach-avoidance conflict" under uncertainty. *Human Vaccines & Immunotherapeutics, 18*(1), 1–6. https://doi.org/10.1080/21645515.2021.1967038

Eichner, M., Schwehm, M., Duerr, H., Witschi, M., Koch, D., Brockmann, S., et al. (2009). Antiviral prophylaxis during pandemic influenza may increase drug resistance. *BMC Infectious Diseases, 9*, article 4. https://doi.org/10.1186/1471-2334-9-4

Frederick, J., Brown, A., Cummings, D., Gaydos, C., Gibert, C., Gorse, G., et al. (2018). Protecting healthcare personnel in outpatient settings: The influence of mandatory versus nonmandatory influenza vaccination policies on workplace absenteeism during multiple respiratory virus seasons. *Infection Control & Hospital Epidemiology, 39*, 452–461. https://doi.org/10.1017/ice.2018.9

Godlee, F., Smith, J., & Marcovitch, H. (2011). Wakefield's article linking MMR vaccine and autism was fraudulent. *British Medical Journal, 342*, c7452. https://doi.org/10.1136/bmj.c7452

Gouglas, D., Le, T., Henderson, K., Kaloudis, A., Danielsen, T., Hammersland, N., et al. (2018). Estimating the cost of vaccine developent against epidemic infectious diseases: A cost minimisation study. *Lancet Global Health, 6*(12), e1386–e1396. https://doi.org/10.1016/S2214-109X(18)30346-2

Han, P., Zikmund-Fisher, B., Duarte, C., Knaus, M., Black, A., Scherer, A., et al. (2018). Communication of scientific uncertainty about a novel pandemic health threat: Ambiguity aversion and its mechanisms. *Journal of Health Communication, 23*(5), 435–444. https://doi.org/10.1080/10810730.2018.1461961

Heagerty, J. J. (1919). Influenza and vaccination. *Canadian Medical Association Journal, 9*, 226–228.

Henderson, P. (1965). Smallpox and patriotism: The Norfolk riots, 1768–1769. *Virginia Magazine of History & Biography, 73*(4), 413–424.

Holder, J. (2023). Tracking coronavirus vaccinations around the world. *New York Times*. https://www.nytimes.com/interactive/2021/world/covid-vaccinations-tracker.html

Hornsey, M. J., Harris, E. A., & Fielding, K. S. (2018). The psychological roots of anti-vaccination attitudes: A 24-nation investigation. *Health Psychology, 37*, 307–315. https://doi.org/10.1037/hea0000586

Huang, Y., Huang, X., & Yu, R. (2023). The effectiveness of nonfinancial interventions and monetary incentives on COVID-19 vaccination: A meta-analysis. *Health Psychology, 42*(6), 411–424. https://doi.org/10.1037/hea0001288

Jefferson, T., Dooley, L., Ferroni, E., Al-Ansary, L. A., van Driel, M. L., Bawazeer, G. A., et al. (2023). Physical interventions to interrupt or reduce the spread of respiratory viruses. *Cochrane Database of Systematic Reviews*, CD006207. https://doi.org/10.1002/14651858.CD006207.pub6

Lang, J., Erickson, W. W., & Jing-Schmidt, Z. (2021). #MaskOn! #MaskOff! Digital polarization of mask-wearing in the United States during COVID-19. *PLOS ONE, 16*(4), e0250817. https://doi.org/10.1371/journal.pone.0250817

Leibovitch, E. C., & Jacobson, S. (2016). Vaccinations for neuroinfectious disease: A global health priority. *Neurotherapeutics, 13*(3), 562–570. https://doi.org/10.1007/s13311-016-0453-3

Lewin, K. (1935). *A dynamic theory of personality*. McGraw-Hill.

Lukich, N., Kekewich, M., & Roth, V. (2018). Should influenza vaccination be mandatory for healthcare workers? *Healthcare Management Forum, 31*, 214–217. https://doi.org/10.1177/0840470418794209

Macdonald, B. (2021). Attitudes to COVID-19 vaccinations. *OurWorldInData.org*. https://ourworldindata.org/attitudes-to-covid-vaccinations

MacIntyre, C. R., Chughtai, A. A., Fisman, D., & Greenhalgh, T. (2023). Yes, masks reduce the risk of spreading COVID, despite a review saying they don't. *The Conversation*. https://theconversation.com/yes-masks-reduce-the-risk-of-spreading-covid-despite-a-review-saying-they-dont-198992

Mattie, H. J. (2023). Men in tights: Charles de Lorme (1584–1678) and the first plague costume. *European Journal for the History of Medicine and Health*. https://doi.org/10.1163/26667711-BJA10033

Megiddo, I., Drabik, D., Bedford, T., Morton, A., Wesseler, J., & Laxminarayan, R. (2019). Investing in antibiotics to alleviate future catastrophic outcomes: What is the value of having an effective antibiotic to mitigate pandemic influenza? *Health Economics, 28*, 556–571. https://doi.org/10.1002/hec.3867

Milkman, K., Patel, M., Gandhi, L., Graci, H., Gromet, D., Ho, H., et al. (2021). A megastudy of text-based nudges encouraging patients to get vaccinated at an upcoming doctor's appointment. *PNAS, 118*(20), article e2101165118. https://doi.org/10.1073/pnas.2101165118

Morens, D. M., Taubenberger, J. K., & Fauci, A. S. (2008). Predominant role of bacterial pneumonia as a cause of death in pandemic influenza: Implications for pandemic influenza preparedness. *Journal of Infectious Diseases, 198*, 962–970. https://doi.org/10.1086/591708

Morens, D. M., Taubenberger, J. K., Folkers, G. K., & Fauci, A. S. (2010). Pandemic influenza's 500th anniversary. *Clinical Infectious Diseases, 51*, 1442–1444. https://doi.org/10.1086/657429

Murayama, H., Takagi, Y., Tsuda, H., & Kato, Y. (2023). Applying nudge to public health policy: Practical examples and tips for designing nudge interventions. *International Journal of Environmental Research and Public Health, 20*(5), article 3962. https://doi.org/10.3390/ijerph20053962

Needell, J. D. (1987). The Revolta Contra Vacina of 1904: The revolt against "modernization" in belle-epoque Rio de Janeiro. *Hispanic American Historical Review, 67*(2), 233–269. https://doi.org/10.1215/00182168-67.2.233

Oakland Tribune. (1918, November 9). Commuters without masks are arrested. *Oakland Tribune*, 7. https://newspaperarchive.com/oakland-tribune-nov-09-1918-p-7/

Pettigrew, E. (1983). *The silent enemy: Canada and the deadly flu of 1918*. Western Producer Prairie Books.

Rolleston, J. D. (1933). The smallpox pandemic of 1870–1874. *Proceedings of the Royal Society of Medicine, 27*(2), 177–192.

San Francisco Chronicle. (1918, October 29). Three shot in struggle with mask slacker. *San Francisco Chronicle*, 1. http://hdl.handle.net/2027/spo.0030flu.0009.300

San Francisco Examiner. (1918, October 29). "Mask slackers" given jail sentences, fines. *San Francisco Examiner*, 13. http://hdl.handle.net/2027/spo.5710flu.0009.175

Sawchuk, L. A., & Tripp, L. (2021). Managing an epidemic in imperfect times: Encampment and immunity passes in 19th century Gibraltar. *BMJ Global Health, 6*(8), article e006713. https://doi.org/10.1136/bmjgh-2021-006713

Siu, J. Y. (2016). Qualitative study on the shifting sociocultural meanings of the facemask in Hong Kong since the severe acute respiratory syndrome (SARS) outbreak: Implications for infection control in the post-SARS era. *International Journal for Equity in Health, 15*, article 73. https://doi.org/10.1186/s12939-016-0358-0

Skegg, D., Gluckman, P., Boulton, G., Hackmann, H., Karim, S., Piot, P., et al. (2021). Future scenarios for the COVID-19 pandemic. *Lancet, 397*(10276), 777–778. https://doi.org/10.1016/S0140-6736(21)00424-4

Statistics Canada. (2010). *Community Health Survey*. http://www.statcan.gc.ca/daily-quotidien/100719/dq100719beng.htm

SteelFisher, G. K., Blendon, R. J., Ward, J. R. M., Rapoport, R., Kahn, E. B., & Kohl, K. S. (2012). Public response to the 2009 influenza A H1N1 pandemic: A polling study in five countries. *Lancet Infectious Diseases, 12*, 845–850. https://doi.org/10.1016/S1473-3099(12)70206-2

Taha, S., Matheson, K., & Anisman, H. (2013). The 2009 H1N1 influenza pandemic: The role of threat, coping, and media trust on vaccination intentions in Canada. *Journal of Health Communication, 18*, 278–290. https://doi.org/10.1080/10810730.2012.727960

Taylor, S., & Asmundson, G. J. G. (2021). Negative attitudes about facemasks during the COVID-19 pandemic: The dual importance of perceived ineffectiveness and psychological reactance. *PLOS ONE, 16*(2), article e0246317. https://doi.org/10.1371/journal.pone.0246317

Taylor, S., Landry, C. A., Paluszek, M. M., Groenewoud, R., Rachor, G. S., & Asmundson, G. J. G. (2020). A proactive approach for managing COVID-19: The importance of understanding the motivational roots of vaccination hesitancy for SARS-CoV2. *Frontiers in Psychology, 11*, article 575950. https://doi.org/10.3389/fpsyg.2020.575950

Thaler, R. H., & Sunstein, C. R. (2008). *Nudge: Improving decisions about heath, wealth, and happiness*. Yale University Press.

Townsend, G. L. (1965). The plague doctor. *Journal of the History of Medicine and Allied Sciences, 20*, 276–277.

Vandenbos, G. R. (Ed.). (2007). *APA dictionary of psychology*. American Psychological Association.

Wakefield, A. J., Murch, S. H., Anthony, A., Linnell, J., Casson, D. M., Malik, M., et al. (1998). RETRACTED: Ileal-lymphoid-nodular hyperplasia, non-specific colitis, and pervasive developmental disorder in children. *Lancet, 351*(9103), 637–641. https://doi.org/10.1016/S0140-6736(97)11096-0

Wang, T. L., Jing, L., & Bocchini, J. A., Jr. (2017). Mandatory influenza vaccination for all healthcare personnel: A review on justification, implementation and effectiveness. *Current Opinion in Pediatrics, 29*, 606–615. https://doi.org/10.1097/MOP.0000000000000527

WHO. (2012). Vaccines against influenza WHO position paper. *Weekly Epidemiological Record, 87*, 461–476.

WHO. (2019). Ten threats to global health in 2019. https://www.who.int/emergencies/ten-threats-to-global-health-in-2019

Wolfe, R. M., & Sharp, L. K. (2002). Anti-vaccinationists past and present. *BMJ (Clinical Research Ed.), 325*(7361), 430–432. https://doi.org/10.1136/bmj.325.7361.430

Yaqub, O., Castle-Clarke, S., Sevdalis, N., & Chataway, J. (2014). Attitudes to vaccination: A critical review. *Social Science & Medicine, 112*, 1–11. https://doi.org/10.1016/j.socscimed.2014.04.018

Chapter 6

Alonso, M., & Hackney, D. (2020, April 5). Churches hold Palm Sunday services despite state bans on gatherings. *CNN News*. https://www.cnn.com/2020/04/05/us/church-services-palm-sunday-coronavirus-trnd/index.html

Andrew, J., & Baker, M. (2021). The general data protection regulation in the age of surveillance capitalism. *Journal of Business Ethics, 168*(3), 565–578. https://doi.org/10.1007/s10551-019-04239-z

Anonymous. (1665). *The shutting up infected houses as it is practised in England soberly debated*. Sine Nomine.

Anonymous. (1721). *The late dreadful plague at Marseilles compared with that terrible plague in London in the year 1665*. Parker.

Atlanta Constitution. (1918, October 15). Protest is made by theater men. *Atlanta Constitution*, 1. http://hdl.handle.net/2027/spo.7520flu.0016.257

Baltimore Sun. (1918, October 19). Closing the churches and keeping open the saloons. *Baltimore Sun*, 6. http://hdl.handle.net/2027/spo.4550flu.0000.554

Barry, J. M. (2020). The steep costs of "herd immunity." *New York Times, 170*, A27.

Becker, K. M. (2020). More than 200 COVID-19 cases linked to Fitchburg church. *NBC News*. https://www.nbcboston.com/news/local/more-than-200-covid-19-cases-linked-to-fitchburg-church/2225433/?amp

Bentotahewa, V., Hewage, C., & Williams, J. (2021). Solutions to big data privacy and security challenges associated with COVID-19 surveillance systems. *Frontiers in Big Data, 4*, article 645204. https://doi.org/10.3389/fdata.2021.645204

Berkman, B. E. (2008). Mitigating pandemic influenza: The ethics of implementing a school closure policy. *Journal of Public Health Management and Practice, 14*, 372–378. https://doi.org/10.1097/01.PHH.0000324566.72533.0b

Blackwell, T. (2022). These doctors and COVID-19 experts are pushing for quicker return to pre-pandemic normal. *National Post*. https://nationalpost.com/health/covid-19-urgency-of-normal

Boghurst, W. (1666). *Loimographia: The great plague of London in the year 1665*. Shaw & Sons.

Brooks, S., Webster, R., Smith, L., Woodland, L., Wessely, S., Greenberg, N., et al. (2020). The psychological impact of quarantine and how to reduce it: Rapid review of the evidence. *Lancet, 395*(10227), 912–920. https://doi.org/10.1016/S0140-6736(20)30460-8

Byrne, J. P. (2006). *Daily life during the Black Death*. Greenwood.

Carmichael, A. G. (1986). *Plague and the poor in renaissance Florence*. Cambridge University Press.

CBC News. (2020, November 29). B.C. church fined $2.3.k for violating COVID-19 ban on worship services. *CBC News*. https://www.cbc.ca/news/canada/british-columbia/b-c-church-fined-2-3k-for-violating-covid-19-ban-on-worship-services-1.5821450

CBS News. (2020, November 26). Supreme court bars New York's COVID limits on religious house of worship attendance. *CBS News*. https://www.cbsnews.com/news/supreme-court-new-york-covid-restrictions-religious-house-of-worship/?ftag=CNM-00-10aab4i&_amp=1*19d7cr2*s_vid*YW1wLXhWd3BRcFlIeExKOWpvT3czWmxoTUE.

Charleston News and Courier. (1918, October 30). Calls for opening of local churches. *Charleston News and Courier*, 8. http://hdl.handle.net/2027/spo.8860flu.0001.688

Chicago Herald and Examiner. (1918, October 5). Police given order to war on influenza. *Chicago Herald and Examiner*, 11. http://hdl.handle.net/2027/spo.1480flu.0001.841

Chicago Tribune. (1918, October 19). All who peril health of city to be arrested. *Chicago Tribune*, 13. http://hdl.handle.net/2027/spo.2920flu.0012.292

Cincinnati Enquirer. (1918, October 26). "Don't open!" is drastic command. *Cincinnati Enquirer*, 8.

Cleveland Plain Dealer. (1918, October 24). Protest saloon hours. *Cleveland Plain Dealer*, 8. http://hdl.handle.net/2027/spo.9070flu.0002.709

Crane, M. A., Shermock, K. M., Omer, S. B., & Romley, J. A. (2021). Change in reported adherence to nonpharmaceutical interventions during the COVID-19 pandemic, April-November 2020. *JAMA, 325*(9), 883–885. https://doi.org/10.1001/jama.2021.0286

D'Amore, R. (2020, February 11). "Yes, this drone is speaking to you": How China is reportedly enforcing coronavirus rules. *Global News*. https://globalnews.ca/news/6535353/china-coronavirus-drones-quarantine/

Davis, B. M., Markel, H., Navarro, A., Wells, E., Monto, A. S., & Aiello, A. E. (2015). The effect of reactive school closure on community influenza-like illness counts in the state of Michigan during the 2009 H1N1 pandemic. *Clinical Infectious Diseases, 60*, e90–e97. https://doi.org/10.1093/cid/civ182

Duca, L. A., Coyle, J., McCabe, C., & McLean, C. A. (2020). COVID-19 incidence, by urban-rural classification — United States, January 22-October 31, 2020. *Morbidity and Mortality Weekly Report, 69*(46), p. 1753. https://doi.org/10.15585/mmwr.mm6946a6

Evening Star. (1918a, October 28). Opposes further church closing. *Evening Star*, 18. http://hdl.handle.net/2027/spo.4980flu.0011.894

Evening Star. (1918b, October 15). Pastors protest closing churches. *Evening Star*, 28. http://hdl.handle.net/2027/spo.5280flu.0011.825

Ferretti, L., Wymant, C., Kendall, M., Zhao, L., Nurtay, A., Abeler-Dörner, L., et al. (2020). Quantifying SARS-CoV-2 transmission suggests epidemic control with digital contact tracing. *Science, 368*(6491), article eabb6936. https://doi.org/10.1126/science.abb6936

Finkelstein, S., Prakash, S., Nigmatulina, K., Klaiman, T., & Larson, R. (2010). Pandemic influenza: Non-pharmaceutical interventions and behavioral changes that may save lives. *International Journal of Health Management and Information, 1*, 1–18.

Foucault, M. (1979). *Discipline and punish: The birth of the prison*. Vintage Books.

French, M., & Monahan, T. (2020). Dis-ease surveillance: How might surveillance studies address COVID-19? *Surveillance and Society, 18*(1), 1–11. https://doi.org/10.24908/ss.v18i1.13985

Gasser, U., Ienca, M., Scheibner, J., Sleigh, J., & Vayena, E. (2020). Digital tools against COVID-19: Taxonomy, ethical challenges, and navigation aid. *Lancet Digital Health, 2*(8), e425–e434. https://doi.org/10.1016/S2589-7500(20)30137-0

Hart, R. (2020). Fauci attacks herd immunity declaration embraced by White House as "total nonsense." *Forbes.* https://www.forbes.com/sites/roberthart/2020/2010/2015/fauci-attacks-herd-immunity-declaration-embraced-by-white-house-as-total-nonsense/?sh=2032c2024d2026ca2458d

Hassandoust, F., Akhlaghpour, S., & Johnston, A. C. (2021). Individuals' privacy concerns and adoption of contact tracing mobile applications in a pandemic: A situational privacy calculus perspective. *Journal of the American Medical Informatics Association, 28*(3), 463–471. https://doi.org/10.1093/jamia/ocaa240

Haug, N., Geyrhofer, L., Londei, A., Dervic, E., Desvars-Larrive, A., Loreto, V., et al. (2020). Ranking the effectiveness of worldwide COVID-19 government interventions. *Nature Human Behaviour, 4*(12), 1303–1312. https://doi.org/10.1038/s41562-020-01009-0

House, T., Baguelin, M., Van Hoek, A., White, P., Sadique, Z., Eames, K., et al. (2011). Modelling the impact of local reactive school closures on critical care provision during an influenza pandemic. *Proceedings of the Royal Society B: Biological Sciences, 278,* 2753–2760. https://doi.org/10.1098/rspb.2010.2688

Kawaguchi, R., Miyazono, M., Noda, T., Takayama, Y., Sasai, Y., & Iso, H. (2009). Influenza (H1N1) 2009 outbreak and school closure, Osaka Prefecture, Japan. *Emerging Infectious Diseases, 15,* article 1685. https://doi.org/10.3201/eid1510.091029

Kleitman, S., Fullerton, D., Zhang, L., Blanchard, M., Lee, J., Stankov, L., et al. (2021). To comply or not comply? A latent profile analysis of behaviours and attitudes during the COVID-19 pandemic. *PLOS ONE, 16*(7), article e0255268. https://doi.org/10.1371/journal.pone.0255268

Kokkoris, M. D., & Kamleitner, B. (2020). Would you sacrifice your privacy to protect public health? Prosocial responsibility in a pandemic paves the way for digital surveillance. *Frontiers in Psychology, 11,* article 578618. https://doi.org/10.3389/fpsyg.2020.578618

Kovac, A. (2020). 10 arrested, over 140 tickets given as thousands protest in Montreal against pandemic public health measures. *CTV News.* https://montreal.ctvnews.ca/10-arrested-over-140-tickets-given-as-thousands-protest-in-montreal-against-pandemic-public-health-measures-1.5346328

Kovac, A., & Greig, K. (2021). Quebec couple hit with curfew-violation fine after wife walks husband on a leash. *CTV News.* https://montreal.ctvnews.ca/quebec-couple-hit-with-curfew-violation-fine-after-wife-walks-husband-on-a-leash-1.5262178

Kulldorff, M., Gupta, S., & Bhattacharya, J. (2020). Great Barrington declaration. https://gbdeclaration.org

Labine, J. (2021). GraceLife church holds secret service after AHS fenced facility for violating public health orderss. *Edmonton Journal.* https://edmontonjournal.com/news/local-news/gracelife-church-holds-secret-service-after-ahs-fenced-facility-for-violating-public-health-orders#:~:text=GraceLife%20Church%20held%20an%20in,violating%20COVID%2D19%20health%20orders.&text=During%20the%20service%2C%20Coates%20described,%E2%80%9Cjailed%E2%80%9D%20the%20church's%20facility

Mackowiak, P. A., & Sehdev, P. S. (2002). The origin of quarantine. *Clinical Infectious Diseases, 35,* 1071–1072. https://doi.org/10.1086/344062

Maharaj, S., & Kleczkowski, A. (2012). Controlling epidemic spread by social distancing: Do it well or not at all. *BMC Public Health, 12,* article 679. https://doi.org/10.1186/1471-2458-12-679

Majeed, A. (2022). Technical analysis of contact tracing platform developed by Google–Apple for constraining the spread of COVID-19. *ISPRS International Journal of Geo-Information, 11*(11), article 539. https://doi.org/10.3390/ijgi11110539

Miljure, B. (2021). Protesters gather in downtown Vancouver for rally against COVID-19 restrictions. *CTV News.* https://bc.ctvnews.ca/protesters-gather-in-downtown-vancouver-for-rally-against-covid-19-restrictions-1.5317487

Mitchell, T., Dee, D., Phares, C., Lipman, H., Gould, L., Kutty, P., et al. (2011). Non-pharmaceutical interventions during an outbreak of 2009 pandemic influenza A (H1N1) virus infection at a large public university, April-May 2009. *Clinical Infectious Diseases, 52*(Suppl 1), S138–S145. https://doi.org/10.1093/cid/ciq056

Moon, M. J. (2020). Fighting COVID-19 with agility, transparency, and participation: Wicked policy problems and new governance challenges. *Public Administration Review, 80*(4), 651–656. https://doi.org/10.1111/puar.13214

Nature. (2020). COVID-19 digital apps need due diligence. *Nature, 580,* p. 563.

Nay, O. (2020). Can a virus undermine human rights? *Lancet Public health, 5*(5), e238–e239. https://doi.org/10.1016/S2468-2667(20)30092-X

Neufeld, M., Lachenmeier, D. W., Ferreira-Borges, C., & Rehm, J. (2020). Is alcohol an "essential good" During COVID-19? Yes, but only as a disinfectant! *Alcoholism, Clinical and Experimental Research, 44*(9), 1906–1909. https://doi.org/10.1111/acer.14417

New Orleans Times-Picayune. (1918, November 10). Rev. Dr. Barr raps health board head. *New Orleans Times-Picayune,* C10. http://hdl.handle.net/2027/spo.7800flu.0007.087

Newark Evening News. (1918, October 10). Rev. C. H. Wells writes Gillen; church to close under protest. *Newark Evening News,* 5. http://hdl.handle.net/2027/spo.1810flu.0007.181

Nicholson, B., & Martins, N. (2021). Owner of Rio Theatre says B.C. restaurant industry gets special treatment under COVID-19. *News 1130.* https://www.citynews1130.com/2021/01/12/rio-theatre-bc-restaurant-industry-special-treatment

Nikolaeva, A., & Versnel, J. (2022). Analytical observational study evaluating global pandemic preparedness and the effectiveness of early COVID-19 responses in Ethiopia, Nigeria, Singapore, South Korea, Sweden, Taiwan, UK and USA. *BMJ Open, 12*(2), article e053374. https://doi.org/10.1136/bmjopen-2021-053374

Nuzzo, A., Tan, C. O., Raskar, R., DeSimone, D. C., Kapa, S., & Gupta, R. (2020). Universal shelter-in-place versus advanced automated contact tracing and targeted isolation: A case for 21st-century technologies for SARS-CoV-2 and future pandemics. *Mayo Clinic Proceedings, 95*(9), 1898–1905. https://doi.org/10.1016/j.mayocp.2020.06.027

Pan-Canadian Public Health Network. (2016). *Canadian pandemic influenza preparedness.* Canadian Government Information Digital Preservation Network.

Philadelphia Inquirer. (1918, October 18). Pastors protest church closing. *Philadelphia Inquirer,* 15. http://hdl.handle.net/2027/spo.0000flu.0008.000

Quinn, M. (2020, December 3). Supreme court sides with church challenging California's COVID restrictions. *CBC News.* https://www.cbsnews.com/amp/news/supreme-court-covid-restrictions-california-church/

Rocky Mountain News. (1918, November 23). Theater men protest ban. *Rocky Mountain News,* 7. http://hdl.handle.net/2027/spo.6090flu.0003.906

Rose, C. (2018). Plague and violence in early modern Italy. *Renaissance Quarterly, 71*(3), 1000–1035. https://doi.org/10.1086/699602

Rosenberg, C. E. (1987). *The cholera years: The United States in 1832, 1849, and 1866.* University of Chicago Press.

Salt Lake Tribune. (1918, December 11). Board protests school closing. *Salt Lake Tribune,* 2. http://hdl.handle.net/2027/spo.4240flu.0009.424

Salter, P. (2020). At least 30 jailed for curfew violations late Monday, early Tuesday. *Lincoln Journal Star*. https://journalstar.com/news/local/crime-and-courts/at-least-30-jailed-for-curfew-violations-late-monday-early-tuesday/article_e7a11dea-75a3-5897-82f7-f67c0b63667b.html

Slack, P. (1985). *The impact of plague in Tudor and Stuart England*. Routledge.

Spokane Daily Chronicle. (1918, October 29). Wholesome fear of influenza is needed by city. *Spokane Daily Chronicle*, 1.

St. Paul Daily News. (1918, October 20). School officials may face arrest. *St. Paul Daily News*, 1 and 5. http://hdl.handle.net/2027/spo.9610flu.0010.169

SteelFisher, G. K., Blendon, R. J., Ward, J. R. M., Rapoport, R., Kahn, E. B., & Kohl, K. S. (2012). Public response to the 2009 influenza A H1N1 pandemic: A polling study in five countries. *Lancet Infectious Diseases*, *12*, 845–850. https://doi.org/10.1016/S1473-3099(12)70206-2

Storr, V. H., Haeffele, S., Lofthouse, J. K., & Grube, L. E. (2021). Essential or not? Knowledge problems and COVID-19 stay-at-home orders. *Southern Economic Journal*, *87*(4), 1229–1249. https://doi.org/10.1002/soej.12491

Tan, S. B., Chiu-Shee, C., & Duarte, F. (2022). From SARS to COVID-19: Digital infrastructures of surveillance and segregation in exceptional times. *Cities*, *120*, article 103486. https://doi.org/10.1016/j.cities.2021.103486

Taylor, S., Paluszek, M., Landry, C., Rachor, G. S., & Asmundson, G. J. G. (2020). Worry, avoidance, and coping during the COVID-19 pandemic: A comprehensive network analysis. *Journal of Anxiety Disorders*, *76*, article 102327. https://doi.org/10.1016/j.janxdis.2020.102327

Taylor, S., Rachor, G. S., & Asmundson, G. J. G. (2022). Who develops pandemic fatigue? Insights from latent class analysis. *PLOS ONE*, *17*(11), article e0276791. https://doi.org/10.1371/journal.pone.0276791

Tognotti, E. (2013). Lessons from the history of quarantine, from plague to influenza A. *Emerging Infectious Diseases*, *19*(2), 254–259. https://doi.org/10.3201/eid1902.120312

Tomes, N. (2010). "Destroyer and teacher": Managing the masses during the 1918–1919 influenza pandemic. *Public Health Reports*, *125 (Suppl. 3)*, 48–62. https://doi.org/10.1177/00333549101250S308

Túri, G., & Virág, A. (2021). Experiences and lessons learned from COVID-19 pandemic management in South Korea and the V4 Countries. *Tropical Medicine and Infectious Disease*, *6*(4), article 201. https://doi.org/10.3390/tropicalmed6040201

Weisgarber, M. (2021). Vancouver restaurant owner defying public health order banning indoor dining. *CTV News*. https://bc.ctvnews.ca/vancouver-restaurant-owner-defying-public-health-order-banning-indoor-dining-1.5372333

WHO. (2010a). Pandemic (H1N1) 2009. https://www.who.int/csr/disease/swineflu/en

WHO. (2010b). What is a pandemic? http://www.who.int/csr/disease/swineflu/frequently_asked_questions/pandemic/en/

WHO. (2020). Pandemic fatigue: Reinvigorating the public to prevent COVID-19. http://apps.who.int/iris/handle/10665/335820?search-result=true&query=pandemic+fatigue&scope=&rpp=335810&sort_by=score&order=desc

Wnuk, A., Oleksy, T., & Domaradzka, A. (2021). Prosociality and endorsement of liberty: Communal and individual predictors of attitudes towards surveillance technologies. *Computers in Human Behavior*, *125*, article 106938. https://doi.org/10.1016/j.chb.2021.106938

Wnuk, A., Oleksy, T., & Maison, D. (2020). The acceptance of Covid-19 tracking technologies: The role of perceived threat, lack of control, and ideological beliefs. *PLOS ONE*, *15*(9), article e0238973. https://doi.org/10.1371/journal.pone.0238973

Worcester Evening Post. (1918, October 4). Theater men protest on new order. *Worcester Evening Post*, 1 and 10. http://hdl.handle.net/2027/spo.6400flu.0012.046

Wu, J., Cowling, B., Lau, E., Ip, D., Ho, L., Tsang, T., et al. (2010). School closure and mitigation of pandemic (H1N1) 2009, Hong Kong. *Emerging Infectious Diseases, 16*, 538–541. https://doi.org/10.3201/eid1603.091216

Xuefei, R. (2022). Urban China and COVID-19: How Chinese cities responded to the pandemic. *Journal of International Affairs, 74*(1), 162–172.

Yamey, G. (2020). How not to fight COVID-19. *Time, 196*(16/17), 27–28.

Yoon, K. (2021). Digital dilemmas in the (post-)pandemic state: Surveillance and information rights in South Korea. *Journal of Digital Media & Policy, 12*(1), 67–80. https://doi.org/10.1386/jdmp_00048_1

Yost, A. B., Behrend, T. S., Howardson, G., Darrow, J. B., & Jensen, J. M. (2019). Reactance to electronic surveillance: A test of antecedents and outcomes. *Journal of Business and Psychology, 34*(1), 71–86. https://doi.org/10.1007/s10869-018-9532-2

Yuan, E. J. (2021). Governing risk society: The socio-technological experiences of China and South Korea in the COVID-19 pandemic. *Asian Journal of Communication, 31*(5), 322–336. https://doi.org/10.1080/01292986.2021.1913620

Zuboff, S. (2019). *The age of surveillance capitalism*. Profile Books.

Chapter 7

Agence France-Presse. (2021). Former U.S. CDC head thinks coronavirus came from Chinese lab, has no evidence. https://www.ctvnews.ca/health/coronavirus/former-u-s-cdc-head-thinks-coronavirus-came-from-chinese-lab-has-no-evidence-1.5364208

Akkermans, J. (2021a). Dutch Covid riots add to political tension ahead of elections. *Bloomberg.com*. https://www.bnnbloomberg.ca/dutch-covid-riots-add-to-political-tension-ahead-of-elections-1.1553981

Akkermans, J. (2021b). Netherlands has worst riots in four decades over Covid curbs. *Bloomberg.com*. https://www.bloomberg.com/news/articles/2021-01-26/dutch-covid-riots-add-to-political-tension-ahead-of-elections

Aljazeera. (2020). Protests against new coronavirus measures in Italy turn violent. *Aljazeera*. https://www.aljazeera.com/news/2020/10/27/protests-flare-up-in-italy-against-new-coronavirus-restrictions

Aloisi, A., & De Stefano, V. (2022). Essential jobs, remote work and digital surveillance: Addressing the COVID-19 pandemic panopticon. *International Labour Review, 161*(2), 289–314. https://doi.org/10.1111/ilr.12219

Amarasingam, A., Carvin, S., & Phillips, K. (2021). *Anti-lockdown activity: Canada country profile*. Institute for Strategic Dialogue.

Annár, D. (2020). Budapest dormitory damaged by students with a hammer. *Daily News Hungary*. https://dailynewshungary.com/budapest-dormitory-damaged-by-students-with-a-hammer/.

August, M. (2020). The 1918 flu pandemic killed hundreds of thousands of Americans. The White House never said a word about it. *Time*. https://time.com/5877129/1918-pandemic-white-house/

Ayoubkhani, D., Khunti, K., Nafilyan, V., Maddox, T., Humberstone, B., Diamond, I., et al. (2021). Epidemiology of post-COVID syndrome following hospitalisation with coronavirus: A retrospective cohort study. *British Medical Journal, 372*, article 693. https://doi.org/10.1136/bmj.n693

Baio, A. (2024). Democrats blast Republicans for "fuelling a political agenda" with Covid report and push back on lab leak claim. *The Independent*. https://www.independent.co.uk/news/world/americas/us-politics/house-democrats-republicans-covid-report-b2658172.html

Barrett, E. (2022). Pepper spray, tow trucks, and Bitcoin seizures: How Canada finally ended the weeks-long Freedom Convoy protests in Ottawa. *Fortune.com*. https://fortune.com/2022/02/21/canada-ottawa-freedom-convoy-protest-ends-truckers-arrest-covid-vaccine-mandate/

Bartusevičius, H., Bor, A., Jørgensen, F., & Petersen, M. B. (2021). The psychological burden of the COVID-19 pandemic is associated with antisystemic attitudes and political violence. *Psychological Science, 32*(9), 1391–1403. https://doi.org/10.1177/09567976211031847

Bayramoğlu, Y. (2021). Border panic over the pandemic: Mediated anxieties about migrant sex workers and queers during the AIDS crises in Turkey. *Ethnic and Racial Studies, 44*(9), 1589–1606. https://doi.org/10.1080/01419870.2021.1881141

BBC News. (2020). Coronavirus: Armed protesters enter Michigan statehouse. *BBC News*. https://www.bbc.com/news/world-us-canada-52496514

BBC News. (2022). Pressure grows on Boris Johnson after Partygate report. https://www.bbc.com/news/uk-politics-61645661

Bensadoun, E. (2021). The Canadian politicians who travelled over the holidays during a coronavirus pandemic. *Global News*. https://globalnews.ca/news/7551438/canadian-politicians-vacation-coronavirus/

Berkowitz, L. (1989). Frustration-aggression hypothesis: Examination and reformulation. *Psychological Bulletin, 106*, 59–73. https://doi.org/10.1037/0033-2909.106.1.59

Bhuiyan, A., Sakib, N., Pakpour, A., Griffiths, M., & Mamun, M. (2020). COVID-19-related suicides in Bangladesh due to lockdown and economic factors: Case study evidence from media reports. *International Journal of Mental Health and Addiction, 19*, 2110–2115. https://doi.org/10.1007/s11469-020-00307-y

Bird, M. D., Arispe, S., Muñoz, P., & Freier, L. F. (2023). Trust, social protection, and compliance: Moral hazard in Latin America during the COVID-19 pandemic. *Journal of Economic Behavior & Organization, 206*, 279–295. https://doi.org/10.1016/j.jebo.2022.12.010

Blackburn, A. M., Han, H., Jeftić, A., Stöckli, S., Gelpí, R., Acosta-Ortiz, A. M., et al. (2024). Predictors of compliance with COVID-19 guidelines across countries: The role of social norms, moral values, trust, stress, and demographic factors. *Current Psychology, 43*(19), 17939–17955. https://doi.org/10.1007/s12144-023-05281-x

Blair, R. A., Morse, B. S., & Tsai, L. L. (2017). Public health and public trust: Survey evidence from the Ebola Virus Disease epidemic in Liberia. *Social Science & Medicine, 172*, 89–97. https://doi.org/10.1016/j.socscimed.2016.11.016

Bliss, M. (1991). *Plague: A story of smallpox in Montreal*. HarperCollins.

Block, R., Jr., Burnham, M., Kahn, K., Peng, R., Seeman, J., & Seto, C. (2022). Perceived risk, political polarization, and the willingness to follow COVID-19 mitigation guidelines. *Social Science & Medicine, 305*, article 115091. https://doi.org/10.1016/j.socscimed.2022.115091

Bloomberg. (2020, August 29). Berlin protest turns violent. *Bloomberg.com*. https://www.bloomberg.com/news/articles/2020-08-28/texas-hospitalizations-halve-nyc-museums-reopen-virus-update

Bloomberg. (2022a, November 15). Covid lockdowns spark violent protests in China's Guangzhou city. *Bloomberg.com*. https://www.bnnbloomberg.ca/covid-lockdowns-spark-violent-protests-in-china-s-guangzhou-city-1.1846426

Bloomberg. (2022b, November 30). Violent protests flare again in locked-down part of South China. *Bloomberg.com*. https://www.bloomberg.com/news/articles/2022-11-30/violent-protests-flare-again-in-locked-down-part-of-south-china

Bratanic, J., & Kuzmanovic, J. (2020, November 6). Anti-lockdown protest turns violent for first time in Slovenia. Bloomberg.com. https://www.bloomberg.com/news/articles/2020-11-05/anti-lockdown-protest-turns-violent-for-first-time-in-slovenia

Breeden, A. (2021, November 23). French vaccine regulations stir violent protests in Guadeloupe. *New York Times, 171*, A28.

Briggs, A. (1961). Cholera and society in the nineteenth century. *Past & Present, 19*(1), 76–96. https://doi.org/10.1093/past/19.1.76

Bucks, J. (2020, November 1). Italy riots as America sets grim new record. *Mail on Sunday*, 17.

Buguzi, S. (2021). Covid-19: Counting the cost of denial in Tanzania. *BMJ (Clinical Research Ed.), 373*, article n1052. https://doi.org/10.1136/bmj.n1052

Burrell, S., & Gill, G. (2005). The Liverpool cholera epidemic of 1832 and anatomical dissection: Medical mistrust and civil unrest. *Journal of the History of Medicine and Allied Sciences, 60*(4), 478–498. https://doi.org/10.1093/jhmas/jri061

Cao, A., Ueta, M., Uchibori, M., Murakami, M., Kunishima, H., Santosh Kumar, R., et al. (2024). Trust in governments, public health institutions, and other information sources as determinants of COVID-19 vaccine uptake behavior in Japan. *Vaccine, 42*(17), 3684–3692. https://doi.org/10.1016/j.vaccine.2024.04.081

Chandavarkar, R. (1992). Plague panic and epidemic politics in India, 1896–1914. In P. Slack & T. Ranger (Eds.), *Epidemics and ideas: Essays on the historical perception of pestilence* (pp. 203–240). Cambridge University Press. https://doi.org/10.1017/CBO9780511563645.010

Charters, E., & McKay, R. A. (2020). The history of science and medicine in the context of COVID-19. *Centaurus, 62*(2), 223–233. https://doi.org/10.1111/1600-0498.12311

Cheng, C. (2004). To be paranoid is the standard? Panic responses to SARS out-break in the Hong Kong Special Administrative Region. *Asian Perspective, 28*, 67–98. https://doi.org/10.1353/apr.2004.0034

Christensen, S. R., Pilling, E. B., Eyring, J. B., Dickerson, G., Sloan, C. D., & Magnusson, B. M. (2020). Political and personal reactions to COVID-19 during initial weeks of social distancing in the United States. *PLOS ONE, 15*(9), article e0239693. https://doi.org/10.1371/journal.pone.0239693

Cohn, S. K. (2017). Cholera revolts: A class struggle we may not like. *Social History, 42*, 162–180. https://doi.org/10.1080/03071022.2017.1290365

Cohn, S. K., & Kutalek, R. (2016). Historical parallels, Ebola virus disease and cholera: Understanding community distrust and social violence with epidemics. *PLOS Currents, 8*. https://doi.org/10.1371/currents.outbreaks.aa1f2b60e8d43939b43fbd93e1a63a94

Coletta, A., Berger, M., & Simon, M. F. (2022, February 19). Police close in on Ottawa's "Freedom Convoy" protests. *Washington Post*, 11.

Connor, T. (2020, October 1). NYPD arrests leader of violent ultra-orthodox COVID protest: Heshy Tischler will be charged with inciting a riot and unlawful imprisonment after a journalist was assaulted. *Daily Beast*. https://www.thedailybeast.com/nypd-arrests-heshy-tischler-leader-of-violent-ultra-orthodox-covid-protest

Czeisler, M., Lane, R., Petrosky, E., Wiley, J., Christensen, A., Njai, R., et al. (2020). Mental health, substance use, and suicidal ideation during the COVID-19 pandemic — United States, June 24–30, 2020. *Morbidity and Mortality Weekly Report, 69*(32), 1049–1057. https://doi.org/10.15585/mmwr.mm6932a1

Davis, L., & Macfarlane, J. (2021, November 21). Violent Covid-19 protests erupt. *ABC World News Sunday*.

Delaporte, F. (1986). *Disease and civilization: The cholera in Paris, 1832.* MIT Press.

Devine, D., Valgarðsson, V., Smith, J., Jennings, W., Scotto Di Vettimo, M., Bunting, H., et al. (2024). Political trust in the first year of the COVID-19 pandemic: A meta-analysis of 67 studies. *Journal of European Public Policy, 31*(3), 657–679. https://doi.org/10.1080/13501763.2023.2169741

Di Donato, V., & Dewan, A. (2020). Protesters clash with police in northern Italy as anger mounts over Covid-19 restrictions. *CNN*. https://edition.cnn.com/2020/10/27/europe/italy-coronavirus-protests-intl/index.html

Erlanger, S. (2021, November 23). Anger fills Europe's streets as lockdowns spread. *New York Times*, A1 and A8.

Evans, R. J. (1988). Epidemics and revolutions: Cholera in nineteenth-century Europe. *Past & Present, 120*, 123–146.

Falkenbach, M., & Greer, S. L. (2021). Denial and distraction: How the populist radical right responds to COVID-19. *International Journal of Health Policy and Management, 10*(9), 578–580. https://doi.org/10.34172/ijhpm.2020.141

Farokhi, Z. (2022). Making freedom great again: Conspiracy theories, affective nostalgia and alignment, and the right-wing base grammars of the #Freeedomconvoy. *Global Media Journal: Canadian Edition, 14*(1), 67–92.

Flores, A., Cole, J., Dickert, S., Eom, K., Jiga-Boy, G., Kogut, T., et al. (2022). Politicians polarize and experts depolarize public support for COVID-19 management policies across countries. *PNAS, 119*(3), article e2117543119. https://doi.org/10.1073/pnas.2117543119

Freeman, D., Waite, F., Rosebrock, L., Petit, A., Causier, C., East, A., et al. (2022). Coronavirus conspiracy beliefs, mistrust, and compliance with government guidelines in England. *Psychological Medicine, 52*(2), 251–263. https://doi.org/10.1017/S0033291720001890

Fruehwirth, J. C., Biswas, S., & Perreira, K. M. (2021). The Covid-19 pandemic and mental health of first-year college students: Examining the effect of Covid-19 stressors using longitudinal data. *PLOS ONE, 16*(3), article e0247999. https://doi.org/10.1371/journal.pone.0247999

Ghitis, F. (2021, January 28). The Netherlands' violent anti-lockdown protests are a bad omen. *World Politics Review*. https://www.worldpoliticsreview.com/the-netherlands-lockdown-riots-are-a-bad-omen/

Gordon, B. (2020, February 29). The dark history of the official "Keep calm and carry on" advice. *Daily Telegraph*, 29.

Gostin, L. O. (2022). Life after the COVID-19 pandemic. *JAMA Health Forum, 3*(2), article e220323. https://doi.org/10.1001/jamahealthforum.2022.0323

Gravlee, C. C. (2020). Systematic racism, chronic health inequalities, and COVID-19: A syndemic in the making? *American Journal of Human Biology, 32*(5), article e23482. https://doi.org/10.1002/ajhb.23482

Green, J. N., & Skidmore, T. E. (2021). *Brazil: Five centuries of change* (3rd ed.). Oxford University Press.

Grimaud, J., & Legagneur, F. (2011). Community beliefs and fears during a cholera outbreak in Haiti. *Intervention: International Journal of Mental Health, Psychosocial Work & Counselling in Areas of Armed Conflict, 9*(1), 26–34. https://doi.org/10.1097/WTF.0b013e3283453ef2

Hanau, S. (2021). Heshy Tischler sentenced to 10 days community service for inciting riot. *The Jerusalem Post*. https://www.jpost.com/diaspora/heshy-tischler-sentenced-to-10-days-community-service-for-inciting-riot-667565

Hegland, A., Zhang, A. L., Zichettella, B., & Pasek, J. (2022). A partisan pandemic: How COVID-19 was primed for polarization. *Annals of the American Academy of Political and Social Science, 700*(1), 55–72. https://doi.org/10.1177/00027162221083686

Hier, S. P. (2021). A moral panic in reverse? Implicatory denial and COVID-19 pre-crisis risk communication in Canada. *Canadian Journal of Communication, 46*(3), 505–521. https://doi.org/10.22230/cjc.2021v46n3a3981

Hookham, M. (2020, September 27). Nine police injured as violence flares again at Covid-deniers protest. *Mail on Sunday*, 15.

Husna, S. (2021). Denial attitude and behavior as a response to the COVID-19 pandemic: A qualitative study. *Humanitas, 18*(2), 153–163. https://doi.org/10.26555/humanitas.v18i2.19173

Ilsøe, T. M., & Clante, C. (2021). Six people sentenced after Men in Black demos. *Danish Broadcasting Corporation*. https://www.dr.dk/nyheder/indland/overblik-seks-personer-doemt-efter-men-black-demoer#:~:text=Kun%20to%20ud%20af%20tre,efter%20den%20s%C3%A6rlige%20corona%2Dparagraf

Imperato, P. J., Imperato, G. H., & Imperato, A. C. (2015). The second world cholera pandemic (1826–1849) in the kingdom of the two Sicilies with special reference to the towns of San Prisco and Forio d'Ischia. *Journal of Community Health, 40*(6), 1224–1286. https://doi.org/10.1007/s10900-015-0089-y

Jha, A. (2022). Why do the rich get richer—even during global crises? *Al Jazeera*. https://www.aljazeera.com/features/2022/12/27/why-do-the-rich-get-richer-even-during-global

Kalichman, S. C. (2014). The psychology of AIDS denialism. *European Psychologist, 19*(1), 13–22. https://doi.org/10.1027/1016-9040/a000175

Karimi, F. (2020). Before Trump, another US president downplayed a pandemic and was infected. *CNN*. https://www.cnn.com/2020/10/03/us/woodrow-wilson-coronavirus-trnd/index.html

Keith, T. (2020). Trump says he downplayed coronavirus threat in U.S. to avert panic. *NPR*. https://www.npr.org/2020/09/11/911828384/trump-says-he-downplayed-coronavirus-threat-in-u-s-to-avert-panic

Keogh, G., & Franey, J. (2021, November 22). Europe gripped by violent protests over fresh wave of Covid restrictions. *Daily Mail*, 24.

Kishi, R., Pavlik, M., Bynum, E., Miller, A., Goos, C., Satre, J., et al. (2021). ACLED 2020: The year in review. https://acleddata.com/acleddatanew/wp-content/uploads/2021/08/ACLED_Annual-Report-2020_Upd2021.pdf

Kruglanski, A. W., Ellenberg, M., Szumowska, E., Molinario, E., Speckhard, A., Leander, N. P., et al. (2023). Frustration-aggression hypothesis reconsidered: The role of significance quest. *Aggressive Behavior, 49*(5), 445–468. https://doi.org/10.1002/ab.22092

Kvetenadze, T. (2021, November 21). Violent protests against Covid lockdowns—35,000 in Brussels—continue in Europe. *Forbes.com*. https://www.forbes.com/sites/teakvetenadze/2021/2011/2021/violent-protests-against-covid-lockdowns-35000-in-brussels-continue-in-europe/?sh=31093e35005a32254

Le, P., Misra, S., Hagen, D., Wang, S., Li, T., Brenneke, S., et al. (2023). Coronavirus disease (COVID-19) related discrimination and mental health in five US Southern cities. *Stigma and Health, 8*(1), 133–137. https://doi.org/10.1037/sah0000351

McCoy, J., Rahman, T., & Somer, M. (2018). Polarization and the global crisis of democracy: Common patterns, dynamics, and pernicious consequences for democratic polities. *American Behavioral Scientist, 62*(1), 16–42. https://doi.org/10.1177/0002764218759576

Meade, T. (1986). "Civilizing Rio de Janeiro": The public health campaign and the riot of 1904. *Journal of Social History, 20*(2), 301–322. https://doi.org/10.1353/jsh/20.2.301

Merriman, S. (2021, November 21). Europe rocked by riots as strict lockdowns return to stop virus. *Mail on Sunday*, 6.

Ministry of Foreign Affairs of the People's Republic of China. (2020). Reality check of US allegations against China on COVID-19. https://www.fmprc.gov.cn/mfa_eng/gjhdq_665435/3376_665447/3432_664920/3434_664924/202005/t20200510_587462.html

Moore, S. E., Wierenga, K. L., Prince, D. M., Gillani, B., & Mintz, L. J. (2021). Disproportionate impact of the COVID-19 pandemic on perceived social support, mental health and somatic symptoms in sexual and gender minority populations. *Journal of Homosexuality, 68*(4), 577–591. https://doi.org/10.1080/00918369.2020.1868184

Morales, A., & Konotey-Ahulu, O. (2020, March 20). Large-scale rioting unlikely in U.K., virus committee says. *Bloomberg.com*. https://www.bnnbloomberg.ca/large-scale-rioting-unlikely-in-u-k-virus-committee-says-1.1409482

Morton, R. (2021, October 6). "Fascist" anti-vax riot sparks COVID outbreak in Australia—with Rupert Murdoch's help. *Daily Beast.* https://www.thedailybeast.com/fascist-anti-vax-riot-sparks-covid-outbreak-in-australiawith-rupert-murdochs-help

Needell, J. D. (1987). The Revolta Contra Vacina of 1904: The revolt against "modernization" in belle-epoque Rio de Janeiro. *Hispanic American Historical Review, 67*(2), 233–269. https://doi.org/10.1215/00182168-67.2.233

Nixon, G. (2022). How the flouting of COVID-19 restrictions by leaders damages credibility and trust. *CBC News.* https://www.cbc.ca/news/world/covid-pandemic-leaders-behaviour-damage-1.6315350

Parets, M. (1651). *A journal of the plague year: The diary of the Barcelona tanner Miquel Parets 1651* (J. S. Amelang, Trans. & Ed., 1991). Oxford University Press.

Pennycook, G., McPhetres, J., Bago, B., & Rand, D. G. (2022). Beliefs about COVID-19 in Canada, the United Kingdom, and the United States: A novel test of political polarization and motivated reasoning. *Personality and Social Psychology Bulletin, 48*(5), 750–765. https://doi.org/10.1177/01461672211023652

Pettigrew, E. (1983). *The silent enemy: Canada and the deadly flu of 1918.* Western Producer Prairie Books.

Potegal, M. (2023). Are reactions to frustrative nonreward in other animals a model for human anger? Neurobehavioral implications and therapeutic applications. *Behavioral Neuroscience, 137*(6), 364–372. https://doi.org/10.1037/bne0000574

Rosenberg, C. E. (1987). *The cholera years: The United States in 1832, 1849, and 1866.* University of Chicago Press.

Scott, J. (2021, September 20). Anti-vaccination protests force Melbourne construction shutdown. *Bloomberg.com.* https://www.bloomberg.com/news/articles/2021-2009-2020/melbourne-shuts-down-construction-amid-anti-vaccination-protests

Select Subcommittee on the Coronavirus Pandemic. (2024). *After action review of the COVID-19 pandemic: The lessons learned and a path forward.* U.S. House of Representatives.

Select Subcommittee on the Coronavirus Pandemic: Democrats. (2024). *Partisan probes over pandemic prevention and preparedness: Select subcommittee Republicans spent the 118th Congress putting politics over people and public health.* Author.

Seputyte, M. (2021, October 10). Lithuanian anti-vax protest turns violent with one cop injured. *Bloomberg.com.* https://www.bloomberg.com/news/articles/2021-2008-2010/thousands-of-anti-vax-protesters-block-parliament-in-lithuania

Skafida, V., & Heins, E. (2024). Trust in COVID-19 information sources and vaccination status: Exploring social inequalities and differences within the four United Kingdom nations using a representative survey. *Journal of Health Services Research & Policy, 29*(3), 153–162. https://doi.org/10.1177/13558196241227749

Slack, P. (1985). *The impact of plague in Tudor and Stuart England.* Routledge.

Snowden, F. M. (2019). *Epidemics and society: From the Black Death to the present.* Yale University Press.

Staiano, J. (2008). The impact of plague on human behavior in seventeenth century Europe. *ESSAI, 6*(1), article 46, https://dc.cod.edu/essai/vol46/iss41/46/

Taylor, S., & Asmundson, G. J. G. (2021). Negative attitudes about facemasks during the COVID-19 pandemic: The dual importance of perceived ineffectiveness and psychological reactance. *PLOS ONE, 16*(2), article e0246317. https://doi.org/10.1371/journal.pone.0246317

Thanthong-Knight, S. (2020, March 29). Prisoners riot in Thailand reportedly over fears of coronavirus. *Bloomberg.com.* https://www.bnnbloomberg.ca/prisoners-riot-in-thailand-reportedly-over-fears-of-coronavirus-2021.1414202

The Guardian. (2022). Covid lockdown protests break out in western China after deadly fire. *The Guardian.* https://www.theguardian.com/world/2022/nov/26/covid-lockdown-protests-break-out-in-western-china-after-deadly-fire

The Local. (2021). Nine arrested in Denmark after violent anti-lockdown demo. *The Local*. https://www.thelocal.dk/20210110/nine-arrested-in-denmark-after-anti-lockdown-violence/

Todd, F. M. (1909). *Eradicating plague from San Francisco: Report of the Citizens' Health Committee and an account of its work*. Murdock & Co.

Total Slovenia News. (2020). Violence between protesters and police in Ljubljana. *Total Slovenia News*. https://www.total-slovenia-news.com/politics/7264-violence-between-protesters-police-in-ljubljana-videos

Wallace, J., Goldsmith-Pinkham, P., & Schwartz, J. L. (2023). Excess death rates for republican and democratic registered voters in Florida and Ohio during the COVID-19 pandemic. *JAMA Internal Medicine*, *183*(9), 916–923. https://doi.org/10.1001/jamainternmed.2023.1154

Walsh, N. P., Shelley, J., Duwe, E., & Bonnett, W. (2020). Bolsonaro calls coronavirus a "little flu." Inside Brazil's hospitals, doctors know the horrifying reality. *CNN*. https://www.cnn.com/2020/05/23/americas/brazil-coronavirus-hospitals-intl/index.html

Washer, P. (2010). *Emerging infectious diseases and society*. Palgrave Macmillan.

Westfall, S. (2022, February 9). Here's what you need to know about the "Freedom Convoy" in Canada. *The Washington Post*. https://www.washingtonpost.com/world/2022/2002/2007/freedom-convoy-ottawa-canada-vaccine/

Wharton, J. (2021, August 22). Chaos as lockdown protests hit Australia. *Mail on Sunday*, 25.

Willems, M. (2021, November 23). EU Covid crisis unleashes riots over vaccines. *City A.M. (London)*, 17.

Winter, H., Gerster, L., Helmer, J., & Baaken, T. (2021). *Disinformation overdose: A study of the crisis of trust among vaccine sceptics and anti-vaxxers*. Institute for Strategic Dialogue.

Yaylali, E., Erdogan, Z. M., Calisir, F., Gokengin, D., Korten, V., Tabak, F., et al. (2023). Modeling the future of HIV in Turkey: Cost-effectiveness analysis of improving testing and diagnosis. *PLOS ONE*, *18*(6), article e0286254. https://doi.org/10.1371/journal.pone.0286254

Young, I. (2020). Vancouver protesters call coronavirus fake news and say distancing rule should be defied, appalling health authorities. *The Star*. https://www.thestar.com.my/tech/tech-news/2020/04/14/vancouver-protesters-call-coronavirus-fake-news-and-say-distancing-rule-should-be-defied-appalling-health-authorities

Yu, V., & Davidson, H. (2022). Anti-lockdown protests spread across China amid growing anger at zero-Covid strategy. *The Guardian*. https://www.theguardian.com/world/2022/nov/27/anti-lockdown-protests-spread-across-china-amid-growing-anger-at-zero-covid-strategy

Chapter 8

ABC News. (2020). Prime Minister Scott Morrison says there is no need for panic buying. https://www.abc.net.au/news/2020-06-26/prime-minister-scott-morrison-says-no-need-for-panic-buying/12398700?nw=0

Aberth, J. (2010). *From the brink of the apocalypse: Confronting famine, war, plague, and death in the later middle ages* (2nd ed.). Routledge.

Aghababaeian, H., Hamdanieh, L., & Ostadtaghizadeh, A. (2020). Alcohol intake in an attempt to fight COVID-19: A medical myth in Iran. *Alcohol*, *88*, 29–32. https://doi.org/10.1016/j.alcohol.2020.07.006

Allen, V., & Ellicott, C. (2020, October 10). Salute to the COVID heroes. *Daily Mail*, 1.

Anonymous. (1721). *The late dreadful plague at Marseilles compared with that terrible plague in London in the year 1665*. Parker.

Anonymous. (1849). Fear a cause of epidemics. *New England Botanic, Medical & Surgical Journal*, 3(5), 84–86.

Associated Press. (2021). India's crematoriums overwhelmed as COVID-19 patients scramble for medical help. *Associated Press*. https://www.cbc.ca/news/world/india-covid19-patients-creamatorium-1.6001536

Atlanta Constitution. (1918, October 18). Sulfur in shoes will check the "flu," asserts physician. *Atlanta Constitution*, 5, http://hdl.handle.net/2027/spo.4520flu.0016.254

Barauskaitė, D., Gineikienė, J., & Fennis, B. M. (2022). Saved by the past? Disease threat triggers nostalgic consumption. *Psychology & Marketing*, 39(8), 1433–1450. https://doi.org/10.1002/mar.21663

Bauman, A., Shepherd, L., & Ding, M. (2020). Does nicotine protect us against coronavirus? The Conversation. https://theconversation.com/does-nicotine-protect-us-against-coronavirus-137488

Bellieni, C. V. (2020). Nurses and doctors heroes? A risky myth of the COVID19 era. *Nursing Reports*, 10(2), 37–40. https://doi.org/10.3390/nursrep10020006

Bentzen, J. S. (2021). In crisis, we pray: Religiosity and the COVID-19 pandemic. *Journal of Economic Behavior & Organization*, 192, 541–583. https://doi.org/10.1016/j.jebo.2021.10.014

Boghurst, W. (1666). *Loimographia: The great plague of London in the year 1665*. Shaw & Sons.

Boguszewski, R., Makowska, M., Bożewicz, M., & Podkowińska, M. (2020). The COVID-19 Pandemic's impact on religiosity in Poland. *Religions*, 11, article 646. https://doi.org/10.3390/rel11120646

Bonanno, G. A., & Diminich, E. D. (2013). Positive adjustment to adversity—Trajectories of minimal-impact resilience and emergent resilience. *Journal of Child Psychology and Psychiatry*, 54, 378–401. https://doi.org/10.1111/jcpp.12021

Boulton, M., Garnett, A., & Webster, F. (2021). A Foucauldian discourse analysis of media reporting on the nurse-as-hero during COVID-19. *Nursing Inquiry*, 29(3), article e12471. https://doi.org/10.1111/nin.12471

Briggs, A. (1961). Cholera and society in the nineteenth century. *Past & Present*, 19(1), 76–96. https://doi.org/10.1093/past/19.1.76

Brune, K. (1997). The early history of non-opioid analgesics. *Acute Pain*, 1, 33–40.

Buckley, T. (2021). The family behind the Covid bleach cure was making a fortune. *Bloomberg*. https://www.bloomberg.com/news/features/2021-06-29/covid-bleach-cure-how-operation-quack-hack-took-down-the-genesis-ii-church

Buguzi, S. (2021). Covid-19: Counting the cost of denial in Tanzania. *BMJ (Clinical Research Ed.)*, 373, article n1052. https://doi.org/10.1136/bmj.n1052

Busari, S., & Adebayo, B. (2020). Nigeria records chloroquine poisoning after Trump endorses it for coronavirus treatment. *CNN*. https://www.cnn.com/2020/03/23/africa/chloroquine-trump-nigeria-intl/index.html

Butcher, T. (1855). *"Mordichim": Recollections of cholera in the Barbados, during the middle of the year 1854*. Partidge, Oakey, & Co.

Byck, D. (2020). You can now buy Anthony Fauci swag. *The Washingtonian*. https://www.washingtonian.com/2020/03/27/you-can-now-buy-anthony-fauci-swag/

Byrne, J. P. (2006). *Daily life during the Black Death*. Greenwood.

Byrne, J. P. (2012). *Encyclopedia of the Black Death*. ABC-CLIO.

CBS News. (2020). Grocery stores seeing second wave of panic buying. https://www.cbs19news.com/story/42933419/grocery-stores-seeing-second-wave-of-panic-buying

Chai, P. R., Ferro, E. G., Kirshenbaum, J. M., Hayes, B. D., Culbreth, S. E., Boyer, E. W., et al. (2020). Intentional hydroxychloroquine overdose treated with high-dose diazepam: An increasing concern in the COVID-19 pandemic. *Journal of Medical Toxicology*, 16, 314–320. https://doi.org/10.1007/s13181-020-00790-8

Chary, M. A., Overbeek, D. L., Papadimoulis, A., Sheroff, A., & Burns, M. M. (2021). Geospatial correlation between COVID-19 health misinformation and poisoning with household cleaners in the Greater Boston Area. *Clinical Toxicology, 59*, 320–325. https://doi.org/10.1080/15563650.2020.1811297

Chaya, L. (2021). Canadian doctor debunks "detoxx" advice for anti-vaxxers. *National Post.* https://nationalpost.com/news/canadian-doctor-debunks-detoxx-advice-for-anti-vaxxers-who-get-a-shot-under-mandate

Chen, S., Bi, K., Sun, P., & Bonanno, G. A. (2022). Psychopathology and resilience following strict COVID-19 lockdowns in Hubei, China: Examining person- and context-level predictors for longitudinal trajectories. *American Psychologist, 77*(2), 262–275. https://doi.org/10.1037/amp0000958

Cheng, C. (2004). To be paranoid is the standard? Panic responses to SARS out-break in the Hong Kong Special Administrative Region. *Asian Perspective, 28*, 67–98. https://doi.org/10.1353/apr.2004.0034

Cheng, C., & Cheung, M. W. (2005). Psychological responses to outbreak of severe acute respiratory syndrome: A prospective, multiple time-point study. *Journal of Personality, 73*, 261–285. https://doi.org/10.1111/j.1467-6494.2004.00310.x

Cheng, C., Ying, W., Ebrahimi, O. V., & Wong, K. F. E. (2024). Coping style and mental health amid the first wave of the COVID-19 pandemic: A culture-moderated meta-analysis of 44 nations. *Health Psychology Review, 18*(1), 141–164. https://doi.org/10.1080/17437199.2023.2175015

Clark, D. (2020). Trump suggests "injection" of disinfectant to beat coronavirus and "clean" the lungs. *NBC News.* https://www.nbcnews.com/politics/donald-trump/trump-suggests-injection-disinfectant-beat-coronavirus-clean-lungs-n1191216

CNN. (2020). "It's crazy": Panic buying forces stores to limit purchases of toilet paper and masks. https://www.cnn.com/2020/03/06/business/coronavirus-global-panic-buying-toilet-paper/index.html

Cortez, M. F. (2020). CDC warns against drinking hand sanitizer amid reports of deaths. *Bloomberg.* https://www.bloomberg.com/news/articles/2020-08-05/cdc-warns-against-drinking-hand-sanitizer-amid-reports-of-deaths

Cox, C. L. (2020). "Healthcare Heroes": Problems with media focus on heroism from healthcare workers during the COVID-19 pandemic. *Journal of Medical Ethics, 46*(8), 510–513. https://doi.org/10.1136/medethics-2020-106398

Daily Mail. (2021, June 12). Saluting Covid heroes. *Daily Mail,* 24.

DeFranza, D., Lindow, M., Harrison, K., Mishra, A., & Mishra, H. (2021). Religion and reactance to COVID-19 mitigation guidelines. *American Psychologist, 76*(5), 744–754. https://doi.org/10.1037/amp0000717

Dennis, A., & Ogden, J. (2022). Nostalgia, gratitude, or optimism: The impact of a two-week intervention on well-being during Covid-19. *Journal of Happiness Studies, 23*, 2613–2634. https://doi.org/10.1007/s10902-022-00513-6

Deutsche Welle. (2020). Coronavirus: German minister warns against new wave of panic-buying. https://www.dw.com/en/coronavirus-german-minister-warns-against-new-wave-of-panic-buying/a-55316406.

Dezecache, G. (2015). Human collective reactions to threat. *WIREs Cognitive Science, 6*, 209–219. https://doi.org/10.1002/wcs.1344

Doino, W. (2020). The best saints to pray to during a pandemic. *Catholic Herald.* https://catholicherald.co.uk/the-best-saints-to-pray-to-during-a-pandemic/

Elliott, C. (2024). *Pox Romana: The plague that shook the Roman world.* Princeton Universtiy Press.

Evans, H., & Bartholomew, R. E. (2009). *Outbreak! The encyclopedia of extraordinary social behavior.* Anomalist Books.

Fatima, H., Oyetunji, T., Mishra, S., Sinha, K., Olorunsogbon, O., Akande, O., et al. (2022). Religious coping in the time of COVID-19 pandemic in India and Nigeria: Finding of a cross-national community survey. *International Journal of Social Psychiatry, 68*(2), 309–315. https://doi.org/10.1177/0020764020984511

Fiquepron, M. R. (2018). Places, attitudes and moments during the epidemics: Representations of yellow fever and cholera in the city of Buenos Aires, 1867–1871. *História, Ciências, Saúde, 25*(2), 1–16. https://doi.org/10.1590/S0104-59702018000200003

Fitchburg Daily Sentinel. (1918, September 26). Camphor gum bags about as effective as rabbit foot. *Fitchburg Daily Sentinel*, 7.

Frankenbach, J., Wildschut, T., Juhl, J., & Sedikides, C. (2020). Does neuroticism disrupt the psychological benefits of nostalgia? A meta-analytic test. *European Journal of Personality, 35*(2), 249–266. https://doi.org/10.1002/per.2276

Freckelton, I. (2020). COVID-19: Fear, quackery, false representations and the law. *International Journal of Law and Psychiatry, 72*, article 101611. https://doi.org/10.1016/j.ijlp.2020.101611

Fullana, M. A., Hidalgo-Mazzei, D., Vieta, E., & Radua, J. (2020). Coping behaviors associated with decreased anxiety and depressive symptoms during the COVID-19 pandemic and lockdown. *Journal of Affective Disorders, 275*, 80–81. https://doi.org/10.1016/j.jad.2020.06.027

Galatzer-Levy, I. R., Huang, S. H., & Bonanno, G. A. (2018). Trajectories of resilience and dysfunction following potential trauma: A review and statistical evaluation. *Clinical Psychology Review, 63*, 41–55. https://doi.org/10.1016/j.cpr.2018.05.008

Gammon, S., & Ramshaw, G. (2021). Distancing from the present: Nostalgia and leisure in lockdown. *Leisure Sciences, 43*(1–2), 131–137. https://doi.org/10.1080/01490400.2020.1773993

Garrido, S. (2018). The influence of personality and coping style on the affective outcomes of nostalgia: Is nostalgia a healthy coping mechanism or rumination? *Personality and Individual Differences, 120*, 259–264. https://doi.org/10.1016/j.paid.2016.07.021

Gecewicz, C. (2020). Few Americans say their house of worship is open, but a quarter say their faith has grown amid pandemic. *Pew Research Center*. https://www.pewresearch.org/fact-tank/2020/04/30/few-americans-say-their-house-of-worship-is-open-but-a-quarter-say-their-religious-faith-has-grown-amid-pandemic/

Gilmour, J., Machin, T., Brownlow, C., & Jeffries, C. (2020). Facebook-based social support and health: A systematic review. *Psychology of Popular Media, 9*(3), 328–346. https://doi.org/10.1037/ppm0000246

Glendinning, M. (2020). Two Calgary fashion brands have created t-shirts to celebrate Canada's public health heroines. *Fashion Magazine*. https://fashionmagazine.com/style/theresa-tam-bonnie-henry-deena-hinshaw-t-shirts/

Götmann, A., & Bechtoldt, M. N. (2021). Coping with COVID-19: Longitudinal analysis of coping strategies and the role of trait mindfulness in mental well-being. *Personality and Individual Differences, 175*, article 110695. https://doi.org/10.1016/j.paid.2021.110695

Gowen, B. S. (1907). Some aspects of pestilences and other epidemics. *American Journal of Psychology, 18*(1), 1–60. https://doi.org/10.2307/1412171

Grasso, A., Resnati, C., Lanza, A., Berrino, L., & Villani, R. (2021). Toxicovigilance during COVID-19: Attention to poisoning related to disinfection. *Minerva Anestesiologica, 87*, 251–252. https://doi.org/10.23736/S0375-9393.20.15010-7

Greenberg, J., Helm, P. J., Landau, M. J., & Solomon, S. (2020). Dwelling forever in the house of the Lord: On the terror management function of religion. In K. E. Vail & C. Routledge (Eds.), *The science of religion, spirituality, and existentialism* (pp. 3–20). Elsevier.

Halpern, J. J. (2021). The influence of cognitive heuristics and biases on palliative social workers' support of patient and caregiver decision making: The pulse oximeter buying trend during the COVID-19 pandemic. *Journal of Social Work in End-of-Life & Palliative Care, 17*(2–3), 186–197. https://doi.org/10.1080/15524256.2021.1910108

Harden, L. M., Kent, S., Pittman, Q. J., & Roth, J. (2015). Fever and sickness behavior: Friend or foe? *Brain, Behavior, and Immunity, 50,* 322–333. https://doi.org/10.1016/j.bbi.2015.07.012

Heidari, M., & Sayfouri, N. (2022). COVID-19 and alcohol poisoning: A fatal competition. *Disaster Medicine and Public Health Preparedness, 16*(5), 2179–2181. https://doi.org/10.1017/dmp.2021.89

Henderson, D. A. (2009). *Smallpox: The death of a disease.* Prometheus.

Henry, N., Parthiban, S., & Farroha, A. (2021). The effect of COVID-19 lockdown on the incidence of deliberate self-harm injuries presenting to the emergency room. *International Journal of Psychiatry in Medicine, 56*(4), 266–277. https://doi.org/10.1177/0091217420982100

Higgins, C. (2020). Why we shouldn't be calling our healthcare workers "heroes." *The Guardian.* https://www.theguardian.com/commentisfree/2020/may/27/healthcare-workers-heros-language-heroism

Holmes, T. J. (2021, April 2). Covid vaccine hero. *Good Morning America.* https://search.ebscohost.com/login.aspx?direct=true&AuthType=shib&db=bwh&AN=149889305&site=ehost-live&scope=site&custid=s5672194

Honigsbaum, M. (2010). The great dread: Cultural and psychological impacts and responses to the "Russian" influenza in the United Kingdom, 1889–1893. *Social History of Medicine, 23*(2), 299–319. https://doi.org/10.1093/shm/hkq011

Hymes, R. (2014). A hypothesis on the east Asian beginnings of the *Yersinia pestis* polytomy. In M. Green (Ed.), *Pandemic diseases in the medieval world: Rethinking the Black Death* (pp. 285–308). ARC Medieval Press.

Iezzoni, L. (1999). *Influenza 1918: The worst epidemic in American history.* TV Books.

Infurna, F. J., & Jayawickreme, E. (2019). Fixing the growth illusion: New directions for research in resilience and posttraumatic growth. *Current Directions in Psychological Science, 28*(2), 152–158. https://doi.org/10.1177/0963721419827017

Jovančević, A., & Milićević, N. (2020). Optimism-pessimism, conspiracy theories and general trust as factors contributing to COVID-19 related behavior—A cross-cultural study. *Personality and Individual Differences, 167,* article 110216. https://doi.org/10.1016/j.paid.2020.110216

Kan, W., Ma, B., & Lin, G. (2011). Sulfur fumigation processing of traditional Chinese medicinal herbs: Beneficial or detrimental? *Frontiers in Pharmacology, 2,* article 84. https://doi.org/10.3389/fphar.2011.00084

Kaur, H. (2020). People are buying pulse oximeters to try and detect coronavirus at home. Do you need one? *CNN.* https://www.cnn.com/2020/04/26/health/pulse-oximeters-coronavirus-wellness-scn-trnd/index.html

Keane, M., & Neal, T. (2020). Consumer panic in the COVID-19 pandemic. *Journal of Econometrics, 220*(1), 86–105. https://doi.org/10.1016/j.jeconom.2020.07.045

Kell, K. T. (1965). Tobacco in folk cures in Western society. *Journal of American Folklore, 78*(308), 99–114. https://doi.org/10.2307/538277

Kinsella, E. L., Ritchie, T. D., & Igou, E. R. (2015). Lay perspectives on the social and psychological functions of heroes. *Frontiers in Psychology, 6,* article 130. https://doi.org/10.3389/fpsyg.2015.00130

Knapp, A. (2020). The original plandemic: Unmasking the eerily familiar conspiracy theories behind the Russian flu of 1889. *Forbes.* https://www.forbes.com/sites/alexknapp/2020/05/15/the-original-plandemic-unmasking-the-eerily-parallel-conspiracy-theories-behind-the-russian-flu-of-1889/?sh=71fe578250d5

Lancet. (1890). The influenza epidemic. *Lancet, 1*(3463), p. 88.

Lancet. (1892). Carlill v. the Carbolic Smoke-Ball Company. *Lancet, 140*(3593), p. 102. https://doi.org/10.1016/S0140-6736(01)91779-9

Lazarus, R. S. (1991). *Emotion and adaptation*. Oxford University Press.
Le Roux, G., Sinno-Tellier, S., Puskarczyk, E., Labadie, M., von Fabeck, K., Pélissier, F., et al. (2021). Poisoning during the COVID-19 outbreak and lockdown: Retrospective analysis of exposures reported to French poison control centres. *Clinical Toxicology, 59*(9), 832–839. https://doi.org/10.1080/15563650.2021.1874402
Lebin, J. A., Ma, A., Mudan, A., & Smollin, C. G. (2021). Fatal ingestion of sodium chlorite used as hand sanitizer during the COVID-19 pandemic. *Clinical Toxicology, 59*(3), 265–266. https://doi.org/10.1080/15563650.2020.1798981
Lehrer, P. M., & Woolfolk, R. L. (2021). *Principles and practice of stress management* (4th ed.). Guilford.
Leichtenstern, O. (1905). Influenza and dengue. In J. Mannaberg & O. Leichtenstern (Eds.), *Malaria, influenza and dengue* (pp. 521–716). Saunders.
Leunissen, J., Wildschut, T., Sedikides, C., & Routledge, C. (2021). The hedonic character of nostalgia: An integrative data analysis. *Emotion Review, 13*(2), 139–156. https://doi.org/10.1177/1754073920950455
Levitan, R. (2020). The infection that's silently killing coronavirus patients: This is what I learned during 10 days of treating COVID pneumonia at Bellevue Hospital. *New York Times*. https://www.nytimes.com/2020/04/20/opinion/sunday/coronavirus-testing-pneumonia.html
Lewin, K. (1935). *A dynamic theory of personality*. McGraw-Hill.
Lipworth, W. (2020). Beyond duty: Medical "heroes" and the COVID-19 pandemic. *Journal of Bioethical Inquiry, 17*(4), 723–730. https://doi.org/10.1007/s11673-020-10065-0
Liu, X. S., Shi, Y., Xue, N. I., & Shen, H. (2022). The impact of time pressure on impulsive buying: The moderating role of consumption type. *Tourism Management, 91*, article 104505. https://doi.org/10.1016/j.tourman.2022.104505
Loeb, L. (2005). Beating the flu: Orthodox and commercial responses to influenza in Britain, 1889–1919. *Social History of Medicine, 18*(2), 203–224. https://doi.org/10.1093/sochis/hki030
Luther, M. (1527). Whether one may flee from a deadly plague. In J. J. Pelikan, H. C. Oswald, & H. T. Lehmann (Eds.), *Luther's works* (Vol. 43, pp. 119–138). Fortress.
Lytvynenko, J. (2020). Here's a running list of the latest hoaxes spreading about the coronavirus. *BuzzFeed News*. https://www.buzzfeednews.com/article/janelytvynenko/coronavirus-fake-news-disinformation-rumors-hoaxes
Marsh, C. (2020). In an age of COVID villains, an unlikely hero has emerged: B.C.'s Dr. Bonnie Henry. *National Post*. https://nationalpost.com/news/in-an-age-of-covid-villains-an-unlikely-hero-has-emerged-b-c-s-dr-bonnie-henry
McKay, K., Wayland, S., Ferguson, D., Petty, J., & Kennedy, E. (2021). "At least until the second wave comes ..": A Twitter analysis of the NHS and COVID-19 between March and June 2020. *International Journal of Environmental Research and Public Health, 18*(8), article 3943. https://doi.org/10.3390/ijerph18083943
McMeekin, J., & Shah, A. (2020). FDA protects patients and consumers from fraud during COVID-19. https://www.fda.gov/news-events/fda-voices/fda-protects-patients-and-consumers-fraud-during-covid-19#:~:text=To%20proactively%20identify%20and%20neutralize,during%20the%20COVID%2D19%20pandemic
Mead, R. (1744). *A discourse on the plague* (9th ed.). Millar.
Milwaukee Sentinel. (1918, September 22). Says worry can cause Spanish influenza. *Milwaukee Sentinel*, 6.
Mohammed, S., Peter, E., Killackey, T., & Maciver, J. (2021). The "nurse as hero" discourse in the COVID-19 pandemic: A poststructural discourse analysis. *International Journal of Nursing Studies, 117*, article 103887. https://doi.org/10.1016/j.ijnurstu.2021.103887
Myer, J. S. (1912). *Life and letters of Dr. William Beaumont*. Mosby.

New York American. (1918, October 20). Many patients furnished soup. *New York American*, L5.

Nitschke, J., Forbes, P., Ali, N., Cutler, J., Apps, M., Lockwood, P., et al. (2020). Resilience during uncertainty? Greater social connectedness during Covid-19 lockdown is associated with reduced distress and fatigue. *British Journal of Health Psychology*, 26(2), 553–569. https://doi.org/10.1111/bjhp.12485

Osikoya, B. (2020). A fake claim that cocaine cures the coronavirus is spreading online, and the French government was forced to tell people that it won' t. *Business Insider*. https://www.businessinsider.com/coronavirus-cocaine-cure-fake-spreads-rebutted-by-french-government-2020-3

Park, C. L., Finkelstein-Fox, L., Russell, B. S., Fendrich, M., Hutchison, M., & Becker, J. (2021). Americans' distress early in the COVID-19 pandemic: Protective resources and coping strategies. *Psychological Trauma: Theory, Research, Practice and Policy*, 13(4), 422–431. https://doi.org/10.1037/tra0000931

Patanavanich, R., Siripoon, T., Amponnavarat, S., & Glantz, S. A. (2023). Active smokers are at higher risk of COVID-19 death: A systematic review and meta-analysis. *Nicotine & Tobacco Research*, 25(2), 177–184. https://doi.org/10.1093/ntr/ntac085

Pearse, R. (2017). John of Ephesus describes the Justinianic plague. https://www.roger-pearse.com/weblog/2017/05/10/john-of-ephesus-describes-the-justinianic-plague/

Pettigrew, E. (1983). *The silent enemy: Canada and the deadly flu of 1918*. Western Producer Prairie Books.

Pew Research Center. (2020). Most Americans say coronavirus outbreak has impacted their lives. *Pew Research Center*. https://www.pewresearch.org/social-trends/2020/03/30/most-americans-say-coronavirus-outbreak-has-impacted-their-lives/

Pigaiani, Y., Zoccante, L., Zocca, A., Arzenton, A., Menegolli, M., Fadel, S., et al. (2020). Adolescent lifestyle behaviors, coping strategies and subjective wellbeing during the COVID-19 pandemic: An online student survey. *Healthcare*, 8(4), article 472. https://doi.org/10.3390/healthcare8040472

Reuters. (2021). Plan to ban people from leaving their homes triggers panic buying in Ho Chi Minh City. *The Strait Times*. https://www.straitstimes.com/asia/se-asia/panic-buying-in-vietnams-ho-chi-minh-city-before-tighter-covid-19-lockdown

Rimmer, A. (2021). Covid-19: Drop the hero narrative and support doctors' mental health, says charity. *BMJ (Clinical Research Ed.)*, 372, article n337. https://doi.org/10.1136/bmj.n337

Robins, N. (2005). *Copeland's cure: Homeopathy and the war between conventional and alternative medicine*. Knopf.

Rochester Times-Union. (1918, October 17). Must get food to victims of "flu" at home. *Rochester Times-Union*, 9.

Rocky Mountain News. (1918, November 23). Influenza germs hates smoke city bacteriologist declares. *Rocky Mountain News*, 6. http://hdl.handle.net/2027/spo.8980flu.0003.898

Romas, J. A., & Sharma, M. (2022). *Practical stress management: A comprehensive workbook (8th ed.)*. Academic Press.

Rosenberg, C. E. (1987). *The cholera years: The United States in 1832, 1849, and 1866*. University of Chicago Press.

Schoch-Spana, M. (2004). Lessons from the 1918 pandemic influenza: Psychosocial consequences of a catastrophic outbreak of disease. In R. J. Ursano, A. E. Norwood, & C. S. Fullerton (Eds.), *Bioterrorism: Psychological and public health interventions* (pp. 38–55). Cambridge University Press.

Schuster, M., Stein, B., Jaycox, L., Collins, R., Marshall, G., Elliott, M., et al. (2001). A national survey of stress reactions after the September 11, 2001, terrorist attacks. *New England Journal of Medicine*, 345(20), 1507–1512. https://doi.org/10.1056/NEJM200111153452024

Sedikides, C., & Wildschut, T. (2018). Finding meaning in nostalgia. *Review of General Psychology, 22*(1), 48–61. https://doi.org/10.1037/gpr0000109

Seeger, C. L. (1832). *A lecture on the epidemic cholera.* Wright.

Sefidbakht, S., Lotfi, M., Jalli, R., Moghadami, M., Sabetian, G., & Iranpour, P. (2020). Methanol toxicity outbreak: When fear of COVID-19 goes viral. *Emergency Medicine Journal, 37,* p. 416. https://doi.org/10.1136/emermed-2020-209886

Skog, F., & Lundström, R. (2022). Heroes, victims, and villains in news media narratives about COVID-19. Analysing moralising discourse in Swedish newspaper reporting during the Spring of 2020. *Social Science & Medicine, 294,* article 114718. https://doi.org/10.1016/j.socscimed.2022.114718

Slack, P. (1985). *The impact of plague in Tudor and Stuart England.* Routledge.

Soltaninejad, K. (2020). Methanol mass poisoning outbreak: A consequence of COVID-19 pandemic and misleading messages on social media. *International Journal of Occupational and Environmental Medicine, 11,* 148–150. https://doi.org/10.34172/ijoem.2020.1983

Sommerlad, A., Marston, L., Huntley, J., Livingston, G., Lewis, G., Steptoe, A., et al. (2021). Social relationships and depression during the COVID-19 lockdown: Longitudinal analysis of the COVID-19 social study. *Psychological Medicine, 52*(15), 3381–3390. https://doi.org/10.1017/S0033291721000039

Spocchia, G. (2021). DeSantis sells anti-Fauci t-shirts as Florida Covid death toll hits 38,000. *The Independent.* https://www.independent.co.uk/news/world/americas/us-politics/ron-desantis-merch-covid-florida-b1884009.html

Taylor, S. (2019). *The psychology of pandemics: Preparing for the next global outbreak of infectious disease.* Cambridge Scholars Publishing.

Taylor, S. (2021). Understanding and managing pandemic-related panic buying. *Journal of Anxiety Disorders, 78,* article 102364. https://doi.org/10.1016/j.janxdis.2021.102364

Taylor, S., Landry, C. A., Paluszek, M. M., Fergus, T. A., McKay, D., & Asmundson, G. J. G. (2020). Covid stress syndrome: Concept, structure, and correlates. *Depression and Anxiety, 37,* 706–714. https://doi.org/10.1002/da.23071

Taylor, S., Landry, C. A., Rachor, G. S., Paluszek, M. M., & Asmundson, G. J. G. (2020). Fear and avoidance of healthcare workers: An important, under-recognized form of stigmatization during the COVID-19 pandemic. *Journal of Anxiety Disorders, 75,* article 102289. https://doi.org/10.1016/j.janxdis.2020.102289

Taylor, S., Paluszek, M., Rachor, G. S., McKay, D., & Asmundson, G. J. G. (2021). Substance use and abuse, COVID-19-related distress, and disregard for social distancing: A network analysis. *Addictive Behaviors, 114,* article 106754. https://doi.org/10.1016/j.addbeh.2020.106754

Taylor, S. E. (2011). Social support: A review. In H. S. Friedman (Ed.), *The Oxford handbook of health psychology* (pp. 189–214). Oxford University Press.

The Guardian. (1909, March 11). Influenza again! *The Guardian,* 4.

Van Lange, P. A. M., & Columbus, S. (2021). Vitamin S: Why is social contact, even with strangers, so important to well-being? *Current Directions in Psychological Science, 30*(3), 267–273. https://doi.org/10.1177/09637214211002538

van Westen-lagerweij, N. A., Meijer, E., Meeuwsen, E. G., Chavannes, N. H., Willemsen, M. C., & Croes, E. A. (2021). Are smokers protected against SARS-CoV-2 infection (COVID-19)? The origins of the myth. *Primary Care Respiratory Medicine, 31*(1), article 10. https://doi.org/10.1038/s41533-021-00223-1

Vandenbos, G. R. (Ed.). (2007). *APA dictionary of psychology.* American Psychological Association.

Veer, I., Riepenhausen, A., Zerban, M., Wackerhagen, C., Puhlmann, L., Engen, H., et al. (2021). Psycho-social factors associated with mental resilience in the Corona lockdown. *Translational Psychiatry, 11*(1), article 67. https://doi.org/10.1038/s41398-020-01150-4

Verplanken, B. (2012). When bittersweet turns sour: Adverse effects of nostalgia on habitual worriers. *European Journal of Social Psychology, 42*(3), 285–289. https://doi.org/10.1002/ejsp.1852

Wear, A. (1999). Fear, anxiety and the plague in early modern England. In J. R. Hinnells & R. Porter (Eds.), *Religion, health and suffering* (pp. 339–363). Routledge.

Weiss, K. J., & Dube, A. R. (2021). What ever happened to nostalgia (the diagnosis)? *Journal of Nervous and Mental Disease, 209*(9), 622–627. https://doi.org/10.1097/NMD.0000000000001349

Weiss, S. (2020). Inside the infodemic: Coronavirus in the age of wellness. *New Statesman.* https://www.newstatesman.com/politics/health/2020/02/inside-infodemic-coronavirus-age-wellness

Wildschut, T., & Sedikides, C. (2001). Psychology and nostalgia: Toward a functional approach. In M. H. Jacobsen (Ed.), *Intimations of nostalgia* (pp. 110–128). Bristol University Press.

Wildschut, T., & Sedikides, C. (2022). Benefits of nostalgia in vulnerable populations. *European Review of Social Psychology, 34*(1), 44–91. https://doi.org/10.1080/10463283.2022.2036005

Wilson, J. M., Iannarone, M., & Wang, C. (2009). Media reporting of the emergence of the 1968 influenza pandemic in Hong Kong: Implications for modern-day situational awareness. *Disaster Medicine & Public Health Preparedness, 3*(Suppl 2), S148–S153. https://doi.org/10.1097/DMP.0b013e3181abd603

Wilson, S., Boorstein, M., Hernndez, A., & Rozsa, L. (2020). Coronavirus creates conflict for churches, where gatherings can be dangerous but also provide solace. *Washington Post.* https://www.washingtonpost.com/national/coronavirus-church-services-outbreak/2020/04/05/7f5b63cc-7773-11ea-90ad-819caa48d39f_story.html?utm_source=twitter&utm_medium=social&utm_campaign=wp_main

Wong, A. (2020). COVID-19 and toxicity from potential treatments: Panacea or poison. *Emergency Medicine Australasia, 32*, 697–699. https://doi.org/10.1111/1742-6723.13537

Chapter 9

Anonymous. (1721). *The late dreadful plague at Marseilles compared with that terrible plague in London in the year 1665.* Parker.

Baltimore Sun. (1918, November 6). Flee to hills from "flu." *Baltimore Sun*, 2.

Bandura, A. (1986). *Social foundations of thought and action: A social cognitive theory.* Prentice-Hall.

Barbarossa, M. V., Bogya, N., Dénes, A., Röst, G., Varma, H. V., & Vizi, Z. (2021). Fleeing lockdown and its impact on the size of epidemic outbreaks in the source and target regions - a COVID-19 lesson. *Scientific Reports, 11*(1), 9233. https://doi.org/10.1038/s41598-021-88204-9

Barrett, J. (2020). Tourist towns say, "Please stay away," during coronavirus lockdowns. *Wall Street Journal.* https://www.wsj.com/articles/tourist-towns-say-please-stay-away-during-coronavirus-lockdowns-11586165401?mod=article_inline

Boghurst, W. (1666). *Loimographia: The great plague of London in the year 1665.* Shaw & Sons.

Burns, J. F. (1994a, October 7). As the plague ebbs, India is overcome by guilt. *New York Times, 144*, 2.

Burns, J. F. (1994b, October 1). India's city of plague: A caldron of urban ills. *New York Times, 144*, A1.

Burns, J. F. (1994c, September 26). Refugees fleeing plague carry it south to Bombay. *New York Times, 144*, A1.

Burns, J. F. (1994d, October 1). Thousands return to Indian city hit by outbreak of plague. *New York Times, 144*, 8.

Butcher, T. (1855). *"Mordichim": Recollections of cholera in the Barbados, during the middle of the year 1854*. Partidge, Oakey, & Co.
Byrne, J. P. (2006). *Daily life during the Black Death*. Greenwood.
Byrne, J. P. (2012). *Encyclopedia of the Black Death*. ABC-CLIO.
Chander, R., Murugesan, M., Ritish, D., Damodharan, D., Arunachalam, V., Parthasarathy, R., et al. (2021). Addressing the mental health concerns of migrant workers during the COVID-19 pandemic: An experiential account. *International Journal of Social Psychiatry, 67*(7), 826–829. https://doi.org/10.1177/0020764020937736
Chen, Z. L., Zhang, Q., Lu, Y., Guo, Z. M., Zhang, X., Zhang, W. J., et al. (2020). Distribution of the COVID-19 epidemic and correlation with population emigration from Wuhan, China. *Chinese Medical Journal, 133*(9), 1044–1050. https://doi.org/10.1097/cm9.0000000000000782
Chinazzi, M., Davis, J. T., Ajelli, M., Gioannini, C., Litvinova, M., Merler, S., et al. (2020). The effect of travel restrictions on the spread of the 2019 novel coronavirus (COVID-19) outbreak. *Science, 368*(6489), 395–400. https://doi.org/10.1126/science.aba9757
Cohn, S. K. (2018). *Epidemics: Hate and compassion from the plague of Athens to AIDS*. Oxford University Press.
Crampton, T. (2003). As SARS rages, Hong Kong orders a quarantine. *New York Times*. https://www.nytimes.com/2003/04/01/news/as-sars-rages-hong-kong-orders-a-quarantine.html
D'Irsay, S. (1927). Defense reactions during the Black Death, 1348–1349. *Annals of Medical History, 9*, 169–179.
De Groot, J. H. B., Semin, G. R., & Smeets, M. A. M. (2014). I can see, hear, and smell your fear: Comparing olfactory and audiovisual media in fear communication. *Journal of Experimental Psychology: General, 143*, 825–834. https://doi.org/10.1037/a0033731
Debiec, J., & Olsson, A. (2017). Social fear learning: From animal models to human function. *Trends in Cognitive Sciences, 21*, 546–555. https://doi.org/10.1016/j.tics.2017.04.010
Dekker, T. (1625). *A rod for run-awayes*. J. Trundle.
Delaporte, F. (1986). *Disease and civilization: The cholera in Paris, 1832*. MIT Press.
Dutt, A. K., Akhtar, R., & McVeigh, M. (2006). Surat plague of 1994 re-examined. *Southeast Asian Journal of Tropical Medicine and Public Health, 37*(4), 755–760.
Elliott, C. (2024). *Pox Romana: The plague that shook the Roman world*. Princeton University Press.
Epstein, J. M., Parker, J., Cummings, D., & Hammond, R. A. (2008). Coupled contagion dynamics of fear and disease: Mathematical and computational explorations. *PLOS ONE, 3*(12), article e3955. https://doi.org/10.1371/journal.pone.0003955
Errett, N. A., Sauer, L. M., & Rutkow, L. (2020). An integrative review of the limited evidence on international travel bans as an emerging infectious disease disaster control measure. *Journal of Emergency Management, 18*(1), 7–14. https://doi.org/10.5055/jem.2020.0446
Fiquepron, M. R. (2018). Places, attitudes and moments during the epidemics: Representations of yellow fever and cholera in the city of Buenos Aires, 1867–1871. *História, Ciências, Saúde, 25*(2), 1–16. https://doi.org/10.1590/S0104-59702018000200003
Garza, R. P. (2008). *Understanding plague: The medical and imaginative texts of medieval Spain*. Peter Lang.
Gettleman, J., Raj, S., & Yasir, S. (2021, April 14). In India, a second wave of Covid-19 prompts a new exodus from the cities. *New York Times*, A7. https://www.nytimes.com/2021/04/14/world/asia/india-covid-migration.html
Grépin, K. A., Aston, J., & Burns, J. (2023). Effectiveness of international border control measures during the COVID-19 pandemic: A narrative synthesis of published systematic reviews. *Philosophical Transactions: Series A, Mathematical, Physical, and Engineering Sciences, 381*(2257), 20230134. https://doi.org/10.1098/rsta.2023.0134

Gump, B. B., & Kulik, J. A. (1997). Stress, affiliation, and emotional contagion. *Journal of Personality and Social Psychology, 72*, 305–319.

Hajari, N. (2020). India's grim coronavirus exodus has some ugly echoes. *Bloomberg Opinion*. https://www.bloomberg.com/opinion/articles/2020-04-01/india-s-grim-coronavirus-exodus-has-some-ugly-echoes

Hatfield, E., Cacioppo, J. T., & Rapson, R. L. (1994). *Emotional contagion*. Cambridge University Press.

Hatfield, E., Carpenter, M., & Rapson, R. L. (2014). Emotional contagion as a precursor to collective emotions. In C. von Scheve & M. Salmela (Eds.), *Collective emotions: Perspectives from psychology, philosophy, and sociology* (pp. 108–122). Oxford University Press. https://doi.org/10.1093/acprof:oso/9780199659180.003.0008

Hatfield, E., Paige, S., & Rapson, R. L. (2020). Emotional contagion, intimate intercultural relationships, and intercultural training. In D. Landis & D. P. S. Bhawuk (Eds.), *The Cambridge handbook of intercultural training* (4th ed., pp. 640–657). Cambridge University Press. https://doi.org/10.1017/9781108854184.028

Haug, N., Geyrhofer, L., Londei, A., Dervic, E., Desvars-Larrive, A., Loreto, V., et al. (2020). Ranking the effectiveness of worldwide COVID-19 government interventions. *Nature Human Behaviour, 4*(12), 1303–1312. https://doi.org/10.1038/s41562-020-01009-0

Keogh, G. (2020, March 30). The virus vigilantes. *Daily Mail*, 8.

Kephale, R. (1665). *Medela pestilentiae*. Samuel Speed.

Kinetz, E. (2020). Where did they go? Millions fled Wuhan, China, before coronavirus lockdown. *Global News*. https://globalnews.ca/news/6527152/coronavirus-lockdown-wuhan/

Kotoky, A. (2021). Wealthy Indians flee by private jet as virus infections spiral. *Bloomberg.com*. https://www.bloomberg.com/news/articles/2021-04-26/wealthy-indians-flee-by-private-jet-as-virus-infections-spiral#:~:text=India's%20mounting%20crisis%20surrounding%20a,the%20country%20by%20private%20jet.&text=%E2%80%9CWhoever%20can%20afford%20to%20take,worldwide%20since%20the%20pandemic%20began

Kumar, K., Singh, P., Shouan, A., & Singh, S. M. (2021). The exodus of migrant workers during the coronavirus disease 2019 (COVID-19) pandemic in India: Thematic findings on emotional concerns. *Open Journal of Psychiatry & Allied Sciences, 12*(1), 68–69. https://doi.org/10.5958/2394-2061.2021.00005.7

Luther, M. (1527). Whether one may flee from a deadly plague. In J. J. Pelikan, H. C. Oswald, & H. T. Lehmann (Eds.), *Luther's works* (Vol. 43, pp. 119–138). Fortress.

Malatzky, C., Gillespie, J., Couch, D. L., & Cosgrave, C. (2020). Why place matters: A rurally-orientated analysis of COVID-19's differential impacts. *Social Sciences & Humanities Open, 2*(1), article 100063. https://doi.org/10.1016/j.ssaho.2020.100063

Mawson, A. R. (2005). Understanding mass panic and other collective responses to threat and disaster. *Psychiatry: Interpersonal and Biological Processes, 68*(2), 95–113. https://doi.org/10.1521/psyc.2005.68.2.95

Pang, Z., Zhang, Z., Zhu, C., & Wang, J. (2022). Spill-over effect of Wuhan travel ban on population flow in the outbreak stage of COVID-19 in China. *Cities, 120*, 103404. https://doi.org/10.1016/j.cities.2021.103404

Parets, M. (1651). *A journal of the plague year: The diary of the Barcelona tanner Miquel Parets 1651* (J. S. Amelang, Trans. & Ed., 1991). Oxford University Press.

Patil, S. S., & Chaukimath, S. P. (2020). COVID-19: Mass exodus of migrant workers in India, are we staring at a mental health crisis? *Industrial Psychiatry Journal, 29*(2), 360–361. https://doi.org/10.4103/ipj.ipj_102_20

Pearse, R. (2017). John of Ephesus describes the Justinianic plague. https://www.roger-pearse.com/weblog/2017/05/10/john-of-ephesus-describes-the-justinianic-plague/

Pomfret, J. (2003, April 24). Thousands flee Beijing, fearing SARS. *Washington Post*, A20. https://www.washingtonpost.com/archive/politics/2003/04/24/thousands-flee-beijing-fearing-sars/da04ce95-058d-408c-ad97-a8f2017e4058/

Ramalingaswami, V. (2001). Psychosocial effects of the 1994 plague outbreak in Surat, India. *Military Medicine*, 166(12, Suppl 2), 29–30.

Rosenberg, C. E. (1987). *The cholera years: The United States in 1832, 1849, and 1866*. University of Chicago Press.

Sen, S. R., & Pandya, D. (2021, April 20). New virus wave sparks fresh worker exodus from India's cities. *Bloomberg.com*, April 20. https://www.bloomberg.com/news/articles/2021-04-20/new-virus-wave-sparks-fresh-worker-exodus-from-india-s-cities

Shiraef, M. A., Friesen, P., Feddern, L., & Weiss, M. A. (2022). Did border closures slow SARS-CoV-2? *Scientific Reports*, 12(1), 1709. https://doi.org/10.1038/s41598-022-05482-7

Sinha, H. (2000). Plague: A challenge for urban crisis management. *Journal of Contingencies & Crisis Management*, 8(1), 42–54. https://doi.org/10.1111/1468-5973.00123

Slack, P. (1985). *The impact of plague in Tudor and Stuart England*. Routledge.

Snowden, F. M. (2019). *Epidemics and society: From the Black Death to the present*. Yale University Press.

Stanford, P. (2020). "Visitors go home": Fear and loathing in UK holiday villages. *The Telegraph*. https://www.telegraph.co.uk/family/life/visitors-go-home-fear-loathing-uk-holiday-villages/

Stewart, B. (2020). COVID-19 travel advisories create tensions in B.C. tourist towns. *CBC News*. https://www.cbc.ca/news/canada/british-columbia/pandemic-bc-alberta-tourism-tensions-1.5599998

Wear, A. (1999). Fear, anxiety and the plague in early modern England. In J. R. Hinnells & R. Porter (Eds.), *Religion, health and suffering* (pp. 339–363). Routledge.

Wear, A. (2015). Making us as cruel as dogs: Plague in 16th and 17th century England. *Lancet*, 385(9986), 2456–2457. https://doi.org/10.1016/S0140-6736(15)61129-1

Chapter 10

Abeysinghe, S., & White, K. (2010). Framing disease: The avian influenza pandemic in Australia. *Health Sociology Review*, 19, 369–381. https://doi.org/10.5172/hesr.2010.19.3.369

Adebayo, G., Neumark, Y., Gesser-Edelsburg, A., Abu Ahmad, W., & Levine, H. (2017). Zika pandemic online trends, incidence and health risk communication: A time trend study. *BMJ Global Health*, 2, e000296. https://doi.org/10.1136/bmjgh-2017-000296

Ahmed, S., & Rasul, M. E. (2022). Social media news use and COVID-19 misinformation engagement: Survey study. *Journal of Medical Internet Research*, 24(9), e38944. https://doi.org/10.2196/38944

Allington, D., McAndrew, S., Moxham-Hall, V. L., & Duffy, B. (2021). Media usage predicts intention to be vaccinated against SARS-CoV-2 in the US and the UK. *Vaccine*, 39(18), 2595–2603. https://doi.org/10.1016/j.vaccine.2021.02.054

Bago, B., Rand, D. G., & Pennycook, G. (2020). Fake news, fast and slow: Deliberation reduces belief in false (but not true) news headlines. *Journal of Experimental Psychology: General*, 149(8), 1608–1613. https://doi.org/10.1037/xge0000729

BBC News. (2021). YouTube removes Bolsonaro videos for Covid misinformation. *BBC News*. https://www.bbc.com/news/world-latin-america-57923862

Bebbington, K., MacLeod, C., Ellison, T. M., & Fay, N. (2017). The sky is falling: Evidence of a negativity bias in the social transmission of information. *Evolution and Human Behavior*, 38(1), 92–101. https://doi.org/10.1016/j.evolhumbehav.2016.07.004

Bienenstock, E. J., Bonacich, P., & Oliver, M. (1990). The effect of network density and homogeneity on attitude polarization. *Social Networks, 12*(2), 153–172. https://doi.org/10.1016/0378-8733(90)90003-R

Bora, K., Das, D., Barman, B., & Borah, P. (2018). Are internet videos useful sources of information during global public health emergencies? A case study of YouTube videos during the 2015–16 Zika virus pandemic. *Pathogens and Global Health, 112*, 320–328. https://doi.org/10.1080/20477724.2018.1507784

Brady, W. J., Gantman, A. P., & Van Bavel, J. J. (2020). Attentional capture helps explain why moral and emotional content go viral. *Journal of Experimental Psychology: General, 149*(4), 746–756. https://doi.org/10.1037/xge0000673

Brauer, M., Judd, C. M., & Gliner, M. D. (1995). The effects of repeated expressions on attitude polarization during group discussions. *Journal of Personality and Social Psychology, 68*(6), 1014–1029. https://doi.org/10.1037/0022-3514.68.6.1014

Bronstein, M. V., Pennycook, G., Bear, A., Rand, D. G., & Cannon, T. D. (2019). Belief in fake news is associated with delusionality, dogmatism, religious fundamentalism, and reduced analytic thinking. *Journal of Applied Research in Memory and Cognition, 8*(1), 108–117. https://doi.org/10.1016/j.jarmac.2018.09.005

Brown, D. K., Yoo, J., & Johnson, T. J. (2019). Spreading Ebola panic: Newspaper and social media coverage of the 2014 Ebola health crisis. *Health Communication, 34*(8), 811–817. https://doi.org/10.1080/10410236.2018.1437524

Butler, K. (2021). The mother of conspiracies. *Mother Jones, 46*(1), 55–58.

CBC News. (2022). B.C. doctor accused of spreading COVID-19 misinformation suspended from practice. *CBC News*. https://www.cbc.ca/news/canada/british-columbia/b-c-doctor-suspended-for-spreading-covid-19-misinformation-1.6400737.

Center for Countering Digital Hate. (2021). The disinformation dozen: Why platforms must act on twelve leading online anti-vaxxers. https://252f2edd-1c8b-49f5-9bb2-cb57bb47e4ba.filesusr.com/ugd/f4d9b9_b7cedc0553604720b7137f8663366ee5.pdf

Chinese Embassy. (2020). Sixteen COVID-19 rumors and facts about China. http://ug.china-embassy.gov.cn/eng/xwdt/202004/t20200429_6944209.htm.

Clayton, K., Blair, S., Busam, J., Forstner, S., Glance, J., Green, G., et al. (2020). Real solutions for fake news? Measuring the effectiveness of general warnings and fact-check tags in reducing belief in false stories on social media. *Political Behavior, 42*, 1073–1095. https://doi.org/10.1007/s11109-019-09533-0

Corner, A., Whitmarsh, L., & Xenias, D. (2012). Uncertainty, scepticism and attitudes towards climate change: Biased assimilation and attitude polarisation. *Climatic Change, 114*(3), 463–478. https://doi.org/10.1007/s10584-012-0424-6

Craig, M., & Vijaykumar, S. (2023). One dose is not enough: The beneficial effect of corrective COVID-19 information is diminished if followed by misinformation. *Social Media + Society, 9*(2), article 1298. https://doi.org/10.1177/20563051231161298

Datareportal. (2024). Global social media statistics. https://datareportal.com/social-media-users

Davey, G. C., Hampton, J., Farrell, J., & Davidson, S. (1992). Some characteristics of worrying: Evidence for worrying and anxiety as separate constructs. *Personality and Individual Differences, 13*, 133–147. https://doi.org/10.1016/0191-8869(92)90036-O

Devine, A., Boluk, K., & Devine, F. (2017). Managing social media during a crisis: A conundrum for event managers. *Event Management, 21*, 375–389. https://doi.org/10.3727/152599517X14998876105729

Dorfman, A. (2022). The futility of censorship. *New York Review of Books*. https://www.nybooks.com/articles/2022/04/07/the-futility-of-censorship-dangerous-ideas-eric-berkowitz/?printpage=true

Dorr, A. (2001). Media literacy. In N. J. Smelser & P. B. Baltes (Eds.), *International encyclopedia of the social & behavioral sciences* (pp. 9494–9497). Pergamon. https://doi.org/10.1016/B0-08-043076-7/04354-0

Ecker, U., Lewandowsky, S., Cook, J., Schmid, P., Fazio, L., Brashier, N., et al. (2022). The psychological drivers of misinformation belief and its resistance to correction. *Nature Reviews Psychology, 1*(1), 13–29. https://doi.org/10.1038/s44159-021-00006-y

Evanega, S., Lynas, M., Adams, J., & Smolenyak, K. (2020). *Coronavirus misinformation: Quantifying sources and themes in the COVID-19 "infodemic."* Cornell Alliance for Science.

Fiquepron, M. R. (2018). Places, attitudes and moments during the epidemics: Representations of yellow fever and cholera in the city of Buenos Aires, 1867–1871. *História, Ciências, Saúde, 25*(2), 1–16. https://doi.org/10.1590/S0104-59702018000200003

Forsyth, D. R. (2020). Group-level resistance to health mandates during the COVID-19 pandemic: A groupthink approach. *Group Dynamics: Theory, Research, and Practice, 24*(3), 139–152. https://doi.org/10.1037/gdn0000132

Furey, A. (2021). Why this nurse chose firing over a vaccine. *National Post*. https://nationalpost.com/opinion/why-this-nurse-chose-firing-over-a-vaccine-full-comment-with-anthony-furey

Garza, R. P. (2008). *Understanding plague: The medical and imaginative texts of medieval Spain*. Peter Lang.

Gruner, S., & Kruger, F. (2021). Infodemics: Do healthcare professionals detect corona-related false news stories better than students? *PLOS ONE, 16*, e0247517. https://doi.org/10.1371/journal.pone.0247517

Guadagno, R. E., Rempala, D. M., Murphy, S., & Okdie, B. M. (2013). What makes a video go viral? An analysis of emotional contagion and Internet memes. *Computers in Human Behavior, 29*(6), 2312–2319. https://doi.org/10.1016/j.chb.2013.04.016

Guess, A. M., Lerner, M., Lyons, B., Montgomery, J., Nyhan, B., Reifler, J., et al. (2020). A digital media literacy intervention increases discernment between mainstream and false news in the United States and India. *PNAS, 117*(27), 15536–15545. https://doi.org/10.1073/pnas.1920498117

Gvirsman, S. D. (2014). It's not that we don't know, it's that we don't care: Explaining why selective exposure polarizes attitudes. *Mass Communication & Society, 17*(1), 74–97. https://doi.org/10.1080/15205436.2013.816738

Herhalt, C. (2021). Ontario regulator says anti-COVID-19 vaccine doctor can no longer practice medicine. *CP24*. https://www.cp24.com/news/ontario-regulator-says-anti-covid-19-vaccine-doctor-can-no-longer-practice-medicine-1.5642086?cache=yes%2Fweather-7.623929%3FclipId%3D89530

Hirst, L. F. (1953). *The conquest of plague*. Clarendon.

Honigsbaum, M. (2010). The great dread: Cultural and psychological impacts and responses to the "Russian" influenza in the United Kingdom, 1889–1893. *Social History of Medicine, 23*(2), 299–319. https://doi.org/10.1093/shm/hkq011

Kempińska-Mirosławska, B., & Woźniak-Kosek, A. (2013). The influenza epidemic of 1889–90 in selected European cities—a picture based on the reports of two Poznań daily newspapers from the second half of the nineteenth century. *Medical Science Monitor, 19*, 1131–1141. https://doi.org/10.12659/MSM.889469

Kim, M., & Choi, Y. (2017). Risk communication: The roles of message appeal and coping style. *Social Behavior & Personality, 45*, 773–784. https://doi.org/10.2224/sbp.6327

Kirkey, S. (2023). Ontario doctors give up licences after complaints over COVID vaccine exemptions, misinformation. *National Post*. https://nationalpost.com/news/canada/doctors-resign-licences-covid-19-vaccine-exemptions-misinformation

Klemm, C., Das, E., & Hartmann, T. (2016). Swine flu and hype: A systematic review of media dramatization of the H1N1 influenza pandemic. *Journal of Risk Research, 19*, 1–20. https://doi.org/10.1080/13669877.2014.923029

Kreps, S. E., & Kriner, D. L. (2022). The COVID-19 infodemic and the efficacy of interventions intended to reduce misinformation. *Public Opinion Quarterly, 86*(1), 162–175. https://doi.org/10.1093/poq/nfab075

Kucharski, A. (2020). Misinformation on the coronavirus might be the most contagious thing about it. *The Guardian.* https://www.theguardian.com/commentisfree/2020/feb/08/misinformation-coronavirus-contagious-infections

Lancet. (1890). The influenza epidemic. *Lancet, 1*(3463), p. 88.

Lazaruk, S. (2022). COVID-19: About 2,500 B.C. health-care workers lost jobs over refusal to vaccinate. *Vancouver Sun.* https://vancouversun.com/news/local-news/about-2500-health-care-workers-lost-jobs-over-refusal-to-vaccinate

Lazer, D., Baum, M., Benkler, Y., Berinsky, A., Greenhill, K., Menczer, F., et al. (2018). The science of fake news. *Science, 359*(6380), 1094–1096. https://doi.org/10.1126/science.aao2998

Lee, J., & Bissell, K. (2024). Correcting vaccine misinformation on social media: The inadvertent effects of repeating misinformation within such corrections on COVID-19 vaccine misperceptions. *Current Psychology*, 1–13. https://doi.org/10.1007/s12144-024-05651-z

Lewandowsky, S., Cook, J., Ecker, U., Albarracín, D., Amazeen, M. A., Kendeou, P., et al. (2020). The debunking handbook. https://sks.to/db2020

London Evening News and Post. (1892, January 7). The influenza plague. *London Evening News and Post*, 3. https://newspaperarchive.com/london-evening-news-and-post-jan-07-1892-p-3/

Long, V. J. E., Koh, W. S., Saw, Y. E., & Liu, J. C. (2021). Vulnerability to rumours during the COVID-19 pandemic in Singapore. *Annals of the Academy of Medicine, Singapore, 50*(3), 232–240. https://doi.org/10.47102/annals-acadmedsg.2020523

Martel, C., Pennycook, G., & Rand, D. G. (2020). Reliance on emotion promotes belief in fake news. *Cognitive Research: Principles and Implications, 5*(1), article 47. https://doi.org/10.1186/s41235-020-00252-3

McPherson, M., Smith-Lovin, L., & Cook, J. M. (2001). Birds of a feather: Homophily in social networks. *Annual Review of Sociology, 27*, 415–444. https://doi.org/10.1146/annurev.soc.27.1.415

Miller, S. M. (1989). Cognitive informational styles in the process of coping with threat and frustration. *Advances in Behaviour Research and Therapy, 11*, 223–234. https://doi.org/10.1016/0146-6402(89)90026-X

Miller, S. M. (1996). Monitoring and blunting of threatening information: Cognitive interference and facilitation in the coping process. In I. G. Sarason, G. R. Pierce, & B. R. Sarason (Eds.), *Cognitive interference: Theories, methods, and findings.* (pp. 175–190). Erlbaum.

Miller, S. M., Fang, C. Y., Diefenbach, M. A., & Bales, C. B. (2001). Tailoring psychosocial interventions to the individual's health information-processing style: The influence of monitoring versus blunting in cancer risk and disease. In A. Baum & B. L. Andersen (Eds.), *Psychosocial interventions for cancer.* (pp. 343–362). American Psychological Association. https://doi.org/10.1037/10402-018

Miller, S. M., Fleisher, L., Roussi, P., Buzaglo, J., Schnoll, R., Slater, E., Raysor, S., & Popa-Mabe, M. (2005). Facilitating informed decision making about breast cancer risk and genetic counseling among women calling the NCI's cancer information service. *Journal of Health Communication, 10*, 119–136. https://doi.org/10.1080/07366290500265335

Mitchell, G. (2021). Covid-denier and anti-vaxxer nurse struck off register by NMC. *Nursing Times*. https://www.nursingtimes.net/news/professional-regulation/covid-denier-and-anti-vaxxer-nurse-struck-off-register-by-nmc-04-06-2021/

Modgil, S., Singh, R. K., Gupta, S., & Dennehy, D. (2021). A confirmation bias view on social media induced polarisation during Covid-19. *Information Systems Frontiers, 26*, 417–441. https://doi.org/10.1007/s10796-021-10222-9

Muzzatti, S. L. (2005). Bits of falling sky and global pandemics: Moral panic and Severe Acute Respiratory Syndrome (SARS). *Illness, Crisis, & Loss, 13*, 117–128. https://doi.org/10.1177/105413730501300203

Nerlich, B., & Halliday, C. (2007). Avian flu: The creation of expectations in the interplay between science and the media. *Sociology of Health & Illness, 29*, 46–65. https://doi.org/10.1111/j.1467-9566.2007.00517.x

Palmer, J. (2020). Don't blame bat soup for the coronavirus. *Foreign Policy*. https://foreignpolicy.com/2020/01/27/coronavirus-covid19-dont-blame-bat-soup-for-the-virus/

Pennycook, G., McPhetres, J., Zhang, Y., Lu, J. G., & Rand, D. G. (2020). Fighting COVID-19 misinformation on social media: Experimental evidence for a scalable accuracy-nudge intervention. *Psychological Science, 31*(7), 770–780. https://doi.org/10.1177/0956797620939054

Pennycook, G., & Rand, D. G. (2019). Lazy, not biased: Susceptibility to partisan fake news is better explained by lack of reasoning than by motivated reasoning. *Cognition, 188*, 39–50. https://doi.org/10.1016/j.cognition.2018.06.011

Pennycook, G., & Rand, D. G. (2020). Who falls for fake news? The roles of bullshit receptivity, overclaiming, familiarity, and analytic thinking. *Journal of Personality, 88*(2), 185–200. https://doi.org/10.1111/jopy.12476

Pennycook, G., & Rand, D. G. (2021). The psychology of fake news. *Trends in Cognitive Sciences, 25*(5), 388–402. https://doi.org/10.1016/j.tics.2021.02.007

Pilkington, E., & Glenza, J. (2019). Facebook under pressure to halt rise of anti-vaccination groups. *The Guardian*. https://www.theguardian.com/technology/2019/feb/12/facebook-anti-vaxxer-vaccination-groups-pressure-misinformation?CMP=share_btn_link

Procopius. (551 AD). *History of the wars: Book II* (H. B. Dewing, Trans., 1914). Heinemann.

Ritchie, J. (2021). Alberta premier facing criticism for Wuhan bat soup comments in year-end interview. *City News*. https://calgary.citynews.ca/2021/12/24/kenney-criticism-wuhan-bat-soup/

Roozenbeek, J., Schneider, C. R., Dryhurst, S., Kerr, J., Freeman, A. L. J., Recchia, G., et al. (2020). Susceptibility to misinformation about COVID-19 around the world. *Royal Society Open Science, 7*(10), 201199. https://doi.org/10.1098/rsos.201199

Rothkopf, D. J. (2003, May 11). When the buzz bites back. *Washington Post*, B01. http://www1.udel.edu/globalagenda/2004/student/readings/infodemic.html

Rozsa, M. (2020). Fox News host claims coronavirus outbreak was caused by Chinese people "eating raw bats and snakes." *Salon*. https://www.salon.com/2020/03/03/fox-news-host-claims-coronavirus-outbreak-was-caused-by-chinese-people-eating-raw-bats-and-snakes/

Rubenking, B. (2019). Emotion, attitudes, norms and sources: Exploring sharing intent of disgusting online videos. *Computers in Human Behavior, 96*, 63–71. https://doi.org/10.1016/j.chb.2019.02.011

Rubin, G. J., Amlôt, R., Page, L., & Wessely, S. (2009). Public perceptions, anxiety, and behaviour change in relation to the Swine flu outbreak: Cross sectional telephone survey. *British Medical Journal, 339*, article b2651. https://doi.org/10.1136/bmj.b2651

Scheirer, W. (2020). A pandemic of bad science. *Bulletin of the Atomic Scientists, 76*(4), 175–184. https://doi.org/10.1080/00963402.2020.1778361

Scherer, L., McPhetres, J., Pennycook, G., Kempe, A., Allen, L., Knoepke, C., et al. (2021). Who is susceptible to online health misinformation? A test of four psychosocial hypotheses. *Health Psychology, 40*(4), 274–284. https://doi.org/10.1037/hea0000978

Sharma, M., Yadav, K., Yadav, N., & Ferdinand, K. C. (2017). Zika virus pandemic-analysis of Facebook as a social media health information platform. *American Journal of Infection Control, 45*, 301–302. https://doi.org/10.1016/j.ajic.2016.08.022

Shen-Berro, J. (2020). Sen. Cornyn: China to blame for coronavirus, because "people ate bats." *NBC News*. https://www.nbcnews.com/news/asian-america/sen-cornyn-china-blame-coronavirus-because-people-eat-bats-n1163431

Sørensen, K., Van den Broucke, S., Fullam, J., Doyle, G., Pelikan, J., Slonska, Z., et al. (2012). Health literacy and public health: A systematic review and integration of definitions and models. *BMC Public Health, 12*, article 80. https://doi.org/10.1186/1471-2458-12-80

Sperry, E. (2018). Lord have mercy on us: Broadsides and London plague life. *Sixteenth Century Journal, 49*(1), 95–113. https://doi.org/10.1086/SCJ4901005

Stern, J. (2016). Radicalization to extremism and mobilization to violence: What have we learned and what can we do about it? *Annals of the American Academy of Political and Social Science, 668*(1), 102–117. https://doi.org/10.1177/0002716216673807

Strekalova, Y. A. (2017). Health risk information engagement and amplification on social media: News about an emerging pandemic on Facebook. *Health Education & Behavior, 44*, 332–339. https://doi.org/10.1177/1090198116660310

Stuart, J., & Cady, N. J. (2023). Examining approaches to encourage Covid-19 vaccination on social media. *Social and Personality Psychology Compass, 17*(11), article e12866. https://doi.org/10.1111/spc3.12866

Tang, L., Bie, B., Park, S.-E., & Zhi, D. (2018). Social media and outbreaks of emerging infectious diseases: A systematic review of literature. *American Journal of Infection Control, 46*, 962–972. https://doi.org/10.1016/j.ajic.2018.02.010

Taylor, S. (2019). *The psychology of pandemics: Preparing for the next global outbreak of infectious disease*. Cambridge Scholars Publishing.

Taylor, S., Landry, C. A., Paluszek, M. M., Fergus, T. A., McKay, D., & Asmundson, G. J. G. (2020). Covid stress syndrome: Concept, structure, and correlates. *Depression and Anxiety, 37*, 706–714. https://doi.org/10.1002/da.23071

Thomas, E. (2021). *Australia's fragmented, conspiracy-focused anti-lockdown movement*. Institute for Strategic Dialogue.

Weiss, S. (2020). Inside the infodemic: Coronavirus in the age of wellness. *New Statesman*. https://www.newstatesman.com/politics/health/2020/02/inside-infodemic-coronavirus-age-wellness

WHO. (2020). Managing the COVID-19 infodemic: Promoting healthy behaviours and mitigating the harm from misinformation and disinformation. https://www.who.int/news/item/23-09-2020-managing-the-covid-19-infodemic-promoting-healthy-behaviours-and-mitigating-the-harm-from-misinformation-and-disinformation

WHO. (2022). Coronavirus disease (COVID-19) advice for the public: Mythbusters. https://www.who.int/emergencies/diseases/novel-coronavirus-2019/advice-for-public/myth-busters

Wong, J., Yi, P. X., Quek, F. Y. X., Lua, V. Y. Q., Majeed, N. M., & Hartanto, A. (2024). A four-level meta-analytic review of the relationship between social media and well-being: A fresh perspective in the context of Covid-19. *Current Psychology, 43*, 14972–14986. https://doi.org/10.1007/s12144-022-04092-w

Yun, G., Morin, D., Park, S., Joa, C., Labbe, B., Lim, J., et al. (2016). Social media and flu: Media Twitter accounts as agenda setters. *International Journal of Medical Informatics, 91*, 67–73. https://doi.org/10.1016/j.ijmedinf.2016.04.009

Zhou, L. (2020). "Sorry about the tasty bat": Chinese online host apologies for travel show dining advice as Wuhan virus spreads. *South China Morning Post*. https://www.scmp.com/news/china/society/article/3047683/sorry-about-tasty-bat-chinese-online-host-apologises-travel-show

Zhuo, Q., Cui, C., Liang, H., Bai, Y., Hu, Q., Hanum, A., et al. (2021). Cross-cultural adaptation, validity and reliability of the Chinese version of Miller Behavioral Style Scale. *Health and Quality of Life Outcomes*, 19, article 86. https://doi.org/10.1186/s12955-021-01717-9

Chapter 11

Abel, M., Byker, T., & Carpenter, J. (2021). Socially optimal mistakes? Debiasing COVID-19 mortality risk perceptions and prosocial behavior. *Journal of Economic Behavior & Organization*, 183, 456–480. https://doi.org/10.1016/j.jebo.2021.01.007

Abu-Rumaileh, M. A., Alsharif, N. M., Abdulelah, M., Mueting, S., & Bader, H. (2021). You only find what you look for: Anchor bias during the COVID-19 pandemic. *Cureus*, 13(6), article e15416. https://doi.org/10.7759/cureus.15416

Arntz, A., Rauner, M., & Van den Hout, M. (1995). "If I feel anxious, there must be danger": Ex-consequentia reasoning in inferring danger in anxiety disorders. *Behaviour Research and Therapy*, 33(8), 917–925. https://doi.org/10.1016/0005-7967(95)00032-S

Bahnik, S., Englich, B., Strack, F. (2017). Anchoring effect. In R. F. Pohl (Ed.), *Cognitive illusions: Intriguing phenomena in thinking, judgment and memory* (2nd ed.) (pp. 223–241). Routledge.

Banerjee, R., Bhattacharya, J., & Majumdar, P. (2021). Exponential-growth prediction bias and compliance with safety measures related to COVID-19. *Social Science & Medicine*, 268, article113473. https://doi.org/10.1016/j.socscimed.2020.113473

Baumgaertner, E., & Rainey, J. (2020). Trump administration ended pandemic early-warning program to detect coronaviruses. *LA Times*. https://www.latimes.com/science/story/2020-04-02/coronavirus-trump-pandemic-program-viruses-detection

Béna, J., Rihet, M., Carreras, O., & Terrier, P. (2023). Repetition could increase the perceived truth of conspiracy theories. *Psychonomic Bulletin & Review*, 30(6), 2397–2406. https://doi.org/10.3758/s13423-023-02276-4

Benoît, J.-P., & Dubra, J. (2019). Apparent bias: What does attitude polarization show? *International Economic Review*, 60(4), 1675–1703. http://www.jstor.org/stable/45220819

Bhula, S., Osorio, L., Shah, G., & Patel, A. (2022). A lesson on anchoring bias during a pandemic: A case presentation. *Chest*, 162(Suppl 4), A901.

Bixter, M. T., & Luhmann, C. C. (2021). The social contagion of temporal discounting in small social networks. *Cognitive Research: Principles and Implications*, 6(1), article 13. https://doi.org/10.1186/s41235-020-00249-y

Blank, H. (2024). Looking back on the COVID-19 pandemic: Hindsight and outcome bias. In M. K. Miller (Ed.), *The social science of the COVID-19 pandemic: A call to action for researchers* (pp. 488–499). Oxford University Press. https://doi.org/10.1093/oso/9780197615133.003.0038

Botzen, W. J. W., Duijndam, S. J., Robinson, P. J., & van Beukering, P. (2022). Behavioral biases and heuristics in perceptions of COVID-19 risks and prevention decisions. *Risk Analysis*, 42(12), 2671–2690. https://doi.org/10.1111/risa.13882

Brashier, N. M., & Marsh, E. J. (2020). Judging truth. *Annual Review of Psychology*, 71, 499–515. https://doi.org/10.1146/annurev-psych-010419-050807

Byrne, K. A., Six, S. G., Anaraky, R. G., Harris, M. W., & Winterlind, E. L. (2021). Risk-taking unmasked: Using risky choice and temporal discounting to explain COVID-19 preventative behaviors. *PLOS ONE, 16*(5), article e0251073. https://doi.org/10.1371/journal.pone.0251073

Calluso, C., Devetag, M. G., & Donato, C. (2021). "I feel therefore I decide": Effect of negative emotions on temporal discounting and probability discounting. *Brain Sciences, 11*, article 1407. https://doi.org/10.3390/brainsci11111407

Casey, S. (2018). A cup of tea, a Bex and a good lie down. *Australian Pharmacist.* https://www.australianpharmacist.com.au/cup-of-tea-bex-good-lie-down/

Critchfield, T. S., & Kollins, S. H. (2001). Temporal discounting: Basic research and the analysis of socially important behavior. *Journal of Applied Behavior Analysis, 34*(1), 101–122. https://doi.org/10.1901/jaba.2001.34-101

Croskerry, P., Singhal, G., & Mamede, S. (2013a). Cognitive debiasing 1: Origins of bias and theory of debiasing. *BMJ Quality & Safety, 22*(Suppl 2), ii58–ii64. https://doi.org/10.1136/bmjqs-2012-001712

Croskerry, P., Singhal, G., & Mamede, S. (2013b). Cognitive debiasing 2: Impediments to and strategies for change. *BMJ Quality & Safety, 22*(Suppl 2), ii65–ii72. https://doi.org/10.1136/bmjqs-2012-001713

Daniel, M., Khandelwal, S., Santen, S. A., Malone, M., & Croskerry, P. (2017). Cognitive debiasing strategies for the emergency department. *AEM Education and Training, 1*(1), 41–42. https://doi.org/10.1002/aet2.10010

De Neys, W. (2018). Dual process theory 2.0: An introduction. In W. De Neys (Ed.), *Dual process theory 2.0.* (pp. 1–4). Routledge.

Dechêne, A., Stahl, C., Hansen, J., & Wänke, M. (2010). The truth about the truth: A meta-analytic review of the truth effect. *Personality and Social Psychology Review, 14*, 238–257.

Dryhurst, S., Schneider, C. R., Kerr, J., Freeman, A. L. J., Recchia, G., van der Bles, A. M., et al. (2020). Risk perceptions of COVID-19 around the world. *Journal of Risk Research, 23*(7–8), 994–1006. https://doi.org/10.1080/13669877.2020.1758193

Ecker, U., Lewandowsky, S., Cook, J., Schmid, P., Fazio, L., Brashier, N., et al. (2022). The psychological drivers of misinformation belief and its resistance to correction. *Nature Reviews Psychology, 1*(1), 13–29. https://doi.org/10.1038/s44159-021-00006-y

Frederick, S., Loewenstein, G., & O'Donoghue, T. (2002). Time discounting and time preference: A critical review. *Journal of Economic Literature, 40*(2), 351–401. https://doi.org/10.1257/002205102320161311

Freitas-Lemos, R., Tomlinson, D. C., Yeh, Y.-H., Dwyer, C. L., Dai, H. D., Leventhal, A., et al. (2023). Can delay discounting predict vaccine hesitancy 4-years later? A study among US young adults. *Preventive Medicine Reports, 35*, article 102280. https://doi.org/https://doi.org/10.1016/j.pmedr.2023.102280

Frost, K., Frank, E., & Maibach, E. (1997). Relative risk in the news media: A quantification of misrepresentation. *American Journal of Public Health, 87*, 842–845.

Giroux, M. E., Derksen, D. G., Coburn, P. I., & Bernstein, D. M. (2023). Hindsight bias and COVID-19: Hindsight was not 20/20 in 2020. *Journal of Applied Research in Memory and Cognition, 12*(1), 105–115. https://doi.org/10.1037/mac0000033

Halilova, J. G., Fynes-Clinton, S., Green, L., Myerson, J., Wu, J., Ruggeri, K., et al. (2022). Short-sighted decision-making by those not vaccinated against COVID-19. *Scientific Reports, 12*(1), article 11906. https://doi.org/10.1038/s41598-022-15276-6

Harada, T., Watari, T., Miyagami, T., Watanuki, S., Shimzu, T., & Hiroshige, J. (2020). COVID blindness: Delayed diagnosis of aseptic meningitis in the COVID-19 era. *European Journal of Case Reports in Internal Medicine, 7*(11), article 1940. https://doi.org/10.12890/2020_001940

Johnson, H. M., & Seifert, C. M. (1994). Sources of the continued influence effect: When misinformation in memory affects later inferences. *Journal of Experimental Psychology: Learning, Memory, and Cognition, 20*(6), 1420–1436. https://doi.org/10.1037/0278-7393.20.6.1420

Kahneman, D. (2011). *Thinking, fast and slow.* Farrar, Strauss, Giroux.

Kahneman, D., Sibony, O., & Sunstein, C. R. (2021). *Noise: A flaw in human judgment.* Little, Brown Spark.

Kahneman, D., & Tversky, A. (1973). On the psychology of prediction. *Psychological Review, 80*(4), 237–251.

Lammers, J., Crusius, J., & Gast, A. (2020). Correcting misperceptions of exponential coronavirus growth increases support for social distancing. *PNAS, 117*(28), 16264–16266. https://doi.org/10.1073/pnas.2006048117

Lee, J., & Bissell, K. (2024). Correcting vaccine misinformation on social media: The inadvertent effects of repeating misinformation within such corrections on COVID-19 vaccine misperceptions. *Current Psychology,* 1–13. https://doi.org/10.1007/s12144-024-05651-z

Lewandowsky, S., Cook, J., Ecker, U., Albarracín, D., Amazeen, M. A., Kendeou, P., et al. (2020). The debunking handbook. https://sks.to/db2020

Li, T., & Jager, W. (2023). How availability heuristic, confirmation bias and fear may drive societal polarisation: An opinion dynamics simulation of the case of COVID-19 vaccination. *Journal of Artificial Societies and Social Simulation, 26*(4), article 2. https://doi.org/10.18564/jasss.5135

Lloyd, A., McKay, R., Hartman, T. K., Vincent, B. T., Murphy, J., Gibson-Miller, J., et al. (2021). Delay discounting and under-valuing of recent information predict poorer adherence to social distancing measures during the COVID-19 pandemic. *Scientific Reports, 11*(1), article 19237.

Loewenstein, G., & Prelec, D. (1992). Anomalies in intertemporal choice: Evidence and an interpretation. *Quarterly Journal of Economics, 107*(2), 573–597. https://doi.org/10.2307/2118482

Lommen, M. J. J., Engelhard, I. M., van den Hout, M. A., & Arntz, A. (2013). Reducing emotional reasoning: An experimental manipulation in individuals with fear of spiders. *Cognition and Emotion, 27*(8), 1504–1512. https://doi.org/10.1080/02699931.2013.795482

Ludolph, R., & Schulz, P. J. (2017). Debiasing health-related judgments and decision making: A systematic review. *Medical Decision Making, 38*(1), 3–13. https://doi.org/10.1177/0272989X17716672

Ly, D. P., Shekelle, P. G., & Song, Z. (2023). Evidence for anchoring bias during physician decision-making. *JAMA Internal Medicine, 183*(8), 818–823. https://doi.org/10.1001/jamainternmed.2023.2366

Madison, A. A., Way, B. M., Beauchaine, T. P., & Kiecolt-Glaser, J. K. (2021). Risk assessment and heuristics: How cognitive shortcuts can fuel the spread of COVID-19. *Brain, Behavior, and Immunity, 94,* 6–7. https://doi.org/10.1016/j.bbi.2021.02.023

Malthouse, E. (2023). Confirmation bias and vaccine-related beliefs in the time of COVID-19. *Journal of Public Health, 45*(2), 523–528. https://doi.org/10.1093/pubmed/fdac128

Martel, C., Pennycook, G., & Rand, D. G. (2020). Reliance on emotion promotes belief in fake news. *Cognitive Research: Principles and Implications, 5*(1), article 47. https://doi.org/10.1186/s41235-020-00252-3

McNeil, D. G. (2019). U.S. shuts project meant to find the next Ebola. *New York Times, 169*(58495), D1–D3. https://www.nytimes.com/2019/10/25/health/predict-usaid-viruses.html

Meppelink, C. S., Smit, E. G., Fransen, M. L., & Diviani, N. (2019). "I was right about vaccination": Confirmation bias and health literacy in online health information seeking. *Journal of Health Communication, 24*(2), 129–140. https://doi.org/10.1080/10810730.2019.1583701

Mercier, H. (2017). Confirmation bias – myside bias. In R. F. Pohl (Ed.), *Cognitive illusions: Intriguing phenomena in thinking, judgment and memory (2nd ed.)* (pp. 99–114). Routledge.

Milman, O. (2020, April 3). Trump administration cut pandemic early warning program in September. *The Guardian.* https://www.theguardian.com/world/2020/apr/03/trump-scrapped-pandemic-early-warning-program-system-before-coronavirus

Misuraca, R., Teuscher, U., Scaffidi Abbate, C., Ceresia, F., Roccella, M., Parisi, L., et al. (2022). Can we do better next time? Italians' response to the COVID-19 emergency through a heuristics and biases lens. *Behavioral Sciences, 12*(2), article 39. https://doi.org/10.3390/bs12020039

Mussweiler, T., Strack, F., & Pfeiffer, T. (2000). Overcoming the inevitable anchoring effect: Considering the opposite compensates for selective accessibility. *Personality and Social Psychology Bulletin, 26*(9), 1142–1150. https://doi.org/10.1177/01461672002611010

Nickerson, R. S. (1998). Confirmation bias: A ubiquitous phenomenon in many guises. *Review of General Psychology, 2*(2), 175–220. https://doi.org/10.1037/1089-2680.2.2.175

Nisbett, R. E., & Ross, L. (1980). *Human inference: Strategies and shortcomings of social judgment.* Prentice-Hall.

O'Sullivan, E. D., & Schofield, S. J. (2018). Cognitive bias in clinical medicine. *Journal of the Royal College of Physicians of Edinburgh, 48*(3), 225–232.

Özdemir, İ., & Kuru, E. (2023). Investigation of cognitive distortions in panic disorder, generalized anxiety disorder and social anxiety disorder. *Journal of Clinical Medicine, 12*(19), article 6351. https://doi.org/10.3390/jcm12196351

Paredes-Mealla, M., Martínez-Borba, V., Miragall, M., García-Palacios, A., Baños, R. M., & Suso-Ribera, C. (2022). Is there evidence that emotional reasoning processing underlies emotional disorders in adults? A systematic review. *Current Psychology, 42,* 28738–28754. https://doi.org/10.1007/s12144-022-03884-4

Patel, N., Ilyas, S., Mobin, N., & Tokarski, M. (2021). Anchoring bias during the COVID-19 pandemic. *Chest, 160*(Suppl 4), 456A. https://doi.org/10.1016/j.chest.2021.07.448

Pendleton, D. (2020). History suggests the handshake will survive the pandemic. *Bloomberg.com.* https://www.bloomberg.com/news/articles/2020-06-05/history-of-kissing-suggests-handshakes-will-survive-the-pandemic?embedded-checkout=true

Pillai, R. M., & Fazio, L. K. (2021). The effects of repeating false and misleading information on belief. *WIREs Cognitive Science, 12*(6), e1573. https://doi.org/10.1002/wcs.1573

Pohl, R. F. (2017). Cognitive illusions. In R. F. Pohl (Ed.), *Cognitive illusions: Intriguing phenomena in thinking, judgment and memory* (2nd ed.) (pp. 3–21). Routledge.

Pohl, R. F., & Erdfelder, E. (2017). Hindsight bias. In R. F. Pohl (Ed.), *Cognitive illusions: Intriguing phenomena in thinking, judgment and memory* (2nd ed.) (pp. 424–445). Routledge.

Pyszczynski, T., & Greenberg, J. (1987). Toward an integration of cognitive and motivational perspectives on social inference: A biased hypothesis-testing model. In L. Berkowitz (Ed.), *Advances in experimental social psychology* (Vol. 20., pp. 297–340). Academic Press. https://doi.org/10.1016/S0065-2601(08)60417-7

Rehana, R. W., & Huda, N. (2021). A common heuristic in medicine: Anchoring. *Annals of Medical and Health Sciences Research, 11,* 1461–1463.

Remmerswaal, D., Huijding, J., Bouwmeester, S., Brouwer, M., & Muris, P. (2014). Cognitive bias in action: Evidence for a reciprocal relation between confirmation bias and fear in children. *Journal of Behavior Therapy and Experimental Psychiatry, 45*(1), 26–32. https://doi.org/10.1016/j.jbtep.2013.07.005

Renner, C. H. (2017). Validity effect. In R. F. Pohl (Ed.), *Cognitive illusions: Intriguing phenomena in thinking, judgment and memory* (2nd ed.) (pp. 242–255). Routledge.

Saposnik, G., Redelmeier, D., Ruff, C. C., & Tobler, P. N. (2016). Cognitive biases associated with medical decisions: A systematic review. *BMC Medical Informatics and Decision Making, 16*(1), article 138. https://doi.org/10.1186/s12911-016-0377-1

Schmidt, C. (2020). Why the coronavirus slipped past disease detectives. Scientific American. https://www.scientificamerican.com/article/why-the-coronavirus-slipped-past-disease-detectives/

Sherman, S. J., Cialdini, R. B., Schwartzman, D. F., & Reynolds, K. D. (2002). Imagining can heighten or lower the perceived likelihood of contracting a disease: The mediating effect of ease of imagery. In T. Gilovich, D. Griffin, & D. Kahneman (Eds.), *Heuristics and biases: The psychology of intuitive judgment* (pp. 98–102). Cambridge University Press.

Slovic, P., & Peters, E. (2006). Risk perception and affect. *Current Directions in Psychological Science, 15*(6), 322–325. https://doi.org/10.1111/j.1467-8721.2006.00461.x

Stango, V., & Zinman, J. (2009). Exponential growth bias and household finance. *Journal of Finance, 64*(6), 2807–2849. https://doi.org/10.1111/j.1540-6261.2009.01518.x

Taylor, S. (2000). *Understanding and treating panic disorder: Cognitive-behavioural approaches.* Wiley.

Taylor, S., Landry, C. A., Paluszek, M. M., Fergus, T. A., McKay, D., & Asmundson, G. J. G. (2020). Covid stress syndrome: Concept, structure, and correlates. *Depression and Anxiety, 37*, 706–714. https://doi.org/10.1002/da.23071

Thucydides. (411 BC). *The history of the Peloponnesian War* (R. Crawley, Trans., 2009). Project Gutenberg. www.gutenberg.org

Tversky, A., & Kahneman, D. (1973). Availability: A heuristic for judging frequency and probability. *Cognitive Psychology, 5*, 207–232.

Tversky, A., & Kahneman, D. (1974). Judgment under uncertainty: Heuristics and biases. *Science, 185*, 1124–1131.

Unkelbach, C., & Koch, A. (2019). Gullible but functional? Information repetition and the formation of beliefs. In J. P. Forgas & R. P. Baumeister (Eds.), *The social psychology of gullibility: Fake news, conspiracy theories, and irrational beliefs* (pp. 42–60). Routledge.

Unkelbach, C., & Speckmann, F. (2021). Mere repetition increases belief in factually true COVID-19-related information. *Journal of Applied Research in Memory and Cognition, 10*(2), 241–247. https://doi.org/10.1016/j.jarmac.2021.02.001

van der Linden, S. (2022). Misinformation: Susceptibility, spread, and interventions to immunize the public. *Nature Medicine, 28*(3), 460–467. https://doi.org/10.1038/s41591-022-01713-6

Vellani, V., Zheng, S., Ercelik, D., & Sharot, T. (2023). The illusory truth effect leads to the spread of misinformation. *Cognition, 236*, article 105421. https://doi.org/10.1016/j.cognition.2023.105421

Xu, S., Coman, I. A., Yamamoto, M., & Najera, C. J. (2023). Exposure effects or confirmation bias? Examining reciprocal dynamics of misinformation, misperceptions, and attitudes toward COVID-19 vaccines. *Health Communication, 38*(10), 2210–2220. https://doi.org/10.1080/10410236.2022.2059802

Young, M. E., Norman, G. R., & Humphreys, K. R. (2008). Medicine in the popular press: The influence of the media on perceptions of disease. *PLOS ONE, 3*(10), e3552. https://doi.org/10.1371/journal.pone.0003552

Zamora, M., Osian, O., & Crimi, E. (2023). Anchoring bias in the era of Covid-19 pandemia. *Annals of Clinical and Medical Case Reports, 11*(3), 1–6.

Zhang, X., Wu, Z., & He, Q. (2023). A mini-review on how the COVID-19 pandemic affected intertemporal choice. *Psychoradiology, 3*, article kkad0210. https://doi.org/10.1093/psyrad/kkad021

Chapter 12

A Physician of New Orleans. (1854). *History of the yellow fever in New Orleans.* C. W. Kenworthy.

Achinstein, S. (1992). Plagues and publication: Ballads and the representation of disease in the English Renaissance. *Criticism, 34*(1), 27–49. http://www.jstor.org/stable/23113580

Agence France-Presse. (2021). Former U.S. CDC head thinks coronavirus came from Chinese lab, has no evidence, https://www.ctvnews.ca/health/coronavirus/former-u-s-cdc-head-thinks-coronavirus-came-from-chinese-lab-has-no-evidence-1.5364208

Ahmed, W., Downing, J., Tuters, M., & Knight, P. (2020). Four experts investigate how the 5G corinavirus conspiracy theory began. *The Conversation.* https://theconversation.com/four-experts-investigate-how-the-5g-coronavirus-conspiracy-theory-began-139137

Allington, D., Duffy, B., Wessely, S., Dhavan, N., & Rubin, J. (2021). Health-protective behaviour, social media usage and conspiracy belief during the COVID-19 public health emergency. *Psychological Medicine, 51*(10), 1763–1769. https://doi.org/10.1017/S003329172000224X

Allport, G., & Postman, L. (1947). *The psychology of rumor.* Holt.

Alper, S., Bayrak, F., & Yilmaz, O. (2021). Psychological correlates of Covid-19 conspiracy beliefs and preventive measures: Evidence from Turkey. *Current Psychology, 40,* 5708–5717. https://doi.org/10.1007/s12144-020-00903-0

Ang, A. (2003). Chinese turning to occult to fight SARS. *Associated Press.* https://www.theintelligencer.com/news/article/Chinese-Turning-to-Occult-to-Fight-SARS-10576743.php

Anonymous. (1721). *The late dreadful plague at Marseilles compared with that terrible plague in London in the year 1665.* Parker.

Anonymous. (1849). Fear a cause of epidemics. *New England Botanic, Medical & Surgical Journal, 3*(5), 84–86.

Barry, J. M. (2005). 1918 revisited: Lessons and suggestions for further inquiry. In S. L. Knobler, Mack, A., Mahmoud, A., Lemon, S. M. (Eds.), *The threat of pandemic influenza: Are we ready?* (pp. 58–68). National Academies Press.

Barry, J. M. (2018). *The great influenza.* Penguin Random House.

BBC. (2020). Coronavirus: WHO chief warns against "trolls and conspiracy theories." *BBC News.* https://www.bbc.com/news/world-51429400

Benoiston de Châteauneuf, L.-F., Chevallier, J.-B., Devaux, L., Millot, L., Parent-Duchâtelet, A., Petit de Maurienne, A., et al. (1834). *Rapport sur la marche et les effets du choléra-morbus dans Paris et les communes rurales du département de la Seine.* Imprimerie Royale.

Bertin, P., Nera, K., & Delouvée, S. (2020). Conspiracy beliefs, rejection of vaccination, and support for hydroxychloroquine: A conceptual replication-extension in the COVID-19 pandemic context. *Frontiers in Psychology, 11,* article 565128. https://doi.org/10.3389/fpsyg.2020.565128

Biddlestone, M., Green, R., & Douglas, K. M. (2020). Cultural orientation, power, belief in conspiracy theories, and intentions to reduce the spread of COVID-19. *British Journal of Social Psychology, 59*(3), 663–673. https://doi.org/10.1111/bjso.12397

Bierwiaczonek, K., Kunst, J. R., & Pich, O. (2020). Belief in COVID-19 conspiracy theories reduces social distancing over time. *Applied Psychology, 12*(4), 1270–1285. https://doi.org/10.1111/aphw.12223

Bonnet, J. (1858). *Letters of John Calvin (vol. 1).* Presbyterian Board of Publication.

Bruder, M., Haffke, P., Neave, N., Nouripanah, N., & Imhoff, R. (2013). Measuring individual differences in generic beliefs in conspiracy theories across cultures: Conspiracy Mentality

Questionnaire. *Frontiers in Psychology*, 4, article 225. https://doi.org/10.3389/fpsyg.2013.00225

Buckels, E. E., Trapnell, P. D., & Paulhus, D. L. (2014). Trolls just want to have fun. *Personality and Individual Differences*, 67, 97–102. https://doi.org/10.1016/j.paid.2014.01.016

Burrell, S., & Gill, G. (2005). The Liverpool cholera epidemic of 1832 and anatomical dissection: Medical mistrust and civil unrest. *Journal of the History of Medicine and Allied Sciences*, 60(4), 478–498. https://doi.org/10.1093/jhmas/jri061

Butcher, T. (1855). *"Mordichim": Recollections of cholera in the Barbados, during the middle of the year 1854*. Partridge, Oakey, & Co.

Carmichael, A. G. (1986). *Plague and the poor in renaissance Florence*. Cambridge University Press.

Chan, A. (2024). Why the pandemic probably started in a lab, in 5 key points. *New York Times*. https://www.nytimes.com/interactive/2024/06/03/opinion/covid-lab-leak.html

Chan, H.-W., Chiu, C. P.-Y., Zuo, S., Wang, X., Liu, L., & Hong, Y. (2021). Not-so-straightforward links between believing in COVID-19-related conspiracy theories and engaging in disease-preventive behaviours. *Humanities and Social Sciences Communications*, 8(1), article 104. https://doi.org/10.1057/s41599-021-00781-2

Cheng, C., & Cheung, M. W. (2005). Psychological responses to outbreak of severe acute respiratory syndrome: A prospective, multiple time-point study. *Journal of Personality*, 73, 261–285. https://doi.org/10.1111/j.1467-6494.2004.00310.x

Cichocka, A., Marchlewska, M., & Golec de Zavala, A. (2016). Does self-love or self-hate predict conspiracy beliefs? Narcissism, self-esteem, and the endorsement of conspiracy theories. *Social Psychological and Personality Science*, 7, 157–166. https://doi.org/10.1177/1948550615616170

CNN. (2022). CNN is only US outlet living through Shanghai lockdown. See what it's like. *CNN*. https://www.cnn.com/videos/world/2022/04/12/shanghai-covid-lockdown-supply-shortage-culver-dnt-ebof-vpx.cnn

Cohn, S. K. (2012). Pandemics: Waves of disease, waves of hate from the Plague of Athens to A.I.D.S. *Historical Research*, 85(230), 535–555. https://doi.org/10.1111/j.1468-2281.2012.00603.x

Cohn, S. K. (2017). Cholera revolts: A class struggle we may not like. *Social History*, 42, 162–180. https://doi.org/10.1080/03071022.2017.1290365

Cohn, S. K., & Kutalek, R. (2016). Historical parallels, Ebola virus disease and cholera: Understanding community distrust and social violence with epidemics. *PLOS Currents*, 8. https://doi.org/10.1371/currents.outbreaks.aa1f2b60e8d43939b43fbd93e1a63a94

Craft, S., Ashley, S., & Maksl, A. (2017). News media literacy and conspiracy theory endorsement. *Communication and the Public*, 2, 388–401. https://doi.org/10.1177/2057047317725539

Crist, C. (2020). FBI says COVID-19 charity fraud in increasing. *WebMD* News. https://www.webmd.com/lung/news/20201101/fbi-says-covid-19-charity-fraud-is-increasing

Crosby, A. W. (2003). *America's forgotten pandemic: The influenza of 1918* (2nd ed.). Cambridge University Press.

Cunha, B. A. (2004). The cause of the plague of Athens: Plague, typhoid, typhus, smallpox, or measles? *Infectious Disease Clinics of North America*, 18(1), 29–43. https://doi.org/10.1016/s0891-5520(03)00100-4

DiFonzo, N., & Bordia, P. (2007). *Rumor psychology: Social and organizational approaches*. American Psychological Association.

Douglas, K. M., Sutton, R. M., & Cichocka, A. (2017). The psychology of conspiracy theories. *Current Directions in Psychological Science*, 26, 538–542. https://doi.org/10.1177/0963721417718261

Douglas, K. M., Uscinski, J. E., Sutton, R. M., Cichocka, A., Nefes, T., Ang, C., et al. (2019). Understanding conspiracy theories. *Political Psychology, 40*, 3–35. https://doi.org/10.1111/pops.12568

Duplaga, M. (2020). The determinants of conspiracy beliefs related to the COVID-19 pandemic in a nationally representative sample of internet users. *International Journal of Environmental Research and Public Health, 17*(21), article 7818. https://doi.org/10.3390/ijerph17217818

Earnshaw, V. A., Eaton, L. A., Kalichman, S. C., Brousseau, N. M., Hill, E. C., & Fox, A. B. (2020). COVID-19 conspiracy beliefs, health behaviors, and policy support. *Translational Behavioral Medicine, 10*(4), 850–856. https://doi.org/10.1093/tbm/ibaa090

Ecker, U., Lewandowsky, S., Cook, J., Schmid, P., Fazio, L., Brashier, N., et al. (2022). The psychological drivers of misinformation belief and its resistance to correction. *Nature Reviews Psychology, 1*(1), 13–29. https://doi.org/10.1038/s44159-021-00006-y

Eichelberger, L. (2007). SARS and New York's Chinatown: The politics of risk and blame during an epidemic of fear. *Social Science & Medicine, 65*, 1284–1295.

Freeman, D., Waite, F., Rosebrock, L., Petit, A., Causier, C., East, A., et al. (2022). Coronavirus conspiracy beliefs, mistrust, and compliance with government guidelines in England. *Psychological Medicine, 52*(2), 251–263. https://doi.org/10.1017/S0033291720001890

Galliford, N., & Furnham, A. (2017). Individual difference factors and beliefs in medical and political conspiracy theories. *Scandinavian Journal of Psychology, 58*, 422–428. https://doi.org/10.1111/sjop.12382

Gallotti, R., Valle, F., Castaldo, N., Sacco, P., & De Domenico, M. (2020). Assessing the risks of "infodemics" in response to COVID-19 epidemics. *Nature Human Behaviour, 4*(12), 1285–1293. https://doi.org/10.1038/s41562-020-00994-6

Garry, J., Ford, R., & Johns, R. (2022). Coronavirus conspiracy beliefs, mistrust, and compliance: Taking measurement seriously. *Psychological Medicine, 52*(14), 3116–3126. https://doi.org/10.1017/S0033291720005164

Georgiou, N., Delfabbro, P., & Balzan, R. (2020). COVID-19-related conspiracy beliefs and their relationship with perceived stress and pre-existing conspiracy beliefs. *Personality and Individual Differences, 166*, article 110201. https://doi.org/10.1016/j.paid.2020.110201

Grimaud, J., & Legagneur, F. (2011). Community beliefs and fears during a cholera outbreak in Haiti. *Intervention: International Journal of Mental Health, Psychosocial Work & Counselling in Areas of Armed Conflict, 9*(1), 26–34. https://doi.org/10.1097/WTF.0b013e3283453ef2

Hassan, S., & Caven-Atack, J. (2020). Anti-Semitism in cults and hate groups. In H. S. Moffic, J. R. Peteet, A. Hankir, & M. V. Seeman (Eds.), *Anti-semitism and psychiatry: Recognition, prevention, and interventions.* (pp. 295–305). Springer Nature Switzerland AG. https://doi.org/10.1007/978-3-030-37745-8_23

Havey, N. F. (2020). Partisan public health: How does political ideology influence support for COVID-19 related misinformation? *Journal of Computational Social Science, 3*, 319–342. https://doi.org/10.1007/s42001-020-00089-2

Hecker, J. F. C. (1844). *Epidemics of the middle ages* (B. G. Babington, Trans.). Woodfall.

Heller, J. (2015). Rumors and realities: Making sense of HIV/AIDS conspiracy narratives and contemporary legends. *American Journal of Public Health, 105*, e43–e50.

Hirst, L. F. (1953). *The conquest of plague.* Clarendon.

Imhoff, R., & Lamberty, P. (2018). How paranoid are conspiracy believers? Toward a more fine-grained understanding of the connect and disconnect between paranoia and belief in conspiracy theories. *European Journal of Social Psychology, 48*(7), 909–926. https://doi.org/10.1002/ejsp.2494

Jacobs, A., Perpetua, S., Sreeharsha, V., McNeil, D. G., & Tavernise, S. (2016). Conspiracy theories about Zika spread through Brazil with the virus. New York Times, *165*(57145), A6.

Johnson, N. (2006). *Britain and the 1918-19 influenza pandemic.* Routledge.
Jolley, D., & Douglas, K. M. (2017). Prevention is better than cure: Addressing anti-vaccine conspiracy theories. *Journal of Applied Social Psychology, 47,* 459–469. https://doi.org/10.1111/jasp.12453
Klofstad, C. A., Uscinski, J. E., Connolly, J. M., & West, J. P. (2019). What drives people to believe in Zika conspiracy theories? *Palgrave Communications, 5*(1), article 36. https://doi.org/10.1057/s41599-019-0243-8
Kowalski, J., Marchlewska, M., Molenda, Z., Górska, P., & Gawęda, Ł. (2020). Adherence to safety and self-isolation guidelines, conspiracy and paranoia-like beliefs during COVID-19 pandemic in Poland - associations and moderators. *Psychiatry Research, 294,* article 113540. https://doi.org/10.1016/j.psychres.2020.113540
Kumar, S. (1995). Confirmation of Indian plague outbreak? *Lancet, 345*(8947), 443. https://doi.org/10.1016/S0140-6736(95)90415-8
Lahrach, Y., & Furnham, A. (2017). Are modern health worries associated with medical conspiracy theories? *Journal of Psychosomatic Research, 99,* 89–94. https://doi.org/10.1016/j.jpsychores.2017.06.004
Lantian, A., Muller, D., Nurra, C., & Douglas, K. M. (2017). "I know things they don't know!": The role of need for uniqueness in belief in conspiracy theories. *Social Psychology, 48,* 160–173. https://doi.org/10.1027/1864-9335/a000306
Lee, J. D. (2014). *An epidemic of rumors: How stories shape our perception of disease.* University Press of Colorado.
Lewandowsky, S., & Cook, J. (2020). *The conspiracy theory handbook.* http://sks.to/conspiracy
Lewandowsky, S., Cook, J., Ecker, U., & van der Linden, S. (2020). How to spot COVID-19 conspiracy theories. https://www.climatechangecommunication.org/wp-content/uploads/2020/05/How-to-Spot-COVID-19-Conspiracy-Theories.pdf
Lewandowsky, S., Oberauer, K., & Gignac, G. E. (2013). NASA faked the moon landing—therefore, (climate) science is a hoax: An anatomy of the motivated rejection of science. *Psychological Science, 24,* 622–633. https://doi.org/10.1177/0956797612457686
Lynas, M. (2020). COVID: Top 10 current conspiracy theories. https://allianceforscience.cornell.edu/blog/2020/04/covid-top-10-current-conspiracy-theories/
Lytvynenko, J. (2020). Here's a running list of the latest hoaxes spreading about the coronavirus. BuzzFeed News. https://www.buzzfeednews.com/article/janelytvynenko/coronavirus-fake-news-disinformation-rumors-hoaxes
Mallapaty, S. (2024). Wuhan lab samples hold no close relatives to virus behind COVID. *Nature.* https://www.nature.com/articles/d41586-024-03982-2
March, E. (2019). Psychopathy, sadism, empathy, and the motivation to cause harm: New evidence confirms malevolent nature of the Internet Troll. *Personality and Individual Differences, 141,* 133–137. https://doi.org/10.1016/j.paid.2019.01.001
Marchlewska, M., Cichocka, A., & Kossowska, M. (2018). Addicted to answers: Need for cognitive closure and the endorsement of conspiracy beliefs. *European Journal of Social Psychology, 48,* 109–117. https://doi.org/10.1002/ejsp.2308
Marinthe, G., Brown, G., Delouvée, S., & Jolley, D. (2020). Looking out for myself: Exploring the relationship between conspiracy mentality, perceived personal risk, and COVID-19 prevention measures. *British Journal of Health Psychology, 25*(4), 957–980. https://doi.org/10.1111/bjhp.12449
Mayhew, H. (1865). *London labour and the London poor (vol. 1).* Griffin, Bohn, & Co.
Merriam-Webster. (2021). *Merriam-Webster dictionary.* https://www.merriam-webster.com/dictionary

Miller, J. M. (2020). Do COVID-19 conspiracy theory beliefs form a monological belief system? *Canadian Journal of Political Science, 53*(2), 319–326. https://doi.org/10.1017/S0008423920000517

Morens, D. M., Folkers, G. K., & Fauci, A. S. (2008). Emerging infections: A perpetual challenge. *Lancet Infectious Diseases, 8*, 710–719. https://doi.org/10.1016/S1473-3099(08)70256-1

Morris, E. (2020). *Edison*. Random House.

Moulding, R., Nix-Carnell, S., Schnabel, A., Nedeljkovic, M., Burnside, E., Lentini, A., et al. (2016). Better the devil you know than a world you don't? Intolerance of uncertainty and worldview explanations for belief in conspiracy theories. *Personality and Individual Differences, 98*, 345–354. https://doi.org/10.1016/j.paid.2016.04.060

New York Herald (European Edition). (1890, January 31). The very latest. *New York Herald (European Edition)*, 2.

New York Times. (1918, September 19). Think influenza came in U-boat. *New York Times*, 11.

Nohl, J. (1926). *The Black Death: A chronical of the plague*. Allen & Unwin.

Oliver, J. E., & Wood, T. (2014). Medical conspiracy theories and health behaviors in the United States. *JAMA Internal Medicine, 174*, 817–818. https://doi.org/10.1001/jamainternmed.2014.190

Oxford, J. S. (2000). Influenza A pandemics of the 20th century with special reference to 1918: Virology, pathology and epidemiology. *Reviews in Medical Virology, 10*(2), 119–133. https://doi.org/10.1002/(SICI)1099-1654(200003/04)10:2<119::AID-RMV272>3.0.CO;2-O

Parets, M. (1651). *A journal of the plague year: The diary of the Barcelona tanner Miquel Parets 1651* (J. S. Amelang, Trans. & Ed., 1991). Oxford University Press.

Parsons, S., Simmons, W., Shinhoster, F., & Kilburn, J. (1999). A test of the grapevine: An empirical examination of conspiracy theories among African Americans. *Sociological Spectrum, 19*, 201–222. https://doi.org/10.1080/027321799280235

Quick, J. D. (2018). *The end of epidemics: The looming threat and how to stop it*. St. Martin's Press.

Rabbani, G. H., & Greenough, W. B. (1999). Food as a vehicle of transmission of cholera. *Journal of Diarrhoeal Diseases Resarch, 17*(1), 1–9.

Rahman, S. A. (2020). Coronavirus rumors spark communal violence in India. *VOA News*. https://www.voanews.com/a/covid-19-pandemic_coronavirus-rumors-spark-communal-violence-india/6192466.html

Romer, D., & Jamieson, K. H. (2020). Conspiracy theories as barriers to controlling the spread of COVID-19 in the U.S. *Social Science & Medicine, 263*, article 113356. https://doi.org/10.1016/j.socscimed.2020.113356

Roos, D. (2021). How 5 of history's worst pandemics finally ended. https://www.history.com/news/pandemics-end-plague-cholera-black-death-smallpox

Rosenberg, C. E. (1987). *The cholera years: The United States in 1832, 1849, and 1866*. University of Chicago Press.

Ruiz, J. B., & Bell, R. A. (2021). Predictors of intention to vaccinate against COVID-19: Results of a nationwide survey. *Vaccine, 39*(7), 1080–1086. https://doi.org/10.1016/j.vaccine.2021.01.010

Sallam, M., Dababseh, D., Eid, H., Al-Mahzoum, K., Al-Haidar, A., Taim, D., et al. (2021). High rates of COVID-19 vaccine hesitancy and its association with conspiracy beliefs: A study in Jordan and Kuwait among other Arab countries. *Vaccines, 9*(1), article 42. https://doi.org/10.3390/vaccines9010042

Sallam, M., Dababseh, D., Yaseen, A., Al-Haidar, A., Ababneh, N., Bakri, F., et al. (2020). Conspiracy beliefs are associated with lower knowledge and higher anxiety levels regarding COVID-19 among students at the University of Jordan. *International Journal of*

Environmental Research and Public Health, 17(14), article 4915. https://doi.org/10.3390/ijerph17144915

Schellack, N., Strydom, M., Pepper, M., Herd, C., Hendricks, C., Bronkhorst, E., et al. (2022). Social media and COVID-19-perceptions and public deceptions of Ivermectin, Colchicine and Hydroxychloroquine: Lessons for future pandemics. *Antibiotics, 11*(4), article 445. https://doi.org/10.3390/antibiotics11040445

Schoch-Spana, M. (2004). Lessons from the 1918 pandemic influenza: Psychosocial consequences of a catastrophic outbreak of disease. In R. J. Ursano, A. E. Norwood, & C. S. Fullerton (Eds.), *Bioterrorism: Psychological and public health interventions* (pp. 38–55). Cambridge University Press.

Sest, N., & March, E. (2017). Constructing the cyber-troll: Psychopathy, sadism, and empathy. *Personality and Individual Differences, 119*, 69–72. https://doi.org/10.1016/j.paid.2017.06.038

Shepherd, K. (2020). A man thought aquarium cleaner with the same name as the anti-viral drug chloroquine would prevent coronavirus. It killed him. *Washington Post*. https://www.washingtonpost.com/nation/2020/03/24/coronavirus-chloroquine-poisoning-death/

Shibutani, T. (1966). *Improvised news: A sociological study of rumor*. Bobbs-Merrill.

Slack, P. (1985). *The impact of plague in Tudor and Stuart England*. Routledge.

Smallman, S. (2015). Whom do you trust? Doubt and conspiracy theories in the 2009 influenza pandemic. *Journal of International & Global Studies, 6*, 1–24.

Statista. (2019). To what extent to do believe in the conspiracy theory that 9/11 was an inside job? https://www.statista.com/statistics/959504/belief-september-11-inside-job-conspiracy-us/

Swami, V., Voracek, M., Stieger, S., Tran, U. S., & Furnham, A. (2014). Analytic thinking reduces belief in conspiracy theories. *Cognition, 133*, 572–585. https://doi.org/10.1016/j.cognition.2014.08.006

Swift, A. (2013). *Majority in U.S. still believe JFK killed in a conspiracy*. Gallup. https://news.gallup.com/poll/165893/majority-believe-jfk-killed-conspiracy.aspx

Taylor, A. (2020). Experts debunk fringe theory linking China's coronavirus to weapons research. *Washington Post*. https://www.washingtonpost.com/world/2020/01/29/experts-debunk-fringe-theory-linking-chinas-coronavirus-weapons-research/

Taylor, S. (2019). *The psychology of pandemics: Preparing for the next global outbreak of infectious disease*. Cambridge Scholars Publishing.

Taylor, S. (2022). The psychology of pandemics. *Annual Review of Clinical Psychology, 18*, 581–609. https://doi.org/10.1146/annurev-clinpsy-072720-020131

Taylor, S., & Asmundson, G. J. G. (2021). Negative attitudes about facemasks during the COVID-19 pandemic: The dual importance of perceived ineffectiveness and psychological reactance. *PLOS ONE, 16*(2), article e0246317. https://doi.org/10.1371/journal.pone.0246317

Taylor, S., Paluszek, M., Landry, C., Rachor, G. S., & Asmundson, G. J. G. (2020). Worry, avoidance, and coping during the COVID-19 pandemic: A comprehensive network analysis. *Journal of Anxiety Disorders, 76*, article 102327. https://doi.org/10.1016/j.janxdis.2020.102327

The Straits Times. (2020). Taiwan accuses Chinese Internet trolls of sowing coronavirus panic. *The Straits Times*. https://www.straitstimes.com/asia/east-asia/taiwan-accuses-chinese-trolls-of-sowing-coronavirus-panic

Thomas, E. (2021). *Australia's fragmented, conspiracy-focused anti-lockdown movement*. Institute for Strategic Dialogue.

Thucydides. (431 BC). *The history of the Peloponnesian War* (R. Crawley, Trans., 2009). Project Gutenberg. www.gutenberg.org

Tobin, M. J. (2022). Fiftieth anniversary of uncovering the Tuskegee Syphilis Study: The story and timeless lessons. *American Journal of Respiratory and Critical Care Medicine, 205*(10), 1145–1158. https://doi.org/10.1164/rccm.202201-0136SO

Turner, P. A. (1993). *I heard it through the gravevine: Rumor in African American culture.* University of California Press.

van Prooijen, J.-W., Etienne, T. W., Kutiyski, Y., & Krouwel, A. P. M. (2023). Conspiracy beliefs prospectively predict health behavior and well-being during a pandemic. *Psychological Medicine, 53*(6), 2514–2521. https://doi.org/10.1017/S0033291721004438

van Prooijen, J.-W., & van Vugt, M. (2018). Conspiracy theories: Evolved functions and psychological mechanisms. *Perspectives on Psychological Science, 13*, 770–788. https://doi.org/10.1177/1745691618774270

Waldersee, V. (2019). Which science-based conspiracy theories do Britons believe? *YouGov.* https://yougov.co.uk/topics/science/articles-reports/2019/04/25/which-science-based-conspiracy-theories-do-britons

Weigmann, K. (2018). The genesis of a conspiracy theory: Why do people believe in scientific conspiracy theories and how do they spread? *EMBO Reports, 19*(4), e45935. https://doi.org/10.15252/embr.201845935

Wong, C. S. (1987). *An illustrated cycle of Chinese festivities in Malaysia and Singapore.* Jack Chia-MPH.

Wood, M. J. (2018). Propagating and debunking conspiracy theories on Twitter during the 2015–2016 Zika virus outbreak. *Cyberpsychology, Behavior, and Social Networking, 21*, 485–490. https://doi.org/10.1089/cyber.2017.0669

Wu, H. (2021). China pushes conspiracy theories on COVID origin, vaccines. *US News.* https://www.usnews.com/news/world/articles/2021-01-25/china-pushes-fringe-theories-on-pandemic-origins-virus

Wyrobisz, A. (2000). Misericordia pestis tempore. Attitudes and behaviour during pestilences in early modern Poland (16th-18th centuries). *Acta Poloniae Historica, 81*, 165–181.

Young, I. (2020). Panic at the Costco: Coronavirus, a bogus photo and the contagion of fear behind Vancouver's supermarket stampede. *South China Morning Post.* https://www.scmp.com/news/china/society/article/3065292/panic-costco-coronavirus-bogus-photo-and-contagion-fear-behind

Zimmer, S. M., & Burke, D. S. (2009). Historical perspective—Emergence of influenza A (H1N1) viruses. *New England Journal of Medicine, 361*(3), 279–285. https://doi.org/10.1056/NEJMra0904322

Chapter 13

Abramowitz, J. S., & Braddock, A. E. (2011). *Hypchondriasis and health anxiety.* Hogrefe & Huber.

American Psychiatric Association. (2022). *Diagnostic and statistical manual of mental disorders* (5th ed., text rev.). Author.

Anand, N., Sharma, M., Thakur, P., Mondal, I., Sahu, M., Singh, P., et al. (2021). Doomsurfing and doomscrolling mediate psychological distress in Covid-19 lockdown: Implications for awareness of cognitive biases. *Perspectives in Psychiatric Care, 58*, 170–172. https://doi.org/10.1111/ppc.12803

Asmundson, G. J. G., & Taylor, S. (2005). *It's not all in your head: How worrying about your health could be making you sick—and what you can do about it.* Guilford.

Barsky, A. J., & Klerman, G. L. (1983). Overview: Hypochondriasis, bodily complaints, and somatic styles. *American Journal of Psychiatry, 140*, 273–283. https://doi.org/10.1176/ajp.140.3.273

Bobevski, I., Clarke, D. M., & Meadows, G. (2016). Health anxiety and its relationship to disability and service use: Findings from a large epidemiological survey. *Psychosomatic Medicine, 78,* 13–25. https://doi.org/10.1097/PSY.0000000000000252

Borkovec, T. D., Robinson, E., Pruzinsky, T., & DePree, J. A. (1983). Preliminary exploration of worry: Some characteristics and processes. *Behaviour Research and Therapy, 21*(1), 9–16. https://doi.org/10.1016/0005-7967(83)90121-3

Burton, R. (1652). *The anatomy of melancholy (6th ed.).* Crips & Lloyd.

Cassiday, K. L. (2022). *Freedom from health anxiety: Understand and overcome obsessive worry about your health or someone else's and find peace of mind.* New Harbinger.

Côté, G., O'Leary, T., Barlow, D. H., Strain, J. J., Salkovskis, P. M., Warwick, H. M. C., et al. (1996). Hypochondriasis. In T. A. Widiger, A. J. Frances, H. A. Pincus, R. Ross, M. B. First, & W. W. Davis (Eds.), *DSM-IV sourcebook (vol. 2)* (pp. 933–947). American Psychiatric Association.

Easterling, D. V., & Leventhal, H. (1989). Contribution of concrete cognition to emotion: Neutral symptoms as elicitors of worry about cancer. *Journal of Applied Psychology, 74,* 787–796. https://doi.org/10.1037/0021-9010.74.5.787

Eilenberg, T., Frostholm, L., Schroder, A., Jensen, J. S., & Fink, P. (2015). Long-term consequences of severe health anxiety on sick leave in treated and untreated patients: Analysis alongside a randomised controlled trial. *Journal of Anxiety Disorders, 32,* 95–102. https://doi.org/10.1016/j.janxdis.2015.04.001

Gilles, I., Bangerter, A., Clémence, A., Green, E., Krings, F., Staerklé, C., et al. (2011). Trust in medical organizations predicts pandemic (H1N1) 2009 vaccination behavior and perceived efficacy of protection measures in the Swiss public. *European Journal of Epidemiology, 26,* 203–210. https://doi.org/10.1007/s10654-011-9577-2

Goodwin, R., Gaines, S. O., Myers, L., & Neto, F. (2009). Initial psychological reactions to swine flu. *International Journal of Behavioral Medicine, 18,* 88–92. https://doi.org/10.1007/s12529-010-9083-z

Hedman, E., Lekander, M., Karshikoff, B., Ljótsson, B., Axelsson, E., & Axelsson, J. (2016). Health anxiety in a disease-avoidance framework: Investigation of anxiety, disgust and disease perception in response to sickness cues. *Journal of Abnormal Psychology, 125,* 868–878. https://doi.org/10.1037/abn0000195

Imataki, O., & Uemura, M. (2021). Psychogenic fever due to worry about COVID-19: A case report. *Clinical Case Reports, 9*(8), article e04560. https://doi.org/10.1002/ccr3.4560

James, A., & Wells, A. (2002). Death beliefs, superstitious beliefs and health anxiety. *British Journal of Clinical Psychology, 41*(1), 43–53. https://doi.org/10.1348/014466502163787

Jones, J. H., & Salathé, M. (2009). Early assessment of anxiety and behavioral response to novel swine-origin influenza A(H1N1). *PLOS ONE, 4*(12), article e8032. https://doi.org/10.1371/journal.pone.0008032

Kanadiya, M. K., & Sallar, A. M. (2011). Preventive behaviors, beliefs, and anxieties in relation to the swine flu outbreak among college students aged 18–24 years. *Journal of Public Health, 19,* 139–145. https://doi.org/10.1007/s10389-010-0373-3

Knapp, S., & Vandecreek, L. (1989). Fear of AIDS: Its meaning and implications for clinical practice. *Journal of Contemporary Psychotherapy, 19*(3), 239–247. https://doi.org/10.1007/BF00946034

Lucock, M. P., White, C., Peake, M. D., & Morley, S. (1998). Biased perception and recall of reassurance in medical patients. *British Journal of Health Psychology, 3,* 237–243. https://doi.org/10.1111/j.2044-8287.1998.tb00570.x

Nakamura, K., & Morrison, S. F. (2022). Central sympathetic network for thermoregulatory responses to psychological stress. *Autonomic Neuroscience: Basic & Clinical, 237,* article 102918. https://doi.org/10.1016/j.autneu.2021.102918

Norris, A. L., & Marcus, D. K. (2014). Cognition in health anxiety and hypochondriasis: Recent advances. *Current Psychiatry Reviews, 10*, 44–49. https://doi.org/10.2174/1573400509666131119004151

Olivier, B. (2015). Psychogenic fever, functional fever, or psychogenic hyperthermia? *Temperature, 2*(3), 324–325. https://doi.org/10.1080/23328940.2015.1071701

Pennebaker, J. W. (1982). *The psychology of physical symptoms*. Springer.

Rubin, G. J., Amlôt, R., Page, L., & Wessely, S. (2009). Public perceptions, anxiety, and behaviour change in relation to the Swine flu outbreak: Cross sectional telephone survey. *British Medical Journal, 339*, article b2651. https://doi.org/10.1136/bmj.b2651

Salkovskis, P. M., & Warwick, H. M. C. (2001). Meaning, misinterpretations, and medicine: A cognitive-behavioral approach to understanding health anxiety and hypochondriasis. In V. Starcevic, D. R. Lipsitt, V. Starcevic, & D. R. Lipsitt (Eds.), *Hypochondriasis: Modern perspectives on an ancient malady* (pp. 202–222). Oxford University Press.

Singh, S., Kaur, P., & Singh, G. (2013). Study to assess the awareness, perception and myths regarding swine flu among educated common public in Patiala district. *International Journal of Research & Development of Health, 1*(2), 54–60.

Steinbrook, R. (1985). The Times poll: Majority see their risk of contracting AIDS as low. *Los Angeles Times*. https://www.latimes.com/archives/la-xpm-1985-12-18-mn-26846-story.html

Sunderland, M., Newby, J. M., & Andrews, G. (2013). Health anxiety in Australia: prevalence, comorbidity, disability and service use. *British Journal of Psychiatry, 202*, 56–61. https://doi.org/10.1192/bjp.bp.111.103960

Taylor, S. (2021). COVID Stress Syndrome: Clinical and nosological considerations. *Current Psychiatry Reports, 23*, article 19. https://doi.org/10.1007/s11920-021-01226-y

Taylor, S., & Asmundson, G. J. G. (2004). *Treating health anxiety*. Guilford.

Taylor, S., & Asmundson, G. J. G. (2017). Treatment of health anxiety. In E. Storch, J. S. Abramowitz, & D. McKay (Eds.), *Handbook of obsessive-compulsive disorders: Vol. 2: Obsessive-compulsive related disorders* (pp. 977–989). Wiley.

Taylor, S., Paluszek, M., Landry, C., Rachor, G. S., & Asmundson, G. J. G. (2020). Worry, avoidance, and coping during the COVID-19 pandemic: A comprehensive network analysis. *Journal of Anxiety Disorders, 76*, article 102327. https://doi.org/10.1016/j.janxdis.2020.102327

Tyrer, H. (2013). *Tackling health anxiety: A CBT handbook*. RCPsych Publications.

Tyrer, P., & Tyrer, H. (2018). Health anxiety: Detection and treatment. *British Journal of Psychiatry Advances, 24*, 66–72. https://doi.org/10.1192/bja.2017.5

Wells, A., & Hackmann, A. (1993). Imagery and core beliefs in health anxiety: Contents and origins. *Behavioural and Cognitive Psychotherapy, 21*, 265–273. https://doi.org/10.1017/S1352465800010511

Wheaton, M. G., Abramowitz, J. S., Berman, N. C., Fabricant, L. E., & Olatunji, B. O. (2012). Psychological predictors of anxiety in response to the H1N1 (swine flu) pandemic. *Cognitive Therapy and Research, 36*, 210–218. https://doi.org/10.1007/s10608-011-9353-3

Wheaton, M. G., Berman, N. C., Franklin, J. C., & Abramowitz, J. S. (2010). Health anxiety: Latent structure and associations with anxiety-related psychological processes. *Journal of Psychopathology and Behavioral Assessment, 32*, 565–574. https://doi.org/10.1007/s10862-010-9179-4

Williams, L., Rasmussen, S., Kleczkowski, A., Maharaj, S., & Cairns, N. (2015). Protection motivation theory and social distancing behaviour in response to a simulated infectious disease epidemic. *Psychology, Health & Medicine, 20*, 832–837. https://doi.org/10.1080/13548506.2015.1028946

Wilson, R., & Veale, D. (2022). *Overcoming health anxiety (2nd ed.)*. Robinson.

Witthöft, M., Kerstner, T., Ofer, J., Mier, D., Rist, F., Diener, C., et al. (2016). Cognitive biases in pathological health anxiety: The contribution of attention, memory, and evaluation processes. *Clinical Psychological Science, 4*, 464–479. https://doi.org/10.1177/2167702615593474

Wong, L. P., & Sam, I. C. (2011). Knowledge and attitudes in regard to pandemic influenza A(H1N1) in a multiethnic community of Malaysia. *International Journal of Behavioral Medicine, 18*, 112–121. https://doi.org/10.1007/s12529-010-9114-9

Chapter 14

A Physician of New Orleans. (1854). *History of the yellow fever in New Orleans*. C. W. Kenworthy.

Aberth, J. (2010). *From the brink of the apocalypse: Confronting famine, war, plague, and death in the later middle ages* (2nd ed.). Routledge.

Alterisio, H. (2020). Psychologist's dark humor group brings light to dark times. *Eagle Tribune*. https://www.eagletribune.com/psychologists-dark-humor-group-brings-light-to-dark-times/article_2fe5eaee-3a28-5fef-b383-957a4304ae5b.html

Amici, P. (2020). Humor in the age of COVID-19 lockdown: An explorative qualitative study. *Psychiatria Danubina, 32*(Suppl 1), 15–20.

Archambeau, N. (2011). Healing options during the plague: Survivor stories from a fourteenth-century canonization inquest. *Bulletin of the History of Medicine, 85*(4), 531–559. https://doi.org/10.1353/bhm.2011.0081

Bailey, T., & Walter, T. (2016). Funerals against death. *Mortality, 21*(2), 149–166. https://doi.org/10.1080/13576275.2015.1071344

Becker, E. (1973). *The denial of death*. Simon & Schuster.

Bélanger, J. J., Faber, T., & Gelfand, M. J. (2013). Supersize my identity: When thoughts of contracting swine flu boost one's patriotic identity. *Journal of Applied Social Psychology, 43*(Suppl 1), E153–E155.

Burke, B. L., Kosloff, S., & Landau, M. J. (2013). Death goes to the polls: A meta-analysis of mortality salience effects on political attitudes. *Political Psychology, 34*(2), 183–200. https://doi.org/10.1111/pops.12005

Carrigan, J. A. (1963). Impact of epidemic yellow fever on life in Louisiana. *Louisiana History, 4*(1), 5–34.

Chew, C., & Eysenbach, G. (2010). Pandemics in the age of Twitter: Content analysis of Tweets during the 2009 H1N1 outbreak. *PLOS ONE, 5*, articlee14118. https://doi.org/10.1371/journal.pone.0014118

Clissold, E., Nylander, D., Watson, C., & Ventriglio, A. (2020). Pandemics and prejudice. *International Journal of Social Psychiatry, 66*(5), 421–423. https://doi.org/10.1177/0020764020937873

Correia, A. M. (2018). Coimbra's response to the 1918-1919 influenza epidemic, seen from the viewpoint of a local newspaper. *História, Ciências, Saúde-Manguinhos, 25*(3), 1–16. https://doi.org/10.1590/S0104-59702018000400005

D'Irsay, S. (1927). Defense reactions during the Black Death, 1348-1349. *Annals of Medical History, 9*, 169–179.

Davis, J. T., & Perry, S. L. (2021). White Christian nationalism and relative political tolerance for racists. *Social Problems, 68*(3), 513–534. https://doi.org/10.1093/socpro/spaa002

De Bow's Review. (1853). The plague in the south-west. *De Bow's Review, 15*, 595–635.

Dundes, A. (1987). At ease, disease—AIDS jokes as sick humor. *American Behavioral Scientist, 30*(3), 72–81. https://doi.org/10.1177/000276487030003006

Engle, J. (2020). Is it OK to laugh during dark times? *New York Times.* https://www.nytimes.com/2020/04/29/learning/is-it-ok-to-laugh-during-dark-times.html

Fiquepron, M. R. (2018). Places, attitudes and moments during the epidemics: Representations of yellow fever and cholera in the city of Buenos Aires, 1867-1871. *História, Ciências, Saúde, 25*(2), 1–16. https://doi.org/10.1590/S0104-59702018000200003

Fritz, H. L., Russek, L. N., & Dillon, M. M. (2017). Humor use moderates the relation of stressful life events with psychological distress. *Personality and Social Psychology Bulletin, 43*(6), 845–859. https://doi.org/10.1177/0146167217699583

Garza, R. P. (2008). *Understanding plague: The medical and imaginative texts of medieval Spain.* Peter Lang.

Goldenberg, J. L., & Arndt, J. (2008). The implications of death for health: A terror management health model for behavioral health promotion. *Psychological Review, 115,* 1032–1053. https://doi.org/10.1037/a0013326

Gowen, B. S. (1907). Some aspects of pestilences and other epidemics. *American Journal of Psychology, 18*(1), 1–60. https://doi.org/10.2307/1412171

Greenberg, J., Pyszczynski, T., & Solomon, S. (1986). The causes and consequences of a need for self-esteem: A terror management theory. In R. F. Baumeister (Ed.), *Public self and private self* (pp. 189–212). Springer-Verlag.

Greenberg, J., Solomon, S., & Arndt, J. (2008). A basic but uniquely human motivation: Terror management. In J. Y. Shah & W. L. Gardner (Eds.), *Handbook of motivation science* (pp. 114–134). Guilford.

Hecker, J. F. C. (1844). *Epidemics of the middle ages* (B. G. Babington, Trans.). Woodfall.

Hsee, C. K., & Ruan, B. (2016). The Pandora effect: The power and peril of curiosity. *Psychological Science, 27*(5), 659–666. https://doi.org/10.1177/0956797616631733

Juhl, J. (2019). Terror management theory: A theory of psychological well-being. In C. Routledge & M. Vess (Eds.), *Handbook of terror management theory* (pp. 303–324). Academic Press. https://doi.org/10.1016/B978-0-12-811844-3.00013-5

King, F. (1918, October 11). Spanish "flu fence" has advantages; will be a life saver in face powder. *San Francisco Examiner,* 6. http://hdl.handle.net/2027/spo.6010flu.0009.2106

Kuiper, N. A. (2012). Humor and resiliency: Towards a process model of coping and growth. *Europe's Journal of Psychology, 8*(3), 475–491. https://doi.org/10.5964/ejop.v8i3.464

Lee, J. D. (2014). *An epidemic of rumors: How stories shape our perception of disease.* University Press of Colorado.

Lee, M. (2021). Christian nationalism is worse than you think. *Chistianity Today.* https://www.christianitytoday.com/ct/podcasts/quick-to-listen/christian-nationalism-capitol-riots-trump-podcast.html

McDonald, M. (2011). *The Armageddon factor: The rise of Christian nationalism in Canada.* Vintage Canada.

McGee, L. (2022). Boris Johnson apologizes for attending Downing Street "bring your own booze" party during lockdown. *CNN.* https://www.cnn.com/2022/01/12/uk/boris-johnson-pmqs-downing-street-party-intl-gbr/index.html

Michel, C. (2017). How Russia became the leader of the global Christian right. *Politico.* https://www.politico.com/magazine/story/2017/02/how-russia-became-a-leader-of-the-worldwide-christian-right-214755/

Munson, K. (2021). Laughter in dark times. *Utah State Magazine.* https://utahstatemagazine.usu.edu/health/laughter-in-dark-times/

Parets, M. (1651). *A journal of the plague year: The diary of the Barcelona tanner Miquel Parets 1651* (J. S. Amelang, Trans. & Ed., 1991). Oxford University Press.

Pepys, S. (1669). *The diary of Samual Pepys.* Knopf (republished in 2018).

Perchtold, C., Weiss, E., Rominger, C., Feyaerts, K., Ruch, W., Fink, A., et al. (2019). Humorous cognitive reappraisal: More benign humour and less "dark" humour is affiliated with more adaptive cognitive reappraisal strategies. *PLOS ONE, 14*(1), article e0211618. https://doi.org/10.1371/journal.pone.0211618

Perry, S. L., Whitehead, A. L., & Grubbs, J. B. (2020). Culture wars and COVID-19 conduct: Christian nationalism, religiosity, and Americans' behavior during the coronavirus pandemic. *Journal for the Scientific Study of Religion, 59*(3), 405–416. https://doi.org/10.1111/jssr.12677

Perry, S. L., Whitehead, A. L., & Grubbs, J. B. (2021). Prejudice and pandemic in the promised land: How white Christian nationalism shapes Americans' racist and xenophobic views of COVID-19. *Ethnic and Racial Studies, 44*(5), 759–772. https://doi.org/10.1080/01419870.2020.1839114

Perry, S. L., Whitehead, A. L., & Grubbs, J. B. (2022). "I don't want everybody to vote": Christian nationalism and restricting voter access in the United States. *Sociological Forum, 37*(1), 4–26. https://doi.org/10.1111/socf.12776

Procopius. (551 AD). *History of the wars: Book II* (H. B. Dewing, Trans, 1914). Heinemann.

Pyszczynski, T., Kesebir, P., & Lockett, M. (2019). A terror management theory perspective on human motivation. In R. M. Ryan (Ed.), *The Oxford handbook of human motivation* (2nd ed.) (pp. 67–88). Oxford University Press.

Pyszczynski, T., Lockett, M., Greenberg, J., & Solomon, S. (2021). Terror management theory and the COVID-19 pandemic. *Journal of Humanistic Psychology, 61*(2), 173–189. https://doi.org/10.1177/0022167820959488

Reynolds, C. (2022). Transport Canada fines passengers on Sunwing party flight. *Globe and Mail.* https://www.theglobeandmail.com/business/article-transport-canada-fines-passengers-on-sunwing-party-flight-2/

Rowe, A., & Regehr, C. (2010). Whatever gets you through today: An examination of cynical humor among emergency service professionals. *Journal of Loss and Trauma, 15*(5), 448–464. https://doi.org/10.1080/15325024.2010.507661

Saiya, N. (2022a). *The global politics of Jesus: A Christian case for church-state separation.* Oxford University Press.

Saiya, N. (2022b). Why Christian nationalism is a growing problem. *ABC Religion & Ethics.* https://www.abc.net.au/religion/christian-nationalism-is-a-global-problem/13968062

Samson, A. C., & Gross, J. J. (2012). Humour as emotion regulation: The differential consequences of negative versus positive humour. *Cognition and Emotion, 26*(2), 375–384. https://doi.org/10.1080/02699931.2011.585069

Scrivner, C. (2021). The psychology of morbid curiosity: Development and initial validation of the Morbid Curiosity Scale. *Personality and Individual Differences, 183*, article 111139. https://doi.org/10.1016/j.paid.2021.111139

Shults, F. L., Lane, J. E., Wildman, W. J., Diallo, S., Lynch, C. J., & Gore, R. (2018). Modelling terror management theory: Computer simulations of the impact of mortality salience on religiosity. *Religion, Brain & Behavior, 8*(1), 77–100. https://doi.org/10.1080/2153599X.2016.1238846

Slack, P. (1985). *The impact of plague in Tudor and Stuart England.* Routledge.

Sorokin, P. A. (1942). *Man and society in calamity.* Routledge.

Steel, D. (1918). Plague writing: From Boccaccio to Camus. *Journal of European Studies, 11*, 88–110.

Thucydides. (411 BC). *The history of the Peloponnesian War* (R. Crawley trans., 2009). Project Gutenberg, www.gutenberg.org

Weeks, A. (1918, October 23). "Oh, my gauze," sneeze signal. *Detroit News*, 1–2. https://doi.org/http://hdl.handle.net/2027/spo.6990flu.0011.996

Chapter 15

A Physician of New Orleans. (1854). *History of the yellow fever in New Orleans*. C. W. Kenworthy.

Aarøe, L., Petersen, M. B., & Arceneaux, K. (2017). The behavioral immune system shapes political intuitions: Why and how individual differences in disgust sensitivity underlie opposition to immigration. *American Political Science Review, 111*, 277–294. https://doi.org/10.1017/S0003055416000770

Ackerman, J. M., Hill, S. E., & Murray, D. R. (2018). The behavioral immune system: Current concerns and future directions. *Social and Personality Psychology Compass, 12*, 57–70. https://doi.org/10.1111/spc3.12371

Alexander, B. (2009). Amid swine flu outbreak, racism goes viral. *NBC News*. https://www.nbcnews.com/id/wbna30467300

Anonymous. (1721). *The late dreadful plague at Marseilles compared with that terrible plague in London in the year 1665*. Parker.

Arnold, C. (2018). "Eat more onions!": Desperate and massively debatable medical advice from 1918. *Lapham's Quarterly*. https://www.laphamsquarterly.org/roundtable/eat-more-onions

Atlani-Duault, L., Mercier, A., Rousseau, C., Guyot, P., & Moatti, J. P. (2015). Blood libel rebooted: Traditional scapegoats, online media, and the H1N1 epidemic. *Culture, Medicine and Psychiatry, 39*, 43–61. https://doi.org/10.1007/s11013-014-9410-y

Bradley, R. (1721). *The plague at Marseilles consider'd (3rd ed.)*. Mears.

Brand, J., McKay, D., Wheaton, M. G., & Abramowitz, J. S. (2013). The relationship between obsessive compulsive beliefs and symptoms, anxiety and disgust sensitivity, and Swine flu fears. *Journal of Obsessive-Compulsive and Related Disorders, 2*, 200–206. https://doi.org/10.1016/j.jocrd.2013.01.007

Burton, R. (1652). *The anatomy of melancholy (6th ed.)*. Crips & Lloyd.

Carrigan, J. A. (1994). *Saffron scourge: A history of yellow fever in Louisiana, 1796-1905*. University of Southwestern Louisiana.

Chapin, C. V. (1906). The fetich [sic] of disinfection. *JAMA, 47*(8), 574–580. https://doi.org/10.1001/jama.1906.25210080026002f

Cohn, S. K. (2012). Pandemics: Waves of disease, waves of hate from the Plague of Athens to A.I.D.S. *Historical Research, 85*(230), 535–555. https://doi.org/10.1111/j.1468-2281.2012.00603.x

Cohn, S. K. (2017). Plague violence and abandonment from the Black Death to the early moden period. *Annales de Demographie Historique, 134*(2), 39–61. https://doi.org/10.3917/adh.134.0039

Cox, R. C., Jessup, S. C., Luber, M. J., & Olatunji, B. O. (2020). Pre-pandemic disgust proneness predicts increased coronavirus anxiety and safety behaviors: Evidence for a diathesis-stress model. *Journal of Anxiety Disorders, 76*, 102315. https://doi.org/10.1016/j.janxdis.2020.102315

Curtis, V., de Barra, M., & Aunger, R. (2011). Disgust as an adaptive system for disease avoidance behaviour. *Philosophical Transactions of the Royal Society: Series B: Biological Sciences, 366*, 389–401. https://doi.org/10.1098/rstb.2010.0117

Díaz, R., & Cova, F. (2021). Reactance, morality, and disgust: The relationship between affective dispositions and compliance with official health recommendations during the Covid-19 pandemic. *Cognition and Emotion, 36*(1), 120–136. https://doi.org/10.1080/02699931.2021.1941783

Duncan, L. A., & Schaller, M. (2009). Prejudicial attitudes toward older adults may be exaggerated when people feel vulnerable to infectious disease: Evidence and implications. *Analyses of Social Issues and Public Policy, 9*, 97–115. https://doi.org/10.1111/j.1530-2415.2009.01188.x

Duncan, L. A., Schaller, M., & Park, J. H. (2009). Perceived vulnerability to disease: Development and validation of a 15-item self-report instrument. *Personality and Individual Differences*, 47, 541–546. https://doi.org/10.1016/j.paid.2009.05.001

Echols, E. C. (1961). *Herodian of Antioch's history of the Roman Empire*. University of California Press.

Elias, A., Ben, J., Mansouri, F., & Paradies, Y. (2021). Racism and nationalism during and beyond the COVID-19 pandemic. *Ethnic and Racial Studies*, 44(5), 783–793. https://doi.org/10.1080/01419870.2020.1851382

Elliott, C. (2024). *Pox Romana: The plague that shook the Roman world*. Princeton University Press.

Ellis, R. (2017). Disinfecting the mail: Disease, panic, and the post office department in nineteenth-century America. *Information & Culture*, 52(4), 436–461. https://doi.org/10.7560/IC52403

Faulkner, J., Schaller, M., Park, J. H., & Duncan, L. A. (2004). Evolved disease-avoidance mechanisms and contemporary xenophobic attitudes. *Group Processes and Intergroup Behavior*, 7, 333–353. https://doi.org/10.1177/1368430204046142

Gilles, I., Bangerter, A., Clémence, A., Green, E., Krings, F., Mouton, A., et al. (2013). Collective symbolic coping with disease threat and othering: A case study of avian influenza. *British Journal of Social Psychology*, 52, 83–102. https://doi.org/10.1111/j.2044-8309.2011.02048.x

Ginzburg, C. (2004). *Ecstasies: Deciphering the witches' sabbath*. University of Chicago Press.

Goetz, A. R., Lee, H., Cougle, J. R., & Turkel, J. E. (2013). Disgust propensity and sensitivity: Differential relationships with obsessive–compulsive symptoms and behavioral approach task performance. *Journal of Obsessive Compulsive and Related Disorders*, 2, 412–419. https://doi.org/10.1016/j.jocrd.2013.07.006

Gong, M., Dong, H., Tang, Y., Huang, W., & Lu, F. (2020). Effects of aromatherapy on anxiety: A meta-analysis of randomized controlled trials. *Journal of Affective Disorders*, 274, 1028–1040. https://doi.org/10.1016/j.jad.2020.05.118

Green, E. G., Krings, F., Staerklé, C., Bangerter, A., Clémence, A., Wagner-Egger, P., et al. (2010). Keeping the vermin out: Perceived disease threat and ideological orientations as predictors of exclusionary immigration attitudes. *Journal of Community Applied Social Psychology*, 20, 299–316. https://doi.org/dx.doi.org/10.1002/casp.1037

Haidt, J., McCauley, C., & Rozin, P. (1994). Individual differences in sensitivity to disgust: A scale sampling seven domains of disgust elicitors. *Personality and Individual Differences*, 16(5), 701–713. https://doi.org/10.1016/0191-8869(94)90212-7

Hirst, L. F. (1953). *The conquest of plague*. Clarendon.

Hodges, N., & Quincy, J. (1720). *Loimologia: Or, an historical account of the plague in London in 1665 with precautionary directions against the like contagion*. Bell.

Holmes, C. (2011). What we can learn about racism from the swine flu scare. *Huffington Post*. https://www.huffpost.com/entry/what-can-we-learn-about-r_n_203602

Inì, M. (2021). Materiality, quarantine and contagion in the early modern mediterranean. *Social History of Medicine*, 34(4), 1161–1184. https://doi.org/10.1093/shm/hkaa124

Institute for Strategic Dialogue. (2021). *The rise of antisemitism online during the pandemic: A study of French and German content*. Publications Office of the European Union.

Joffe, H. (1999). *Risk and the "other."* Cambridge University Press.

Joffe, H., Washer, P., & Solberg, C. (2011). Public engagement with emerging infectious disease: The case of MRSA in Britain. *Psychology & Health*, 26, 667–683. https://doi.org/10.1080/08870441003763238

Kephale, R. (1665). *Medela pestilentiae*. Samuel Speed.

King, A. (2022). Medieval Islamicate aromatherapy: Medical perspectives on aromatics and perfumes. *Senses & Society*, 17(1), 37–51. https://doi.org/10.1080/17458927.2021.2020606

Lee, W. (1869). *Daniel Defoe: His life, and recently discovered writings* (Vol. 2). Hotten.
Literary Digest. (1918a, October 12). How to fight Spanish influenza. *Literary Digest, 59*, 13–14.
Literary Digest. (1918b, December 7). Is the influenza a Chinese plague? *Literary Digest, 59*, 26–27.
Maclean's. (2009). "Devil's dung" protects against Swine flu. *Maclean's, 122*(37), 46.
Makhanova, A., Miller, S. L., & Maner, J. K. (2015). Germs and the out-group: Chronic and situational disease concerns affect intergroup categorization. *Evolutionary Behavioral Sciences, 9*, 8–19. https://doi.org/10.1037/ebs0000028
Man, S. (2020). Anti-Asian violence and US imperialism. *Race & Class, 62*(2), 24–33. https://doi.org/10.1177/0306396820949779
Markel, H. (2004). *When germs travel: Six major epidemics that have invaded America since 1900 and the fears they have unleashed*. Pantheon.
McCauley, M., Minsky, S., & Viswanath, K. (2013). The H1N1 pandemic: Media frames, stigmatization and coping. *BMC Public Health, 13*, article 1116. https://doi.org/10.1186/1471-2458-13-1116
Montreal Daily Herald. (1885, October 22). Beware of odorless disinfectants!! *Montreal Daily Herald*, 1.
Mussell, J. (2007). Pandemic in print: The spread of influenza in the fin de siècle. *Endeavour, 31*(1), 12–17. https://doi.org/10.1016/j.endeavour.2007.01.008
Navarrete, C. D., & Fessler, D. M. T. (2006). Disease avoidance and ethnocentrism: The effects of disease vulnerability and disgust sensitivity on intergroup attitudes. *Evolution and Human Behavior, 27*, 270–282. https://doi.org/10.1016/j.evolhumbehav.2005.12.001
Nelkin, D., & Gilman, S. L. (1988). Placing blame for devastating disease. *Social Research, 55*, 362–378.
Nemeroff, C. (1995). Magical thinking about illness virulence: Conceptions of germs from "safe" versus "dangerous" others. *Health Psychology, 14*, 147–151. https://doi.org/10.1037/0278-6133.14.2.147
New World. (1840). The plague at Alexandria. *New World, 1*(9), p. 141.
New York Times. (1918, September 19). Think influenza came in U-boat. *New York Times*, 11.
Newitz, A. (2021). What social distancing looked like in 1666. *New York Times*. https://www.nytimes.com/2020/03/29/opinion/covid-plague-samuel-pepys.html
Nick, I. M. (2021). In the name of hate: An editorial note on the role geographically marked names for COVID-19 have played in the pandemic of anti-Asian violence. *Names: A Journal of Onomastics, 69*(2), 1–10. https://doi.org/10.5195/names.2021.2276
Oaten, M., Stevenson, R. J., & Case, T. I. (2009). Disgust as a disease avoidance mechanism. *Psychological Bulletin, 135*, 303–321. https://doi.org/10.1037/a0014823
Olivarius, K. (2019). Immunity, capital, and power in antebellum New Orleans. *American Historical Review, 124*(2), 425–455. https://doi.org/10.1093/ahr/rhz176
Parets, M. (1651). *A journal of the plague year: The diary of the Barcelona tanner Miquel Parets 1651* (J. S. Amelang, Trans. & Ed., 1991). Oxford University Press.
Park, J. H., Faulkner, J., & Schaller, M. (2003). Evolved disease-avoidance processes and contemporary anti-social behavior: Prejudicial attitudes and avoidance of people with physical disabilities. *Journal of Nonverbal Behavior, 27*, 65–87. https://doi.org/10.1023/A:1023910408854
Park, J. H., Schaller, M., & Crandall, C. S. (2007). Pathogen-avoidance mechanisms and the stigmatization of obese people. *Evolution and Human Behavior, 28*, 410–414. https://doi.org/10.1016/j.evolhumbehav.2007.05.008
Perry, A. W. (1873). Yellow fever and the results of disinfection in New Orleans. *Clinic, 5*(21), 243–244.

Pringle, H. (2015). How Europeans brought sickness to the New World. *Science*. http://www.sciencemag.org/news/2015/2006/how-europeans-brought-sickness-new-world

Quick, J. D. (2018). *The end of epidemics: The looming threat and how to stop it*. St. Martin's Press.

Rast, C., Woronko, S., Jessup, S. C., & Olatunji, B. O. (2023). Treatment of disgust in specific emotional disorders. *Bulletin of the Menninger Clinic, 87*, 5–30. https://doi.org/10.1521/bumc.2023.87.suppA.5

Rozin, P., Haidt, J., & McCauley, C. R. (2008). Disgust. In M. Lewis, J. M. Haviland-Jones, & L. F. Barrett (Eds.), *Handbook of emotions* (3rd ed.) (pp. 757–776). Guilford.

Schaller, M., & Park, J. H. (2011). The behavioral immune system (and why it matters). *Current Directions in Psychological Science, 20*, 99–103. https://doi.org/10.1177/0963721411402596

Shook, N. J., Sevi, B., Lee, J., Oosterhoff, B., & Fitzgerald, H. N. (2020). Disease avoidance in the time of COVID-19: The behavioral immune system is associated with concern and preventative health behaviors. *PLOS ONE, 15*(8), article e0238015. https://doi.org/10.1371/journal.pone.0238015

Spirit of The Times. (1848). Disinfectants, and rival professors. *Spirit of The Times, 18*(38), p. 447.

Sternberg, G. M. (1900). *Disinfection and individual prophylaxis against infectious dieases*. Berlin Printing Co.

Taylor, S. (2019). *The psychology of pandemics: Preparing for the next global outbreak of infectious disease*. Cambridge Scholars Publishing.

Taylor, S., Landry, C. A., Paluszek, M. M., Fergus, T. A., McKay, D., & Asmundson, G. J. G. (2020). Covid stress syndrome: Concept, structure, and correlates. *Depression and Anxiety, 37*, 706–714. https://doi.org/10.1002/da.23071

Todd, F. M. (1909). *Eradicating plague from San Francisco: Report of the Citizens' Health Committee and an account of its work*. Murdock & Co.

Tomes, N. (1999). *The gospel of germs: Men, women, and the microbe in American life*. Harvard University Press.

Tomes, N. (2010). "Destroyer and teacher": Managing the masses during the 1918-1919 influenza pandemic. *Public Health Reports, 125 (Suppl. 3)*, 48–62. https://doi.org/10.1177/00333549101250S308

Troisi, A., Di Cave, D., Carola, V., & Nanni, R. C. (2022). The behavioral immune system in action: Psychological correlates of pathogen disgust sensitivity in healthcare professionals working in a COVID-19 hospital. *Physiology & Behavior, 251*, article 113821. https://doi.org/10.1016/j.physbeh.2022.113821

Von Pettenkofer, M. (1873). What we can do against cholera: Practical instructions concerning what to do to prevent an epidemic as well as how to guard against it during its prevalence. *Public Health Papers and Reports, 1*, 317–335.

Washer, P. (2004). Representations of SARS in the British newspapers. *Social Science and Medicine, 59*, 2561–2571. https://doi.org/10.1016/j.socscimed.2004.03.038

Wheaton, M. G., Abramowitz, J. S., Berman, N. C., Fabricant, L. E., & Olatunji, B. O. (2012). Psychological predictors of anxiety in response to the H1N1 (swine flu) pandemic. *Cognitive Therapy and Research, 36*, 210–218. https://doi.org/10.1007/s10608-011-9353-3

White, A. E., Johnson, K. A., & Kwan, V. S. Y. (2014). Four ways to infect me: Spatial, temporal, social, and probability distance influence evaluations of disease threat. *Social Cognition, 32*, 239–255. https://doi.org/10.1521/soco.2014.32.3.239

White, A. I. (2018). Epidemic orientalism: Social construction and the global management of infectious disease. Ph.D. thesis, Boston University. https://open.bu.edu/bitstream/handle/2144/33196/White_bu_0017E_13746.pdf?sequence=5&isAllowed=y

Yap, D. L., Mandell, C., & Behar, E. (2023). The role of perceived risk in the relationship between disgust sensitivity and COVID-19 vaccine hesitancy. *Cognitive Therapy and Research, 47*, 543–554. https://doi.org/10.1007/s10608-023-10391-8

Chapter 16

Aaj Bikel News. (2022). Haldia's "Maduli Baba" claims Covid-19 patients will recover by using amulets. *Aaj Bikel News.* https://www.youtube.com/watch?v=aIU33i7bp7U

Abramson, L. Y., Metalsky, G. I., & Alloy, L. B. (1989). Hopelessness depression: A theory-based subtype of depression. *Psychological Review, 96*(2), 358–372. https://doi.org/10.1037/0033-295X.96.2.358

Alloy, L. B., Burke, T. A., O'Garro-Moore, J., & Abramson, L. Y. (2018). Cognitive vulnerability to depression and bipolar disorder. In R. L. Leahy (Ed.), *Science and practice in cognitive therapy: Foundations, mechanisms, and applications* (pp. 105–123). Guilford.

Almutairi, A. F., Adlan, A. A., Balkhy, H. H., Abbas, O. A., & Clark, A. M. (2018). "It feels like I'm the dirtiest person in the world.": Exploring the experiences of healthcare providers who survived MERS-CoV in Saudi Arabia. *Journal of Infection and Public Health, 11*(2), 187–191. https://doi.org/10.1016/j.jiph.2017.06.011

Amazon. (2023). Omamori charm for goodbye Covid-19, Japanese shrine lucky amulet, bring good luck and protect, deity fortune, pink. https://www.amazon.sa/-/en/Omamori-Goodbye-Covid-19-Japanese-Protect/dp/B0969QWHCR

Antipov, E. A., & Pokryshevskaya, E. B. (2015). Are buyers of apartments superstitious? Evidence from the Russian real estate market. *Judgment and Decision Making, 10*(6), 590–592. https://doi.org/10.1017/S1930297500007026

Baldwin, M. R. (1993). Toads and plague: The amulet controversy in seventeenth-century medicine. *Bulletin of the History of Medicine, 67*(2), 227–247.

Bax, P. (2014). Ebola survivor shunned as a zombie joins fight against disease. *Bloomberg.com.* https://www.bloomberg.com/news/articles/2014-07-17/ebola-survivor-shunned-as-a-zombie-joins-fight-against-disease?embedded-checkout=true

Bility, M. T., Agarwal, Y., Ho, S., Castronova, I., Beatty, C., Biradar, S., et al. (2020). WITHDRAWN: Can traditional Chinese medicine provide insights into controlling the COVID-19 pandemic: Serpentinization-induced lithospheric long-wavelength magnetic anomalies in proterozoic bedrocks in a weakened geomagnetic field mediate the aberrant transformation of biogenic molecules in COVID-19 via magnetic catalysis. *Science of the Total Environment*, article 142830. https://doi.org/10.1016/j.scitotenv.2020.142830

Bocci, L., & Gordon, P. K. (2007). Does magical thinking produce neutralising behaviour? An experimental investigation. *Behaviour Research and Therapy, 45*(8), 1823–1833. https://doi.org/10.1016/j.brat.2007.02.003

Brabant, M. (2020). How COVID-19 reshapes our views of life, and of loss. *PBS News Hour.* https://www.pbs.org/newshour/show/how-covid-19-reshapes-our-views-of-life-and-of-loss

Brambilla, P., Fagnani, C., Cecchetto, F., Medda, E., Bellani, M., Salemi, M., et al. (2014). Genetic and environmental bases of the interplay between magical ideation and personality. *Psychiatry Research, 215*(2), 453–459. https://doi.org/10.1016/j.psychres.2013.11.021

Brashier, N. M., & Multhaup, K. S. (2017). Magical thinking decreases across adulthood. *Psychology and Aging, 32*(8), 681–688. https://doi.org/10.1037/pag0000208

Burakov, D. (2018). Do discounts mitigate numerological superstitions? Evidence from the Russian real estate market. *Judgment and Decision Making, 13*(5), 467–470. https://doi.org/10.1017/S1930297500008743

Byrne, J. P. (2006). *Daily life during the Black Death.* Greenwood.

Carroll, J. (2007). Thirteen Percent of Americans Bothered to Stay on Hotels' 13th Floor: Most who are bothered would ask for a room on a different floor. *Gallup Poll Briefing*, 5–8. https://search.ebscohost.com/login.aspx?direct=true&AuthType=shib&db=bsu&AN=25077377&site=ehost-live&scope=site&custid=s5672194

Caspi, A., Shmuel, E., & Chajut, E. (2024). A quantitative examination of half-belief in superstition. *Journal of Individual Differences, 45*(1), 16–31. https://doi.org/10.1027/1614-0001/a000401

CDC. (2007). *Crisis and emergency risk communication: Pandemic influenza.* Author.

Christianson, J. P., Fernando, A. B. P., Kazama, A. M., Jovanovic, T., Ostroff, L. E., & Sangha, S. (2012). Inhibition of fear by learned safety signals: A mini-symposium review. *Journal of Neuroscience, 32*(41), 14118–14124. https://doi.org/10.1523/JNEUROSCI.3340-12.2012

Connolly, S. J. (1983). The "Blessed Turf": Cholera and popular panic in Ireland, June 1832. *Irish Historical Studies, 23*(91), 214–232. https://doi.org/10.1017/S0021121400017648

Dauverd, C. (2020). *Church and state in Spanish Italy: Rituals and legitimacy in the Kingdom of Naples.* Cambridge University Press. https://doi.org/10.1017/9781108779555

Eccles, R. (2020). The powerful placebo effect in cough: Relevance to treatment and clinical trials. *Lung, 198*(1), 13–21. https://doi.org/10.1007/s00408-019-00305-5

Eckblad, M., & Chapman, L. J. (1983). Magical ideation as an indicator of schizotypy. *Journal of Consulting and Clinical Psychology, 51*(2), 215–225. https://doi.org/10.1037//0022-006x.51.2.215

Fraser, J. G. (1894). *The golden bough: A study of comparative religion.* Macmillan.

Gorvins. (2016). *People fear making a will tempts fate.* https://www.gorvins.com/news-media/allnews/people-fear-making-will-tempts-fate/

Henry, B. (2020). *"It's extremely lonely": Recovered from COVID-19, but shunned socially. Texas Public Radio.* https://www.tpr.org/bioscience-medicine/2020-06-30/its-extremely-lonely-recovered-from-covid-19-but-shunned-socially

Hoffmann, A., Plotkina, D., Roger, P., & D'Hondt, C. (2022). Superstitious beliefs, locus of control, and feeling at risk in the face of Covid-19. *Personality and Individual Differences, 196*, article 111718. https://doi.org/10.1016/j.paid.2022.111718

Huang, L.-S., & Teng, C.-I. (2009). Development of a Chinese superstitious belief scale. *Psychological Reports, 104*(3), 807–819. https://doi.org/10.2466/pr0.104.3.807-819

Ichino, A. (2022). Vaccine hesitancy and the reluctance to "tempt fate." *Philosophical Psychology, 36*(6), 1080–1101. https://doi.org/10.1080/09515089.2022.2096432

James, A., & Wells, A. (2002). Death beliefs, superstitious beliefs and health anxiety. *British Journal of Clinical Psychology, 41*(1), 43–53. https://doi.org/10.1348/014466502163787

Jones, C. P. (2016). An amulet from London and events surrounding the Antonine Plague. *Journal of Roman Archaeology, 29*(1), 469–472. https://doi.org/10.1017/S1047759400072251

Karcher, N. R., Slutske, W. S., Kerns, J. G., Piasecki, T. M., & Martin, N. G. (2014). Sex differences in magical ideation: A community-based twin study. *Personality Disorders: Theory, Research, and Treatment, 5*(2), 212–219. https://doi.org/10.1037/per0000040

Keinan, G. (2003). Magical thinking as a way of coping with stress. In R. Jacoby & G. Keinan (Eds.), *Between stress and hope: From a disease-centered to a health-centered perspective* (pp. 123–138). Praeger.

Levy, M. (2020). *When life gets us down, Jewish gallows humor can bring us a laugh.* https://reformjudaism.org/blog/when-life-gets-us-down-jewish-gallows-humor-can-bring-us-laugh

Life Magazine. (1908, October 3). The cholera scare in St. Petersburg: Combating the epidemic with amulets and hot tea. *Life Magazine, 78*, 1.

Lobato, E. J. C., & Zimmerman, C. (2018). The psychology of (pseudo)science: Cognitive, social, and cultural factors. In A. B. Kaufman & J. C. Kaufman (Eds.), *Pseudoscience: The conspiracy against science.* (pp. 21–43). MIT Press. https://doi.org/10.7551/mitpress/9780262037426.003.0002

Mackenzie, M. (2022). *Meghan McCain says COVID-19 impacted her mental health. Self.* https://www.self.com/story/meghan-mccain-covid

Malinowski, B. (1955). *Magic, science, and religion*. Doubleday.

Markle, D. T. (2010). The magic that binds us: Magical thinking and inclusive fitness. *Journal of Social, Evolutionary, and Cultural Psychology, 4*(1), 18–33. https://doi.org/10.1037/h0099304

Mobilia Gallery. (2021). *Talisman & amulets: Protective jewelry in the age of COVID*. https://www.mobilia-gallery.com/exhibits/talisman-amulets-protective-jewelry-in-the-age-of-covid/

Nemeroff, C., & Rozin, P. (2000). The makings of the magical mind: The nature and function of sympathetic magical thinking. In K. S. Rosengren, C. N. Johnson, & P. L. Harris (Eds.), *Imagining the impossible: Magical, scientific, and religious thinking in children* (pp. 1–34). Cambridge University Press. https://doi.org/10.1017/CBO9780511571381.002

Nguyen, H. (2018). *Nearly a quarter of Americans carry a lucky charm*. https://today.yougov.com/society/articles/21156-nearly-quarter-americans-carry-lucky-charm?redirect_from=%2Ftopics%2Flifestyle%2Farticles-reports%2F2018%2F07%2F11%2Fnearly-quarter-americans-carry-lucky-charm

Nickell, J. (2009). Science and the "miraculous blood." *Center for Inquiry*. https://centerforinquiry.org/blog/science_and_the_miraculous_blood/

Nohl, J. (1926). *The Black Death: A chronical of the plague*. Allen & Unwin.

Nursing Standard. (2004). SARS nurses shunned after recovery. *Nursing Standard, 18*, 4. https://doi.org/10.7748/ns.18.51.4.s4

O'Neil, S. (2020). Coronavirus is killing Lopez Obrador's big plans for Mexico. *Council on Foreign Relations*. https://www.cfr.org/blog/coronavirus-killing-lopez-obradors-big-plans-mexico

Orth, T. (2022). *Which superstitions are Americans most likely to believe?* https://today.yougov.com/society/articles/42425-which-superstitions-are-americans-most-likely-beli

Pearse, R. (2017). *John of Ephesus describes the Justinianic plague*. https://www.roger-pearse.com/weblog/2017/05/10/john-of-ephesus-describes-the-justinianic-plague/

Perry, M. (2014). You think Ebola's bad? Try the Black Death. *Politico*. https://www.politico.com/magazine/story/2014/11/you-think-ebolas-bad-try-the-black-death-112985/

Phiri, P. (2016). As Cholera outbreak surges in Zambia, survivors suffer from widespread myths. *Global Press Journal*. https://globalpressjournal.com/africa/zambia/cholera-outbreak-surges-zambia-survivors-suffer-widespread-myths/

Piskorz, J. (2021). *How the pandemic turned me into a superstitious person*. Refinery29. https://www.refinery29.com/en-gb/superstition-control-mental-health.

Reiner, E. (1960). Plague amulets and house blessings. *Journal of Near Eastern Studies, 19*(2), 148–155.

Reuters. (2020). Blood of Naples saint fails to liquefy in what some see as bad omen. *Reuters*. https://www.reuters.com/article/us-health-coronavirus-italy-san-gennaro-idUSKBN28Q2UY

Risen, J. L. (2016). Believing what we do not believe: Acquiescence to superstitious beliefs and other powerful intuitions. *Psychological Review, 123*(2), 182–207. https://doi.org/10.1037/rev0000017

Risen, J. L., & Gilovich, T. (2008). Why people are reluctant to tempt fate. *Journal of Personality and Social Psychology, 95*(2), 293–307. https://doi.org/10.1037/0022-3514.95.2.293

Roger, P., D'Hondt, C., Plotkina, D., & Hoffmann, A. (2023). Number 19: Another victim of the COVID-19 pandemic? *Journal of Gambling Studies, 39*(3), 1417–1450. https://doi.org/10.1007/s10899-022-10145-3

Rosengren, K. S., & French, J. A. (2013). Magical thinking. In M. Taylor (Ed.), *The Oxford handbook of the development of imagination* (pp. 42–60). Oxford University Press.

Rozin, P., Markwith, M., & Nemeroff, C. (1992). Magical contagion beliefs and fear of AIDS. *Journal of Applied Social Psychology, 22*(14), 1081–1092. https://doi.org/10.1111/j.1559-1816.1992.tb00943.x

Rozin, P., & Nemeroff, C. (2002). Sympathetic magical thinking: The contagion and similarity "heuristics." In T. Gilovich, D. Griffin, & D. Kahneman (Eds.), *Heuristics and biases: The psychology of intuitive judgment* (pp. 201–216). Cambridge University Press.

Rudski, J. M. (2004). The illusion of control, superstitious belief, and optimism. *Current Psychology, 22*(4), 306–315. https://doi.org/10.1007/s12144-004-1036-8

Rudski, J. M., & Edwards, A. (2007). Malinowski goes to college: Factors influencing students' use of ritual and superstition. *Journal of General Psychology, 134*(4), 389–403. https://doi.org/10.3200/GENP.134.4.389-404

Sherman, C. (2021). Mexico's president says he's tested positive for COVID-19. *Associated Press*. https://apnews.com/article/pandemics-marcelo-ebrard-mexico-coronavirus-pandemic-vladimir-putin-7cf4feae9e363d519d5c336202be0ae6

Slack, P. (1985). *The impact of plague in Tudor and Stuart England*. Routledge.

South China Morning Post. (2021). Thai taxi drivers turn to holy amulets to protect them from coronavirus. *South China Morning Post*. https://www.scmp.com/news/asia/southeast-asia/article/3133596/thai-taxi-drivers-turns-holy-amulets-protect-them

Subbotsky, E. (2007). Children's and adults' reactions to magical and ordinary suggestion: Are suggestibility and magical thinking psychologically close relatives? *British Journal of Psychology, 98*(4), 547–574. https://doi.org/10.1348/000712606X166069

Tanakasempipat, P. (2022). COVID to crypto-amulets: Young Thais seek fortune-telling ugrades. *Reuters*. https://www.reuters.com/world/asia-pacific/covid-crypto-amulets-young-thais-seek-fortune-telling-upgrades-2022-04-15/

Taylor, S., & Asmundson, G. J. G. (2004). *Treating health anxiety*. Guilford.

Thomason, S. (2022). Learn the history of amulets and create your own. *University of Alabama at Birmingham News*. https://www.uab.edu/news/arts/item/12569-learn-the-history-of-amulets-and-create-your-own-jan-24

Thucydides. (411 BC). *The history of the Peloponnesian War* (R. Crawley, Trans., 2009). Project Gutenberg. www.gutenberg.org

van Wolferen, J., Inbar, Y., & Zeelenberg, M. (2013). Magical thinking in predictions of negative events: Evidence for tempting fate but not for a protection effect. *Judgment and Decision Making, 8*(1), 45–54.

Vyse, S. (2019). *Superstition: A very short introduction*. Oxford University Press.

Wolff, J. (1692). *Curiosus amuletorum scrutator*. Groschuffius.

Wong, S. H. (2012). Does superstition help? A study of the role of superstitions and death beliefs on death anxiety amongst Chinese undergraduates in Hong Kong. *Omega: Journal of Death & Dying, 65*(1), 55–70. https://doi.org/10.2190/OM.65.1.d

Chapter 17

Alloy, L. B., Burke, T. A., O'Garro-Moore, J., & Abramson, L. Y. (2018). Cognitive vulnerability to depression and bipolar disorder. In R. L. Leahy (Ed.), *Science and practice in cognitive therapy: Foundations, mechanisms, and applications.* (pp. 105–123). Guilford.

Alloy, L. B., & Clements, C. M. (1992). Illusion of control: Invulnerability to negative affect and depressive symptoms after laboratory and natural stressors. *Journal of Abnormal Psychology, 101*(2), 234–245. https://doi.org/10.1037/0021-843X.101.2.234

Ang, A. (2003). Chinese turning to occult to fight SARS. *Associated Press*. https://www.theintelligencer.com/news/article/Chinese-Turning-to-Occult-to-Fight-SARS-10576743.php

Aranguren, M. (2022). Face mask use conditionally decreases compliance with physical distancing rules against COVID-19: Gender differences in risk compensation pattern. *Annals of Behavioral Medicine*, 56(4), 332–346. https://doi.org/10.1093/abm/kaab072

Aranguren, M., Cartaud, A., Cissé, I., & Coello, Y. (2023). People interact closer when a face mask is worn but risk compensation is at best partial. *European Journal of Public Health*, 33(6), 1177–1182. https://doi.org/10.1093/eurpub/ckad161

Bardon, A. (2019). *The truth about denial: Bias and self-deception in science, politics, and religion*. Oxford University Press. https://doi.org/10.1093/oso/9780190062262.003.0001

Barlow, D. H. (2004). *Anxiety and its disorders (2nd ed.)*. Guilford.

Baumeister, R. F., Dale, K., & Sommer, K. L. (1998). Freudian defense mechanisms and empirical findings in modern social psychology: Reaction formation, projection, displacement, undoing, isolation, sublimation, and denial. *Journal of Personality*, 66(6), 1081–1124. https://doi.org/10.1111/1467-6494.00043

Benedetti, F. (2021). *Placebo effects: Understanding the other side of medical care* (3rd ed.). Oxford University Press.

Bogdan, R., Pringle, P. L., Goetz, E. L., & Pizzagalli, D. A. (2012). Perceived stress, anhedonia and illusion of control: Evidence for two mediational models. *Cognitive Therapy and Research*, 36(6), 827–832. https://doi.org/10.1007/s10608-011-9413-8

Carrigan, J. A. (1959). Yellow fever in New Orleans, 1853: Abstractions and realities. *Journal of Southern History*, 25(3), 339–355. https://doi.org/10.2307/2954767

Chan, D. C. N., Wu, A. M. S., & Hung, E. P. W. (2010). Invulnerability and the intention to drink and drive: An application of the theory of planned behavior. *Accident Analysis and Prevention*, 42, 1549–1555. https://doi.org/10.1016/j.aap.2010.03.011

Chapin, C. V. (1906). The fetich [sic] of disinfection. *JAMA*, 47(8), 574–580. https://doi.org/10.1001/jama.1906.25210080026002f

Choi, C. (2020). Groceries need wipe down? *South Florida Times*, 30(50), 1B–2B.

Clapp, T. (1857). *Autobiographical sketches and recollections, during a thirty-five years residence in New Orleans*. Phillips, Sampson & Co.

Cramer, P. (2015). Defense mechanisms: 40 years of empirical research. *Journal of Personality Assessment*, 97(2), 114–122. https://doi.org/10.1080/00223891.2014.947997

D'Irsay, S. (1927). Defense reactions during the Black Death, 1348-1349. *Annals of Medical History*, 9, 169–179.

de Vries, L. P., van de Weijer, M. P., Pelt, D. H. M., Ligthart, L., Willemsen, G., Boomsma, D. I., et al. (2022). Gene-by-crisis interaction for optimism and meaning in life: The effects of the covid-19 pandemic. *Behavior Genetics*, 52(1), 13–25. https://doi.org/10.1007/s10519-021-10081-9

Desrichard, O., Moussaoui, L., & Ofosu, N. (2022). Reduction of precautionary behaviour following vaccination against COVID-19: A test on a British cohort. *Vaccines*, 10(6), article 936. https://doi.org/10.3390/vaccines10060936

Fiedler, K. (2017). Illusory correlation. In R. F. Pohl (Ed.), *Cognitive illusions: Intriguing phenomena in thinking, judgment and memory* (2nd ed.) (pp. 115–133). Routledge.

Freud, A. (1966). *The ego and the mechanisms of defence*. Routledge.

Gallaher, T. J., Pollock, A. M., & Draine, W. (1855). Report made to the Medical Society of Alleghany County, Pa., on the epidemic cholera which prevailed in Pittsburgh during the months of September and October, 1854. *American Journal of Medical Sciences*, 58, 334–352.

Gerrard, M., & Warner, T. D. (1994). Comparison of Marine and college women's HIV/AIDS-relevant sexual behaviors. *Journal of Applied Social Psychology, 24*(11), 959–980. https://doi.org/10.1111/j.1559-1816.1994.tb02368.x

Goldman, E. (2020). Exaggerated risk of transmission of COVID-19 by fomites. *Lancet Infectious Disease, 20*, 892–893. https://doi.org/10.1016/S1473-3099(20)30561-2

Guenther, B., Galizzi, M. M., & Sanders, J. G. (2021). Heterogeneity in risk-taking during the COVID-19 pandemic: Evidence from the UK lockdown. *Frontiers in Psychology, 12*, article 643653. https://doi.org/10.3389/fpsyg.2021.643653

Hall, P. A., Meng, G., Sakib, M. N., Quah, A. C. K., Agar, T., & Fong, G. T. (2023). Do the vaccinated perform less distancing, mask wearing and hand hygiene? A test of the risk compensation hypothesis in a representative sample during the COVID-19 pandemic. *Vaccine, 41*(27), 4027–4030. https://doi.org/10.1016/j.vaccine.2022.10.028

Hamilton, D. L., & Lickel, B. (2000). Illusory correlation. In A. E. Kazdin (Ed.), *Encyclopedia of psychology* (Vol. 4., pp. 226–227). Oxford University Press. https://doi.org/10.1037/10519-098

Harper's Weekly. (1865). Cholera at Marseilles—fires lighted in the square of the old palace of justice to destroy the pestilence. *Harper's Weekly, 9*(464), 724.

Harvey, R. (1892). A brief sketch of the epidemic of cholera in Srinagar, Kashmir, May-June, 1892. *British Medical Journal, 2*(1650), 345–347. http://www.jstor.org/stable/20177558

Haug, N., Geyrhofer, L., Londei, A., Dervic, E., Desvars-Larrive, A., Loreto, V., et al. (2020). Ranking the effectiveness of worldwide COVID-19 government interventions. *Nature Human Behaviour, 4*(12), 1303–1312. https://doi.org/10.1038/s41562-020-01009-0

Hill, P. L., Duggan, P. M., & Lapsley, D. K. (2012). Subjective invulnerability, risk behavior, and adjustment in early adolescence. *Journal of Early Adolescence, 32*, 489–501. https://doi.org/10.1177/0272431611400304

Hoye, B. (2021). Death bed denials, pandemic "hoax" accusations common in southern Manitoba hospital patients, doctor says. *CBC News.* https://www.cbc.ca/news/canada/manitoba/winkler-doctor-hospital-vaccine-hesitancy-1.6044904

Jefferson, A., Bortolotti, L., & Kuzmanovic, B. (2017). What is unrealistic optimism? *Consciousness and Cognition, 50*, 3–11. https://doi.org/10.1016/j.concog.2016.10.005

Ji, L.-J., Zhang, Z., Usborne, E., & Guan, Y. (2004). Optimism across cultures: In response to the Severe Acute Respiratory Syndrome outbreak. *Asian Journal of Social Psychology, 7*, 25–34. https://doi.org/10.1111/j.1467-839X.2004.00132.x

Jørgensen, F., Lindholt, M. F., Bor, A., & Petersen, M. B. (2021). Does face mask use elicit risk-compensation? Quasi-experimental evidence from Denmark during the SARS-COV-2 pandemic. *European Journal of Public Health, 31*(6), 1259–1265. https://doi.org/10.1093/eurpub/ckab136

Kalichman, S. C. (2018). "HIV does not cause AIDS": A journey into AIDS denialism. In A. B. Kaufman & J. C. Kaufman (Eds.), *Pseudoscience: The conspiracy against science* (pp. 420–440). MIT Press. https://doi.org/10.7551/mitpress/9780262037426.003.0019

Kaspar, K. (2013). Washing one's hands after failure enhances optimism but hampers future performance. *Social Psychological and Personality Science, 4*(1), 69–73. https://doi.org/10.1177/1948550612443267

Kell, K. T. (1965). Tobacco in folk cures in Western society. *Journal of American Folklore, 78*(308), 99–114. https://doi.org/10.2307/538277

Khan, M., & Grisham, J. R. (2018). Wiping your conscience clean: Investigating the Macbeth effect in individuals with high obsessive-compulsive contamination concerns. *Journal of Experimental Psychopathology, 9*(3). https://doi.org/10.1177/2043808718786595

Kihlstrom, J. F. (1987). The cognitive unconscious. *Science, 237*(4821), 1445–1452. https://doi.org/10.1126/science.3629249

Kim, H. K., & Niederdeppe, J. (2013). Exploring optimistic bias and the integrative model of behavioral prediction in the context of a campus influenza outbreak. *Journal of Health Communication, 18*, 206–222. https://doi.org/10.1080/10810730.2012.688247

Kiyingi, M., Nankabirwa, J. I., Sekaggya-Wiltshire, C., Nangendo, J., Kiweewa, J. M., Katahoire, A. R., et al. (2023). Predictors of delayed anti-retroviral therapy initiation among adults referred for HIV treatment in Uganda: A cross-sectional study. *BMC Health Services Research, 23*(1), article 40. https://doi.org/10.1186/s12913-023-09052-z

Kleiman, E. M., Chiara, A. M., Liu, R. T., Jager-Hyman, S. G., Choi, J. Y., & Alloy, L. B. (2017). Optimism and well-being: A prospective multi-method and multi-dimensional examination of optimism as a resilience factor following the occurrence of stressful life events. *Cognition and Emotion, 31*, 269–283. https://doi.org/10.1080/02699931.2015.1108284

Koelle, K., Martin, M. A., Antia, R., Lopman, B., & Dean, N. E. (2022). The changing epidemiology of SARS-CoV-2. *Science, 375*(6585), 1116–1121. https://doi.org/10.1126/science.abm4915

Langer, E. J. (1975). The illusion of control. *Journal of Personality and Social Psychology, 32*, 311–328. https://doi.org/10.1037/0022-3514.32.2.311

Lee, S. W. S., Chen, K., Ma, C., & Hoang, J. (2024). Wipe it off: A meta-analytic review of the psychological consequences and antecedents of physical cleansing. *Psychological Bulletin, 150*(4), 355–398. https://doi.org/10.1037/bul0000421

Leotti, L. A., Iyengar, S. S., & Ochsner, K. N. (2010). Born to choose: The origins and value of the need for control. *Trends in Cognitive Sciences, 14*(10), 457–463. https://doi.org/10.1016/j.tics.2010.08.001

Lewis, D. (2021). COVID-19 rarely spreads through surfaces. *Nature*. https://www.nature.com/articles/d41586-021-00251-4

Liebst, L. S., Ejbye-Ernst, P., de Bruin, M., Thomas, J., & Lindegaard, M. R. (2022). No evidence that mask-wearing in public places elicits risk compensation behavior during the COVID-19 pandemic. *Scientific Reports, 12*(1), 1511. https://doi.org/10.1038/s41598-022-05270-3

Luckman, A., Zeitoun, H., Isoni, A., Loomes, G., Vlaev, I., Powdthavee, N., et al. (2021). Risk compensation during COVID-19: The impact of face mask usage on social distancing. *Journal of Experimental Psychology: Applied, 27*(4), 722–738. https://doi.org/10.1037/xap0000382

Makridakis, S., & Moleskis, A. (2015). The costs and benefits of positive illusions. *Frontiers in Psychology, 6*, article 859. https://doi.org/10.3389/fpsyg.2015.00859

Mantzari, E., Rubin, G. J., & Marteau, T. M. (2020). Is risk compensation threatening public health in the COVID-19 pandemic? *BMJ, 370*, article m2913. https://doi.org/10.1136/bmj.m2913

McColl, K., Martin-Lapoirie, D., Veltri, G. A., Arwidson, P., & Raude, J. (2024). Does vaccination elicit risk compensation? Insights from the COVID-19 pandemic in France. *Health Psychology and Behavioral Medicine, 12*(1), article 2287663. https://doi.org/10.1080/21642850.2023.2287663

Meissner, K., & Linde, K. (2018). Are blue pills better than green? How treatment features modulate placebo effects. *International Review of Neurobiology, 139*, 357–378. https://doi.org/10.1016/bs.irn.2018.07.014

Millest, A., Saeed, S., Symons, C., & Carter, H. (2024). Effect of face-covering use on adherence to other COVID-19 protective behaviours: A systematic review. *PLOS ONE, 19*(4), article e0284629. https://doi.org/10.1371/journal.pone.0284629

Miranda, G. (2021, September 25). "I don't have COVID": Doctor says some COVID patients deny virus, decry vaccines from their deathbed. *USA Today*. Retr https://www.usatoday.com/story/news/nation/2021/09/25/dr-matthew-trunsky-says-some-dying-covid-patients-deny-virus/5866695001/

Morrell, H. E. R., Lapsley, D. K., & Halpern-Felsher, B. L. (2016). Subjective invulnerability and perceptions of tobacco-related benefits predict adolescent smoking behavior. *Journal of Early Adolescence, 36*, 679–703. https://doi.org/10.1177/0272431615578274

Nickerson, R. S. (1998). Confirmation bias: A ubiquitous phenomenon in many guises. *Review of General Psychology, 2*(2), 175–220. https://doi.org/10.1037/1089-2680.2.2.175

O Murchu, E., Marshall, L., Teljeur, C., Harrington, P., Hayes, C., Moran, P., et al. (2022). Oral pre-exposure prophylaxis (PrEP) to prevent HIV: A systematic review and meta-analysis of clinical effectiveness, safety, adherence and risk compensation in all populations. *BMJ Open, 12*(5), article e048478. https://doi.org/10.1136/bmjopen-2020-048478

Patierno, C., Fava, G. A., & Carrozzino, D. (2023). Illness denial in medical disorders: A systematic review. *Psychotherapy & Psychosomatics, 92*(4), 211–226. https://doi.org/10.1159/000531260

Perloff, L. S., & Fetzer, B. K. (1986). Self-other judgments and perceived vulnerability to victimization. *Journal of Personality and Social Psychology, 50*, 502–510. https://doi.org/10.1037/0022-3514.50.3.502

Ravert, R. D., Schwartz, S. J., Zamboanga, B. L., Kim, S. Y., Weisskirch, R. S., & Bersamin, M. (2009). Sensation seeking and danger invulnerability: Paths to college student risk-taking. *Personality and Individual Differences, 47*, 763–768. https://doi.org/10.1016/j.paid.2009.06.017

Rocky Mountain News. (1918, November 23). Influenza germs hates smoke city bacteriologist declares. *Rocky Mountain News*, 6. http://hdl.handle.net/2027/spo.8980flu.0003.898

Rodin, J. (1986). Aging and health: Effects of the sense of control. *Science, 233*, 1271–1276. https://doi.org/10.1126/science.3749877

Salcedo, A. (2021, September 24). Doctor who has lost more than 100 patients to COVID says some deny virus from their death beds: "I don't believe you." *Seattle Times*. https://www.seattletimes.com/nation-world/doctor-who-has-lost-more-than-100-patients-to-covid-says-some-deny-virus-from-their-death-beds-i-dont-believe-you/

Seres, G., Balleyer, A., Cerutti, N., Friedrichsen, J., & Süer, M. (2021). Face mask use and physical distancing before and after mandatory masking: No evidence on risk compensation in public waiting lines. *Journal of Economic Behavior & Organization, 192*, 765–781. https://doi.org/10.1016/j.jebo.2021.10.032

Sharot, T., Korn, C. W., & Dolan, R. J. (2011). How unrealistic optimism is maintained in the face of reality. *Nature Neuroscience, 14*, 1475–1479. https://doi.org/10.1038/nn.2949

Shiloh, S., Peleg, S., & Nudelman, G. (2023). Core self-evaluations as resilience and risk factors of psychological distress during the COVID-19 pandemic. *Psychology, Health & Medicine, 28*(1), 95–109. https://doi.org/10.1080/13548506.2022.2030480

Shukla, S., Mishra, S. K., & Rai, H. (2021). Optimistic bias, risky behavior, and social norms among Indian college students during COVID-19. *Personality and Individual Differences, 183*, article 111076. https://doi.org/10.1016/j.paid.2021.111076

Simões, R. A. G., Benvenuti, M. F. L., Rodrigues, A., Coutinho, S. P., Muñoz, M. Á., & Bizarro, L. (2020). Persistence of repeated self-reported illusion of control as a product of action and outcome association in productive and preventive scenarios. *Psychological Research, 84*(5), 1184–1197. https://doi.org/10.1007/s00426-019-01147-9

Smith, M. D. (2016). The specter of cholera in nineteenth-century Cincinnati. *Ohio Valley History, 16*(2), 21–40.

Staiano, J. (2008). The impact of plague on human behavior in seventeenth century Europe. *ESSAI, 6*(1), article 46, https://dc.cod.edu/essai/vol46/iss41/46/.

Sun, L., Chen, L., Chen, W., Zhang, M., Yang, M., Mo, L., et al. (2022). Association between health behaviours and the COVID-19 vaccination: Risk compensation among healthcare workers in Taizhou, China. *Human Vaccines & Immunotherapeutics, 18*(1), article 2029257. https://doi.org/10.1080/21645515.2022.2029257

Taha, S., Matheson, K., & Anisman, H. (2013). The 2009 H1N1 influenza pandemic: The role of threat, coping, and media trust on vaccination intentions in Canada. *Journal of Health Communication, 18*, 278–290. https://doi.org/10.1080/10810730.2012.727960

Taylor, S., Fong, A., & Asmundson, G. J. G. (2021). Predicting the severity of symptoms of the COVID stress syndrome from personality traits: A prospective network analysis. *Frontiers in Psychology, 12*, article 632227. https://doi.org/10.3389/fpsyg.2021.632227

Taylor, S. E. (2011). Positive illusions: How ordinary people become extaordinary. In M. Gernsbacher, R. W. Pew, L. M. Hough, & J. R. Pomerantz (Eds.), *Psychology and the real world: Essays illustrating fundamental contributions to society* (pp. 224–228). Worth.

Taylor, S. E., & Brown, J. D. (1988). Illusion and well-being: A social psychological perspective on mental health. *Psychological Bulletin, 103*, 193–210. https://doi.org/10.1037/0033-2909.103.2.193

Taylor, S. E., & Brown, J. D. (1994). Positive illusions and well-being revisited: Separating fact from fiction. *Psychological Bulletin, 116*, 21–27. https://doi.org/10.1037/0033-2909.116.1.21

Thompson, D. (2020). Hygiene theater is a huge waste of time. *The Atlantic.* https://www.theatlantic.com/ideas/archive/2020/07/scourge-hygiene-theater/614599/

Thompson, S. C. (2017). Illusions of control. In R. F. Pohl (Ed.), *Cognitive illusions: Intriguing phenomena in thinking, judgment and memory* (2nd ed.) (pp. 134–149). Routledge.

Thorpe, A., Fagerlin, A., Drews, F. A., Shoemaker, H., & Scherer, L. D. (2022). Self-reported health behaviors and risk perceptions following the COVID-19 vaccination rollout in the USA: An online survey study. *Public Health, 208*, 68–71. https://doi.org/10.1016/j.puhe.2022.05.007

Tomes, N. (1997). Moralizing the microbe: The germ theory and the moral construction of behavior in the late-nineteenth-century antituberculosis movement. In A. M. Brandt & P. Rozin (Eds.), *Morality and health* (pp. 271–294). Taylor & Frances/Routledge.

Tomes, N. (1999). *The gospel of germs: Men, women, and the microbe in American life.* Harvard University Press.

Villegas, P. (2020, November 16). South Dakota nurse says many patients deny the coronavirus exists—right up until death. *Washington Post.* https://www.washingtonpost.com/health/2020/11/16/south-dakota-nurse-coronavirus-deniers/?utm_campaign=wp_post_most&utm_medium=email&utm_source=newsletter&wpisrc=nl_most&carta-url=https%3A%2F%2Fs2.washingtonpost.com%2Fcar-ln-tr%2F2ccba14%2F5fb401589d2fda0efb6af332%2F5ead92119bbc0f3a78cf15ed%2F11%2F72%2F82c0c70595648b78a5f6dbe6bcb26515

Wadud, Z., Rahman, S. M., & Enam, A. (2022). Face mask mandates and risk compensation: An analysis of mobility data during the COVID-19 pandemic in Bangladesh. *BMJ Global Health, 7*(1), article e006803. https://doi.org/10.1136/bmjgh-2021-006803

Wallerstein, R. S. (1967). Development and metapsychology of the defense organization of the ego. *Journal of the American Psychoanalytic Association, 15*, 130–149.

Wear, A. (2015). Making us as cruel as dogs: Plague in 16th and 17th century England. *Lancet, 385*(9986), 2456–2457. https://doi.org/10.1016/S0140-6736(15)61129-1

Weinstein, N. D. (1980). Unrealistic optimism about future life events. *Journal of Personality and Social Psychology, 39*, 806–820. https://doi.org/10.1037/0022-3514.39.5.806

Wootton, R. E., Davis, O. S. P., Mottershaw, A. L., Wang, R. A. H., & Haworth, C. M. A. (2017). Genetic and environmental correlations between subjective wellbeing and experience of life events in adolescence. *European Child & Adolescent Psychiatry, 26*(9), 1119–1127. https://doi.org/10.1007/s00787-017-0997-8

Xu, A. J., Schwarz, N., & Zwick, R. (2012). Washing away your (good or bad) Luck: Physical cleansing affects risk-taking behavior. *Journal of Experimental Psychology: General, 141*(1), 26–30. https://doi.org/10.1037/a0023997

Yan, Y., Bayham, J., Richter, A., & Fenichel, E. P. (2021). Risk compensation and face mask mandates during the COVID-19 pandemic. *Scientific Reports, 11*(1), article 3174. https://doi.org/10.1038/s41598-021-82574-w

Yang, M.-G., Wang, L.-J., Xu, L.-Y., Ke, M., & Sun, L.-X. (2023). Health behaviours among travellers regarding risk compensation following COVID-19 vaccination in Taizhou, China. *Canadian Journal of Infectious Diseases & Medical Microbiology, 2023*, article 1329291. https://doi.org/10.1155/2023/1329291

Zhong, C.-B., & Liljenquist, K. (2006). Washing away your sins: Threatened morality and physical cleansing. *Science, 313*(5792), 1451–1452. https://doi.org/10.1126/science.1130726

Zweig, D. (2020, November 19). Are COVID patients gasping "It isn't real" as they die? *Wired.* https://www.wired.com/story/are-covid-patients-gasping-it-isnt-real-as-they-die/

Chapter 18

Acar-Burkay, S., Fennis, B. M., & Warlop, L. (2014). Trusting others: The polarization effect of need for closure. *Journal of Personality and Social Psychology, 107*(4), 719–735. https://doi.org/10.1037/a0037022

Altemeyer, B. (1996). *The authoritarian specter.* Harvard University Press.

Altemeyer, B. (2009). *The authoritarians.* Cherry Hill Publishing.

Arnáez, S., García Soriano, G., López Santiago, J., & Belloch, A. (2021). Illness related intrusive thoughts and illness anxiety disorder. *Psychology and Psychotherapy: Theory, Research and Practice, 94*(1), 63–80. https://doi.org/10.1111/papt.12267

Asmundson, G. J. G., Taylor, S., & Cox, B. J. (2001). *Health anxiety.* Wiley.

Azarpanah, H., Farhadloo, M., Vahidov, R., & Pilote, L. (2021). Vaccine hesitancy: Evidence from an adverse events following immunization database, and the role of cognitive biases. *BMC Public Health, 21*(1), article 1686. https://doi.org/10.1186/s12889-021-11745-1

Baker, M. N., & Merkley, E. (2023). Dynamic role of personality in explaining COVID-19 vaccine hesitancy and refusal. *Frontiers in Psychology, 14*, article 1163570. https://doi.org/10.3389/fpsyg.2023.1163570

Baldner, C., Jaume, L. C., Pierro, A., & Kruglanski, A. W. (2019). The epistemic bases of prejudice: The role of need for cognitive closure. *Testing, Psychometrics, Methodology in Applied Psychology, 26*(3), 447–461. https://doi.org/10.4473/TPM26.3.9

Ball, H., & Wozniak, T. R. (2022). Why do some Americans resist COVID-19 prevention behavior? An analysis of issue importance, message fatigue, and reactance regarding COVID-19 messaging. *Health Communication, 37*(14), 1812–1819. https://doi.org/10.1080/10410236.2021.1920717

Barlow, D. H., Farchione, T. J., Sauer-Zavala, S., Latin, H. M., Ellard, K. K., Bullis, J. R., et al. (2017). *Unified protocol for transdiagnostic treatment of emotional disorders* (2nd ed.). Guilford.

Bartone, P. T., McDonald, K., Hansma, B. J., & Solomon, J. (2022). Hardiness moderates the effects of COVID-19 stress on anxiety and depression. *Journal of Affective Disorders, 317*, 236–244. https://doi.org/10.1016/j.jad.2022.08.045

Bench, S. W., & Lench, H. C. (2019). Boredom as a seeking state: Boredom prompts the pursuit of novel (even negative) experiences. *Emotion, 19*, 242–254. https://doi.org/10.1037/emo0000433

Bilewicz, M., Bulska, D., Winiewski, M., & Fritsche, I. (2023). Obedience to authorities is not unconditional: Differential effects of COVID-19 threat on three facets of RWA in Poland and Germany. *Social & Personality Psychology Compass, 17*(9), article e12800. https://doi.org/10.1111/spc3.12800

Birrell, J., Meares, K., Wilkinson, A., & Freeston, M. (2011). Toward a definition of intolerance of uncertainty: A review of factor analytical studies of the Intolerance of Uncertainty Scale. *Clinical Psychology Review, 31*, 1198–1208. https://doi.org/10.1016/j.cpr.2011.07.009

Bish, A., & Michie, S. (2010). Demographic and attitudinal determinants of protective behaviours during a pandemic: A review. *British Journal of Health Psychology, 15*, 797–824. https://doi.org/10.1348/135910710X485826

Blakey, S. M., & Abramowitz, J. S. (2017). Psychological predictors of health anxiety in response to the Zika virus. *Journal of Clinical Psychology in Medical Settings, 24*, 270–278. https://doi.org/10.1007/s10880-017-9514-y

Blakey, S. M., & Deacon, B. J. (2015). If a safety aid is present, there must be danger: The paradoxical effects of hand sanitizer during a contamination exposure task. *Journal of Experimental Psychopathology, 6*, 264–277. https://doi.org/10.5127/jep.040814

Boelen, P. A., & Carleton, R. N. (2012). Intolerance of uncertainty, hypochondriacal concerns, obsessive-compulsive symptoms, and worry. *Journal of Nervous and Mental Disease, 200*, 208–213. https://doi.org/10.1097/NMD.0b013e318247cb17

Boettcher, H., Sandage, S., Latin, H. M., & Barlow, D. H. (2019). Transdiagnostic treatments for enhancing positive affect and well-being. In J. Gruber (Ed.), *Oxford handbook of positive emotion and psychopathology* (pp. 525–538). Oxford University Press.

Bonanno, G. A., & Diminich, E. D. (2013). Positive adjustment to adversity—Trajectories of minimal-impact resilience and emergent resilience. *Journal of Child Psychology and Psychiatry, 54*, 378–401. https://doi.org/10.1111/jcpp.12021

Booth, R. W., & Sharma, D. (2021). Biased probability estimates in trait anxiety and trait depression are unrelated to biased availability. *Journal of Behavior Therapy and Experimental Psychiatry, 73*, article 101672. https://doi.org/10.1016/j.jbtep.2021.101672

Bottesi, G., Ghisi, M., Sica, C., & Freeston, M. H. (2017). Intolerance of uncertainty, not just right experiences, and compulsive checking: Test of a moderated mediation model on a non-clinical sample. *Comprehensive Psychiatry, 73*, 111–119. https://doi.org/10.1016/j.comppsych.2016.11.014

Boylan, J., Seli, P., Scholer, A. A., & Danckert, J. (2021). Boredom in the COVID-19 pandemic: Trait boredom proneness, the desire to act, and rule-breaking. *Personality and Individual Differences, 171*, article 110387. https://doi.org/10.1016/j.paid.2020.110387

Brandes, C. M., Herzhoff, K., Smack, A. J., & Tackett, J. L. (2019). The p factor and the n factor: Associations between the general factors of psychopathology and neuroticism in children. *Clinical Psychological Science, 7*, 1266–1284. https://doi.org/10.1177/2167702619859332

Brehm, J. W. (1966). *A theory of psychological reactance*. Academic.

Brehm, S. S., & Brehm, J. W. (1981). *Psychological reactance: A theory of freedom and control*. Academic.

Brosch, K., Meller, T., Pfarr, J.-K., Stein, F., Schmitt, S., Ringwald, K., et al. (2022). Which traits predict elevated distress during the Covid-19 pandemic? Results from a large, longitudinal cohort study with psychiatric patients and healthy controls. *Journal of Affective Disorders, 297*, 18–25. https://doi.org/10.1016/j.jad.2021.10.017

Brosowsky, N. P., Van Tilburg, W., Scholer, A. A., Boylan, J., Seli, P., & Danckert, J. (2021). Boredom proneness, political orientation and adherence to social-distancing in the pandemic. *Motivation and Emotion, 45*(5), 631–640. https://doi.org/10.1007/s11031-021-09888-0

Brun, C., Akinyemi, A., Houtin, L., Zerhouni, O., Monvoisin, R., & Pinsault, N. (2022). Intolerance of uncertainty and attitudes towards vaccination impact vaccinal decision while perceived uncertainty does not. *Vaccines, 10*(10), article 1742. https://doi.org/10.3390/vaccines10101742

Campbell, W. K., Bonacci, A. M., Shelton, J., Exline, J. J., & Bushman, B. J. (2004). Psychological entitlement: Interpersonal consequences and validation of a self-report measure. *Journal of Personality Assessment, 83*(1), 29–45, https://doi.org/10.1207/s15327752jpa15328301_15327704.

Cheng, C., & Cheung, M. W. (2005). Psychological responses to outbreak of severe acute respiratory syndrome: A prospective, multiple time-point study. *Journal of Personality, 73*, 261–285. https://doi.org/10.1111/j.1467-6494.2004.00310.x

Cloninger, C. R. (1994). Temperament and personality. *Current Opinion in Neurobiology, 4*, 266–273. https://doi.org/10.1016/0959-4388(94)90083-3

Costa, P. T., & McCrae, R. R. (1987). Neuroticism, somatic complaints, and disease: Is the bark worse than the bite? *Journal of Personality, 55*, 299–316. https://doi.org/10.1111/j.1467-6494.1987.tb00438.x

Costa, P. T., & McCrae, R. R. (2005). *NEO Personality Inventory-3 professional manual*. Psychological Assessment Resources.

Costello, T. H., Bowes, S. M., Stevens, S. T., Waldman, I. D., Tasimi, A., & Lilienfeld, S. O. (2022). Clarifying the structure and nature of left-wing authoritarianism. *Journal of Personality and Social Psychology, 122*(1), 135–170. https://doi.org/10.1037/pspp0000341

Crawford, J. T., Brandt, M. J., Inbar, Y., Chambers, J. R., & Motyl, M. (2017). Social and economic ideologies differentially predict prejudice across the political spectrum, but social issues are most divisive. *Journal of Personality and Social Psychology, 112*, 383–412. https://doi.org/10.1037/pspa0000074

Cukrowicz, K. C., Poindexter, E. K., & Joiner, T. E., Jr. (2011). Cognitive behavioral approaches to the treatment of narcissistic personality disorder. In W. K. Campbell & J. D. Miller (Eds.), *The handbook of narcissism and narcissistic personality disorder: Theoretical approaches, empirical findings, and treatments* (pp. 457–465). Wiley.

De Landsheer, C., & Walburg, V. (2022). Links between rational and irrational beliefs, trait anxiety and fear of COVID-19. *Psychologie Française, 67*(3), 305–316. https://doi.org/10.1016/j.psfr.2022.06.005

Deason, G., & Dunn, K. (2022). Authoritarianism and perceived threat from the novel coronavirus. *International Journal of Psychology, 57*(3), 341–351. https://doi.org/10.1002/ijop.12836

Díaz, R., & Cova, F. (2021). Reactance, morality, and disgust: The relationship between affective dispositions and compliance with official health recommendations during the Covid-19 pandemic. *Cognition and Emotion, 36*(1), 120–136. https://doi.org/10.1080/02699931.2021.1941783

Drody, A. C., Hicks, L. J., & Danckert, J. (2022). Boredom proneness and rule-breaking: A persistent relation one year into the COVID-19 pandemic. *Behavioral Sciences, 12*(8), article 251. https://doi.org/10.3390/bs12080251

Dugas, M. J., & Robichaud, M. (2007). *Cognitive-behavioral treatment for generalized anxiety disorder: From science to practice*. Routledge.

Duplaga, M., & Grysztar, M. (2021). The association between future anxiety, health literacy and the perception of the COVID-19 pandemic: A cross-sectional study. *Healthcare, 9*(1), article 43. https://doi.org/10.3390/healthcare9010043

Epishin, V. E., Salikhova, A. B., Bogacheva, N. V., Bogdanova, M. D., & Kiseleva, M. G. (2020). Mental health and the COVID-19 pandemic: Hardiness and meaningfulness reduce negative effects on psychological well-being. *Psychology in Russia: State of the Art, 13*(4), 75–88. https://doi.org/10.11621/pir.2020.0405

Fan, D., Li, C., Zhu, N., Wang, T., & Kong, F. (2022). Trait resilience and subjective well-being in emerging adulthood: A two-wave longitudinal study. *Current Psychology, 42*, 26200–26206. https://doi.org/10.1007/s12144-022-03727-2

Färber, F., & Rosendahl, J. (2020). Trait resilience and mental health in older adults: A meta-analytic review. *Personality and Mental Health, 14*(4), 361–375. https://doi.org/10.1002/pmh.1490

Farmer, R., & Sundberg, N. D. (1986). Boredom proneness—The development and correlates of a new scale. *Journal of Personality Assessment, 50*, 4–17. https://doi.org/10.1207/s15327752jpa5001_2

Fergus, T. A. (2015). Anxiety sensitivity and intolerance of uncertainty as potential risk factors for cyberchondria: A replication and extension examining dimensions of each construct. *Journal of Affective Disorders, 184*, 305–309. https://doi.org/10.1016/j.jad.2015.06.017

Fergus, T. A., Bardeen, J. R., & Orcutt, H. K. (2015). Examining the specific facets of distress tolerance that are relevant to health anxiety. *Journal of Cognitive Psychotherapy, 29*, 32–44. https://doi.org/10.1891/0889-8391.29.1.32

Ferguson, E. (2000). Hypochondriacal concerns and the five-factor model of personality. *Journal of Personality, 68*, 705–724. https://doi.org/10.1111/1467-6494.00113

Fernández, R. S., Crivelli, L., Guimet, N. M., Allegri, R. F., & Pedreira, M. E. (2020). Psychological distress associated with COVID-19 quarantine: Latent profile analysis, outcome prediction and mediation analysis. *Journal of Affective Disorders, 277*, 75–84. https://doi.org/10.1016/j.jad.2020.07.133

Fournier, J., Wright, A., Tackett, J., Uliaszek, A., Pilkonis, P., Manuck, S., et al. (2019). Decoupling personality and acute psychiatric symptoms in a depressed sample and a community sample. *Clinical Psychological Science, 7*, 566–581. https://doi.org/10.1177/2167702618813989

Fox, C. R., & Tversky, A. (1995). Ambiguity aversion and comparative ignorance. *Quarterly Journal of Economics, 110*(3), 585–603. https://doi.org/10.2307/2946693

Frank, S. J., Jackson-Walker, S., Marks, M., Van Egeren, L. A., Loop, K., & Olson, K. (1998). From the laboratory to the hospital, adults to adolescents, and disorders to personality: The case of psychological reactance. *Journal of Clinical Psychology, 54*, 361–381. https://doi.org/10.1002/(SICI)1097-4679(199804)54:3<361::AID-JCLP6>3.0.CO;2-S

Frost, R. O., & Steketee, G. (2002). *Cognitive approaches to obsessions and compulsions: Theory, assessment, and treatment.* Elsevier.

Gentes, E. L., & Ruscio, A. M. (2011). A meta-analysis of the relation of intolerance of uncertainty to symptoms of generalized anxiety disorder, major depressive disorder, and obsessive–compulsive disorder. *Clinical Psychology Review, 31*, 923–933. https://doi.org/10.1016/j.cpr.2011.05.001

Giancola, M., Palmiero, M., & D'Amico, S. (2023). Dark Triad and Covid-19 vaccine hesitancy: The role of conspiracy beliefs and risk perception. *Current Psychology, 43*, 16808–16820. https://doi.org/10.1007/s12144-023-04609-x

Gillman, A. S., Scharnetzki, L., Boyd, P., Ferrer, R. A., Klein, W. M. P., & Han, P. K. J. (2023). Perceptions and tolerance of uncertainty: Relationship to trust in COVID-19 health information and vaccine hesitancy. *Journal of Behavioral Medicine, 46*(1), 40–53. https://doi.org/10.1007/s10865-022-00302-9

Golec de Zavala, A., Bierwiaczonek, K., Baran, T., Keenan, O., & Hase, A. (2021). The COVID-19 pandemic, authoritarianism, and rejection of sexual dissenters in Poland. *Psychology of Sexual Orientation and Gender Diversity, 8*(2), 250–260. https://doi.org/10.1037/sgd0000446

Götz, F. M., Gvirtz, A., Galinsky, A. D., & Jachimowicz, J. M. (2020). How personality and policy predict pandemic behavior: Understanding sheltering-in-place in 55 countries at the onset of COVID-19. *American Psychologist*, 76(1), 39–49. https://doi.org/10.1037/amp0000740

Green, J. S., & Teachman, B. A. (2013). Predictive validity of explicit and implicit threat overestimation in contamination fear. *Journal of Obsessive-Compulsive and Related Disorders*, 2, 1–8. https://doi.org/10.1016/j.jocrd.2012.09.002

Hartman, T., Stocks, T., McKay, R., Gibson-Miller, J., Levita, L., Martinez, A., et al. (2021). The authoritarian dynamic during the COVID-19 pandemic: Effects on nationalism and anti-immigrant sentiment. *Social Psychological and Personality Science*, 12(7), 1274–1285. https://doi.org/10.1177/1948550620978023

Hatemi, P. K., & Fazekas, Z. (2023). The role of grandiose and vulnerable narcissism on mask wearing and vaccination during the COVID-19 pandemic. *Current Psychology*, 42(22), article 19185. https://doi.org/10.1007/s12144-022-03080-4

Horwood, S., Anglim, J., Bereznicki, H., & Wood, J. K. (2023). Well-being during the coronavirus pandemic: The effect of big five personality and COVID-19 beliefs and behaviors. *Social and Personality Psychology Compass*, 17(7), articlee12744. https://doi.org/10.1111/spc3.12744

Hu, T., Zhang, D., & Wang, J. (2015). A meta-analysis of the trait resilience and mental health. *Personality and Individual Differences*, 76, 18–27. https://doi.org/10.1016/j.paid.2014.11.039

Irmak, C., Murdock, M. R., & Kanuri, V. K. (2020). When consumption regulations backfire: The role of political ideology. *Journal of Marketing Research*, 57, 966–984. https://doi.org/10.1177/0022243720919709

Jessup, S. C., Knowles, K. A., & Olatunji, B. O. (2022). Linking the estimation of threat and COVID-19 fear and safety behavior use: Does intolerance of uncertainty matter? *International Journal of Cognitive Therapy*, 15(4), 479–491. https://doi.org/10.1007/s41811-022-00148-8

Karataş, Z., & Tagay, Ö. (2021). The relationships between resilience of the adults affected by the Covid pandemic in Turkey and Covid-19 fear, meaning in life, life satisfaction, intolerance of uncertainty and hope. *Personality and Individual Differences*, 172, article 110592. https://doi.org/10.1016/j.paid.2020.110592

Karwowski, M., Groyecka, A., Bialek, M., Lebuda, I., Sorokowska, A., & Sorokowski, P. (2020). When in danger, turn right: Does COVID-19 threat promote social conservatism and right-wing presidential candidates? *Human Ethology*, 35, 37–48. https://doi.org/10.22330/he/35/037-048

Kashdan, T. B., & Rottenberg, J. (2010). Psychological flexibility as a fundamental aspect of health. *Clinical Psychology Review*, 30, 467–480. https://doi.org/10.1016/j.cpr.2010.03.001

Kavčič, T., Avsec, A., & Zager Kocjan, G. (2021). Psychological functioning of Slovene adults during the COVID-19 pandemic: Does resilience matter? *Psychiatric Quarterly*, 92(1), 207–216. https://doi.org/10.1007/s11126-020-09789-4

Kendler, K. S., & Prescott, C. A. (2006). *Genes, environment, and psychopathology*. Guilford.

Keren, G., & Gerritsen, L. E. M. (1999). On the robustness and possible accounts of ambiguity aversion. *Acta Psychologica*, 103(1-2), 149–172. https://doi.org/10.1016/S0001-6918(99)00034-7

Khosravi, M., Amali, M., Jalili, F., & Ghiasi, Z. (2022). Prevalence and associated factors of personal protective measures among the southeastern Iranian population during the COVID-19 pandemic. *Electronic Journal of General Medicine*, 19(3), article em367. https://doi.org/10.29333/ejgm/11833

Kobasa, S. C. (1979). Stressful life events, personality and health: An inquiry into hardiness. *Journal of Personality and Social Psychology, 37*, 1–11. https://doi.org/10.1037/0022-3514.37.1.1

Köhne, S., Engert, V., & Rosendahl, J. (2022). Stability of resilience in times of the Covid-19 pandemic. *Personality and Mental Health, 17*(1), 55–66. https://doi.org/10.1002/pmh.1560

Kruglanski, A. W. (1989). *Lay epistemics and human knowledge: Cognitive and motivational bases*. Plenum.

Kruglanski, A. W., & Fishman, S. (2009). The need for cognitive closure. In M. R. Leary & R. H. Hoyle (Eds.), *Handbook of individual differences in social behavior* (pp. 343–353). Guilford.

Kunicki, Z. J., & Harlow, L. L. (2020). Towards a higher-order model of resilience. *Social Indicators Research, 151*(1), 329–344. https://doi.org/10.1007/s11205-020-02368-x

Lau, J. T. F., Kim, J. H., Tsui, H. Y., & Griffiths, S. (2008). Perceptions related to bird-to-human avian influenza, influenza vaccination, and use of face mask. *Infection, 36*, 434–443. https://doi.org/10.1007/s15010-008-7277-y

Lauriola, M., Mosca, O., Trentini, C., Foschi, R., Tambelli, R., & Carleton, R. N. (2018). The Intolerance and Uncertainty Inventory: Validity and comparison of scoring methods to assess individuals screening positive for anxiety and depression. *Frontiers in Psychology, 9*, article 388. https://doi.org/10.3389/fpsyg.2018.00388

Lewing, C. A., & Caraway, S. J. (2019). Psychological reactance as a motivation in psychopathy. *Personality and Individual Differences, 139*, 355–359. https://doi.org/10.1016/j.paid.2018.12.007

Liang, L., Li, C., Meng, C., Guo, X., Lv, J., Fei, J., & Mei, S. (2022). Psychological distress and internet addiction following the COVID-19 outbreak: Fear of missing out and boredom proneness as mediators. *Archives of Psychiatric Nursing, 40*, 8–14. https://doi.org/10.1016/j.apnu.2022.03.007

Linnemann, P., Wellmann, J., Berger, K., & Teismann, H. (2020). Effects of age on trait resilience in a population-based cohort and two patient cohorts. *Journal of Psychosomatic Research, 136*, article 110170. https://doi.org/10.1016/j.jpsychores.2020.110170

Llera, S. J., & Newman, M. G. (2020). Worry impairs the problem-solving process: Results from an experimental study. *Behaviour Research and Therapy, 135*, article 103759. https://doi.org/10.1016/j.brat.2020.103759

Lo Presti, S., Mattavelli, G., Canessa, N., & Gianelli, C. (2022). Risk perception and behaviour during the COVID-19 pandemic: Predicting variables of compliance with lockdown measures. *PLOS ONE, 17*(1), article e0262319. https://doi.org/10.1371/journal.pone.0262319

Lu, Y.-C., Shu, B.-C., Chang, Y.-Y., & Lung, F.-W. (2006). The mental health of hospital workers dealing with severe acute respiratory syndrome. *Psychotherapy and Psychosomatics, 75*, 370–375. https://doi.org/10.1159/000095443

Ma, Y., Dixon, G., & Hmielowski, J. (2019). Psychological reactance from reading basic facts on climate change: The role of prior views and political identification. *Environmental Communication, 13*, 71–86. https://doi.org/10.1080/17524032.2018.1548369

Maddi, S. R. (2013). *Hardiness: Turning stressful circumstances into resilient growth*. Springer.

Maher, P. J., Roth, J., Griffin, S., Foran, A., Jay, S., McHugh, C., et al. (2022). Pandemic threat and group cohesion: National identification in the wake of Covid-19 is associated with authoritarianism. *Journal of Social Psychology, 163*(6), 789–805. https://doi.org/10.1080/00224545.2021.2024122

Manson, J. H. (2020). Right-wing authoritarianism, left-wing authoritarianism, and pandemic-mitigation authoritarianism. *Personality and Individual Differences, 167*, article 110251. https://doi.org/10.1016/j.paid.2020.110251

Marchlewska, M., Cichocka, A., & Kossowska, M. (2018). Addicted to answers: Need for cognitive closure and the endorsement of conspiracy beliefs. *European Journal of Social Psychology, 48,* 109–117. https://doi.org/10.1002/ejsp.2308

McGowan, S. K., Behar, E., & Luhmann, M. (2016). Examining the relationship between worry and sleep: A daily process approach. *Behavior Therapy, 47*(4), 460–473. https://doi.org/10.1016/j.beth.2015.12.003

Molton, I. R., Koelmel, E., Curran, M., von Geldern, G., Ordway, A., & Alschuler, K. N. (2019). Pilot intervention to promote tolerance for uncertainty in early multiple sclerosis. *Rehabilitation Psychology, 64*(3), 339–350. https://doi.org/10.1037/rep0000275

Muris, P., Merckelbach, H., & van Spauwen, I. (2003). The emotional reasoning heuristic in children. *Behaviour Research and Therapy, 41*(3), 261–272. https://doi.org/10.1016/S0005-7967(02)00005-0

Neville, L., Fisk, G. M., & Ens, K. (2024). Psychological entitlement and conspiracy beliefs: Evidence from the Covid-19 pandemic. *Journal of Social Psychology.* https://doi.org/10.1080/00224545.2023.2292626

Ngo, A., Petrides, K. V., & Vernon, P. A. (2023). To vaccinate or not to vaccinate? The role of personality. *Personality and Individual Differences, 213,* article 112300. https://doi.org/10.1016/j.paid.2023.112300

Norr, A. M., Albanese, B. J., Oglesby, M. E., Allan, N. P., & Schmidt, N. B. (2015). Anxiety sensitivity and intolerance of uncertainty as potential risk factors for cyberchondria. *Journal of Affective Disorders, 174,* 64–69. https://doi.org/10.1016/j.jad.2014.11.023

Nürnberger, P., von Lewinski, D., Rothenhäusler, H., Braun, C., Reinbacher, P., Kolesnik, E., et al. (2022). A biopsychosocial model of severe fear of COVID-19. *PLOS ONE, 17*(2), article e0264357. https://doi.org/10.1371/journal.pone.0264357

O'Bryan, E. M., & McLeish, A. C. (2017). An examination of the indirect effect of intolerance of uncertainty on health anxiety through anxiety sensitivity physical concerns. *Journal of Psychopathology and Behavioral Assessment, 39,* 715–722. https://doi.org/10.1007/s10862-017-9613-y

Obsessive-Compulsive Cognitions Working Group. (2005). Psychometric validation of the obsessive belief questionnaire and interpretation of intrusions inventory—part 2: Factor analyses and testing of a brief version. *Behaviour Research and Therapy, 43,* 1527–1542. https://doi.org/10.1016/j.brat.2004.07.010

Ojalehto, H. J., Abramowitz, J. S., Hellberg, S. N., Butcher, M. W., & Buchholz, J. L. (2021). Predicting COVID-19-related anxiety: The role of obsessive-compulsive symptom dimensions, anxiety sensitivity, and body vigilance. *Journal of Anxiety Disorders, 83,* article 102460. https://doi.org/10.1016/j.janxdis.2021.102460

Oral, M., & Karakurt, N. (2022). The impact of psychological hardiness on intolerance of uncertainty in university students during the COVID-19 pandemic. *Journal of Community Psychology, 50*(8), 3574–3589. https://doi.org/10.1002/jcop.22856

Passini, S. (2022). Songs and flags: Concern for COVID-19 and submission to authority. *Personality and Individual Differences, 185,* article 111251. https://doi.org/10.1016/j.paid.2021.111251

Payne, L. A., Ellard, K. K., Farchione, T. J., & Barlow, D. H. (2021). Emotional disorders: A unified protocol for transdiagnostic treatment. In D. H. Barlow (Ed.), *Clinical handbook of psychological disorders: A step-by-step treatment manual (6th ed.)* (pp. 217–256). Guilford.

Pazhoohi, F., & Kingstone, A. (2021). Associations of political orientation, xenophobia, right-wing authoritarianism, and concern of COVID-19: Cognitive responses to an actual pathogen threat. *Personality and Individual Differences, 182,* article 111081. https://doi.org/10.1016/j.paid.2021.111081

Peng, Y. (2022). Politics of COVID-19 vaccine mandates: Left/right-wing authoritarianism, social dominance orientation, and libertarianism. *Personality and Individual Differences, 194*, article 111661. https://doi.org/10.1016/j.paid.2022.111661

Prichard, E. C., & Turner, K. A. (2023). Authoritarianism, psychopathy, and resistance to wearing masks during the COVID-19 pandemic: A partial replication and extension of key findings. *Frontiers in Psychology, 13*, article 1049660. https://doi.org/10.3389/fpsyg.2022.1049660

Querstret, D., & Cropley, M. (2013). Assessing treatments used to reduce rumination and/or worry: A systematic review. *Clinical Psychology Review, 33*(8), 996–1009. https://doi.org/10.1016/j.cpr.2013.08.004

Rains, S. A. (2013). The nature of psychological reactance revisited: A meta-analytic review. *Human Communication Research, 39*, 47–73. https://doi.org/10.1111/j.1468-2958.2012.01443.x

Reagu, S., Jones, R. M., & Alabdulla, M. (2023). COVID-19 vaccine hesitancy and personality traits: Results from a large national cross-sectional survey in Qatar. *Vaccines, 11*(1), article 189. https://doi.org/10.3390/vaccines11010189

Regan, T., Harris, B., Van Loon, M., Nanavaty, N., Schueler, J., Engler, S., et al. (2020). Does mindfulness reduce the effects of risk factors for problematic smartphone use? Comparing frequency of use versus self-reported addiction. *Addictive Behaviors, 108*, article 106435. https://doi.org/10.1016/j.addbeh.2020.106435

Rettie, H., & Daniels, J. (2020). Coping and tolerance of uncertainty: Predictors and mediators of mental health during the COVID-19 pandemic. *American Psychologist, 76*(3), 427–437. https://doi.org/10.1037/amp0000710

Robichaud, M. (2013). Cognitive behavior therapy targeting intolerance of uncertainty: Application to a clinical case of Generalized Anxiety Disorder. *Cognitive and Behavioral Practice, 20*(3), 251–263. https://doi.org/10.1016/j.cbpra.2012.09.001

Rose, K. C., & Anastasio, P. A. (2014). Entitlement is about "others," narcissism is not: Relations to sociotropic and autonomous interpersonal styles. *Personality and Individual Differences, 59*, 50–53. https://doi.org/10.1016/j.paid.2013.11.004

Rosenberg, B. D., & Siegel, J. T. (2018). A 50-year review of psychological reactance theory: Do not read this article. *Motivation Science, 4*, 281–300. https://doi.org/10.1037/mot0000091

Rosser, B. A. (2018). Intolerance of uncertainty as a transdiagnostic mechanism of psychological difficulties: A systematic review of evidence pertaining to causality and temporal precedence. *Cognitive Therapy and Research, 43*, 438–463. https://doi.org/10.1007/s10608-018-9964-z

Sabatini, S., Kaufmann, M., Fadda, M., Tancredi, S., Noor, N., Van Der Linden, B. W. A., et al. (2023). Factors associated with COVID-19 non-vaccination in Switzerland: A nationwide study. *International Journal of Public Health, 68*, article 1605852. https://doi.org/10.3389/ijph.2023.1605852

Sauer-Zavala, S., Fournier, J., Jarvi Steele, S., Woods, B., Wang, M., Farchione, T., et al. (2021). Does the unified protocol really change neuroticism? Results from a randomized trial. *Psychological Medicine, 51*(14), 2378–2387. https://doi.org/10.1017/S0033291720000975

Saulnier, K. G., Koscinski, B., Volarov, M., Accorso, C., Austin, M. J., Suhr, J. A., et al. (2022). Anxiety sensitivity and intolerance of uncertainty are unique and interactive risk factors for COVID-19 safety behaviors and worries. *Cognitive Behaviour Therapy, 51*(3), 217–228. https://doi.org/10.1080/16506073.2021.1976819

Schmit, A., Schurr, T., Frajo-Apor, B., Pardeller, S., Plattner, B., Tutzer, F., et al. (2024). Long-term impact of resilience and extraversion on psychological distress during the COVID-19 pandemic: A longitudinal investigation among individuals with and without mental health disorders. *Frontiers in Psychiatry, 15*, article 1304491. https://doi.org/10.3389/fpsyt.2024.1304491

Schut, A. J., Castonguay, L. G., & Borkovec, T. D. (2001). Compulsive checking behaviors in generalized anxiety disorder. *Journal of Clinical Psychology, 57*(6), 705–715. https://doi.org/10.1002/jclp.1043

Shihata, S., McEvoy, P. M., Mullan, B. A., & Carleton, R. N. (2016). Intolerance of uncertainty in emotional disorders: What uncertainties remain? *Journal of Anxiety Disorders, 41*, 115–124. https://doi.org/10.1016/j.janxdis.2016.05.001

Smirnov, O., & Hsieh, P.-H. (2022). COVID-19, climate change, and the finite pool of worry in 2019 to 2021 Twitter discussions. *PNAS, 119*(43), 1–8. https://doi.org/10.1073/pnas.2210988119

Smith, B. W., Kay, V. S., Hoyt, T. V., & Bernard, M. L. (2009). Predicting the anticipated emotional and behavioral responses to an avian flu outbreak. *American Journal of Infection Control, 37*, 371–380. https://doi.org/10.1016/j.ajic.2008.08.007

Smrdu, M., Kuder, A., Turk, E., Čelik, T., Šet, J., & Kralj-Fišer, S. (2023). COVID-19 pandemic and lockdown: Associations with personality and stress components. *Psychological Reports, 126*(2), 727–758. https://doi.org/10.1177/00332941211043451

Soveri, A., Karlsson, L. C., Mäki, K. O., Holford, D., Fasce, A., Schmid, P., et al. (2024). Trait reactance as psychological motivation to reject vaccination: Two longitudinal studies and one experimental study. *Applied Psychology: Health & Well-Being, 16*(2), 597–614. https://doi.org/10.1111/aphw.12506

Spielberger, C. D. (1979). *Understanding stress and anxiety*. Harper & Row.

Subica, A. M., Allen, J. G., Frueh, B. C., Elhai, J. D., & Fowler, J. C. (2016). Disentangling depression and anxiety in relation to neuroticism, extraversion, suicide, and self-harm among adult psychiatric inpatients with serious mental illness. *British Journal of Clinical Psychology, 55*, 349–370. https://doi.org/10.1111/bjc.12098

Swickert, R. J., Rosentreter, C. J., Hittner, J. B., & Mushrush, J. E. (2002). Extraversion, social support processes, and stress. *Personality and Individual Differences, 32*(5), 877–891. https://doi.org/10.1016/S0191-8869(01)00093-9

Taha, S., Matheson, K., Cronin, T., & Anisman, H. (2014). Intolerance of uncertainty, appraisals, coping, and anxiety: The case of the 2009 H1N1 pandemic. *British Journal of Health Psychology, 19*, 592–605. https://doi.org/10.1111/bjhp.12058

Talkovsky, A. M., & Norton, P. J. (2016). Intolerance of uncertainty and transdiagnostic group cognitive behavioral therapy for anxiety. *Journal of Anxiety Disorders, 41*, 108–114. https://doi.org/10.1016/j.janxdis.2016.05.002

Taylor, S. (2017). *Clinician's guide to PTSD (2nd ed.)*. Guilford.

Taylor, S. (2019a). Anxiety sensitivity. In J. S. Abramowitz & S. M. Blakey (Eds.), *Clinical handbook of fear and anxiety: Psychological processes and treatment mechanisms*. American Psychological Association.

Taylor, S. (2019b). *The psychology of pandemics: Preparing for the next global outbreak of infectious disease*. Cambridge Scholars Publishing.

Taylor, S., & Asmundson, G. J. G. (2004). *Treating health anxiety*. Guilford.

Taylor, S., & Asmundson, G. J. G. (2021). Negative attitudes about facemasks during the COVID-19 pandemic: The dual importance of perceived ineffectiveness and psychological reactance. *PLOS ONE, 16*(2), article e0246317. https://doi.org/10.1371/journal.pone.0246317

Taylor, S., Fong, A., & Asmundson, G. J. G. (2021). Predicting the severity of symptoms of the COVID stress syndrome from personality traits: A prospective network analysis. *Frontiers in Psychology, 12*, article 632227. https://doi.org/10.3389/fpsyg.2021.632227

Taylor, S., Landry, C. A., Paluszek, M. M., Fergus, T. A., McKay, D., & Asmundson, G. J. G. (2020). Covid stress syndrome: Concept, structure, and correlates. *Depression and Anxiety, 37*, 706–714. https://doi.org/10.1002/da.23071

Taylor, S., Paluszek, M., Landry, C., Rachor, G. S., & Asmundson, G. J. G. (2021). Predictors of distress and coping during pandemic-related self isolation: The relative importance of personality traits and beliefs about personal threat. *Personality and Individual Differences, 176*, article 110779. https://doi.org/10.1016/j.paid.2021.110779

Taylor, S., Rachor, G. S., & Asmundson, G. J. G. (2022). Who develops pandemic fatigue? Insights from latent class analysis. *PLOS ONE, 17*(11), article e0276791. https://doi.org/10.1371/journal.pone.0276791

Telaku, N., Musliu, A., Cana, L., Han, H., & Zharku, L. (2022). The relationship between personality traits and compliance with the COVID-19 preventive measures in Kosovo. *Psych, 4*(4), 856–867. https://doi.org/10.3390/psych4040063

Thibodeau, M., Carleton, R. N., McEvoy, P. M., Zvolensky, M., Brandt, C., Boelen, P., et al. (2015). Developing scales measuring disorder-specific intolerance of uncertainty (DSIU): A new perspective on transdiagnostic. *Journal of Anxiety Disorders, 31*, 49–57. https://doi.org/10.1016/j.janxdis.2015.01.006

Timulak, L., Richards, D., Bhandal-Griffin, L., Healy, P., Azevedo, J., Connon, G., et al. (2022). Effectiveness of the internet-based Unified Protocol transdiagnostic intervention for the treatment of depression, anxiety and related disorders in a primary care setting: a randomized controlled trial. *Trials, 23*(1), article 721. https://doi.org/10.1186/s13063-022-06551-y

Todd, F. M. (1909). *Eradicating plague from San Francisco: Report of the Citizens' Health Committee and an account of its work*. Murdock & Co.

Torbit, L., & Laposa, J. M. (2016). Group CBT for GAD: The role of change in intolerance of uncertainty in treatment outcomes. *International Journal of Cognitive Therapy, 9*(4), 356–368. https://doi.org/10.1521/ijct_2016_09_17

Turk, E., Čelik, T., Smrdu, M., Šet, J., Kuder, A., Gregorič, M., et al. (2023). Adherence to COVID-19 mitigation measures: The role of sociodemographic and personality factors. *Current Psychology, 42*(9), 7771–7787. https://doi.org/10.1007/s12144-021-02051-5

Tybur, J. M., Inbar, Y., Aarøe, L., Barclay, P., Barlow, F., Barra, M., et al. (2016). Parasite stress and pathogen avoidance relate to distinct dimensions of political ideology across 30 nations. *PNAS, 113*, 12408–12413. https://doi.org/10.1073/pnas.1607398113

Vagni, M., Maiorano, T., Giostra, V., Pajardi, D., & Bartone, P. (2022). Emergency stress, hardiness, coping strategies and burnout in health care and emergency response workers during the COVID-19 pandemic. *Frontiers in Psychology, 13*, article 918788. https://doi.org/10.3389/fpsyg.2022.918788

van Dijk, S. D. M., Hanssen, D., Naarding, P., Lucassen, P., Comijs, H., & Oude Voshaar, R. (2016). Big Five personality traits and medically unexplained symptoms in later life. *European Psychiatry, 38*, 23–30. https://doi.org/10.1016/j.eurpsy.2016.05.002

Vint, J., Rachor, G. S., Taylor, S., & Asmundson, G. J. G. (2024). What is COVID-19 anyway? Narcissism and pandemic attitudes and behaviours. *Personality and Individual Differences, 217*, article 112429. https://doi.org/10.1016/j.paid.2023.112429

Waaktaar, T., & Torgersen, S. (2012). Genetic and environmental causes of variation in trait resilience in young people. *Behavior Genetics, 42*(3), 366–377. https://doi.org/10.1007/s10519-011-9519-5

Watson, D., & O'Hara, M. W. (2017). *Understanding the emotional disorders*. Oxford University Press.

Weber, E. U. (2015). Climate change demands behavioral change: What are the challenges? *Social Research, 82*(3), 560–580. https://doi.org/10.1353/sor.2015.0050

Webster, D. M., & Kruglanski, A. W. (1994). Individual differences in need for cognitive closure. *Journal of Personality and Social Psychology, 67*(6), 1049–1062. https://doi.org/10.1037/0022-3514.67.6.1049

Weiss, E. R., Todman, M., Maple, E., & Bunn, R. R. (2022). Boredom in a time of uncertainty: State and trait boredom's associations with psychological health during COVID-19. *Behavioral Sciences, 12*(8), article 298. https://doi.org/10.3390/bs12080298

Wheaton, M. G., Abramowitz, J. S., Berman, N. C., Fabricant, L. E., & Olatunji, B. O. (2012). Psychological predictors of anxiety in response to the H1N1 (swine flu) pandemic. *Cognitive Therapy and Research, 36*, 210–218. https://doi.org/10.1007/s10608-011-9353-3

Wilson, E. J., Abbott, M. J., & Norton, A. R. (2023). The impact of psychological treatment on intolerance of uncertainty in generalized anxiety disorder: A systematic review and meta-analysis. *Journal of Anxiety Disorders, 97*, article 102729. https://doi.org/10.1016/j.janxdis.2023.102729

Xie, X.-F., Stone, E., Zheng, R., & Zhang, R.-G. (2011). The "typhoon eye effect": Determinants of distress during the SARS epidemic. *Journal of Risk Research, 14*, 1091–1107. https://doi.org/10.1080/13669877.2011.571790

Yang, X.-J., Liu, Q.-Q., Lian, S.-L., & Zhou, Z.-K. (2020). Are bored minds more likely to be addicted? The relationship between boredom proneness and problematic mobile phone use. *Addictive Behaviors, 108*, article 106426. https://doi.org/10.1016/j.addbeh.2020.106426

Yao, X., Chan, K. L., Chen, S., & Gao, S. (2024). Associations between psychological flexibility and mental health problems during the Covid-19 pandemic: A three-level meta-analytic review. *Current Psychology*. https://doi.org/10.1007/s12144-024-05628-y

Yunus, F. M., Livet, A., Mahmoud, A., Moore, M., Murphy, C. B., Nogueira-Arjona, R., et al. (2022). Is anxiety sensitivity associated with COVID-19 related distress and adherence among emerging adults? *Psych, 4*(4), 934–951. https://doi.org/10.3390/psych4040069

Zitek, E. M., & Schlund, R. J. (2021). Psychological entitlement predicts noncompliance with the health guidelines of the COVID-19 pandemic. *Personality and Individual Differences, 171*, article 110491. https://doi.org/10.1016/j.paid.2020.110491

Zuffianò, A., Caprara, G., Zamparini, M., Calamandrei, G., Candini, V., Malvezzi, M., et al. (2023). The role of "positivity" and big five traits during the COVID-19 pandemic: An Italian national representative survey. *Journal of Happiness Studies, 24*(8), 2813–2830. https://doi.org/10.1007/s10902-023-00705-8

Chapter 19

Acuff, S. F., Strickland, J. C., Tucker, J. A., & Murphy, J. G. (2022). Changes in alcohol use during COVID-19 and associations with contextual and individual difference variables: A systematic review and meta-analysis. *Psychology of Addictive Behaviors, 36*(1), 1–19. https://doi.org/10.1037/adb0000796

AlDandan, F. N., Aldandan, L. H., Sulais, A. A., Alshaikh, S. T., Alqahtani, A. H., & Khalil, M. S. (2023). The impact of the COVID-19 pandemic on patients with obsessive compulsive disorder (OCD). *Clinical Neuropsychiatry, 20*(4), 358–363. https://doi.org/10.36131/cnfioritieditore20230416

American Psychiatric Association. (1980). *Diagnostic and statistical manual of mental disorders* (3rd ed.). Author.

American Psychiatric Association. (2022). *Diagnostic and statistical manual of mental disorders* (5th ed., text rev.). Author.

Aro, A. R., Henriksson, M., Leinikki, P., & Lönnqvist, J. (1995). Fear of AIDS and suicide in Finland: A review. *AIDS Care, 7*(Suppl 2), S187–S197. https://doi.org/10.1080/09540129550126191

Arora, T., Grey, I., Östlundh, L., Lam, K. B. H., Omar, O. M., & Arnone, D. (2020). The prevalence of psychological consequences of COVID-19: A systematic review and meta-analysis of observational studies. *Journal of Health Psychology, 27*(4), 805–824. https://doi.org/10.1177/1359105320966639

Asmundson, G. J. G., & Taylor, S. (2021). Garbage in, garbage out: The tenuous state of research on PTSD in the context of the COVID-19 pandemic and infodemic. *Journal of Anxiety Disorders, 78*, article 102368. https://doi.org/10.1016/j.janxdis.2021.102368

Bachem, R., & Casey, P. (2018). Adjustment disorder: A diagnosis whose time has come. *Journal of Affective Disorders, 227*, 243–253. https://doi.org/10.1016/j.jad.2017.10.034

Barry, J. M. (2018). *The great influenza*. Penguin Random House.

Batra, K., Pharr, J. R., Kachen, A., Godbey, S., & Terry, E. (2023). Investigating the psychosocial impact of COVID-19 among the sexual and gender minority population: A systematic review and meta-analysis. *LGBT Health, 10*(6), 416–428. https://doi.org/10.1089/lgbt.2022.0249

Bayramoğlu, Y. (2021). Border panic over the pandemic: Mediated anxieties about migrant sex workers and queers during the AIDS crises in Turkey. *Ethnic and Racial Studies, 44*(9), 1589–1606. https://doi.org/10.1080/01419870.2021.1881141

Bello, U. M., Kannan, P., Chutiyami, M., Salihu, D., Cheong, A. M. Y., Miller, T., et al. (2022). Prevalence of anxiety and depression among the general population in Africa during the COVID-19 pandemic: A systematic review and meta-analysis. *Frontiers in Public Health, 10*, article 814981. https://doi.org/10.3389/fpubh.2022.814981

Berger, K. (2020). *Seattle struggles with suicide in late stages of the 1918 flu*. Crosscut. https://crosscut.com/2020/05/seattle-struggled-suicide-late-stages-1918-flu

Bhuiyan, A., Sakib, N., Pakpour, A., Griffiths, M., & Mamun, M. (2020). COVID-19-related suicides in Bangladesh due to lockdown and economic factors: Case study evidence from media reports. *International Journal of Mental Health and Addiction, 19*, 2110–2115. https://doi.org/10.1007/s11469-020-00307-y

Blakey, S. M., & Abramowitz, J. S. (2017). Psychological predictors of health anxiety in response to the Zika virus. *Journal of Clinical Psychology in Medical Settings, 24*, 270–278. https://doi.org/10.1007/s10880-017-9514-y

Blakey, S. M., Reuman, L., Jacoby, R. J., & Abramowitz, J. S. (2015). Tracing "fearbola": Psychological predictors of anxious responding to the threat of Ebola. *Cognitive Therapy and Research, 39*, 816–825. https://doi.org/10.1007/s10608-015-9701-9

Blasco-Belled, A., Tejada-Gallardo, C., Fatsini-Prats, M., & Alsinet, C. (2022). Mental health among the general population and healthcare workers during the Covid-19 pandemic: A meta-analysis of well-being and psychological distress prevalence. *Current Psychology, 43*, 8435–8446. https://doi.org/10.1007/s12144-022-02913-6

Bouton, R. A., Gallaher, P. E., Garlinghouse, P. A., Leal, T., Rosenstein, L. D., & Young, R. K. (1987). Scales for measuring fear of AIDS and homophobia. *Journal of Personality Assessment, 51*(4), 606–614. https://doi.org/10.1207/s15327752jpa5104_13

Bristow, N. K. (2012). *American pandemic: The lost world of the 1918 influenza epidemic*. Oxford University Press.

Bueno-Notivol, J., Gracia-García, P., Olaya, B., Lasheras, I., López-Antón, R., & Santabárbara, J. (2021). Prevalence of depression during the COVID-19 outbreak: A meta-analysis of community-based studies. *International Journal of Clinical and Health Psychology, 21*(1), article 100196. https://doi.org/10.1016/j.ijchp.2020.07.007

Byrne, J. P. (2006). *Daily life during the Black Death*. Greenwood.

Carfi, A., Bernabei, R., & Landi, F. (2020). Persistent symptoms in patients after acute COVID-19. *JAMA, 324*(6), 603–605. https://doi.org/10.1001/jama.2020.12603

CDC. (2024). COVID data tracker. https://covid.cdc.gov/covid-data-tracker/#datatracker-home.

Cénat, J., Blais-Rochette, C., Kokou-Kpolou, C., Noorishad, P., Mukunzi, J., McIntee, S., et al. (2021). Prevalence of symptoms of depression, anxiety, insomnia, posttraumatic stress disorder, and psychological distress among populations affected by the COVID-19 pandemic: A systematic review and meta-analysis. *Psychiatry Research, 295*, article 113599. https://doi.org/10.1016/j.psychres.2020.113599

Chan, S. M., Chiu, F. K., Lam, C. W., Leung, P. Y., & Conwell, Y. (2006). Elderly suicide and the 2003 SARS epidemic in Hong Kong. *International Journal of Geriatric Psychiatry, 21*(2), 113–118. https://doi.org/10.1002/gps.1432

Chau, S., Wong, O., Ramakrishnan, R., Chan, S., Wong, E., Li, P., et al. (2021). History for some or lesson for all? A systematic review and meta-analysis on the immediate and long-term mental health impact of the 2002-2003 Severe Acute Respiratory Syndrome (SARS) outbreak. *BMC Public Health, 21*(1), article 670. https://doi.org/10.1186/s12889-021-10701-3

Chen, J., Farah, N., Dong, R. K., Chen, R. Z., Xu, W., Yin, J., et al. (2021). Mental health during the COVID-19 crisis in Africa: A systematic review and meta-analysis. *International Journal of Environmental Research and Public Health, 18*(20), article 10604. https://doi.org/10.3390/ijerph182010604

Chen, J., Zhang, S. X., Yin, A., & Yáñez, J. A. (2022). Mental health symptoms during the COVID-19 pandemic in developing countries: A systematic review and meta-analysis. *Journal of Global Health, 12*, article 05011. https://doi.org/10.7189/jogh.12.05011

Cheung, Y. T., Chau, P. H., & Yip, P. S. F. (2008). A revisit on older adults suicides and Severe Acute Respiratory Syndrome (SARS) epidemic in Hong Kong. *International Journal of Geriatric Psychiatry, 23*(12), 1231–1238. https://doi.org/10.1002/gps.2056

Chutiyami, M., Cheong, A. M. Y., Salihu, D., Bello, U. M., Ndwiga, D., Maharaj, R., et al. (2022). COVID-19 pandemic and overall mental health of healthcare professionals globally: A meta-review of systematic reviews. *Frontiers in Psychiatry, 12*, article 804525. https://doi.org/10.3389/fpsyt.2021.804525

Clapp, T. (1857). *Autobiographical sketches and recollections, during a thirty-five years residence in New Orleans*. Phillips, Sampson & Co.

Cost, K. T., Crosbie, J., Anagnostou, E., Birken, C. S., Charach, A., Monga, S., et al. (2021). Mostly worse, occasionally better: Impact of Covid-19 pandemic on the mental health of Canadian children and adolescents. *European Child & Adolescent Psychiatry, 31*, 671–684. https://doi.org/10.1007/s00787-021-01744-3

Costa, D., Scharpf, F., Weiss, A., Ayanian, A. H., & Bozorgmehr, K. (2024). Intimate partner violence during COVID-19: Systematic review and meta-analysis according to methodological choices. *BMC Public Health, 24*(1), article 313. https://doi.org/10.1186/s12889-024-17802-9

COVID-19 Mental Disorders Collaborators. (2021). Global prevalence and burden of depressive and anxiety disorders in 204 countries and territories in 2020 due to the COVID-19 pandemic. *Lancet, 398*(10312), 1700–1712. https://doi.org/10.1016/S0140-6736(21)02143-7

Craske, M. G. (2003). *Origins of phobias and anxiety disorders: Why more women than men?* Elsevier.

da Cunha Varella, A. P., Griffin, E., Khashan, A., & Kabir, Z. (2024). Suicide rates before and during the Covid-19 pandemic: A systematic review and meta-analysis. *Social Psychiatry and Psychiatric Epidemiology, 59*. https://doi.org/10.1007/s00127-024-02617-1

Daniali, H., Martinussen, M., & Flaten, M. A. (2023). A global meta-analysis of depression, anxiety, and stress before and during COVID-19. *Health Psychology, 42*(2), 124–138. https://doi.org/10.1037/hea0001259

Darby, R. (2015). Syphilis 1855 and HIV-AIDS 2007: Historical reflections on the tendency to blame human anatomy for the action of micro-organisms. *Global Public Health, 10*(5-6), 573–588. https://doi.org/10.1080/17441692.2014.957231

Davis, H., Assaf, G., McCorkell, L., Wei, H., Low, R., Re'em, Y., et al. (2020). Characterizing Long COVID in an international cohort: 7 months of symptoms and their impact. *Eclinical Medicine, 38*, article 101019. https://doi.org/10.1016/j.eclinm.2021.101019

Demass, T. B., Guadie, A. G., Mengistu, T. B., Belay, Z. A., Melese, A. A., Berneh, A. A., et al. (2023). The magnitude of mortality and its predictors among adult patients admitted to the intensive care unit in Amhara Regional State, Northwest Ethiopia. *Scientific Reports, 13*(1), article 12010. https://doi.org/10.1038/s41598-023-39190-7

Donnelly, M., Grigorian, A., Inaba, K., Kuza, C., Kim, D., Dolich, M., et al. (2021). A dual pandemic: The influence of coronavirus disease 2019 on trends and types of firearm violence in California, Ohio, and the United States. *Journal of Surgical Research, 263*, 24–33. https://doi.org/10.1016/j.jss.2021.01.018

Dsouza, D. D., Quadros, S., Hyderabadwala, Z. J., & Mamun, M. A. (2020). Aggregated COVID-19 suicide incidences in India: Fear of COVID-19 infection is the prominent causative factor. *Psychiatry Research, 290*, article 113145. https://doi.org/10.1016/j.psychres.2020.113145

Duarte, D., El-Hagrassy, M. M., Couto, T. C. E., Gurgel, W., Fregni, F., & Correa, H. (2020). Male and female physician suicidality: A systematic review and meta-analysis. *JAMA Psychiatry, 77*(6), 587–597. https://doi.org/10.1001/jamapsychiatry.2020.0011

Dubé, J. P., Smith, M. M., Sherry, S. B., Hewitt, P. L., & Stewart, S. H. (2021). Suicide behaviors during the COVID-19 pandemic: A meta-analysis of 54 studies. *Psychiatry Research, 301*, article 113998. https://doi.org/10.1016/j.psychres.2021.113998

Duc, T. Q., Chi, V., & Quang, P. N. (2022). Depression prevalence in Vietnam during the Covid-19 pandemic: A systematic review and meta-analysis. *Ethics, Medicine, and Public Health, 23*, article 100806. https://doi.org/10.1016/j.jemep.2022.100806

Dutheil, F., Aubert, C., Pereira, B., Dambrun, M., Moustafa, F., Mermillod, M., et al. (2019). Suicide among physicians and health-care workers: A systematic review and meta-analysis. *PLOS ONE, 14*(12), article e0226361. https://doi.org/10.1371/journal.pone.0226361

Evangeli, M., & Wroe, A. L. (2017). HIV disclosure anxiety: A systematic review and theoretical synthesis. *AIDS and Behavior, 21*(1), 1–11. https://doi.org/10.1007/s10461-016-1453-3

Evening Express. (1918, October 26). Watch out or fluphobia'll catch yuh! *Evening Express*, 23.

Every-Palmer, S., Jenkins, M., Gendall, P., Hoek, J., Beaglehole, B., Bell, C., et al. (2020). Psychological distress, anxiety, family violence, suicidality, and wellbeing in New Zealand during the COVID-19 lockdown: A cross-sectional study. *PLOS ONE, 15*(11), article e0241658. https://doi.org/10.1371/journal.pone.0241658

Fang, Y., Ji, B., Liu, Y., Zhang, J., Liu, Q., Ge, Y., et al. (2022). The prevalence of psychological stress in student populations during the COVID-19 epidemic: A systematic review and meta-analysis. *Scientific Reports, 12*(1), article 12118. https://doi.org/10.1038/s41598-022-16328-7

Farooq, S., Tunmore, J., Wajid Ali, M., & Ayub, M. (2021). Suicide, self-harm and suicidal ideation during COVID-19: A systematic review. *Psychiatry Research, 306*, article 114228. https://doi.org/10.1016/j.psychres.2021.114228

Fineberg, N. A., Van Ameringen, M., Drummond, L., Hollander, E., Stein, D. J., Geller, D., et al. (2020). How to manage obsessive-compulsive disorder (OCD) under COVID-19: A clinician's guide from the International College of Obsessive Compulsive Spectrum Disorders (ICOCS) and the Obsessive-Compulsive and Related Disorders Research Network (OCRN) of the European College of Neuropsychopharmacology. *Comprehensive Psychiatry, 100*, article 152174. https://doi.org/10.1016/j.comppsych.2020.152174

Fiquepron, M. R. (2018). Places, attitudes and moments during the epidemics: Representations of yellow fever and cholera in the city of Buenos Aires, 1867-1871. *História, Ciências, Saúde, 25*(2), 1–16. https://doi.org/10.1590/S0104-59702018000200003

Fruehwirth, J. C., Biswas, S., & Perreira, K. M. (2021). The Covid-19 pandemic and mental health of first-year college students: Examining the effect of Covid-19 stressors using longitudinal data. *PLOS ONE, 16*(3), article e0247999. https://doi.org/10.1371/journal.pone.0247999

Garza, R. P. (2008). *Understanding plague: The medical and imaginative texts of medieval Spain*. Peter Lang.

Geoffroy, M.-C., Chadi, N., Bouchard, S., Fuoco, J., Chartrand, E., Loose, T., et al. (2024). Mental health of Canadian youth: A systematic review and meta-analysis of studies examining changes in depression, anxiety, and suicide-related outcomes during the COVID-19 pandemic. *Canadian Journal of Public Health, 115*, 408–424. https://doi.org/10.17269/s41997-024-00865-x

Giuntella, O., Hyde, K., Saccardo, S., & Sadoff, S. (2021). Lifestyle and mental health disruptions during COVID-19. *PNAS, 118*(9), article e2016632118. https://doi.org/10.1073/pnas.2016632118

Gonçalves-Pereira, J., Oliveira, A., Vieira, T., Rodrigues, A. R., Pinto, M. J., Pipa, S., et al. (2023). Critically ill patient mortality by age: Long-term follow-up (CIMbA-LT). *Annals of Intensive Care, 13*(1), article 7. https://doi.org/10.1186/s13613-023-01102-3

Govender, R. D., Schlebusch, L., & Esterhuizen, T. (2014). Brief suicide preventive intervention in newly diagnosed HIV-positive persons. *African Journal of Psychiatry, 17*(2), 543–547. https://doi.org/10.4172/Psychiatry.1000112

Gowen, B. S. (1907). Some aspects of pestilences and other epidemics. *American Journal of Psychology, 18*(1), 1–60. https://doi.org/10.2307/1412171

Goyal, K., Chauhan, P., Chhikara, K., Gupta, P., & Singh, M. P. (2020). Fear of COVID 2019: First suicidal case in India! *Asian Journal of Psychiatry, 49*, article 101989. https://doi.org/10.1016/j.ajp.2020.101989

Gunnell, D., Appleby, L., Arensman, E., Hawton, K., John, A., Kapur, N., et al. (2020). Suicide risk and prevention during the COVID-19 pandemic. *Lancet Psychiatry, 7*(6), 468–471. https://doi.org/10.1016/S2215-0366(20)30171-1

Hadavi, M., Ghomian, Z., Mohammadi, F., & Sahebi, A. (2023). Workplace violence against health care workers during the COVID-19 Pandemic: A systematic review and meta-analysis. *Journal of Safety Research, 85*, 1–7. https://doi.org/10.1016/j.jsr.2023.01.001

Harrell, J. P., & Wright, L. W., Jr. (1998). The development and validation of the Multicomponent AIDS Phobia Scale. *Journal of Psychopathology and Behavioral Assessment, 20*(3), 201–216. https://doi.org/10.1023/A:1023020617248

Honigsbaum, M. (2009). *Living with Enza: The forgotten story of Britain and the great flu pandemic of 1918*. Macmillan.

Honigsbaum, M. (2010). The great dread: Cultural and psychological impacts and responses to the "Russian" influenza in the United Kingdom, 1889–1893. *Social History of Medicine, 23*(2), 299–319. https://doi.org/10.1093/shm/hkq011

Honigsbaum, M. (2013). "An inexpressible dread": Psychoses of influenza at fin-de-siècle. *Lancet, 381*, 988–989. https://doi.org/10.1016/S0140-6736(13)60701-1

Honigsbaum, M. (2020). Revisiting the 1957 and 1968 influenza pandemics. *Lancet, 395*, 1824–1826. https://doi.org/10.1016/S0140-6736(20)31201-0

Hoots, B. E., Li, J., Hertz, M. F., Esser, M. B., Rico, A., Zavala, E. Y., et al. (2023). Alcohol and other substance use before and during the COVID-19 pandemic among high school students - Youth Risk Behavior Survey, United States, 2021. *MMWR Supplements, 72*(1), 84–92. https://doi.org/10.15585/mmwr.su7201a10

Huang, J., Huang, Z.-T., Sun, X.-C., Chen, T.-T., & Wu, X.-T. (2024). Mental health status and related factors influencing healthcare workers during the COVID-19 pandemic: A systematic review and meta-analysis. *PLOS ONE, 19*(1), article e0289454. https://doi.org/10.1371/journal.pone.0289454

Iob, E., Steptoe, A., & Fancourt, D. (2020). Abuse, self-harm and suicidal ideation in the UK during the COVID-19 pandemic. *British Journal of Psychiatry, 217*, 543–546. https://doi.org/10.1192/bjp.2020.130

Jacob, K. S., John, J. K., Verghese, A., & John, T. J. (1989). The fear of AIDS: Psychiatric symptom or syndrome? *AIDS Care, 1*(1), 35–38. https://doi.org/10.1080/09540128908260232

Jäger, H., Welch, J., & Francis, J. L. (1988). *AIDS phobia: Disease pattern and possibilities of treatment.* Halsted.

Jäger-Collet, B. (1988). The disease pattern in psychological practice. In H. Jäger, Welch, J., & Francis, J. L. (Ed.), *AIDS phobia: Disease pattern and possibilities of treatment* (pp. 71–77). Halstead.

Jahan, I., Ullah, I., Griffiths, M. D., & Mamun, M. A. (2021). COVID-19 suicide and its causative factors among the healthcare professionals: Case study evidence from press reports. *Perspectives in Psychiatric Care, 57*(4), 1707–1711. https://doi.org/10.1111/ppc.12739

Janiri, D., Carfì, A., Kotzalidis, G. D., Bernabei, R., Landi, F., & Sani, G. (2021). Posttraumatic stress disorder in patients after severe COVID-19 infection. *JAMA Psychiatry, 78*, 567–569. https://doi.org/10.1001/jamapsychiatry.2021.0109

John, A., Pirkis, J., Gunnell, D., Appleby, L., & Morrissey, J. (2020). Trends in suicide during the COVID-19 pandemic. *BMJ (Clinical Research Ed.), 371*, article m4352. https://doi.org/10.1136/bmj.m4352

Karamouzian, M., Johnson, C., & Kerr, T. (2020). Public health messaging and harm reduction in the time of COVID-19. *Lancet Psychiatry, 7*(5), 390–391. https://doi.org/10.1016/S2215-0366(20)30144-9

Kidd, J., Jackman, K., Barucco, R., Dworkin, J., Dolezal, C., Navalta, T., et al. (2021). Understanding the impact of the COVID-19 pandemic on the mental health of transgender and gender nonbinary individuals engaged in a longitudinal cohort study. *Journal of Homosexuality, 68*(4), 592–611. https://doi.org/10.1080/00918369.2020.1868185

Kifle, M. E., Aychiluhm, S. B., & Anbesu, E. W. (2024). Global prevalence of intimate partner violence during the COVID-19 pandemic among women: Systematic review and meta-analysis. *BMC Women's Health, 24*(1), article 127. https://doi.org/10.1186/s12905-023-02845-8

Kilian, C., O'Donnell, A., Potapova, N., López-Pelayo, H., Schulte, B., Miquel, L., et al. (2022). Changes in alcohol use during the COVID-19 pandemic in Europe: A meta-analysis of observational studies. *Drug & Alcohol Review, 41*(4), 918–931. https://doi.org/10.1111/dar.13446

Killgore, W. D. S., Cloonan, S. A., Taylor, E. C., Fernandez, F., Grandner, M. A., & Dailey, N. S. (2020). Suicidal ideation during the COVID-19 pandemic: The role of insomnia. *Psychiatry Research, 290*, article 113134. https://doi.org/10.1016/j.psychres.2020.113134

Kim, D.-Y., & Phillips, S. W. (2021). When COVID-19 and guns meet: A rise in shootings. *Journal of Criminal Justice, 73*, article 101783. https://doi.org/10.1016/j.jcrimjus.2021.101783

Knapp, S., & Vandecreek, L. (1989). Fear of AIDS: Its meaning and implications for clinical practice. *Journal of Contemporary Psychotherapy, 19*(3), 239–247. https://doi.org/10.1007/BF00946034

Knoll, C., Watkins, A., & Rothfeld, M. (2020, July 11). I couldn't do anything: The virus and an E.R. doctor's suicide. *New York Times*. https://www.nytimes.com/2020/07/11/nyregion/lorna-breen-suicide-coronavirus.html

Krishnakumar, A., & Verma, S. (2021). Understanding domestic violence in India during COVID-19: A routine activity approach. *Asian Journal of Criminology, 16*, 19–35. https://doi.org/10.1007/s11417-020-09340-1

Kustanti, C. Y., Jen, H. J., Chu, H., Liu, D., Chen, R., Lin, H. C., et al. (2023). Prevalence of grief symptoms and disorders in the time of COVID-19 pandemic: A meta-analysis. *International Journal of Mental Health Nursing, 32*(3), 904–916. https://doi.org/10.1111/inm.13136

Lahav, Y. (2020). Psychological distress related to COVID-19—the contribution of continuous traumatic stress. *Journal of Affective Disorders, 277*, 129–137. https://doi.org/10.1016/j.jad.2020.07.141

Layman, H. M., Thorisdottir, I. E., Halldorsdottir, T., Sigfusdottir, I. D., Allegrante, J. P., & Kristjansson, A. L. (2022). Substance use among youth during the COVID-19 pandemic: A systematic review. *Current Psychiatry Reports, 24*(6), 307–324. https://doi.org/10.1007/s11920-022-01338-z

Lee, H., & Kim, E. (2023). Global prevalence of physical and psychological child abuse during COVID-19: A systematic review and meta-analysis. *Child Abuse & Neglect, 135*, article 105984. https://doi.org/10.1016/j.chiabu.2022.105984

Lee, S. J., Ward, K. P., Lee, J. Y., & Rodriguez, C. M. (2021). Parental social isolation and child maltreatment risk during the COVID-19 pandemic. *Journal of Family Violence, 37*, 813–824. https://doi.org/10.1007/s10896-020-00244-3

Leichtenstern, O. (1905). Influenza and dengue. In J. Mannaberg & O. Leichtenstern (Eds.), *Malaria, influenza and dengue* (pp. 521–716). Saunders.

Logsdail, S., Lovell, K., Warwick, H., & Marks, I. (1991). Behavioural treatment of AIDS-focused illness phobia. *British Journal of Psychiatry, 159*(3), 422–425. https://doi.org/10.1192/bjp.159.3.422

London Standard. (1890, January 6). The influenza epidemic. *London Standard*, 5.

Lundorff, M., Holmgren, H., Zachariae, R., Farver-Vestergaard, I., & O'Connor, M. (2017). Prevalence of prolonged grief disorder in adult bereavement: A systematic review and meta-analysis. *Journal of Affective Disorders, 212*, 138–149. https://doi.org/10.1016/j.jad.2017.01.030

Lundstrom, E. W., Groth, C. P., Harrison, J. E., Hendricks, B., & Smith, G. S. (2023). Excess US firearm mortality during the COVID-19 pandemic stratified by intent and urbanization. *JAMA Network Open, 6*(7), article e2323392. https://doi.org/10.1001/jamanetworkopen.2023.23392

Luo, M., Guo, L., Yu, M., Jiang, W., & Wang, H. (2020). The psychological and mental impact of coronavirus disease 2019 (COVID-19) on medical staff and general public - A systematic review and meta-analysis. *Psychiatry Research, 291*, article 113190. https://doi.org/10.1016/j.psychres.2020.113190

Madigan, S., Korczak, D. J., Vaillancourt, T., Racine, N., Hopkins, W. G., Pador, P., et al. (2023). Comparison of paediatric emergency department visits for attempted suicide, self-harm, and suicidal ideation before and during the COVID-19 pandemic: A systematic review and meta-analysis. *Lancet Psychiatry, 10*(5), 342–351. https://doi.org/10.1016/S2215-0366(23)00036-6

Malas, O., & Tolsá, M.-D. (2022). The COVID-19 pandemic and the obsessive-compulsive phenomena, in the general population and among OCD patients: A systematic review. *European Journal of Mental Health*, *17*(2), 132–148. https://doi.org/10.5708/EJMH.17.2022.2.13

Mamelund, S.-E. (2010). The impact of influenza on mental health in Norway 1872–1929. *Historical influenza pandemics: Lessons learned meeting and workshop, Copenhagen, Denmark* (p. 30).

Mamun, M. A., & Griffiths, M. D. (2020). First COVID-19 suicide case in Bangladesh due to fear of COVID-19 and xenophobia: Possible suicide prevention strategies. *Asian Journal of Psychiatry*, *51*, article 102073. https://doi.org/10.1016/j.ajp.2020.102073

Martin, L., & Kagee, A. (2011). Lifetime and HIV-related PTSD among persons recently diagnosed with HIV. *AIDS and Behavior*, *15*(1), 125–131. https://doi.org/10.1007/s10461-008-9498-6

McDowell, C. P., Herring, M. P., Lansing, J., Brower, C. S., & Meyer, J. D. (2021). Associations between employment changes and mental health: US data from during the COVID-19 pandemic. *Frontiers in Psychology*, *12*, article 631510. https://doi.org/10.3389/fpsyg.2021.631510

McIntyre, R. S., & Lee, Y. (2020). Projected increases in suicide in Canada as a consequence of COVID-19. *Psychiatry Research*, *290*, article 113104. https://doi.org/10.1016/j.psychres.2020.113104

McNally, R. J. (2003). *Remembering trauma*. Harvard University Press.

Metin, A., Erbiçer, E. S., Şen, S., & Çetinkaya, A. (2022). Gender and COVID-19 related fear and anxiety: A meta-analysis. *Journal of Affective Disorders*, *310*, 384–395. https://doi.org/10.1016/j.jad.2022.05.036

Miao, R., Liu, C., Zhang, J., & Jin, H. (2023). Impact of the COVID-19 pandemic on the mental health of children and adolescents: A systematic review and meta-analysis of longitudinal studies. *Journal of Affective Disorders*, *340*, 914–922. https://doi.org/10.1016/j.jad.2023.08.070

Moore, S. E., Wierenga, K. L., Prince, D. M., Gillani, B., & Mintz, L. J. (2021). Disproportionate impact of the COVID-19 pandemic on perceived social support, mental health and somatic symptoms in sexual and gender minority populations. *Journal of Homosexuality*, *68*(4), 577–591. https://doi.org/10.1080/00918369.2020.1868184

Moote, A. L., & Moote, D. C. (2004). *The great plague: The story of London's most deadly year*. Johns Hopkins University Press.

Mortier, P., Vilagut, G., Ferrer, M., Serra, C., Dios Molina, J., L, Ópez-fresneña, N., et al. (2021). Thirty-day suicidal thoughts and behaviors among hospital workers during the first wave of the Spain Covid-19 outbreak. *Depression and Anxiety*, *38*, 528–544. https://doi.org/10.1002/da.23129

Moskowitz, J. T., Hult, J. R., Bussolari, C., & Acree, M. (2009). What works in coping with HIV? A meta-analysis with implications for coping with serious illness. *Psychological Bulletin*, *135*(1), 121–141. https://doi.org/10.1037/a0014210

Mota, N., Weissheimer, J., Ribeiro, M., de Paiva, M., Avilla-Souza, J., Simabucuru, G., et al. (2020). Dreaming during the Covid-19 pandemic: Computational assessment of dream reports reveals mental suffering related to fear of contagion. *PLOS ONE*, *15*(11), article e0242903. https://doi.org/10.1371/journal.pone.0242903

Moutier, C. Y., Myers, M. F., Feist, J. B., Feist, J. C., & Zisook, S. (2021). Preventing clinician suicide: A call to action during the COVID-19 pandemic and beyond. *Academic Medicine*, *96*, 624–628. https://doi.org/10.1097/ACM.0000000000003972

Muris, P., Merckelbach, H., & Clavan, M. (1997). Abnormal and normal compulsions. *Behaviour Research and Therapy, 35*(3), 249–252. https://doi.org/10.1016/S0005-7967(96)00114-3

Nagarajan, R., Krishnamoorthy, Y., Basavarachar, V., & Dakshinamoorthy, R. (2022). Prevalence of post-traumatic stress disorder among survivors of severe COVID-19 infections: A systematic review and meta-analysis. *Journal of Affective Disorders, 299*, 52–59. https://doi.org/10.1016/j.jad.2021.11.040

Nathan, P. E., & Gorman, J. M. (2015). *A guide to treatments that work (4th ed.)*. Oxford University Press.

Necho, M., Tsehay, M., Birkie, M., Biset, G., & Tadesse, E. (2021). Prevalence of anxiety, depression, and psychological distress among the general population during the COVID-19 pandemic: A systematic review and meta-analysis. *International Journal of Social Psychiatry, 67*(7), 892–906. https://doi.org/10.1177/00207640211003121

Nochaiwong, S., Ruengorn, C., Thavorn, K., Hutton, B., Awiphan, R., Phosuya, C., et al. (2021). Global prevalence of mental health issues among the general population during the coronavirus disease-2019 pandemic: A systematic review and meta-analysis. *Scientific Reports, 11*(1), article 10173. https://doi.org/10.1038/s41598-021-89700-8

O'Donnell, M. L., Alkemade, N., Creamer, M., McFarlane, A. C., Silove, D., Bryant, R. A., et al. (2016). A longitudinal study of adjustment disorder after trauma exposure. *American Journal of Psychiatry, 173*, 1231–1238. https://doi.org/10.1176/appi.ajp.2016.16010071

O'Donnell, L., O'Donnell, C. R., Pleck, J. H., Snarey, J., & Rose, R. M. (1987). Psychosocial responses to hospital workers to acquired immune deficiency syndrome (AIDS). *Journal of Applied Social Psychology, 17*, 269–285. https://doi.org/10.1111/j.1559-1816.1987.tb00314.x

Okusaga, O., Yolken, R., Langenberg, P., Lapidus, M., Arling, T., Dickerson, F., et al. (2011). Association of seropositivity for influenza and coronaviruses with history of mood disorders and suicide attempts. *Journal of Affective Disorders, 130*(1), 220–225. https://doi.org/10.1016/j.jad.2010.09.029

Pappa, S., Ntella, V., Giannakas, T., Giannakoulis, V. G., Papoutsi, E., & Katsaounou, P. (2020). Prevalence of depression, anxiety, and insomnia among healthcare workers during the COVID-19 pandemic: A systematic review and meta-analysis. *Brain, Behavior, and Immunity, 88*, 901–907. https://doi.org/10.1016/j.bbi.2020.05.026

Parets, M. (1651). *A journal of the plague year: The diary of the Barcelona tanner Miquel Parets 1651* (J. S. Amelang, Trans. & Ed., 1991). Oxford University Press.

Parker, A. M., Sricharoenchai, T., Raparla, S., Schneck, K. W., Bienvenu, O. J., & Needham, D. M. (2015). Posttraumatic stress disorder in critical illness survivors: A metaanalysis. *Critical Care Medicine, 43*(5), 1121–1129. https://doi.org/10.1097/ccm.0000000000000882

Pelton, M., Ciarletta, M., Wisnousky, H., Lazzara, N., Manglani, M., Ba, D. M., et al. (2021). Rates and risk factors for suicidal ideation, suicide attempts and suicide deaths in persons with HIV: A systematic review and meta-analysis. *General Psychiatry, 34*, article e100247. https://doi.org/10.1136/gpsych-2020-100247

Penninx, B. W. J. H., Benros, M. E., Klein, R. S., & Vinkers, C. H. (2022). How COVID-19 shaped mental health: From infection to pandemic effects. *Nature Medicine, 28*(10), 2027–2037. https://doi.org/10.1038/s41591-022-02028-2

Petry, S. E., Hughes, D., & Galanos, A. (2021). Grief: The epidemic within an epidemic. *American Journal of Hospice & Palliative Care, 38*(4), 419–422. https://doi.org/10.1177/1049909120978796

Piquero, A. R., Jennings, W. G., Jemison, E., Kaukinen, C., & Knaul, F. M. (2021). Domestic violence during the COVID-19 pandemic—Evidence from a systematic review and meta-analysis. *Journal of Criminal Justice, 74*, article 101806. https://doi.org/10.1016/j.jcrimjus.2021.101806

Pirkis, J., Gunnell, D., Shin, S., Del Pozo-Banos, M., Arya, V., Aguilar, P. A., et al. (2022). Suicide numbers during the first 9-15 months of the COVID-19 pandemic compared with pre-existing trends: An interrupted time series analysis in 33 countries. *EClinicalMedicine, 51*, article 101573. https://doi.org/10.1016/j.eclinm.2022.101573

Prati, G., & Mancini, A. D. (2021). The psychological impact of COVID-19 pandemic lockdowns: A review and meta-analysis of longitudinal studies and natural experiments. *Psychological Medicine, 51*, 201–211. https://doi.org/10.1017/S0033291721000015

Procopius. (551 AD). *History of the wars: Book II* (H. B. Dewing, Trans, 1914). Heinemann.

Pugi, D., Angelo, N. L., Ragucci, F., Garcia-Hernandez, M. D., Rosa-Alcázar, A. I., & Pozza, A. (2023). Longitudinal course of obsessive-compulsive symptoms during the COVID-19 pandemic: A systematic review of three years of prospective cohort studies. *Clinical Neuropsychiatry, 20*(4), 293–308. https://doi.org/10.36131/cnfioritieditore20230409

Quinn, A., Grant, J. E., & Chamberlain, S. R. (2022). COVID-19 and resultant restrictions on gambling behaviour. *Neuroscience and Biobehavioral Reviews, 143*, article 104932. https://doi.org/10.1016/j.neubiorev.2022.104932

Rachman, S., & de Silva, P. (1978). Abnormal and normal obsessions. *Behaviour Research and Therapy, 16*(4), 233–248. https://doi.org/10.1016/0005-7967(78)90022-0

Racine, N., McArthur, B. A., Cooke, J. E., Eirich, R., Zhu, J., & Madigan, S. (2021). Global prevalence of depressive and anxiety symptoms in children and adolescents during COVID-19: A meta-analysis. *JAMA Pediatrics, 175*(11), 1142–1150. https://doi.org/10.1001/jamapediatrics.2021.2482

Rafiei, S., Raoofi, S., Pashazadeh Kan, F., Masoumi, M., Doustmehraban, M., Biparva, A. J., et al. (2023). Global prevalence of suicide in patients living with HIV/AIDS: A systematic review and meta-analysis. *Journal of Affective Disorders, 323*, 400–408. https://doi.org/10.1016/j.jad.2022.11.061

Ravens-Sieberer, U., Kaman, A., Erhart, M., Devine, J., Schlack, R., & Otto, C. (2021). Impact of the COVID-19 pandemic on quality of life and mental health in children and adolescents in Germany. *European Child & Adolescent Psychiatry, 31*, 879–889. https://doi.org/10.1007/s00787-021-01726-5

Reger, M. A., Stanley, I. H., & Joiner, T. E. (2020). Suicide mortality and coronavirus disease 2019—A perfect storm? *JAMA Psychiatry, 77*(11), 1093–1094. https://doi.org/10.1001/jamapsychiatry.2020.1060

Remesan, A. K., Sekaran, V. C., Jothikaran, T. A. J., & Ashok, L. (2023). Substance use among emerging adults during the COVID-19 pandemic: A review through the lens of sustainable development goals. *International Journal of Environmental Research and Public Health, 20*(19), article 6834. https://doi.org/10.3390/ijerph20196834

Ren, X., Huang, W., Pan, H., Huang, T., Wang, X., & Ma, Y. (2020). Mental health during the Covid-19 outbreak in China: A meta-analysis. *Psychiatric Quarterly, 91*(4), 1033–1045. https://doi.org/10.1007/s11126-020-09796-5

Rice, G. W. (2005). *Black November: The 1918 influenza pandemic in New Zealand (2nd ed.)*. Canterbury University Press.

Richter, D., Riedel-Heller, S., & Zuercher, S. (2021). Mental health problems in the general population during and after the first lockdown phase due to the SARS-Cov-2 pandemic: Rapid review of multi-wave studies. *Epidemiology and Psychiatric Sciences, 30*, article e27. https://doi.org/10.1017/S2045796021000160

Robillard, R., Daros, A., Phillips, J., Porteous, M., Saad, M., Pennestri, M., et al. (2021). Emerging new psychiatric symptoms and the worsening of pre-existing mental disorders during the COVID-19 pandemic: A Canadian multisite study. *Canadian Journal of Psychiatry, 66*(9), 815–826. https://doi.org/10.1177/0706743720986786

Robinson, E., Sutin, A. R., Daly, M., & Jones, A. (2022). A systematic review and meta-analysis of longitudinal cohort studies comparing mental health before versus during the COVID-19 pandemic in 2020. *Journal of Affective Disorders, 296,* 567–576. https://doi.org/10.1016/j.jad.2021.09.098

Rogers, J., Chesney, E., Oliver, D., Pollak, T., McGuire, P., Fusar-Poli, P., et al. (2020). Psychiatric and neuropsychiatric presentations associated with severe coronavirus infections: A systematic review and meta-analysis with comparison to the COVID-19 pandemic. *Lancet Psychiatry, 7*(7), 611–627. https://doi.org/10.1016/S2215-0366(20)30203-0

Rosa-Alcázar, Á., Parada-Navas, J. L., García-Hernández, M. D., Pozza, A., Tondi, P., & Rosa-Alcázar, A. I. (2023). Severity and changes in OCD dimensions during COVID-19: A two-year longitudinal study. *Brain Sciences, 13*(8), article 1151. https://doi.org/10.3390/brainsci13081151

Salanti, G., Peter, N., Tonia, T., Holloway, A., White, I. R., Darwish, L., et al. (2022). The impact of the COVID-19 pandemic and associated control measures on the mental health of the general population: A systematic review and dose-response meta-analysis. *Annals of Internal Medicine, 175*(11), 1560–1571. https://doi.org/10.7326/m22-1507

Salari, N., Hosseinian-Far, A., Jalali, R., Vaisi-Raygani, A., Rasoulpoor, S., Mohammadi, M., et al. (2020). Prevalence of stress, anxiety, depression among the general population during the COVID-19 pandemic: A systematic review and meta-analysis. *Global Health, 16*(1), article 57. https://doi.org/10.1186/s12992-020-00589-w

Salkovskis, P. M., & Harrison, J. (1984). Abnormal and normal obsessions: A replication. *Behaviour Research and Therapy, 22*(5), 549–552. https://doi.org/10.1016/0005-7967(84)90057-3

Sander, U. (1988). The delusion of being infected. In H. Jäger, Welch, J., & Francis, J. L. (Ed.), *AIDS phobia: Disease pattern and possibilities of treatment* (pp. 7–10). Halstead.

Saunders-Hastings, P. R., & Krewski, D. (2016). Reviewing the history of pandemic influenza: Understanding patterns of emergence and transmission. *Pathogens, 5*(4), article 66. https://doi.org/10.3390/pathogens5040066

Schleimer, J. P., McCort, C. D., Shev, A. B., Pear, V. A., Tomsich, E., De Biasi, A., et al. (2021). Firearm purchasing and firearm violence during the coronavirus pandemic in the United States: A cross-sectional study. *Injury Epidemiology, 8*(1), article 43. https://doi.org/10.1186/s40621-021-00339-5

Sethuraman, U., Kannikeswaran, N., Singer, A., Krouse, C. B., Cloutier, D., Farooqi, A., et al. (2021). Trauma visits to a pediatric emergency department during the COVID-19 quarantine and "stay at home" period. *American Surgeon, 89*(11), 4262–4270. https://doi.org/10.1177/00031348211047497

Shafran, R., Coughtrey, A., & Whittal, M. (2020). Recognising and addressing the impact of COVID-19 on obsessive-compulsive disorder. *Lancet Psychiatry, 7,* 570–572. https://doi.org/10.1016/s2215-0366(20)30222-4

Sharma, L., Balachander, S., Thamby, A., Bhattacharya, M., Kishore, C., Shanbhag, V., et al. (2021). Impact of the COVID-19 pandemic on the short-term course of obsessive-compulsive disorder. *Journal of Nervous and Mental Disease, 209,* 256–264. https://doi.org/10.1097/NMD.0000000000001318

Shear, M. K., & Gribbin, C. E. (2016). Persistent complex bereavement disorder and its treatment. In P. R. Casey & J. J. Strain (Eds.), *Trauma- and stressor-related disorders: A handbook for clinicians* (pp. 133–154). American Psychiatric Publishing.

Shi, L., Que, J., Lu, Z., Gong, Y., Liu, L., Wang, Y., et al. (2021). Prevalence and correlates of suicidal ideation among the general population in China during the COVID-19 pandemic. *European Psychiatry, 64*(1), article e18. https://doi.org/10.1192/j.eurpsy.2021.5

Skilbeck, L., & Byrne, S. (2022). IAPT CBT treatment for PTSD following COVID-19-related intensive care admission—A case study. *The Cognitive Behaviour Therapist, 15,* article e29. https://doi.org/10.1017/S1754470X22000289

Smith, F. B. (1995). The Russian influenza in the United Kingdom, 1889–1894. *Social History of Medicine, 8*(1), 55–73. https://doi.org/10.1093/shm/8.1.55

Sokouti, M., Shafiee-Kandjani, A. R., Sokouti, M., & Sokouti, B. (2023). A meta-analysis of systematic reviews and meta-analyses to evaluate the psychological consequences of COVID-19. *BMC Psychology, 11*(1), article 279. https://doi.org/10.1186/s40359-023-01313-0

Sorokin, P. A. (1942). *Man and society in calamity.* Routledge.

Spokesman Review. (1918, October 18). Cause and treatment of fluphobia. *Spokesman Review,* 14.

Stack, S., & Rockett, I. R. H. (2021). Social distancing predicts suicide rates: Analysis of the 1918 flu pandemic in 43 large cities. *Suicide & Life-Threatening Behavior, 51*(5), 833–835. https://doi.org/10.1111/sltb.12729

Storch, E., Sheu, J., Guzick, A., Schneider, S., Cepeda, S., Rombado, B., et al. (2021). Impact of the COVID-19 pandemic on exposure and response prevention outcomes in adults and youth with obsessive-compulsive disorder. *Psychiatry Research, 295,* article 113597. https://doi.org/10.1016/j.psychres.2020.113597

Sun, S., Cao, W., Ge, Y., Siegel, M., & Wellenius, G. A. (2022). Analysis of firearm violence during the COVID-19 pandemic in the US. *JAMA Network Open, 5*(4), article e229393. https://doi.org/10.1001/jamanetworkopen.2022.9393

Sun, Y., Wu, Y., Fan, S., Santo, T. D., Li, L., Jiang, X., et al. (2023). Comparison of mental health symptoms before and during the COVID-19 pandemic: Evidence from a systematic review and meta-analysis of 134 cohorts. *BMJ, 380,* article e074224. https://doi.org/10.1136/bmj-2022-074224

Suthaharan, P., Reed, E., Leptourgos, P., Kenney, J., Uddenberg, S., Mathys, C., et al. (2021). Paranoia and belief updating during the COVID-19 crisis. *Nature Human Behaviour, 5*(9), 1190–1202. https://doi.org/10.1038/s41562-021-01176-8

Tang, L., Pan, L., Yuan, L., & Zha, L. (2016). Prevalence and related factors of post-traumatic stress disorder among medical staff members exposed to H7N9 patients. *International Journal of Nursing Sciences, 4*(1), 63–67. https://doi.org/10.1016/j.ijnss.2016.12.002

Taylor, S. (2017). *Clinician's guide to PTSD* (2nd ed.). Guilford.

Taylor, S. (2019). *The psychology of pandemics: Preparing for the next global outbreak of infectious disease.* Cambridge Scholars Publishing.

Taylor, S. (2021). COVID Stress Syndrome: Clinical and nosological considerations. *Current Psychiatry Reports, 23,* article 19. https://doi.org/10.1007/s11920-021-01226-y

Taylor, S. (2022). The psychology of pandemics. *Annual Review of Clinical Psychology, 18,* 581–609. https://doi.org/10.1146/annurev-clinpsy-072720-020131

Taylor, S., Landry, C. A., Paluszek, M. M., Fergus, T. A., McKay, D., & Asmundson, G. J. G. (2020a). Covid stress syndrome: Concept, structure, and correlates. *Depression and Anxiety, 37,* 706–714. https://doi.org/10.1002/da.23071

Taylor, S., Landry, C. A., Paluszek, M. M., Fergus, T. A., McKay, D., & Asmundson, G. J. G. (2020b). Development and initial validation of the COVID Stress Scales. *Journal of Anxiety Disorders, 72,* article 102232. https://doi.org/10.1016/j.janxdis.2020.102232

Taylor, S., Paluszek, M., Rachor, G. S., McKay, D., & Asmundson, G. J. G. (2021). Substance use and abuse, COVID-19-related distress, and disregard for social distancing: A network analysis. *Addictive Behaviors, 114,* article 106754. https://doi.org/10.1016/j.addbeh.2020.106754

Teng, Z., Pontes, H. M., Nie, Q., Griffiths, M. D., & Guo, C. (2021). Depression and anxiety symptoms associated with internet gaming disorder before and during the COVID-19 pandemic: A longitudinal study. *Journal of Behavioral Addictions, 10,* 169–180. https://doi.org/10.1556/2006.2021.00016

Tzeng, N., Chung, C., Chang, C., Chang, H., Kao, Y., Chang, S., et al. (2020). What could we learn from SARS when facing the mental health issues related to the COVID-19 outbreak? A nationwide cohort study in Taiwan. *Translational Psychiatry, 10*(1), article 339. https://doi.org/10.1038/s41398-020-01021-y

Verdery, A. M., Smith-Greenaway, E., Margolis, R., & Daw, J. (2020). Tracking the reach of COVID-19 kin loss with a bereavement multiplier applied to the United States. *PNAS, 117*, 17695–17701. https://doi.org/10.1073/pnas.2007476117

Wasserman, I. M. (1992). The impact of epidemic, war, prohibition and media on suicide: United States, 1910-1920. *Suicide and Life-Threatening Behavior, 22*(2), 240–254. https://doi.org/10.1111/j.1943-278X.1992.tb00231.x

Wheaton, M. G., Abramowitz, J. S., Berman, N. C., Fabricant, L. E., & Olatunji, B. O. (2012). Psychological predictors of anxiety in response to the H1N1 (swine flu) pandemic. *Cognitive Therapy and Research, 36*, 210–218. https://doi.org/10.1007/s10608-011-9353-3

WHO. (2019a). ICD-11: Gaming disorder. https://icd.who.int/browse/2024-01/mms/en#1448597234

WHO. (2019b). ICD-11: Prolonged grief disorder. https://icd.who.int/browse11/l-m/en#/http://id.who.int/icd/entity/1183832314

WHO. (2023). Suicide. https://www.who.int/news-room/fact-sheets/detail/suicide

Wiese, A. D., Wojcik, K. D., & Omar, Y. (2022). COVID-19 vaccines and potential implications for COVID-19-specific obsessive-compulsive disorder presentations. *Journal of Cognitive Psychotherapy, 36*(2), 102–111. https://doi.org/10.1891/JCP-2021-0019

Wilson, J. M., Iannarone, M., & Wang, C. (2009). Media reporting of the emergence of the 1968 influenza pandemic in Hong Kong: Implications for modern-day situational awareness. *Disaster Medicine & Public Health Preparedness, 3*(Suppl 2), S148–S153. https://doi.org/10.1097/DMP.0b013e3181abd603

Woolley, I. M. (1963). The 1918 "Spanish Influenza" pandemic in Oregon. *Oregon Historical Quarterly, 64*, 246–258.

Wright, L. W., Jr., Mulick, P. S., & Kincaid, S. B. (2007). Fear of and discrimination against bisexuals, homosexuals, and individuals with AIDS. *Journal of Bisexuality, 6*(4), 71–84. https://doi.org/10.1300/J159v06n04_06

Wu, T., Jia, X., Shi, H., Niu, J., Yin, X., Xie, J., et al. (2021). Prevalence of mental health problems during the COVID-19 pandemic: A systematic review and meta-analysis. *Journal of Affective Disorders, 281*, 91–98. https://doi.org/10.1016/j.jad.2020.11.117

Xie, Y., Xu, E., & Al-Aly, Z. (2022). Risks of mental health outcomes in people with Covid-19: Cohort study. *BMJ, 376*, article e068993. https://doi.org/10.1136/bmj-2021-068993

Xiong, J., Lipsitz, O., Nasri, F., Lui, L., Gill, H., Phan, L., et al. (2020). Impact of COVID-19 pandemic on mental health in the general population: A systematic review. *Journal of Affective Disorders, 277*, 55–64. https://doi.org/10.1016/j.jad.2020.08.001

Xuereb, S., Kim, H. S., Clark, L., & Wohl, M. J. A. (2021). Substitution behaviors among people who gamble during Covid-19 precipitated casino closures. *International Gambling Studies, 21*(3), 411–425. https://doi.org/10.1080/14459795.2021.1903062

Yan, Y., Hou, J., Li, Q., & Yu, N. X. (2023). Suicide before and during the COVID-19 pandemic: A systematic review with meta-analysis. *International Journal of Environmental Research and Public Health, 20*(4), article 3346. https://doi.org/10.3390/ijerph20043346

Yeates, E., Grigorian, A., Barrios, C., Schellenberg, M., Owattanapanich, N., Barmparas, G., et al. (2021). Changes in traumatic mechanisms of injury in Southern California related to COVID-19: Penetrating trauma as a second pandemic. *Journal of Trauma and Acute Care Surgery, 90*(4), 714–721. https://doi.org/10.1002/wmh3.350

Yip, P. S., Cheung, Y. T., Chau, P. H., & Law, Y. W. (2010). The impact of epidemic outbreak: The case of severe acute respiratory syndrome (SARS) and suicide among older adults in Hong Kong. *Crisis, 31*, 86–92. https://doi.org/10.1027/0227-5910/a000015

Yuan, K., Gong, Y., Liu, L., Sun, Y., Tian, S., Wang, Y., et al. (2021). Prevalence of posttraumatic stress disorder after infectious disease pandemics in the twenty-first century, including COVID-19: A meta-analysis and systematic review. *Molecular Psychiatry, 26*(9), 4982–4998. https://doi.org/10.1038/s41380-021-01036-x

Zhang, S., Zhao, Z., Zhang, H., Zhu, Y., Xi, Z., & Xiang, K. (2023). Workplace violence against healthcare workers during the COVID-19 pandemic: A systematic review and meta-analysis. *Environmental Science and Pollution Research International, 30*, 74838–74852. https://doi.org/10.1007/s11356-023-27317-2

Zheng, J., Morstead, T., Sin, N., Klaiber, P., Umberson, D., Kamble, S., et al. (2021). Psychological distress in North America during COVID-19: The role of pandemic-related stressors. *Social Science & Medicine, 270*, article 113687. https://doi.org/10.1016/j.socscimed.2021.113687

Zhou, T., Nguyen, T.-V. T., Zhong, J., & Liu, J. (2020). A COVID-19 descriptive study of life after lockdown in Wuhan, China. *Royal Society Open Science, 7*(9), article 200705. https://doi.org/10.1098/rsos.200705

Zolopa, C., Burack, J. A., O'Connor, R. M., Corran, C., Lai, J., Bomfim, E., et al. (2022). Changes in youth mental health, psychological wellbeing, and substance use during the Covid-19 pandemic: A rapid review. *Adolescent Research Review, 7*, 161–177. https://doi.org/10.1007/s40894-022-00185-6

Chapter 20

Ahmed, H., Patel, K., Greenwood, D., Halpin, S., Lewthwaite, P., Salawu, A., et al. (2020). Long-term clinical outcomes in survivors of severe acute respiratory syndrome and Middle East respiratory syndrome coronavirus outbreaks after hospitalisation or ICU admission: A systematic review and meta-analysis. *Journal of Rehabilitation Medicine, 52*(5), article jrm00063. https://doi.org/10.2340/16501977-2694

Alkodaymi, M., Omrani, O., Fawzy, N., Shaar, B., Almamlouk, R., Riaz, M., et al. (2022). Prevalence of post-acute COVID-19 syndrome symptoms at different follow-up periods: A systematic review and meta-analysis. *Clinical Microbiology and Infection, 28*(5), 657–666. https://doi.org/10.1016/j.cmi.2022.01.014

Altmann, D. M., & Boyton, R. J. (2021). Decoding the unknowns in Long COVID. *BMJ (Clinical Research Ed.), 372*, article n132. https://doi.org/10.1136/bmj.n132

American Psychiatric Association. (2022). *Diagnostic and statistical manual of mental disorders* (5th ed., text rev.). Author.

Andreasson, A., Wicksell, R. K., Lodin, K., Karshikoff, B., Axelsson, J., & Lekander, M. (2018). A global measure of sickness behaviour: Development of the Sickness Questionnaire. *Journal of Health Psychology, 23*(11), 1452–1463. https://doi.org/10.1177/1359105316659917

Antia, R., & Halloran, M. E. (2021). Transition to endemicity: Understanding COVID-19. *Immunity, 54*(10), 2172–2176. https://doi.org/10.1016/j.immuni.2021.09.019

Arumi, A., Bulbena-Cabre, A., & Bulbena, A. (2021). First person account COVID 19 delirium in a doctor: When death stalks the mind. *Frontiers in Psychiatry, 12*, article 626648. https://doi.org/10.3389/fpsyt.2021.626648

Atherton, H., Briggs, T., & Chew-Graham, C. (2021). Long COVID and the importance of the doctor-patient relationship. *British Journal of General Practice, 71*, 54–55. https://doi.org/10.3399/bjgp21X714641

Baldwin, M. R., & Anesi, G. L. (2022). Post-intensive care syndrome in COVID-19 vs non-COVID-19 critical illness survivors: More similar than not? *American Journal of Respiratory and Critical Care Medicine, 205*(10), 1133–1144. https://doi.org/10.1164/rccm.202202-0396ED

Berger, P., & Braude, D. (2021). Post-intensive care syndrome. *Australian Journal of General Practice, 50*(9), 647–649. https://doi.org/10.31128/AJGP-07-20-55491

Boghurst, W. (1666). *Loimographia: The great plague of London in the year 1665.* Shaw & Sons.

Bond, M., Bechter, K., Müller, N., Tebartz van Elst, L., & Meier, U.-C. (2021). A role for pathogen risk factors and autoimmunity in encephalitis lethargica? *Progress in Neuro-Psychopharmacology & Biological Psychiatry, 109*, article 110276. https://doi.org/10.1016/j.pnpbp.2021.110276

Callard, F., & Perego, E. (2021). How and why patients made Long Covid. *Social Science & Medicine, 268*, article 113426. https://doi.org/10.1016/j.socscimed.2020.113426

Ceban, F., Kulzhabayeva, D., Rodrigues, N. B., Di Vincenzo, J. D., Gill, H., Subramaniapillai, M., et al. (2023). COVID-19 vaccination for the prevention and treatment of long COVID: A systematic review and meta-analysis. *Brain, Behavior, and Immunity, 111*, 211–229. https://doi.org/10.1016/j.bbi.2023.03.022

Charlevoix County Herald. (1919, October 17). Bares secrets of sleep sickness: Chicago man recovers and tells his experiences. *Charlevoix County Herald*, 12.

Chen, C., Haupert, S. R., Zimmermann, L., Shi, X., Fritsche, L. G., & Mukherjee, B. (2022). Global prevalence of post-coronavirus disease 2019 (COVID-19) condition or Long COVID: A meta-analysis and systematic review. *Journal of Infectious Diseases, 226*(9), 1593–1607. https://doi.org/10.1093/infdis/jiac136

Chen, X., Laurent, S., Onur, O., Kleineberg, N., Fink, G., Schweitzer, F., et al. (2021). A systematic review of neurological symptoms and complications of COVID-19. *Journal of Neurology, 268*(2), 392–402. https://doi.org/10.1007/s00415-020-10067-3

Chicoyneau, F. (1721). *A succinct account of the plague at Marseilles: Its symptoms and the methods and medicines used for curing it.* Buckley.

Collantes, M. E. V., Espiritu, A. I., Sy, M. C. C., Anlacan, V. M. M., & Jamora, R. D. G. (2021). Neurological manifestations in COVID-19 infection: A systematic review and meta-analysis. *Canadian Journal of Neurological Sciences, 48*(1), 66–76. https://doi.org/10.1017/cjn.2020.146

Copeland, R. S. (1923, April 24). What sleeping sickness is and what is known about it. *Logansport Pharos Tribune*, 6.

Corrard, F., Copin, C., Wollner, A., Elbez, A., Derkx, V., Bechet, S., et al. (2017). Sickness behavior in feverish children is independent of the severity of fever. An observational, multicenter study. *PLOS ONE, 12*, article e0171670. https://doi.org/10.1371/journal.pone.0171670

Creighton, C. (1891). *A history of epidemics in Britain.* Cambridge University Press.

Dantzer, R. (2009). Cytokine, sickness behavior, and depression. *Immunology and Allergy Clinics of North America, 29*, 247–264. https://doi.org/10.1016/j.iac.2009.02.002

Dantzer, R., O'Connor, J. C., Freund, G. C., Johnson, R. W., & Kelley, K. W. (2008). From inflammation to sickness and depression: When the immune system subjugates the brain. *Nature Reviews Neuroscience, 9*, 46–57. https://doi.org/10.1038/nrn2297

De Mertens, C. (1799). *An account of the plague which raged at Moscow, in 1771.* Rivington.

Favas, T., Dev, P., Chaurasia, R., Chakravarty, K., Mishra, R., Joshi, D., et al. (2020). Neurological manifestations of COVID-19: A systematic review and meta-analysis of proportions. *Neurological Sciences, 41*(12), 3437–3470. https://doi.org/10.1007/s10072-020-04801-y

Fernandez-de-las-peñas, C., Notarte, K. I., Macasaet, R., Velasco, J. V., Catahay, J. A., Ver, A. T., et al. (2024). Persistence of post-COVID symptoms in the general population two years after SARS-CoV-2 infection: A systematic review and meta-analysis. *Journal of Infection, 88*(2), 77–88. https://doi.org/10.1016/j.jinf.2023.12.004

Giordano, A., Schwarz, G., Cacciaguerra, L., Esposito, F., & Filippi, M. (2020). COVID-19: Can we learn from encephalitis lethargica? *Lancet Neurology, 19*(7), p. 570. https://doi.org/10.1016/S1474-4422(20)30189-7

Guo, Y., Lin, J., Wu, T., Zhou, T., & Mu, Y. (2023). Risk factors for delirium among hospitalized adults with COVID-19: A systematic review and meta-analysis of cohort studies. *International Journal of Nursing Studies, 148,* article 104602. https://doi.org/10.1016/j.ijnurstu.2023.104602

Halani, S., Tombindo, P. E., O'Reilly, R., Miranda, R. N., Erdman, L. K., Whitehead, C., et al. (2021). Clinical manifestations and health outcomes associated with Zika virus infections in adults: A systematic review. *PLOS Neglected Tropical Diseases, 15*(7), article e0009516. https://doi.org/10.1371/journal.pntd.0009516

Harapan, B. N., & Yoo, H. J. (2021). Neurological symptoms, manifestations, and complications associated with severe acute respiratory syndrome coronavirus 2 (SARS-CoV-2) and coronavirus disease 19 (COVID-19). *Journal of Neurology, 268,* 3059–3071. https://doi.org/10.1007/s00415-021-10406-y

Hart, B. L. (1988). Biological basis of the behavior of sick animals. *Neuroscience and Biobehavioral Reviews, 12*(2), 123–137. https://doi.org/10.1016/s0149-7634(88)80004-6

Hodges, N., & Quincy, J. (1720). *Loimologia: Or, an historical account of the plague in London in 1665 with precautionary directions against the like contagion.* Bell.

Hoffman, L. A., & Vilensky, J. A. (2017). Encephalitis lethargica: 100 years after the epidemic. *Brain, 140*(8), 2246–2251. https://doi.org/10.1093/brain/awx177

Hogan, C., & Wilkins, E. (2011). Neurological complications in HIV. *Clinical Medicine, 11*(6), 571–575. https://doi.org/10.7861/clinmedicine.11-6-571

Honigsbaum, M. (2013). "An inexpressible dread": Psychoses of influenza at fin-de-siècle. *Lancet, 381,* 988–989. https://doi.org/10.1016/S0140-6736(13)60701-1

Inoue, S., Hatakeyama, J., Kondo, Y., Hifumi, T., Sakuramoto, H., Kawasaki, T., et al. (2019). Post-intensive care syndrome: Its pathophysiology, prevention, and future directions. *Acute Medicine & Surgery, 6*(3), 233–246. https://doi.org/10.1002/ams2.415

Jelliffe, S. E. (1918). Nervous and mental disturbances of influenza. *New York Medical Journal, 108,* 725–728.

Kephale, R. (1665). *Medela pestilentiae.* Samuel Speed.

King, A. (2020). An uncommon cold. *New Scientist, 246*(3280), 32–35. https://doi.org/10.1016/S0262-4079(20)30862-9

Kraepelin, E. (1912). *Clinical psychiatry: A text-book for students and physicians (A. R. Diefendorf, trans.).* Macmillan.

Kwek, S., Chew, W., Ong, K., Ng, A., Lee, L., Kaw, G., et al. (2006). Quality of life and psychological status in survivors of severe acute respiratory syndrome at 3 months postdischarge. *Journal of Psychosomatic Research, 60*(5), 513–519. https://doi.org/10.1016/j.jpsychores.2005.08.020

Lasselin, J. (2021). Back to the future of psychoneuroimmunology: Studying inflammation-induced sickness behavior. *Brain, Behavior, & Immunity - Health, 18,* article 100379. https://doi.org/10.1016/j.bbih.2021.100379

LaVergne, S. (2021). How many people get "long COVID" — and who is most at risk? *The Conversation.* https://theconversation.com/how-many-people-get-long-covid-and-who-is-most-at-risk-154331

Leibovitch, E. C., & Jacobson, S. (2016). Vaccinations for neuroinfectious disease: A global health priority. *Neurotherapeutics, 13*(3), 562–570. https://doi.org/10.1007/s13311-016-0453-3

Liang, K., Hui, P., & Green, S. (2024). Postinfectious cough in adults. *Canadian Medical Association Journal, 196*(5), E157. https://doi.org/10.1503/cmaj.231523

Lima Daily News. (1919. March 18). Precaution will keep out malady. *Lima Daily News,* 11.

Ludvigsson, J. F. (2021). Case report and systematic review suggest that children may experience similar long-term effects to adults after clinical COVID-19. *Acta Paediatrica, 110*(3), 914–921. https://doi.org/10.1111/apa.15673

McFarland, D. C., Walsh, L. E., Saracino, R., Nelson, C. J., Breitbart, W., & Rosenfeld, B. (2021). The Sickness Behavior Inventory-Revised: Sickness behavior and its associations with depression and inflammation in patients with metastatic lung cancer. *Palliative & Supportive Care*, *19*(3), 312–321. https://doi.org/10.1017/S1478951520001169

Moldofsky, H., & Patcai, J. (2011). Chronic widespread musculoskeletal pain, fatigue, depression and disordered sleep in chronic post-SARS syndrome: A case-controlled study. *BMC Neurology*, *11*, article 37. https://doi.org/10.1186/1471-2377-11-37

Murray, H., Grey, N., Wild, J., Warnock-Parkes, E., Kerr, A., Clark, D. M., et al., . (2020). Cognitive therapy for posttraumatic stress disorder following critical illness and intensive care unit admission. *The Cognitive Behaviour Therapist*, *13*, article e13. https://doi.org/10.1017/S1754470X2000015X

National Institute for Clinical Excellence. (2020). *COVID-19 rapid guideline: Managing the long-term effects of COVID-19*. Author.

Nature Medicine. (2020). Meeting the challenge of long COVID. *Nature Medicine*, *26*(12), 1803. https://doi.org/10.1038/s41591-020-01177-6

Navis, A. (2023). A review of neurological symptoms in Long COVID and clinical management. *Seminars in Neurology*, *43*(2), 286–296. https://doi.org/10.1055/s-0043-1767781

New Britain Herald. (1920, January 22). Asleep 100 days, music awakes her. *New Britain Herald*, 15.

Ohbe, H., Goto, T., Nakamura, K., Matsui, H., & Yasunaga, H. (2022). Development and validation of early prediction models for new-onset functional impairment at hospital discharge of ICU admission. *Intensive Care Medicine*, *48*, 679–689. https://doi.org/10.1007/s00134-022-06688-z

Ortelli, P., Ferrazzoli, D., Sebastianelli, L., Engl, M., Romanello, R., Nardone, R., et al. (2021). Neuropsychological and neurophysiological correlates of fatigue in post-acute patients with neurological manifestations of COVID-19: Insights into a challenging symptom. *Journal of the Neurological Sciences*, *420*, article 117271. https://doi.org/10.1016/j.jns.2020.117271

Parets, M. (1651). *A journal of the plague year: The diary of the Barcelona tanner Miquel Parets 1651* (J. S. Amelang, Trans. & Ed., 1991). Oxford University Press.

Pearse, R. (2017). John of Ephesus describes the Justinianic plague. https://www.roger-pearse.com/weblog/2017/05/10/john-of-ephesus-describes-the-justinianic-plague/

Pezzini, A., & Padovani, A. (2020). Lifting the mask on neurological manifestations of COVID-19. *Nature Reviews Neurology*, *16*(11), 636–644. https://doi.org/10.1038/s41582-020-0398-3

Philadelphia Inquirer. (1923, March 9). 23 more in New York have sleeping sickness. *Philadelphia Inquirer*, 23.

Procopius. (551 AD). *History of the wars: Book II* (H. B. Dewing, Trans, 1914). Heinemann.

Pun, B., Balas, M., Barnes-Daly, M., Thompson, J., Aldrich, J., Barr, J., et al. (2019). Caring for critically ill patients with the ABCDEF bundle: Results of the ICU Liberation Collaborative in over 15,000 adults. *Critical Care Medicine*, *47*(1), 3–14. https://doi.org/10.1097/ccm.0000000000003482

Ramnarain, D., Aupers, E., den Oudsten, B., Oldenbeuving, A., de Vries, J., & Pouwels, S. (2021). Post intensive care syndrome (PICS): An overview of the definition, etiology, risk factors, and possible counseling and treatment strategies. *Expert Review of Neurotherapeutics*, *21*(10), 1159–1177. https://doi.org/10.1080/14737175.2021.1981289

Ravenholt, R. T., & Foege, W. H. (1982). 1918 influenza, encephalitis lethargica, Parkinsonism. *Lancet*, *2*(8303), 860–864. https://doi.org/10.1016/s0140-6736(82)90820-0

Rayner, D. G., Wang, E., Su, C., Patel, O. D., Aleluya, S., Giglia, A., et al. (2024). Risk factors for Long COVID in children and adolescents: A systematic review and meta-analysis. *World Journal of Pediatrics*, *20*(2), 133–142. https://doi.org/10.1007/s12519-023-00765-z

Rozen, T. D. (2020). Daily persistent headache after a viral illness during a worldwide pandemic may not be a new occurrence: Lessons from the 1890 Russian/Asiatic flu. *Cephalalgia, 40*, 1406–1409. https://doi.org/10.1177/0333102420965132

Shao, S.-C., Lai, C.-C., Chen, Y.-H., Chen, Y.-C., Hung, M.-J., & Liao, S.-C. (2021). Prevalence, incidence and mortality of delirium in patients with COVID-19: A systematic review and meta-analysis. *Age and Ageing, 50*(5), 1445–1453. https://doi.org/10.1093/ageing/afab103

Shattuck, E. C., & Muehlenbein, M. P. (2016). Towards an integrative picture of human sickness behavior. *Brain, Behavior, and Immunity, 57*, 255–262. https://doi.org/10.1016/j.bbi.2016.05.002

Shattuck, E. C., Perrotte, J. K., Daniels, C. L., Xu, X., & Sunil, T. S. (2020). The contribution of sociocultural factors in shaping self-reported sickness behavior. *Frontiers in Behavioral Neuroscience, 14*, article 4. https://doi.org/10.3389/fnbeh.2020.00004

Shorter, E. (2021). The first psychiatric pandemic: Encephalitis lethargica, 1917-27. *Medical Hypotheses, 146*, article 110420. https://doi.org/10.1016/j.mehy.2020.110420

Smith, F. B. (1995). The Russian influenza in the United Kingdom, 1889–1894. *Social History of Medicine, 8*(1), 55–73. https://doi.org/10.1093/shm/8.1.55

Stone, J. K., Berman, S. E., Zheng, W., Wilson, D. R., & Diaz, G. R. (2023). From brain fog to COVID toe: A head-to-toe review of long COVID. *American Journal of Pharmacotherapy & Pharmaceutical Sciences*, 1–17. https://doi.org/10.25259/AJPPS_2023_012

Sudre, C., Murray, B., Varsavsky, T., Graham, M., Penfold, R., Bowyer, R., et al. (2021). Attributes and predictors of Long COVID. *Nature Medicine, 27*, 626–631. https://doi.org/10.1038/s41591-021-01292-y

Taylor, S., & Asmundson, G. J. G. (2004). *Treating health anxiety*. Guilford.

The Hospital. (1897). Influenza and insanity. *The Hospital, 21*(546), 389–390.

The Hospital. (1900). The nervous complications of influenza. *The Hospital, 29*(732), 13–14.

Thucydides. (411 BC). *The history of the Peloponnesian War* (R. Crawley, Trans., 2009). Project Gutenberg. www.gutenberg.org

Tomori, O. (2004). Yellow fever: The recurring plague. *Critical Reviews in Clinical Laboratory Sciences, 41*(4), 391–427. https://doi.org/10.1080/10408360490497474

Turner, E. B. (1919). Discussion on influenza. *Proceedings of the Royal Society of Medicine, 12*, 76–90.

Vink, M., & Vink-Niese, A. (2020). Could cognitive behavioural therapy be an effective treatment for Long COVID and Post COVID-19 Fatigue Syndrome? Lessons from the Qure Study for Q-Fever Fatigue Syndrome. *Healthcare, 8*(4), article 552. https://doi.org/10.3390/healthcare8040552

Washington Evening Star. (1925, October 3). Four-year-old Birdie Lee Bannow calmy wakes from sleep of 3 weeks. *Washington Evening Star*, 12.

Watanabe, A., Iwagami, M., Yasuhara, J., Takagi, H., & Kuno, T. (2023). Protective effect of COVID-19 vaccination against long COVID syndrome: A systematic review and meta-analysis. *Vaccine, 41*(11), 1783–1790. https://doi.org/10.1016/j.vaccine.2023.02.008

Woodrow, M., Carey, C., Ziauddeen, N., Thomas, R., Akrami, A., Lutje, V., et al. (2023). Systematic review of the prevalence of Long COVID. *Open Forum Infectious Diseases, 10*(7), article ofad233. https://doi.org/10.1093/ofid/ofad233

Zakia, H., Pradana, K., & Iskandar, S. (2023). Risk factors for psychiatric symptoms in patients with long COVID: A systematic review. *PLOS ONE, 18*(4), article e0284075. https://doi.org/10.1371/journal.pone.0284075

Zeng, N., Zhao, Y.-M., Yan, W., Li, C., Lu, Q.-D., Liu, L., et al. (2023). A systematic review and meta-analysis of long term physical and mental sequelae of COVID-19 pandemic: Call for research priority and action. *Molecular Psychiatry, 28*(1), 423–433. https://doi.org/10.1038/s41380-022-01614-7

Zheng, C., Chen, X., Sit, C., Liang, X., Li, M., Ma, A., et al. (2024). Effect of physical exercise-based rehabilitation on Long COVID: A systematic review and meta-analysis. *Medicine and Science in Sports and Exercise, 56*(1), 143–154. https://doi.org/10.10.22280907

Zheng, Y.-B., Zeng, N., Yuan, K., Tian, S.-S., Yang, Y.-B., Gao, N., et al. (2023). Prevalence and risk factor for long COVID in children and adolescents: A meta-analysis and systematic review. *Journal of Infection and Public Health, 16*(5), 660–672. https://doi.org/10.1016/j.jiph.2023.03.005

Zhou, Z., Kang, H., Li, S., & Zhao, X. (2020). Understanding the neurotropic characteristics of SARS-CoV-2: From neurological manifestations of COVID-19 to potential neurotropic mechanisms. *Journal of Neurology, 267*(8), 2179–2184. https://doi.org/10.1007/s00415-020-09929-7

Chapter 21

Albu, S., Vallès, M., & Kumru, H. (2023). Diagnostic challenges of functional neurological disorders after Covid-19 disease or vaccination: Case series and review of the literature. *Acta Neurologica Belgica, 123*, 553–564. https://doi.org/10.1007/s13760-022-02140-7

Alonso-Canovas, A., Kurtis, M., Gomez-Mayordomo, V., Macías-García, D., Gutiérrez Viedma, Á., Mondragón Rezola, E., et al. (2023). Functional neurological disorders after COVID-19 and SARS-CoV-2 vaccines: A national multicentre observational study. *Journal of Neurology, Neurosurgery, and Psychiatry, 94*, 776–777. https://doi.org/10.1136/jnnp-2022-330885

Amanzio, M., Cipriani, G. E., & Bartoli, M. (2021). How do nocebo effects in placebo groups of randomized controlled trials provide a possible explicative framework for the COVID-19 pandemic? *Expert Review of Clinical Pharmacology, 14*(4), 439–444. https://doi.org/10.1080/17512433.2021.1900728

American Psychiatric Association. (2022). *Diagnostic and statistical manual of mental disorders* (5th ed., text rev.). Author.

Apiwattanakul, M., Suanprasert, N., Rojana-Udomsart, A., Termglinchan, T., Sinthuwong, C., Tantirittisak, T., et al. (2022). Good recovery of immunization stress-related responses presenting as a cluster of stroke-like events following CoronaVac and ChAdOx1 vaccinations. *PLOS ONE, 17*(8), article e0266118. https://doi.org/10.1371/journal.pone.0266118

Bagarić, B., Jokić-Begić, N., & Sangster Jokić, C. (2022). The nocebo effect: A review of contemporary experimental research. *International Journal of Behavioral Medicine, 29*, 255–265. https://doi.org/10.1007/s12529-021-10016-y

Bloomberg. (2022). *More than 12.7 billion shots given: Covid-19 tracker.* Bloomberg. https://www.bloomberg.com/graphics/covid-vaccine-tracker-global-distribution/

Butler, M., Coebergh, J., Safavi, F., Carson, A., Hallett, M., Michael, B., et al. (2021). Functional neurological disorder after SARS-CoV-2 vaccines: Two case reports and discussion of potential public health implications. *Journal of Neuropsychiatry and Clinical Neurosciences, 33*(4), 345–348. https://doi.org/10.1176/appi.neuropsych.21050116

Butler, M., Tamborska, A., Wood, G., Ellul, M., Thomas, R., Galea, I., et al. (2021). Considerations for causality assessment of neurological and neuropsychiatric complications of SARS-CoV-2 vaccines: From cerebral venous sinus thrombosis to functional neurological disorder. *Journal of Neurology, Neurosurgery, and Psychiatry, 92*, 1144–1151. https://doi.org/10.1136/jnnp-2021-326924

Buttery, J., Madin, S., Crawford, N., Elia, S., La Vincente, S., Hanieh, S., et al. (2008). Mass psychogenic response to human papillomavirus vaccination. *Medical Journal of Australia, 189*(5), 261–262. https://doi.org/10.5694/j.1326-5377.2008.tb02018.x

CDC. (2021). Vaccines and immunizations. https://www.cdc.gov/vaccines/vac-gen/imz-basics.htm#print

Clements, C. J. (2003). Mass psychogenic illness after vaccination. *Drug Safety, 26*(9), 599–604. https://doi.org/10.2165/00002018-200326090-00001

Colloca, L., & Barsky, A. J. (2020). Placebo and nocebo effects. *New England Journal of Medicine, 382*(6), 554–561. https://doi.org/10.1056/NEJMra1907805

D'Argenio, P., Citarella, A., Intorcia, M., & Aversano, G. (1996). An outbreak of vaccination panic. *Vaccine, 14*(13), 1289–1290. https://doi.org/10.1016/s0264-410x(96)00069-2

De Souza, A., Jacques, R., & Mohan, S. (2023). Vaccine-induced functional neurological disorders in the Covid-19 era. *Canadian Journal of Neurological Sciences, 50*(3), 346–350. https://doi.org/10.1017/cjn.2022.48

Demartini, B., Wiedenmann, F., Baccara, A., Nisticò, V., Gambini, O., Elia, A., et al. (2023). A case of functional isolated tongue tremor-like dyskinesia after COVID-19 vaccine. *Psychiatry and Clinical Neurosciences, 77*(2), 122–123. https://doi.org/10.1111/pcn.13477

Dodoo, A., Adjei, S., Couper, M., Hugman, B., & Edwards, R. (2007). When rumours derail a mass deworming exercise. *Lancet, 370,* 465–466. https://doi.org/10.1016/S0140-6736(07)61211-2

Dreger, R. (1992). Hysteria and adverse reactions to Td in a junior high school setting. *British Columbia Health and Disease Surveillance, 1,* 50–54.

Ercoli, T., Lutzoni, L., Orofino, G., Muroni, A., & Defazio, G. (2021). Functional neurological disorder after COVID-19 vaccination. *Neurological Sciences, 42*(10), 3989–3990. https://doi.org/10.1007/s10072-021-05504-8

Espay, A., Aybek, S., Carson, A., Edwards, M., Goldstein, L., Hallett, M., et al. (2018). Current concepts in diagnosis and treatment of functional neurological disorders. *JAMA Neurology, 75*(9), 1132–1141. https://doi.org/10.1001/jamaneurol.2018.1264

Fasano, A., & Daniele, A. (2022). Functional disorders after COVID-19 vaccine fuel vaccination hesitancy. *Journal of Neurology, Neurosurgery, and Psychiatry, 93*(3), 339–340. https://doi.org/10.1136/jnnp-2021-327000

Feldhaus, M. H., Horing, B., Sprenger, C., & Büchel, C. (2021). Association of nocebo hyperalgesia and basic somatosensory characteristics in a large cohort. *Scientific Reports, 11*(1), article 762. https://doi.org/10.1038/s41598-020-80386-y

Fung, W., Sa'di, Q., Katzberg, H., Chen, R., Lang, A. E., Cheung, A. M., et al. (2023). Functional disorders as a common motor manifestation of COVID-19 infection or vaccination. *European Journal of Neurology, 30*(3), 678–691. https://doi.org/10.1111/ene.15630

Gutkin, M., McLean, L., Brown, R., & Kanaan, R. A. (2021). Systematic review of psychotherapy for adults with functional neurological disorder. *Journal of Neurology, Neurosurgery & Psychiatry, 92*(1), 36–44. https://doi.org/10.1136/jnnp-2019-321926

Haas, J., Bender, F., Ballou, S., Kelley, J., Wilhelm, M., Miller, F., et al. (2022). Frequency of adverse events in the placebo arms of COVID-19 vaccine trials: A systematic review and meta-analysis. *JAMA Network Open, 5*(1), article e2143955. https://doi.org/10.1001/jamanetworkopen.2021.43955

Horváth, Á., Köteles, F., & Szabo, A. (2021). Nocebo effects on motor performance: A systematic literature review. *Scandinavian Journal of Psychology, 62*(5), 665–674. https://doi.org/10.1111/sjop.12753

Huang, W. T., Hsu, C. C., Lee, P. I., & Chuang, J. H. (2010). Mass psychogenic illness in nationwide in-school vaccination for pandemic influenza A(H1N1) 2009, Taiwan, November 2009-January 2010. *Euro Surveillance, 15*(21), article 19575. https://doi.org/10.2807/ese.15.21.19575-en

Kennedy, W. P. (1961). The nocebo reaction. *Medical World, 95,* 203–205.

Kern, A., Kramm, C., Witt, C. M., & Barth, J. (2020). The influence of personality traits on the placebo/nocebo response: A systematic review. *Journal of Psychosomatic Research, 128*, article109866. https://doi.org/10.1016/j.jpsychores.2019.109866

Kharabsheh, S., Al-Otoum, H., Clements, J., Abbas, A., Khuri-Bulos, N., Belbesi, A., et al. (2001). Mass psychogenic illness following tetanus-diphtheria toxoid vaccination in Jordan. *Bulletin of the World Health Organization, 79*(8), 764–770.

Khiem, H., Huan, L., Phuong, N., Dang, D., Hoang, D., Phuong, L., et al. (2003). Mass psychogenic illness following oral cholera immunization in Ca Mau City, Vietnam. *Vaccine, 21*(31), 4527–4531. https://doi.org/10.1016/S0264-410X(03)00498-5

Kim, D. D., Kung, C. S., & Perez, D. L. (2021). Helping the public understand adverse events associated with COVID-19 vaccinations: Lessons learned from functional neurological disorder. *JAMA Neurology, 78*(7), 789–790. https://doi.org/10.1001/jamaneurol.2021.1042

Lin, C.-Y., Peng, C.-C., Liu, H.-C., & Chiu, N.-C. (2011). Psychogenic movement disorder after H1N1 influenza vaccination. *Journal of Neuropsychiatry and Clinical Neurosciences, 23*(3), E37–E38. https://doi.org/10.1176/appi.neuropsych.23.3.E37

Loharikar, A., Suragh, T., MacDonald, N., Balakrishnan, M., Benes, O., Lamprianou, S., et al. (2018). Anxiety-related adverse events following immunization (AEFI): A systematic review of published clusters of illness. *Vaccine, 36*(2), 299–305. https://doi.org/10.1016/j.vaccine.2017.11.017

Mao, A., Barnes, K., Sharpe, L., Geers, A., Helfer, S., Faasse, K., et al. (2021). Using positive attribute framing to attenuate nocebo side effects: A cybersickness study. *Annals of Behavioral Medicine, 55*(8), 769–778. https://doi.org/10.1093/abm/kaaa115

Marchetti, R., Gallucci-Neto, J., Kurcgant, D., Proença, I., Valiengo, L., Fiore, L., et al. (2020). Immunization stress-related responses presenting as psychogenic non-epileptic seizures following HPV vaccination in Rio Branco, Brazil. *Vaccine, 38*(43), 6714–6720. https://doi.org/10.1016/j.vaccine.2020.08.044

McMurtry, C. M., Noel, M., Taddio, A., Antony, M. M., Asmundson, G. J. G., Riddell, R. P., et al. (2015). Interventions for individuals with high levels of needle fear: Systematic review of randomized controlled trials and quasi-randomized controlled trials. *Clinical Journal of Pain, 31*(Suppl 10), S109–S123. https://doi.org/10.1097/AJP.0000000000000273

Mennitto, S., Vachon, D. D., Ritz, T., Robillard, P., France, C. R., & Ditto, B. (2022). Social contagion of vasovagal symptoms in blood donors: Interactions with empathy. *Annals of Behavioral Medicine, 56*(6), 645–653. https://doi.org/10.1093/abm/kaab089

Öst, L.-G., & Sterner, U. (1987). Applied tension: A specific behavioral method for treatment of blood phobia. *Behaviour Research and Therapy, 25*, 25–29. https://doi.org/10.1016/0005-7967(87)90111-2

Pan, Y., Kinitz, T., Stapic, M., & Nestoriuc, Y. (2019). Minimizing drug adverse events by informing about the nocebo effect—An experimental study. *Frontiers in Psychiatry, 10*, article e00504. https://doi.org/10.3389/fpsyt.2019.00504

Peiró, E. F., Yáñez, J. L., Carramiñana, I., Rullán, J. V., & Castell, J. (1996). Estudio de un brote de histeria después de la vacunación de hepatitis B. *Medicina Clinica, 107*(1), 1–3.

Peñas, J., de Los Reyes, V., Sucaldito, M., Ballera, J., Hizon, H., Magpantay, R., et al. (2018). Epidemic hysteria following the National School Deworming Day, Zamboanga Peninsula, Philippines, 2015. *Western Pacific Surveillance and Response Journal, 9*(4), 1–6. https://doi.org/10.5365/wpsar.2017.8.1.009

Perez, D. L., Aybek, S., Popkirov, S., Kozlowska, K., Stephen, C. D., Anderson, J., et al. (2021). A review and expert opinion on the neuropsychiatric assessment of motor functional neurological disorders. *Journal of Neuropsychiatry and Clinical Neurosciences, 33*(1), 14–26. https://doi.org/10.1176/appi.neuropsych.19120357

Petrie, K. J., Moss-Morris, R., Grey, C., & Shaw, M. (2004). The relationship of negative affect and perceived sensitivity to symptom reporting following vaccination. *British Journal of Health Psychology, 9*, 101–111. https://doi.org/10.1348/135910704322778759

Petrie, K. J., & Rief, W. (2019). Psychobiological mechanisms of placebo and nocebo effects: Pathways to improve treatments and reduce side effects. *Annual Review of Psychology, 70*, 599–625. https://doi.org/10.1146/annurev-psych-010418-102907

Reis Carneiro, D., & Araújo, R. (2023). Mass "psychogenic transient loss of consciousness" after COVID-19 vaccination. *European Journal of Neurology, 30*(2), 560–561. https://doi.org/10.1111/ene.15639

Reismann, J. L., & Singh, B. (1978). Conversion reactions simulating Guillain-Barré paralysis following suspension of the swine flu vaccination program in the USA. *Australian and New Zealand Journal of Psychiatry, 12*(2), 127–132. https://doi.org/10.3109/00048677809159606

Ryu, J. H., & Baik, J. S. (2010). Psychogenic gait disorders after mass school vaccination of influenza A. *Journal of Movement Disorders, 3*(1), 15–17. https://doi.org/10.14802/jmd.10004

Sanjeev, O. P., Verma, A., Mani, V. E., & Singh, R. K. (2022). COVID-19 vaccine-related functional neurological disorders in the emergency department. *Canadian Journal of Emergency Medicine, 24*(4), 455–456. https://doi.org/10.1007/s43678-022-00272-6

Scamvougeras, A., & Howard, A. (2018). *Understanding and managing somatoform disorders: A guide for clinicians*. AJSK Publishing.

Simas, C., Munoz, N., Arregoces, L., & Larson, H. J. (2019). HPV vaccine confidence and cases of mass psychogenic illness following immunization in Carmen de Bolivar, Colombia. *Human Vaccines & Immunotherapeutics, 15*(1), 163–166. https://doi.org/10.1080/21645515.2018.1511667

Stone, J., & Sharpe, M. (2001). Hoover's sign. Practical Neurology, October, 50–53.

Takahashi, O., Ryuji, S., Setsu, S., & Tsuyoshi, O. (2022). Functional neurological disorders after COVID-19 vaccination: Case series and literature review. *Psychiatry & Clinical Neurosciences, 76*(10), 529–531. https://doi.org/10.1111/pcn.13453

WHO. (2019). *Causality assessment of an adverse event following immunizagion (AEFI): User manual for the revised WHO classification* (2nd ed.). Author.

Wieder, L., Brown, R., Thompson, T., & Terhune, D. B. (2021). Suggestibility in functional neurological disorder: A meta-analysis. *Journal of Neurology, Neurosurgery, and Psychiatry, 92*(2), 150–157. https://doi.org/10.1136/jnnp-2020-323706

Yang, T. U., Kim, H. J., Lee, Y. K., & Park, Y.-J. (2017). Psychogenic illness following vaccination: Exploratory study of mass vaccination against pandemic influenza A (H1N1) in 2009 in South Korea. *Clinical and Experimental Vaccine Research, 6*(1), 31–37. https://doi.org/10.7774/cevr.2017.6.1.31

Yasamy, M. T., Bahramnezhad, A., & Ziaaddini, H. (1999). Postvaccination mass psychogenic illness in an Iranian rural school. *Eastern Mediterranean Health Journal, 5*(4), 710–716.

Zhu, A., & Burke, M. J. (2022). Functional neurologic disorder associated with SARS-CoV-2 vaccination. *Canadian Medical Association Journal, 194*(31), E1086–E1088. https://doi.org/10.1503/cmaj.220039

Chapter 22

Albott, C. S., Wozniak, J. R., McGlinch, B. P., Wall, M. H., Gold, B. S., & Vinogradov, S. (2020). Battle Buddies: Rapid deployment of a psychological resilience intervention for health care workers during the COVID-19 pandemic. *Anesthesia and Analgesia, 131*(1), 43–54. https://doi.org/10.1213/ANE.0000000000004912

Amanvermez, Y., Rahmadiana, M., Karyotaki, E., de Wit, L., Ebert, D., Kessler, R. C., et al. (2023). Stress management interventions for college students: A systematic review and meta-analysis. *Clinical Psychology: Science and Practice, 30*(4), 423–444. https://doi.org/10.1111/cpsp.12342

Bai, Y., Lin, C.-C., Lin, C.-Y., Chen, J.-Y., Chue, C.-M., & Chou, P. (2004). Survey of stress reactions among health care workers involved with the SARS outbreak. *Psychiatric Services, 55*, 1055–1057. https://doi.org/10.1176/appi.ps.55.9.1055

Barlow, D. H. (2021). *Clinical handbook of psychological disorders: A step-by-step treatment manual* (6th ed.). Guilford.

Barlow, D. H., Farchione, T. J., Sauer-Zavala, S., Latin, H. M., Ellard, K. K., Bullis, J. R., et al. (2017). *Unified protocol for transdiagnostic treatment of emotional disorders* (2nd ed.). Guilford.

Batastini, A. B., Paprzycki, P., Jones, A. C. T., & MacLean, N. (2021). Are videoconferenced mental and behavioral health services just as good as in-person? A meta-analysis of a fast-growing practice. *Clinical Psychology Review, 83*, article 101944. https://doi.org/10.1016/j.cpr.2020.101944

Beck, J. S. (2020). *Cognitive therapy: Basics and beyond* (3rd ed.). Guilford.

Berdullas Saunders, S., Gesteira Santos, C., Morán Rodríguez, N., Fernández Hermida, J., Santolaya, F., Sanz Fernández, J., et al. (2020). El teléfono de asistencia psicológica por la COVID-19 del Ministerio de Sanidad y del Consejo General de la Psicología de España: Características y demanda. *Revista Espanola de Salud Publica, 94*(14), e1–e13.

Bilsker, D., & Gilbert, M. (2020). *5RF workbook: Improving resilient coping in paramedic services.* Author.

Binder, F., Mehl, R., Resch, F., Kaess, M., & Koenig, J. (2024). Interventions based on acceptance and commitment therapy for stress reduction in children and adolescents: A systematic review and meta-analysis of randomized controlled trials. *Psychopathology, 57*(3), 202–218. https://doi.org/10.1159/000535048

Boghurst, W. (1666). *Loimographia: The great plague of London in the year 1665.* Shaw & Sons.

Borges, L. M. (2019). A service member's experience of Acceptance and Commitment Therapy for Moral Injury (ACT-MI) via telehealth: "Learning to accept my pain and injury by reconnecting with my values and starting to live a meaningful life." *Journal of Contextual Behavioral Science, 13*, 134–140. https://doi.org/10.1016/j.jcbs.2019.08.002

Borges, L. M., Barnes, S. M., Farnsworth, J. K., Bahraini, N. H., & Brenner, L. A. (2020). A commentary on moral injury among health care providers during the COVID-19 pandemic. *Psychological Trauma: Theory, Research, Practice, and Policy, 12*(S1), S138–S140. https://doi.org/10.1037/tra0000698

Bryant, R. A., Kenny, L., Joscelyne, A., Rawson, N., Maccallum, F., Cahill, C., et al. (2014). Treating prolonged grief disorder: A randomized clinical trial. *JAMA Psychiatry, 71*, 1332–1339. https://doi.org/10.1001/jamapsychiatry.2014.1600

Cheng, P., Casement, M. D., Kalmbach, D. A., Castelan, A. C., & Drake, C. L. (2020). Digital cognitive behavioral therapy for insomnia promotes later health resilience during the coronavirus disease 19 (COVID-19) pandemic. *Sleep, 44*(4), article zsaa258. https://doi.org/10.1093/sleep/zsaa258

Chor, W., Ng, W., Cheng, L., Situ, W., Chong, J., Ng, L., et al. (2020). Burnout amongst emergency healthcare workers during the COVID-19 pandemic: A multi-center study. *American Journal of Emergency Medicine, 46*, 700–702. https://doi.org/10.1016/j.ajem.2020.10.040

Clark, D. A. (2019). *Cognitive-behavioral therapy for OCD and its subtypes* (2nd ed.). Guilford.

Coughtrey, A. E., & Pistrang, N. (2018). The effectiveness of telephone-delivered psychological therapies for depression and anxiety: A systematic review. *Journal of Telemedicine and Telecare, 24*(2), 65–74. https://doi.org/10.1177/1357633X16686547

Crosby, A. W. (2003). *America's forgotten pandemic: The influenza of 1918* (2nd ed.). Cambridge University Press.

D'Ettorre, G., Ceccarelli, G., Santinelli, L., Vassalini, P., Innocenti, G., Alessandri, F., et al. (2021). Post-traumatic stress symptoms in healthcare workers dealing with the COVID-19 pandemic: A systematic review. *International Journal of Environmental Research and Public Health, 18*(2), article 601. https://doi.org/10.3390/ijerph18020601

Dean, W., Talbot, S., & Dean, A. (2019). Reframing clinician distress: Moral injury not burnout. *Federal Practitioner, 36*, 400–402.

Duffy, C. C., Bass, G. A., Fitzpatrick, G., & Doherty, E. M. (2020). What can we learn from the past? Pandemic health care workers' fears, concerns, and needs: A review. *Journal of Patient Safety, 18*(1), 52–57. https://doi.org/10.1097/PTS.0000000000000803

Dugas, M. J., & Robichaud, M. (2007). *Cognitive-behavioral treatment for generalized anxiety disorder: From science to practice.* Routledge.

Elhadi, M., Msherghi, A., Elgzairi, M., Alhashimi, A., Bouhuwaish, A., Biala, M., et al. (2020). Burnout syndrome among hospital healthcare workers during the COVID-19 pandemic and civil war: A cross-sectional study. *Frontiers in Psychiatry, 11*, article 579563. https://doi.org/10.3389/fpsyt.2020.579563

Farnsworth, J. K., Drescher, K. D., Evans, W., & Walser, R. D. (2017). A functional approach to understanding and treating military-related moral injury. *Journal of Contextual Behavioral Science, 6*(4), 391–397. https://doi.org/10.1016/j.jcbs.2017.07.003

Ferreira, M. G., Mariano, L. I., de Rezende, J. V., Caramelli, P., & Kishita, N. (2022). Effects of group Acceptance and Commitment Therapy (ACT) on anxiety and depressive symptoms in adults: A meta-analysis. *Journal of Affective Disorders, 309*, 297–308. https://doi.org/10.1016/j.jad.2022.04.134

Fiest, K. M., Leigh, J., Krewulak, K. D., Plotnikoff, K. M., Kemp, L. G., Ng-Kamstra, J., et al. (2021). Experiences and management of physician psychological symptoms during infectious disease outbreaks: A rapid review. *BMC Psychiatry, 21*(1), article 91. https://doi.org/10.1186/s12888-021-03090-9

Fina, B. A., Wright, E., Rauch, S., Norman, S., Acierno, R., Cuccurullo, L., et al. (2020). Conducting prolonged exposure for PTSD during the COVID-19 pandemic: Considerations for treatment. *Cognitive and Behavioral Practice, 28*(4), 532–542. https://doi.org/10.1016/j.cbpra.2020.09.003

Fiquepron, M. R. (2018). Places, attitudes and moments during the epidemics: Representations of yellow fever and cholera in the city of Buenos Aires, 1867-1871. *História, Ciências, Saúde, 25*(2), 1–16. https://doi.org/10.1590/S0104-59702018000200003

Fischer-Grote, L., Fössing, V., Aigner, M., Fehrmann, E., & Boeckle, M. (2024). Effectiveness of online and remote interventions for mental health in children, adolescents, and young adults after the onset of the COVID-19 pandemic: Systematic review and meta-analysis. *JMIR Mental Health, 11*, article e46637. https://doi.org/10.2196/46637

Gates, P., & Albertella, L. (2016). The effectiveness of telephone counselling in the treatment of illicit drug and alcohol use concerns. *Journal of Telemedicine and Telecare, 22*(2), 67–85. https://doi.org/10.1177/1357633X15587406

Gray, M. J., Schorr, Y., Nash, W., Lebowitz, L., Amidon, A., Lansing, A., et al. (2012). Adaptive disclosure: An open trial of a novel exposure-based intervention for service members with combat-related psychological stress injuries. *Behavior Therapy, 43*, 407–415. https://doi.org/10.1016/j.beth.2011.09.001

Hagerty, S. L., Wielgosz, J., Kraemer, J., Nguyen, H. V., Loew, D., & Kaysen, D. (2020). Best practices for approaching cognitive processing therapy and prolonged exposure during the COVID-19 pandemic. *Journal of Traumatic Stress, 33*(5), 623–633. https://doi.org/10.1002/jts.22583

Haller, M., Norman, S. B., Davis, B. C., Capone, C., Browne, K., & Allard, C. B. (2020). A model for treating COVID-19–related guilt, shame, and moral injury. *Psychological Trauma: Theory, Research, Practice, and Policy, 12*(S1), S174–S176. https://doi.org/10.1037/tra0000742

Hao, X., Qin, Y., Lv, M., Zhao, X., Wu, S., & Li, K. (2023). Effectiveness of telehealth interventions on psychological outcomes and quality of life in community adults during the COVID-19 pandemic: A systematic review and meta-analysis. *International Journal of Mental Health Nursing, 32*(4), 979–1007. https://doi.org/10.1111/inm.13126

Hartzband, P., & Groopman, J. (2020). Physician burnout, interrupted. *New England Journal of Medicine, 382*, 2485–2487. https://doi.org/10.1056/NEJMp2003149

Hayes, S. C., Strosahl, K. D., & Wilson, K. G. (2016). *Acceptance and commitment therapy: The process and practice of mindful change.* Guilford.

He, Z., Chen, J., Pan, K., Yue, Y., Cheung, T., Yuan, Y., et al. (2020). The development of the "COVID-19 Psychological Resilience Model" and its efficacy during the COVID-19 pandemic in China. *International Journal of Biological Sciences, 16*, 2828–2834. https://doi.org/10.7150/ijbs.50127

Held, P., Klassen, B. J., Coleman, J. A., Thompson, K., Rydberg, T. S., & Van Horn, R. (2021). Delivering intensive PTSD treatment virtually: The development of a 2-week intensive cognitive processing therapy–based program in response to COVID-19. *Cognitive and Behavioral Practice, 28*(4), 543–554. https://doi.org/10.1016/j.cbpra.2020.09.002

Ho, S., Kwong-Lo, R., Mak, C., & Wong, J. (2005). Fear of severe acute respiratory syndrome (SARS) among health care workers. *Journal of Consulting and Clinical Psychology, 73*, 344–349. https://doi.org/10.1037/0022-006X.73.2.344

Iglewicz, A., Shear, M. K., Reynolds, C. F., Simon, N., Lebowitz, B., & Zisook, S. (2020). Complicated grief therapy for clinicians: An evidence-based protocol for mental health practice. *Depression and Anxiety, 37*(1), 90–98. https://doi.org/10.1002/da.22965

Jäger, H. (1988). AIDS—psychosocial aspects. In H. Jäger, Welch, J., & Francis, J. L. (Ed.), *AIDS phobia: Disease pattern and possibilities of treatment* (pp. 35–46). Halstead.

Jahan, I., Ullah, I., Griffiths, M. D., & Mamun, M. A. (2021). COVID-19 suicide and its causative factors among the healthcare professionals: Case study evidence from press reports. *Perspectives in Psychiatric Care, 57*(4), 1707–1711. https://doi.org/10.1111/ppc.12739

Jasti, N., Bhargav, H., George, S., Varambally, S., & Gangadhar, B. N. (2020). Tele-yoga for stress management: Need of the hour during the COVID-19 pandemic and beyond? *Asian Journal of Psychiatry, 54*, article 102334. https://doi.org/10.1016/j.ajp.2020.102334

Joyce, S., Shand, F., Tighe, J., Laurent, S. J., Bryant, R. A., & Harvey, S. B. (2018). Road to resilience: A systematic review and meta-analysis of resilience training programmes and interventions. *BMJ Open, 8*(6), article e017858. https://doi.org/10.1136/bmjopen-2017-017858

Kahlon, M., Aksan, N., Aubrey, R., Clark, N., Cowley-Morillo, M., Jacobs, E., et al. (2021). Effect of layperson-delivered, empathy-focused program of telephone calls on loneliness, depression, and anxiety among adults during the COVID-19 pandemic: A randomized clinical trial. *JAMA Psychiatry, 78*(6), 616–622. https://doi.org/10.1001/jamapsychiatry.2021.0113

Knoll, C., Watkins, A., & Rothfeld, M. (2020, July 11). I couldn't do anything: The virus and an E.R. doctor's suicide. *New York Times.* https://www.nytimes.com/2020/07/11/nyregion/lorna-breen-suicide-coronavirus.html

Krzyzaniak, N., Greenwood, H., Scott, A. M., Peiris, R., Cardona, M., Clark, J., & Glasziou, P. (2024). The effectiveness of telehealth versus face-to face interventions for anxiety disorders: A systematic review and meta-analysis. *Journal of Telemedicine and Telecare, 30*(2), 250–261. https://doi.org/10.1177/1357633X211053738

Lee, S. M., Kang, W. S., Cho, A. R., Kim, T., & Park, J. K. (2018). Psychological impact of the 2015 MERS outbreak on hospital workers and quarantined hemodialysis patients. *Comprehensive Psychiatry, 87*, 123–127. https://doi.org/10.1016/j.comppsych.2018.10.003

Literary Digest. (1918). How to fight Spanish influenza. *Literary Digest, 59*(October 12), 13–14.

Litz, B. T., Stein, N., Delaney, E., Lebowitz, L., Nash, W. P., Silva, C., et al. (2009). Moral injury and moral repair in war veterans: A preliminary model and intervention strategy. *Clinical Psychology Review, 29*, 695–706. https://doi.org/10.1016/j.cpr.2009.07.003

Logsdail, S., Lovell, K., Warwick, H., & Marks, I. (1991). Behavioural treatment of AIDS-focused illness phobia. *British Journal of Psychiatry, 159*(3), 422–425. https://doi.org/10.1192/bjp.159.3.422

Macaron, M. M., Segun-Omosehin, O. A., Matar, R. H., Beran, A., Nakanishi, H., Than, C. A., et al. (2023). A systematic review and meta analysis on burnout in physicians during the COVID-19 pandemic: A hidden healthcare crisis. *Frontiers in Psychiatry, 13*, article 1071397. https://doi.org/10.3389/fpsyt.2022.1071397

Malakouti, S. K., Rasouli, N., Rezaeian, M., Nojomi, M., Ghanbari, B., & Shahraki Mohammadi, A. (2020). Effectiveness of self-help mobile telephone applications (apps) for suicide prevention: A systematic review. *Medical Journal of the Islamic Republic of Iran, 34*, article 85. https://doi.org/10.34171/mjiri.34.85

Mathieu, S., Uddin, R., Brady, M., Batchelor, S., Ross, V., Spence, S., et al. (2021). The state of research into youth helplines. *Journal of the American Academy of Child & Adolescent Psychiatry, 60*(10), 1190–1233. https://doi.org/10.1016/j.jaac.2020.12.028

Mollica, R. F., Augusterfer, E. F., Fricchione, G. L., & Graziano, S. (2020). *New self-care protocol: Practice guide for healthcare practitioners and staff.* https://hprtselfcare.org/

Mollica, R. F., Fernando, D. B., & Augusterfer, E. F. (2021). Beyond burnout: Responding to the COVID-19 pandemic challenges to self-care. *Current Psychiatry Reports, 23*, article 21. https://doi.org/10.1007/s11920-021-01230-2

Morell, R. (2020). Reporting and resilience. *Nieman Reports, 74*(3), 40–45.

Morgantini, L., Naha, U., Wang, H., Francavilla, S., Acar, Ö., Flores, J., et al. (2020). Factors contributing to healthcare professional burnout during the COVID-19 pandemic: A rapid turnaround global survey. *PLOS ONE, 15*, article e0238217. https://doi.org/10.1371/journal.pone.0238217

Moutier, C. Y., Myers, M. F., Feist, J. B., Feist, J. C., & Zisook, S. (2021). Preventing clinician suicide: A call to action during the COVID-19 pandemic and beyond. *Academic Medicine, 96*, 624–628. https://doi.org/10.1097/ACM.0000000000003972

Nasirnia Samakoush, A., & Yousefi, N. (2022). The effectiveness of acceptance and commitment therapy on death anxiety, happiness and resilience in the elderly. *Aging Psychology, 8*(2), 149–161.

Nathan, P. E., & Gorman, J. M. (2015). *A guide to treatments that work (4th ed.).* Oxford University Press.

Nejad-Ebrahim Soumee, Z., Tajigharajeh, S., Mousavi, S. E., Nazarali, Z., Bakhshani, N.-M., Nasrabadi, S., et al.. (2024). Group training based on Acceptance and Commitment Therapy for death anxiety and mental health in the older adults: A randomized clinical trial. *Current Psychology.* https://doi.org/10.1007/s12144-024-06801-z

Otared, N., Moharrampour, N. G., Vojoudi, B., & Jahanian Najafabadi, A. (2021). A group-based online Acceptance and Commitment Therapy treatment for depression, anxiety symptoms and quality of life in healthcare workers during COVID-19 pandemic: A randomized controlled trial. *International Journal of Psychology & Psychological Therapy, 21*(3), 399–411.

Paton, N. (2020). Burnout and exhaustion stalk NHS response to Covid-19 second wave. *Occupational Health & Wellbeing, 72*(12), 10–11.

Phoenix Australia. (2020). *Moral stress amongst heathcare workers during COVID-19: A guide to moral injury.* Author.

Ransing, R., Kar, S. K., & Menon, V. (2020). National helpline for mental health during COVID-19 pandemic in India: New opportunity and challenges ahead. *Asian Journal of Psychiatry, 54*, article 102447. https://doi.org/10.1016/j.ajp.2020.102447

Relly, J. E., & Waisbord, S. (2022). Why collective resilience in journalism matters: A call to action in global media development. *Journal of Applied Journalism & Media Studies, 11*(2), 163–188. https://doi.org/10.1386/ajms_00089_1

Resick, P. A., Monson, C. M., & Chard, K. M. (2024). *Cognitive processing therapy for PTSD: A comprehensive therapist manual* (2nd ed.). Guilford.

Rowe-Johnson, M. K., Browning, B., & Scott, B. (2024). Effects of acceptance and commitment therapy on trauma-related symptoms: A systematic review and meta-analysis. *Psychological Trauma: Theory, Research, Practice, and Policy.* https://doi.org/10.1037/tra0001785

Segal, Z., Williams, M., & Teasdale, J. (2018). *Mindfulness-based cognitive therapy for depression* (2nd ed.). Guilford.

Shepherd, K., Golijani-Moghaddam, N., & Dawson, D. L. (2022). ACTing towards better living during COVID-19: The effects of Acceptance and Commitment therapy for individuals affected by COVID-19. *Journal of Contextual Behavioral Science, 23*, 98–108. https://doi.org/10.1016/j.jcbs.2021.12.003

Strudwick, G., Sockalingam, S., Kassam, I., Sequeira, L., Bonato, S., Youssef, A., et al. (2021). Digital interventions to support population mental health in Canada during the COVID-19 pandemic. *JMIR Mental Health, 8*(3), article e26550. https://doi.org/10.2196/26550

Taylor, S. (2019). *The psychology of pandemics: Preparing for the next global outbreak of infectious disease.* Cambridge Scholars Publishing.

Taylor, S., & Asmundson, G. J. G. (2004). *Treating health anxiety.* Guilford.

Taylor, S., Landry, C. A., Rachor, G. S., Paluszek, M. M., & Asmundson, G. J. G. (2020). Fear and avoidance of healthcare workers: An important, under-recognized form of stigmatization during the COVID-19 pandemic. *Journal of Anxiety Disorders, 75*, article 102289. https://doi.org/10.1016/j.janxdis.2020.102289

Varner, C. (2021). Hospitals grappling with nurse exodus. *CMAJ News.* http://cmajnews.com/2021/03/31/nursingretirements-1095934/?utm_source=baytoday.ca&utm_campaign=baytoday.ca&utm_medium=referral

Wahlund, T., Mataix-Cols, D., Olofsdotter Lauri, K., de Schipper, E., Ljótsson, B., Aspvall, K., et al. (2020). Brief online cognitive behavioural intervention for dysfunctional worry related to the COVID-19 Pandemic: A randomised controlled trial. *Psychotherapy and Psychosomatics, 90*, 191–199. https://doi.org/10.1159/000512843

Wallace-Boyd, K., Boggiss, A. L., Ellett, S., Booth, R., Slykerman, R., & Serlachius, A. S. (2023). ACT2COPE: A pilot randomised trial of a brief online acceptance and commitment therapy intervention for people living with chronic health conditions during the COVID-19 pandemic. *Cogent Psychology, 10*(1). https://doi.org/10.1080/23311908.2023.2208916

Wang, J., Wei, H., & Zhou, L. (2020). Hotline services in China during COVID-19 pandemic. *Journal of Affective Disorders, 275*, 125–126. https://doi.org/10.1016/j.jad.2020.06.030

Wang, K., Goldenberg, A., Dorison, C., Miller, J., Uusberg, A., Lerner, J., et al. (2021). A multi-country test of brief reappraisal interventions on emotions during the COVID-19 pandemic. *Nature Human Behaviour, 5*, 1089–1110. https://doi.org/10.1038/s41562-021-01173-x

Ward, B. (2021). Don't blame the pandemic: Healthcare burnout predates it. *Medical Environment Update, 31*(5), 5–6.

Webb, T. L., Miles, E., & Sheeran, P. (2012). Dealing with feeling: A meta-analysis of the effectiveness of strategies derived from the process model of emotion regulation. *Psychological Bulletin, 138*(4), 775–808. https://doi.org/10.1037/a0027600

Wei, E., Segall, J., Linn-Walton, R., Eros-Sarnyai, M., Fattal, O., Toukolehto, O., et al. (2020). Combat stress management and resilience: Adapting Department of Defense combat lessons learned to civilian healthcare during the COVID-19 pandemic. *Health Security, 18*(5), 355–359. https://doi.org/10.1089/hs.2020.0091

WHO. (2019). ICD-11: Burnout. https://icd.who.int/browse11/l-m/en#/http://id.who.int/icd/entity/129180281

WHO. (2020). Pandemic fatigue: Reinvigorating the public to prevent COVID-19. http://apps.who.int/iris/handle/10665/335820?search-result=true&query=pandemic+fatigue&scope=&rpp=335810&sort_by=score&order=desc

Wu, A. W., Connors, C., & Everly, G. S., Jr. (2020). COVID-19: Peer support and crisis communication strategies to promote institutional resilience. *Annals of Internal Medicine, 172*, 822–823. https://doi.org/10.7326/M20-1236

Xiao, X., Zhu, X., Fu, S., Hu, Y., Li, X., & Xiao, J. (2020). Psychological impact of healthcare workers in China during COVID-19 pneumonia epidemic: A multi-center cross-sectional survey investigation. *Journal of Affective Disorders, 274*, 405–410. https://doi.org/10.1016/j.jad.2020.05.081

Yuan, Y. (2021). Mindfulness training on the resilience of adolescents under the COVID-19 epidemic: A latent growth curve analysis. *Personality and Individual Differences, 172*, article110560. https://doi.org/10.1016/j.paid.2020.110560

Zgueb, Y., Bourgou, S., Neffeti, A., Amamou, B., Masmoudi, J., Chebbi, H., et al. (2020). Psychological crisis intervention response to the COVID 19 pandemic: A Tunisian centralised protocol. *Psychiatry Research, 289*, article113042. https://doi.org/10.1016/j.psychres.2020.113042

Chapter 23

Aborode, A., Sukaina, M., Kumar, H., Farooqui, T., Faheem, S., Chahal, P., et al. (2021). Zika virus endemic challenges during COVID-19 pandemic in Africa. *Tropical Medicine & Health, 49*(1), article 82. https://doi.org/10.1186/s41182-021-00372-6

Albom, M. (2009). Hand sanitizer: It's the new bottled water. *Fort Worth Business Press, 25*(41), 35.

Aliche, J. C., Ifeagwazi, C. M., Onyishi, I. E., & Mefoh, P. C. (2019). Presence of meaning in life mediates the relations between social support, posttraumatic growth, and resilience in young adult survivors of a terror attack. *Journal of Loss & Trauma, 24*, 736–749. https://doi.org/10.1080/15325024.2019.1624416

Antia, R., & Halloran, M. E. (2021). Transition to endemicity: Understanding COVID-19. *Immunity, 54*(10), 2172–2176. https://doi.org/10.1016/j.immuni.2021.09.019

Asia Pacific Foundation of Canada. (2023). 2% of Japanese labour force could be "modern-day recluses": Government survey. https://www.asiapacific.ca/publication/2-percent-japanese-labour-force-modern-day-recluses

Asmundson, G. J. G., Paluszek, M. M., & Taylor, S. (2021). Real versus illusory personal growth in reponse to stressors of the COVID-19 pandemic. *Journal of Anxiety Disorders, 81*, article102418. https://doi.org/10.1016/j.janxdis.2021.102418

Barbieri, R., Signoli, M., Chevé, D., Costedoat, C., Tzortzis, S., Aboudharam, G., et al. (2020). Yersinia pestis: The natural history of plague. *Clinical Microbiology Reviews, 34*(1). https://doi.org/10.1128/CMR.00044-19

Bernhard, M., Leuch, C., Kordi, M., Gruebner, O., Matthes, K., Floris, J., et al. (2023). From pandemic to endemic: Spatial-temporal patterns of influenza-like illness incidence in a Swiss canton, 1918-1924. *Economics and Human Biology, 50*, article 101271. https://doi.org/10.1016/j.ehb.2023.101271

Boerner, M., Joseph, S., & Murphy, D. (2020). A theory on reports of constructive (real) and illusory posttraumatic growth. *Journal of Humanistic Psychology, 60*(3), 384–399. https://doi.org/10.1177/0022167817719597

Boston Post. (1918, October 21). Crowds jam all theatres. *Boston Post*, 4. http://hdl.handle.net/2027/spo.7410flu.0001.147

Bower, B. (2020). What will life be like post-pandemic? *Science News, 198*(11), 24–24.

Bowker, J. C., Bowker, M. H., Santo, J. B., Ojo, A. A., Etkin, R. G., & Raja, R. (2019). Severe social withdrawal: Cultural variation in past hikikomori experiences of university students in Nigeria, Singapore, and the United States. *Journal of Genetic Psychology, 180*, 217–230. https://doi.org/10.1080/00221325.2019.1633618

Boyce, J. M., & Pittet, D. (2002). Guideline for hand hygiene in health-care settings: Recommendations of the healthcare infection control practices advisory committee and the HIPAC/SHEA/APIC/IDSA hand hygiene task force. *American Journal of Infection Control, 30*(8), S1–S46. https://doi.org/10.1067/mic.2002.130391

Brüssow, H. (2022). The beginning and ending of a respiratory viral pandemic-lessons from the Spanish flu. *Microbial Biotechnology, 15*(5), 1301–1317. https://doi.org/10.1111/1751-7915.14053

Calhoun, L., & Tedeschi, R. G. (2006). The foundations of posttraumatic growth: An expanded framework. In L. Calhoun & R. G. Tedeschi (Eds.), *Handbook of posttraumatic growth: Research and practice* (pp. 1–23). Routledge.

Cantor, N. (2001). *In the wake of the plague: The Black Death and the world it made*. Free Press.

Carlson, C. J., Bevins, S. N., & Schmid, B. V. (2022). Plague risk in the western United States over seven decades of environmental change. *Global Change Biology, 28*(3), 753–769. https://doi.org/10.1111/gcb.15966

CDC. (2012). *Principles of epidemiology in public health practice (3rd ed.)*. U.S. Department of Health and Human Services.

CDC. (2024). How plague spreads. https://www.cdc.gov/plague/causes/index.html#:~:text=Many%20types%20of%20animals%2C%20such,by%20eating%20other%20infected%20animals

Charters, E., & Heitman, K. (2021). How epidemics end. *Centaurus, 63*(1), 210–224. https://doi.org/10.1111/1600-0498.12370

Chen, R., Sun, C., Chen, J., Jen, H., Kang, X., Kao, C., et al. (2021). A large-scale survey on trauma, burnout, and posttraumatic growth among nurses during the COVID-19 pandemic. *International Journal of Mental Health Nursing, 30*, 102–116. https://doi.org/10.1111/inm.12796

Crosby, A. W. (2003). *America's forgotten pandemic: The influenza of 1918 (2nd ed.)*. Cambridge University Press.

David, I. (2021). The post-pandemic economy will boom - but not for all. *Washington Post*. https://www.washingtonpost.com/opinions/the-post-pandemic-economy-will-boom—but-not-for-all/2021/03/16/d215a5c0-8698-11eb-bfdf-4d36dab83a6d_story.html

Davidson, H. (2023). Child respiratory sickness overloads China's paediatric clinics – reports. *The Guardian*. https://www.theguardian.com/world/2023/nov/29/china-child-respiratory-illness-spike-paediatric-clinics-multiple-pathogens-covid-19-lockdowns-end

Davis, I. M. (2021). SARS-CoV: Lessons learned; opportunities missed for SARS-CoV-2. *Reviews in Medical Virology, 31*(1), article e2152. https://doi.org/https://doi.org/10.1002/rmv.2152

Engelhard, I. M., Lommen, M. J., & Sijbrandij, M. (2015). Changing for better or worse? Posttraumatic growth reported by soldiers deployed to Iraq. *Clinical Psychological Science, 3*, 789–796. https://doi.org/10.1177/216770261454980

Fincher, J. (1989). America's deadly rendezvous with the "Spanish Lady." *Smithsonian Magazine, 19*(10), 132–144.

Floyd, C. J., Joachim, G. E., Boulton, M. L., Zelner, J., & Wagner, A. L. (2022). COVID-19 vaccination and mask wearing behaviors in the United States, August 2020 - June 2021. *Expert Review of Vaccines, 21*(10), 1487–1493. https://doi.org/10.1080/14760584.2022.2104251

Forrester, M. B. (2012). Changes in Texas poison center call patterns in response to H1N1 influenza outbreak. *Texas Public Health Journal, 64*(4), 14–18.

Frazier, P., Tennen, H., Gavian, M., Park, C., Tomich, P., & Tashiro, T. (2009). Does self-reported posttraumatic growth reflect genuine positive change? *Psychological Science, 20*(7), 912–919. https://doi.org/10.1111/j.1467-9280.2009.02381.x

Garcia-Continente, X., Serral, G., López, M. J., Pérez, A., & Nebot, M. (2013). Long-term effect of the influenza A/H1N1 pandemic: Attitudes and preventive behaviours one year after the pandemic. *European Journal of Public Health, 23*(4), 679–681. https://doi.org/10.1093/eurpub/ckt068

Herlihy, D. (1997). *The Black Death and the transformation of the west.* Harvard University Press.

Heung, J., Wong, F., Kwong, E., To, T., & Wong, D. (2005). Severe acute respiratory syndrome outbreak promotes a strong sense of professional identity among nursing students. *Nurse Education Today, 25*(2), 112–118. https://doi.org/10.1016/j.nedt.2004.11.003

Huecker, M., Shreffler, J., & Danzl, D. (2020). COVID-19: Optimizing healthcare provider wellness and posttraumatic growth. *American Journal of Emergency Medicine, 46*, 693–694. https://doi.org/10.1016/j.ajem.2020.08.066

Kang, J. (2021). Retailers couldn't stock hand sanitizer fast enough. Now they can't give it away. *Wall Street Journal.* https://www.wsj.com/articles/america-is-awash-in-hand-sanitizer-11621522829

Karp, A. (2020). Telehealth will remain vital, post-pandemic. *Vision Monday, 34*(4), p. 6.

Kayembe, H., Bompangue, D., Linard, C., Muwonga, J., Moutschen, M., Situakibanza, H., et al. (2022). Modalities and preferred routes of geographic spread of cholera from endemic areas in eastern Democratic Republic of the Congo. *PLOS ONE, 17*(2), article e0263160. https://doi.org/10.1371/journal.pone.0263160

Kenny, C. (2021). *The plague cycle: The unending war between humanity and infectious disease.* Scribner.

Lau, J. T. F., Yang, X., Tsui, H. Y., Pang, E., & Wing, Y. K. (2006). Positive mental health-related impacts of the SARS epidemic on the general public in Hong Kong and their associations with other negative impacts. *Journal of Infection, 53*, 114–124. https://doi.org/10.1016/j.jinf.2005.10.019

Liu, J. J. W., Ein, N., Gervasio, J., Battaion, M., Reed, M., & Vickers, K. (2020). Comprehensive meta-analysis of resilience interventions. *Clinical Psychology Review, 82*, article 101919. https://doi.org/10.1016/j.cpr.2020.101919

MacIntyre, C. R., Nguyen, P., Chughtai, A., Trent, M., Gerber, B., Steinhofel, K., et al. (2021). Mask use, risk-mitigation behaviours and pandemic fatigue during the COVID-19 pandemic in five cities in Australia, the UK and USA: A cross-sectional survey. *International Journal of Infectious Diseases, 106*, 199–207. https://doi.org/10.1016/j.ijid.2021.03.056

Mahmoudi, A., Kryštufek, B., Sludsky, A., Schmid, B. V., Almeida A., Lei, X., et al. (2021). Plague reservoir species throughout the world. *Integrative Zoology, 16*(6), 820–833. https://doi.org/10.1111/1749-4877.12511

Mangelsdorf, J., & Eid, M. (2015). What makes a thriver? Unifying the concepts of posttraumatic and postecstatic growth. *Frontiers in Psychology, 6.* https://doi.org/10.3389/fpsyg.2015.00813

Manning, S., Barry, T., Wilson, N., & Baker, M. (2010). Follow-up study showing postpandemic decline in hand sanitiser use, New Zealand, December 2009. *Eurosurveillance, 15,* article 19466. https://doi.org/10.2807/ese.15.03.19466-en

Mass Market Retailers. (2009). Flu fears jump-start hand sanitizer demand. *Mass Market Retailers, 26*(14), 19.

McCurry, J. (2023). Japan says 1.5m people are living as recluses after Covid. *The Guardian.* https://www.theguardian.com/world/2023/apr/03/japan-says-15-million-people-living-as-recluses-after-covid

McFarland, C., & Alvaro, C. (2000). The impact of motivation on temporal comparisons: Coping with traumatic events by perceiving personal growth. *Journal of Personality and Social Psychology, 79,* 327–343. https://doi.org/10.1037//0022-3514.79.3.327

Peters, J., Bellet, B. W., Jones, P. J., Wu, G. W. Y., Wang, L., & McNally, R. J. (2021). Posttraumatic stress or posttraumatic growth? Using network analysis to explore the relationships between coping styles and trauma outcomes. *Journal of Anxiety Disorders, 78,* article 102359. https://doi.org/10.1016/j.janxdis.2021.102359

Pietrzak, R. H., Tsai, J., & Southwick, S. M. (2021). Association of symptoms of posttraumatic stress disorder with posttraumatic psychological growth among US veterans during the COVID-19 pandemic. *JAMA Network Open, 4,* article e214972. https://doi.org/10.1001/jamanetworkopen.2021.4972

Plaugic, L. (2018). Domestic movie theater attendance hit a 25-year low in 2017. https://www.theverge.com/2018/1/3/16844662/movie-theater-attendance-2017-low-netflix-streaming

PR Newswire. (2020). New research shows baby boomers will continue shopping online post-pandemic, resulting in significant opportunity for retailers. https://www.prweb.com/releases/new_research_shows_baby_boomers_will_continue_shopping_online_post_pandemic_resulting_in_significant_opportunity_for_retailers/prweb17432194.htm

Robins, N. (2005). *Copeland's cure: Homeopathy and the war between conventional and alternative medicine.* Knopf.

Roepke, A. M. (2015). Psychosocial interventions and posttraumatic growth: A meta-analysis. *Journal of Consulting and Clinical Psychology, 83*(1), 129–142. https://doi.org/10.1037/a0036872

Rosenberg, C. E. (1987). *The cholera years: The United States in 1832, 1849, and 1866.* University of Chicago Press.

Ruth, D. E. (1990). Don't shake—salute! *Chicago History, 19*(3/4), 4–23.

Sabrie, G., Buckley, C., Bradsher, K., Wang, V., & Qin, A. (2021). In Wuhan, glimpses of a post-pandemic world. *New York Times.* https://www.nytimes.com/2021/01/22/world/asia/wuhan-china-coronavirus.html

San Francisco Examiner. (1918, November 22). "Flu" mask wearers get "bawling out." *San Francisco Examiner,* 9. http://hdl.handle.net/2027/spo.3020flu.0009.203

Scipioni, J. (2020). White house advisor Dr. Fauci says handshaking needs to stop even when pandemic ands—other experts agree. *CNBC.* https://www.cnbc.com/2020/04/09/dr-anthony-fauci-handshaking-needs-to-stop-even-after-pandemic.html

Shu-Ru, J., & Jiun-Hau, H. (2012). The prevalence of and factors associated with intention to wear a face mask during an influenza-like illness: A comparison between the influenza

A/H1N1 pandemic and the post-pandemic phase. *Taiwan Journal of Public Health, 31,* 570–580.

Singh, S. (2019). The soon to be $200B online food delivery is rapidly changing the global food industry. *Forbes.* https://www.forbes.com/sites/sarwantsingh/2019/09/09/the-soon-to-be-200b-online-food-delivery-is-rapidly-changing-the-global-food-industry/#25473507b1bc

Spinney, L. (2017). *Pale rider: The Spanish flu of 1918 and how it changed the world.* Vintage.

Taku, K., Tedeschi, R. G., Shakespeare-Finch, J., Krosch, D., David, G., Kehl, D., et al. (2021). Posttraumatic growth (PTG) and posttraumatic depreciation (PTD) across ten countries: Global validation of the PTG-PTD theoretical model. *Personality & Individual Differences, 169,* article 110222. https://doi.org/10.1016/j.paid.2020.110222

Tedeschi, R. G., & Calhoun, L. G. (2004). Posttraumatic growth: Conceptual foundations and empirical evidence. *Psychological Inquiry, 15,* 1–18. https://doi.org/10.1207/s15327965pli1501_01

Tedeschi, R. G., & Moore, B. A. (2016). *The posttraumatic growth workbook.* New Harbinger.

Tedeschi, R. G., Shakespeare-Finch, J., Taku, K., & Calhoun, L. G. (2018). *Posttraumatic growth: Theory, research, and applications.* Routledge.

Teo, A. R. (2010). A new form of social withdrawal in Japan: A review of Hikikomori. *International Journal of Social Psychiatry, 56,* 178–185. https://doi.org/10.1177/0020764008100629

Terlep, S. (2021, January 22). Hand sanitizer sales jumped 600% in 2020. Purell maker bets against a post-pandemic collapse. *Wall Street Journal.* https://www.proquest.com/docview/2479655839?accountid=14656&parentSessionId=EIbA0mYIJbkb5C2dRx6zRorCaHiJhWvI%2FAvLLnMsbXk%3D&sourcetype=Newspapers

Tilley, A. (2020). Microsoft will let some staff work from home routinely post-pandemic. *Wall Street Journal.* https://www.wsj.com/articles/microsoft-to-allow-some-employees-to-opt-for-permanent-remote-work-11602269946#:~:text=MSFT%20%2D1.44%25%20is%20going%20to,recent%20months%20will%20be%20enduring.&text=Some%20workers%20will%20be%20able,approved%20by%20managers%2C%20Microsoft%20said

Tomes, N. (1999). *The gospel of germs: Men, women, and the microbe in American life.* Harvard University Press.

U.S. Census Bureau. (2013). Working at home is on the rise. https://www.census.gov/library/visualizations/2013/comm/home_based_workers.html

U.S. Census Bureau. (2014). Online shopping and mail order businesses jump 27 percent, Census Bureau reports. https://www.census.gov/newsroom/press-releases/2014/cb14-102.html

Van Reeth, K., Brown, I. H., & Olsen, C. W. (2012). Influenza virus. In J. J. Zimmerman, L. A. Karriker, A. Ramirez, K. J. Schwartz, & G. W. Stevenson (Eds.), *Diseases of swine* (10th ed.) (pp. 557–571). Wiley-Blackwell.

WHO. (2010). Pandemic (H1N1) 2009. https://www.who.int/csr/disease/swineflu/en/

WHO. (2015a). The Ebola outbreak in Liberia is over. https://www.who.int/mediacentre/news/statements/2015/liberia-ends-ebola/en/.

WHO. (2015b). Ebola transmission in Liberia over. Nation enters 90-day intensive surveillance period. https://www.who.int/mediacentre/news/statements/2015/ebola-transmission-over-liberia/en/

WHO. (2016). Latest Ebola outbreak over in Liberia; West Africa is at zero, but new flare-ups are likely to occur. https://www.who.int/news/item/14-01-2016-latest-ebola-outbreak-over-in-liberia-west-africa-is-at-zero-but-new-flare-ups-are-likely-to-occur#:~:text=likely%20to%20occur-,Latest%20Ebola%20outbreak%20over%20in%20Liberia%3B%20West%20Africa%20is%20at,ups%20are%20likely%20to%20occur&text=Today's%20announcement%20comes%2042%20days,for%20the%20disease%202%20times

WHO. (2023). Statement on the fifteenth meeting of the IHR (2005) Emergency Committee on the COVID-19 pandemic. https://www.who.int/news/item/05-05-2023-statement-on-the-fifteenth-meeting-of-the-international-health-regulations-(2005)-emergency-committee-regarding-the-coronavirus-disease-(covid-19)-pandemic

Wollast, R., Schmitz, M., Bigot, A., Speybroeck, N., Lacourse, É., de la Sablonnière, R., et al. (2023). Trajectories of health behaviors during the COVID-19 pandemic: A longitudinal analysis of handwashing, mask wearing, social contact limitations, and physical distancing. *Psychology & Health*, 1–28. https://doi.org/10.1080/08870446.2023.2278706

Wu, X., Kaminga, A., Dai, W., Deng, J., Wang, Z., Pan, X., et al. (2019). The prevalence of moderate-to-high posttraumatic growth: A systematic review and meta-analysis. *Journal of Affective Disorders*, 243, 408–415. https://doi.org/10.1016/j.jad.2018.09.023

Xu, X., Hu, M., Song, Y., Lu, Z., Chen, Y., Wu, D., et al. (2016). Effect of positive psychological intervention on posttraumatic growth among primary healthcare workers in China: A preliminary prospective study. *Scientific Reports*, 6, article39189. https://doi.org/10.1038/srep39189

Ziegler, P. (2016). *The Black Death*. American Heritage Publishing.

Chapter 24

Aguirre, A. A., Catherina, R., Frye, H., & Shelley, L. (2020). Illicit wildlife trade, wet markets, and COVID-19: Preventing future pandemics. *World Medical & Health Policy*, 12(3), 256–265. https://doi.org/10.1002/wmh3.348

Allen, T., Murray, K., Zambrana-Torrelio, C., Morse, S., Rondinini, C., Di Marco, M., et al. (2017). Global hotspots and correlates of emerging zoonotic diseases. *Nature Communications*, 8(1), article 1124. https://doi.org/10.1038/s41467-017-00923-8

Brom, F., de Hoog, J., Knottnerus, J. A., Mampuys, R., & van der Lippe, T. (2022). Coronavirus disease 2019 scenarios for a long-term strategy under fundamental uncertainty. *Journal of Clinical Epidemiology*, 148, 196–199. https://doi.org/10.1016/j.jclinepi.2022.02.012

Carlson, C., Albery, G., Merow, C., Trisos, C., Zipfel, C., Eskew, E., et al. (2022). Climate change increases cross-species viral transmission risk. *Nature*, 607, 555–562. https://doi.org/10.1038/s41586-022-04788-w

Castillo-Chavez, C., Curtiss, R., Daszak, P., Levin, S., Patterson-Lomba, O., Perrings, C., et al. (2015). Beyond Ebola: Lessons to mitigate future pandemics. *Lancet Global Health*, 3(7), e354–e355. https://doi.org/10.1016/S2214-109X(15)00068-6

CDC. (2007). *Interim pre-pandemic planning guidance: Community strategy for pandemic influenza mitigation in the United States*. Author.

CDC. (2019). 2009 H1N1 pandemic (H1N1 pdm09 virus). https://www.cdc.gov/flu/pandemic-resources/2009-h1n1-pandemic.html#print

Cohn, S. K. (2018). *Epidemics: Hate and compassion from the plague of Athens to AIDS*. Oxford University Press.

Daszak, P. (2021). Lessons from COVID-19 to help prevent future pandemics. *China CDC Weekly*, 3(7), 132–133. https://doi.org/10.46234/ccdcw2021.035

Eschner, K. (2017). The long shadow of the 1976 swine flu vaccine "fiasco." *Smithsonian Magazine*. https://www.smithsonianmag.com/smart-news/long-shadow-1976-swine-flu-vaccine-fiasco-180961994

Fisher, R. (2020). The fiasco of the 1976 "swine flu affair." *BBC Future*. https://www.bbc.com/future/article/20200918-the-fiasco-of-the-us-swine-flu-affair-of-1976

Fumento, M. (2005, November 21). Fuss and feathers: Pandemic panic over the avian flu. *Weekly Standard*. https://fliphtml5.com/hnds/nzhr/basic

Klemm, C., Das, E., & Hartmann, T. (2016). Swine flu and hype: A systematic review of media dramatization of the H1N1 influenza pandemic. *Journal of Risk Research, 19*, 1–20. https://doi.org/10.1080/13669877.2014.923029

Le Bon, G. (1895). *La psychologie des foules*. Alcan.

Marani, M., Katul, G. G., Pan, W. K., & Parolari, A. J. (2021). Intensity and frequency of extreme novel epidemics. *PNAS, 118*(35), article e2105482118. https://doi.org/10.1073/pnas.2105482118

Neustadt, R. E., & Fineberg, H. V. (1983). *The epidemic that never was: Policy-making and the Swine Flu scare*. Vintage.

Nuwer, R. (2020, February 20). Stop wildlife trade to prevent next epidemic, conservationists say. *New York Times, 169*, A8. https://www.nytimes.com/2020/2002/2019/health/coronavirus-animals-markets.html

One Health High Level Expert Panel. (2023). *Prevention of zoonotic spillover*. WHO.

Sandman, P. M. (2009). Pandemics: Good hygiene is not enough. *Nature, 459*, 322–323. https://doi.org/10.1038/459322a

Shah, V., Shah, A., & Joshi, V. (2018). Predicting the origins of next forest-based emerging infectious disease. *Environmental Monitoring & Assessment, 190*(6), article 337. https://doi.org/10.1007/s10661-018-6711-6

Snowden, F. M. (2019). *Epidemics and society: From the Black Death to the present*. Yale University Press.

United Nations. (2022). Population. https://www.un.org/en/global-issues/population#:~:text=The%20world%20population%20is%20projected,surrounding%20these%20latest%20population%20projections

United Nations Department of Economic and Social Affairs. (2024). World population prospects 2024. https://www.un.org/development/desa/pd/world-population-prospects-2024

Welzer, H. (2017). *Climate wars: Why people will be killed in the 21st century*. Polity Press.

WHO. (2005). *WHO checklist for influenza pandemic preparedness planning*. Author.

WHO. (2021a). Live roundtable discussions exploring the future of the COVID-19 pandemic and other infectious threats. https://www.who.int/news-room/events/detail/2021/11/04/default-calendar/live-roundtable-discussions-exploring-the-future-of-the-covid-19-pandemic-and-other-infectious-threats

WHO. (2021b). Preventing the next pandemic. *Bulletin of the World Health Organization, 99*(5), 326–327. https://doi.org/10.2471/BLT.21.020521

WHO. (2022a). *Imagining the future of pandemics and epidemics: A 2022 perspective*. Author.

WHO. (2022b). A WHO Foresight Initiative: Imagining the future of pandemics and epidemics in the next 5 years. *Weekly Epidemiological Record, 97*, 55–59.

Zhu, A., & Zhu, G. (2020). Understanding China's wildlife markets: Trade and tradition in an age of pandemic. *World Development, 136*, article 105108. https://doi.org/10.1016/j.worlddev.2020.105108

Index

For the benefit of digital users, indexed terms that span two pages (e.g., 52–53) may, on occasion, appear on only one of those pages.

Tables, figures, and boxes are indicated by an italic *t*, *f*, and *b* following the paragraph number.

ABCDEF bundle, 239
Acceptance and Commitment Therapy (ACT), 264
acetaminophen, 91
ACT (Acceptance and Commitment Therapy), 264
acute anxiety, vaccination-related, 246
addictive behaviors, mental health and, 227–229
advertising, repetition-induced truth effect and, 127
affect heuristic, 128–129
aging population, 277–278
alcohol consumption
　addictive behavior and, 227–229
　for coping, 90
altruism, for coping, 86–87
ambiguity aversion, intolerance of uncertainty and, 203
The Anatomy of Melancholy (Burton), 157
anchoring bias, 123–124
Anderson, J. B., 17, 40
anger, 229
animals, pandemics spreading by, 12–13
anonymity, trolling and, 146
anti-Asian racism, 177
antibiotics, 53
anticipatory anxiety, 8
Anti-Mask League, 51–52
anti-Mexican racism, during swine flu, 176–177
antipyrine, 87, 91
antisemitism
　Black Death and, 176
　conspiracy theories and, 138
Anti-Vaccination Revolts (Revolta Contra Vacina), 80
antiviral medication, 53
Antonine Plague, *4t*

religious coping during, 93
anxiety, xv. *See also* death anxiety; health anxiety
　affect heuristic and, 128–129
　anticipatory, 8
　COVID-19 pandemic and, 215–218
　depression and, 215–219
　harm avoidance and trait, 200–201
　of HCWs, 218
　during influenza pandemics, 219
　from news media, 100, 112–113
　pandemic lessons learned on, 285–286
　pandemics and, 8–9, 12
　in Russian and Spanish flu pandemics, 219
　sensitivity, 204–205
appearance equals reality, law of similarity, 181–182
applied psychology, xi
approach-avoidance conflicts, for coping, 86–87
aromatic purification, 173–174
asafetida, 173
aspirin poisoning, 91–92
Athens, Plague of, *4t*, 130, 140, 169–170, 238
attitude polarization, media use and, 115–116
authoritarianism, 207–208
availability heuristic, 125–126
avian flu outbreaks, *6t*
　naming, 47
　news media exaggerating danger of, 113

Barcelona, Plague of 1651, 9, 27–28
"bat soup" video, 118
Battle Buddies program, 262–263
behavioral immune system (BIS), xv
　concept of, 171
　disgust sensitivity and, 171, 172–173, 178
　fear triggered by, 175–176

magical thinking, superstitious behavior
and, 188
racism triggered by, 176–177
research on, 178
smells of danger and safety and, 173–175
xenophobia and, 175, 177–178
beliefs about health and disease. *See also* health anxiety
conspiracy theories and, 141–142, 144
dysfunctional, 156–157
maladaptive coping and, 158–160
misinterpretations and, 154–156
selective attention and, 157–158
worry and, 150–151
xenophobia and immunity, 177–178
bereavement, 225
biases. *See also* heuristics
anchoring, 123–124
confirmation, 124–125
denial of disease and self-serving, 196–197
distortions from, 122
exponential growth, 127–128
hindsight, 129
illusory correlations and self-serving, 191–192
judgments shaped by, 122
negativity, law of contagion and, 182
optimism, 189–190
temporal discounting, 130–131, 169
bioweapon conspiracies, 140–141
BIS. *See* behavioral immune system
Black Death, antisemitism and, 176
blame, societal fault lines and, 76–77
Bloomberg Resilience Scale, 42
blunting cognitive style, 111–112
bodily sensations, misinterpretations of, 154–156
Boghurst, William, 62
Bolsonaro, Jair, 74–75
boredom proneness, 209
"brain fog," 235
Brazil, 74–75, 80
buddy systems, for HCW resilience, 262–263
Buenos Aires, 169
burnout, xv
buddy systems for reducing, 262–263
HCW effects of, 261
moral injury and, 260–261
workplace-related, 260
Burton, Robert, 157

bushmeat, 276–277
business closures, objections to, 62–64

Calvin, John, 140
Canada
Freedom Truck Convoy, 78–79
HCW stigmatization in, 32
hero-worshiping for coping in, 95
pandemic-related food insecurity in, 26
Carbolic Smoke Ball, 89
catastrophic thinking, 151
"catch-and-release" lockdowns, 82
causes resemble effects, law of similarity, 181
CBT. *See* cognitive behavioral therapy
censorship, 146–147
challenge, hardiness and, 206
Chapin, Charles V., 194
child abuse, 229–230
China
"bat soup" video and, 118
Chengdu mental health treatment during COVID-19 in, 256–257
COVID-19 pandemic protests in, 79
COVID-19 pandemic stigma in, 32
rumors during SARS in, 134
SARS in Beijing, 2003, 101
surveillance-based health code system of, 68–69
Taiwan and trolling from, 145–146
cholera
conspiracy theories, 80–81
death exposure during, 27–28
desperate pleasures during, 169
disgust from, 18–19
gravediggers, rumors and, 135–136
infodemic during, 117
major historical instances of, 4–8, 4t
negative emotionality during, 84
in New Orleans, 1832-1833, 9–10
over- and under-reactions to, 16–17
protests/riots, 77
PTSD and, 224
religious coping during, 93–94
religious panic in Ireland, 1832 and, 186–187
rumors during, 135
societal change from, 273
unpredictability of, 10
Christian nationalism, 166

chronic fatigue syndrome (myalgic encephalomyelitis), 241
church bell tolling, during plague, 163
church closures, objections to, 62–64
Clapp, Theodore, 9–10, 224
climate change, 277–278
closures, objections to, 62–64
cognitive behavioral model of health anxiety, 154, 155f
cognitive behavioral therapy (CBT)
  for distress vulnerability traits, 210–211
  health anxiety treatment with, 160
  for mental health management, 253–254
  for OCD, 226–227
  online interventions for, 255–256
  personal growth and, 272–273
  telephone hotlines for, 254–255
cognitive closure, need for, 203–204
commitment, hardiness and, 206
communication. *See* risk communication
comprehensive mental health management, 256–257
concealment, disease, 73–74, 82
confirmation bias, 124–125
conflict, xii
  pandemic lessons learned on, 287–288
  psychology of pandemics and, 21
conscientiousness, 210
conservatives, COVID-19 conspiracy theories and, 144
conspiracy entrepreneurs, 145
conspiracy theories. *See also* rumors
  antisemitism and, 138
  bioweapon, 140–141
  cholera, 80–81
  on cover ups, 136
  COVID-19 pandemic, 81, 142, 144
  defense of, 136
  definition of, xv, 133
  element of truth in, 139
  escaped-from-a-lab, 139–140
  5G, 137
  groups spreading, 145
  healthcare, 138–139
  magical thinking and, 188
  managing, 146–148
  nonadherence and belief in, 144
  pharmaceutical industry, 138–139
  protests and, 80–81
  proven true, 147
  psychological characteristics of believers of, 143–144
  repetition-induced truth effect and, 126–127
  during Russian flu, 137
  shadowy elites in, 138
  during Spanish flu, 136
  trolling and, 145–146
  viral behavior of, 137
  widespread belief in, 141–142
  xenophobia and, 138
conspiracy theorists, 145
contagion, law of, 182
control, xii. *See also* illusion of control
  hardiness and, 206
  pandemic lessons learned on, 286–287
  psychology of pandemics and, 20–21
Copeland, Royal S., 40–41, 48–49, 270
coping
  altruism for, 86–87
  approach-avoidance conflicts for, 86–87
  confirmation bias on, 125
  dark humor and, 167–169
  with death anxiety, 22
  desperate and dangerous methods for, 90–92
  during disease outbreaks, 83
  emotion-focused, 84–85
  fads, 96–97
  folk remedies for, 88–89, 92
  hero-worshiping for, 94–95
  illusion of control risks with, 195–196
  maladaptive, 158–160
  nostalgia for, 95–96
  with pandemic fatigue, 259
  panic buying for, 87–88
  problem-focused, 84–85
  quack cures for, 89, 92
  religious, 92–94
  for resilience, 83, 98
  smoking and drinking for, 90
  social support and, 85–86
  superstitious, 187–188
cordon sanitaire, xv, 39
  efficacy of, 105–106
  rumors of, 145
coronaviruses, 3. *See also specific viruses*
  major historical instances of, 6t
  naming, 48
corpse disposal, 10

counter-blame, societal fault lines and, 76–77
cover ups. *See also* conspiracy theories
  conspiracy theories on, 136
  disease concealment and government, 73–74, 82
  Fauci accused of, 76
  social media misinformation on, 114–115
COVID-19 pandemic, xi–xi
  alcohol consumption during, 227
  antiviral medication during, 53
  anxiety and depression during, 215–218
  boredom proneness during, 209
  business closures during, 63
  Chengdu mental health program during, 256–257
  China's surveillance-based health code system and, 68–69
  Christian nationalism and, 166
  church closures during, 63
  conspiracy theories, 81, 142, 144
  declaring end of, 268–269
  delirium during, 237
  denial of disease during, 197
  disease concealment/under-reporting in, 73
  disease-related stigma in, 32
  disgust from, 18–19
  disgust sensitivity during, 172
  disrupted funeral rituals during, 31
  emerging from lockdown after, 271
  emotion-focused coping during, 84–85
  escaped-from-a-lab conspiracies and, 139
  face mask backlash during, 52
  fake news during, 118–119
  fear and anxiety in, 9
  fear-evoking messages during, 45–46
  fleeing, 103–104
  folk remedies for, 88–89
  food insecurity during, 26
  future scenarios of, 279–283, 281*t*
  gambling addiction and, 228
  global research on, xii
  government mistrust and, 74–75
  handwashing during, 193
  HCW stigmatization in, 32
  hero-worshiping of HCWs during, 94–95
  hikikomori syndrome after, 271
  home-use pulse oximeter fad during, 97
  hygiene theater and, 193–194
  immunity documentation during, 56–57
  infodemic and, 117
  interpersonal violence and, 229–230
  intolerance of uncertainty during, 202–203
  kissing, hugging, handshaking after, 270
  lifestyle management during, 85
  maladaptive coping during, 159
  mass psychogenic illness and, 248
  medical misdiagnosis and anchoring bias in, 124
  mental health and social media use during, 115
  monitoring cognitive style in, 112
  mortality salience during, 163
  narcissism, psychological entitlement during, 209–210
  negative emotionality during, 200
  news media stoking anxieties of, 112–113
  nocebo effect and, 250–251
  nonadherence to social distancing during, 64
  nostalgia-seeking during, 95–96
  nudges and mandates during, 57
  OCD and, 226–227
  omens during, 185–186
  online interventions for mental health during, 255–256
  optimism bias during, 190
  over- and under-reactions to, 17
  overview of, 6*t*
  panic buying during, 87
  past pandemics compared to, 19–20
  personal growth and, 272
  poisonings and, 90–91
  political polarization and, 75–76
  price gouging and, 88
  problem-focused coping during, 85
  prolonged grief disorder due to, 225
  protests/riots, 77–80
  psychology of COVID-19, xii, 19–21
  PTSD related to, 222–223
  quack remedies during, 89
  quarantine and lockdown for, 61
  religious coping during, 93–94
  research motivated by, 22–23
  rumors during, 135
  school closures during, 63–64
  shunning survivors during, 183
  social media misinformation on, 115

COVID-19 pandemic (*Continued*)
  societal change from, 273–274
  societal fault lines and stressor distribution in, 77
  South Korea' test-trace-isolate approach to, 69, 70
  substance use during, 227–228
  successful mitigation efforts in, 41–43
  suicide rate during, 230–231
  talismans and, 184
  telephone hotlines for mental health during, 254–255
  temporal discounting during, 130
  in Texas, 2020, 11
  tobacco smoking and risk from, 90
  trait anxiety and harm avoidance during, 201
  traumatic stressors from, 30
  vaccination during, 53, 196
  WHO message inconsistency on face masks in, 25–26
  WHO on pandemic fatigue during, 65
  worry proneness during, 202
  xenophobia during, 94–95
COVID-19 status indicators, 42
COVID Resilience Ranking, 41
COVID stress syndrome, 220
crowds, pandemics spreading by, 12–13
cultural developments, psychology of pandemics and, 278–279

danger
  lack of boundaries between safety and, 17
  omens of, 185–186
  smells of, 173–175
dark humor, 167–169
Daszak, Peter, 131
death
  adapting to exposure to, 28
  exposure as stressor, 27–28
  uncertainty of, 25
death anxiety
  conspiracy theories and, 143
  coping with, 22
  dark humor and, 167–169
  desperate pleasures and, 169–170
  distal defenses for, 164–165
  dysfunctional beliefs and, 157
  morbid curiosity and, 166–167
  mortality salience and, 163

  proximal defenses for, 164
  religious nationalism and, 165–166
  terror management theory for, 162–163
debunking, 120–121
deliberative thinking, 122
delirium, 237–239
Democratic Party, 75–76
denial of disease, 196–197
depression
  anxiety and, 215–219
  COVID-19 pandemic and, 215–218
  of HCWs, 218
  during influenza pandemics, 219
  in Russian and Spanish flu pandemics, 219
desperate pleasures, 169–170
Diagnostic and Statistical Manual of Mental Disorders, Fifth Edition (DSM-5), 29–30, 151, 220
disease concealment, by government, 73–74, 82
disease-related stigma, as stressor, 31–33
disgust, 17
  fear and, 172
  from pandemics, 18–19
  sensitivity, xv, 171, 172–173, 178
  stimuli evoking, 172
disinfection
  hygiene theater and, 194
  uncertainty and, 174–175
disrupted rituals, as source of distress, 30–31
distal defenses, for death anxiety, 164–165
distal factors, 37
distress (emotional distress), xv. *See also* stressors
  disrupted rituals as source of, 30–31
  nonadherence measures provoking, 41
distress vulnerability traits, 199–205
  anxiety sensitivity, 204–205
  CBT for, 210–211
  intolerance of uncertainty, 202–203
  need for cognitive closure, 203–204
  negative emotionality, 199–200
  overestimation of threat, 201
  trait anxiety and harm avoidance, 200–201
  worry proneness, 201–202
"doctor shopping," 159
"doomsurfing/doomscrolling," 159
dose insensitivity, law of contagion and, 182
drinking, for coping, 90

DSM-5 (*Diagnostic and Statistical Manual of Mental Disorders*, Fifth Edition), 29–30, 151, 220
dysfunctional beliefs, 156–157

Ebola outbreaks, 7t
　anticipatory anxiety in, 8
　declaring end of, 268
　government mistrust and, 74
　healthcare conspiracy theories during, 138
　naming, 46
　shunning survivors during, 182–183
　social media misinformation on, 114
economic pressures
　fleeing driven by, 104–105
　protests motivated by, 79
Edison, Thomas, 137
e-health, 254–256
EL (encephalitis lethargica) pandemic, 7t, 48–49, 242–243
emergency declarations, 12
emotional distress. *See* distress
emotional reasoning, 128–129
emotion-focused coping, 84–85
encephalitis lethargica (EL) pandemic, 7t, 48–49, 242–243
endemic, xv, 268
end of pandemics
　emerging from lockdown and, 270–271
　endemicity and, 268
　face masks after, 270
　false and uncertain, 268–269
　handwashing after, 269
　hygiene measures and, 269–270
　kissing, hugging, handshaking after, 270
　personal growth and, 272–273
　physical, 12, 267–268
　social, 12, 267–268
　societal change from, 273–274
"epidemic coma," 48–49
escaped-from-a-lab conspiracies, 139–140
ethanol poisoning, 91
excessive health anxiety, 151–152
exponential growth bias, 127–128

face masks, xv, 38–39, 50
　Anti-Mask League and, 51–52
　contemporary use of, 51
　COVID-19 and WHO inconsistency on, 25–26

COVID-19 pandemic backlash to, 52
　efficacy of, 51
　historical use of, 50
　rise and fall of using, 270
　Spanish flu backlash to, 51–52
fads, coping, 96–97
fake news, 118–119
false alarms, 283–284
fate, tempting, 184–185
Fauci, Anthony, 76, 95
fear, xii, xv
　affect heuristic and, 128–129
　BIS triggering, 175–176
　confirmation bias and, 125
　contagion and fleeing, 103–104
　disgust and, 172
　factors contributing to, 17
　health anxiety and types of, 153–154
　of infection, 219–220
　mental health issues with, 219–222
　pandemic lessons learned on, 285–286
　pandemics and, 8–9, 17–19
　panic buying driven by, 87
　of sexually transmitted diseases, 221–222
　syndromes, 220
fear-evoking messages, 45–46, 49
fellow travelers, 145
filoviruses, 3
firearm violence, 229
5G conspiracy theory, 137
Flagellantism movement, 93
flaviviruses, 3
fleeing
　conflict and, 102–103
　descriptive features of, 101–102
　disease spread from, 99, 101–102
　economic pressures driving, 104–105
　fear contagion triggering, 103–104
　historical advice on, 106–107
　from lockdown threats, 104
　mistrust of government causing, 104–105
　from plague in India, 1994, 100–101
　from SARS in Beijing, 2003, 101
　social factors driving, 105
　societal breakdown from, 102
　travel restrictions against, 105–106
fluoxetine, 160
fluvoxamine, 160
FNDs (functional neurological disorders), 248–250

focused protection, 66–67
folk remedies, 88–89, 92, 191–192
fomites, xv, 58
food insecurity, pandemic-related, 26–27
fragrances, health-promoting, 173–174
Freedom Truck Convoy, Canada, 78–79
frustration, protests and, 79–80
fumigating mail, 174
functional neurological disorders (FNDs), 248–250
funeral rituals, disrupted, 31
future pandemic scenarios, 279–283, *281t*

"gallows humor," 167–168
gambling addiction, 228
Gates, Bill, 138–139
germ theory, xvi
    miasma theory compared to, 36–38
    pandemic-mitigation methods and, 37–38
    on Russian flu pandemic, 37–38
Ghana, 248
government. *See also* politics
    disease concealment/under-reporting by, 73–74, 82
    fleeing driven by mistrust of, 104–105
    trust in, 72, 74–75, 81–82
gravediggers, cholera rumors and, 135–136
Great Barrington Declaration, 66–67
Great Plague of London, 112, 163, 167
grief, prolonged, 225
Guillain Barré syndrome, as vaccination risk, 53
gullibility, conspiracy theories and, 143

H1N1 (influenza A) virus, 139–140
handshaking, after end of pandemics, 270
handwashing, 39, 193, 269
hardiness, 205–206
harm avoidance, trait anxiety and, 200–201
HCWs. *See* healthcare workers
health anxiety
    CBT treating, 160
    cognitive behavioral model of, 154, *155f*
    definition of, 149
    dysfunctional beliefs and, 156–157
    excessive, 151–152
    fear types with, 153–154
    misinterpretations and, 154–156
    psychogenic fever and, 152
    self-help for, 160
    spectrum of, 149–150
    tempting fate and, 184–185
    worries and, 150–151
healthcare conspiracy theories, 138–139
healthcare workers (HCWs)
    anxiety and depression of, 218
    buddy systems for, 262–263
    burnout and moral injury effects on, 261
    face mask shortage concerns for, 25
    hero-worshiping of, 94–95
    resilience enhancement for, 261–263
    stigmatization of, 32
    suicide, 232–233
    workplace violence against, 230
helpless resignation, superstitious coping compared to, 187–188
Hendra virus, 46
Henry, Bonnie, 95
herd immunity, 66–67
hero-worshiping, for coping, 94–95
heuristics. *See also* biases
    affect, 128–129
    availability, 125–126
    distortions from, 122
    judgments shaped by, 122
    repetition-induced truth effect and, 126–127
hikikomori syndrome, 271
hindsight bias, 129
HIV/AIDS pandemic, *7t*
    bioweapon conspiracies and, 141
    denial of disease and, 197
    disease concealment/under-reporting in, 73
    dysfunctional beliefs during, 157–158
    misinterpretations of, 156
    naming, 46–47
    phobia, 221–222
    stigmatization in, 32–33
    suicide rate during, 230
home-use pulse oximeter fad, during COVID-19, 97
hugging, after end of pandemics, 270
hydrogen peroxide poisoning, 91–92
hydroxychloroquine, 91
hygiene measures, 38–39
    end of pandemics and, 269–270
    illusion of control and, 192–193
    nonadherence to, 39–40
hygiene theater, xvi

aromatic purification as, 174
COVID-19 and, 193–194
disinfection and, 194
illusion of control and, 193–195
placebo effects and, 194–195
yellow fever and, 194
hyperthermia, delirium and, 238

illusion of control
coping and risks of, 195–196
denial of disease and, 196–197
factors shaping, 191
false sense of security with, 195
hygiene rituals and, 192–193
hygiene theater and, 193–195
invulnerability and, 190–191
optimism bias and, 189–190
illusory correlations, self-serving biases and, 191–192
immortality projects, 165
immune system, stressors and, 33–34
immunity beliefs, xenophobia and, 177–178
immunity documentation, 56–57
immunization stress reactions
acute anxiety- and stress-reactions, 246
functional neurological disorders, 248–250
management of, 252
mass psychogenic illness, 247–248
nocebo effect and, 250–251
vaccination hesitancy implications of, 251–252
varieties of, 245–246
vasovagal reactions, 246–247
India
COVID-19 pandemic and disrupted funeral rituals in, 31
plague in, 1994, 100–101
rumors during COVID-19 pandemic in, 135
infection fears, 219–220
infection-induced psychopathology
delirium, 237–239
EL pandemic, 242–243
long COVID, 240–241
neuroinvasive pathogens and, 236–237
post-intensive care syndrome, 239
post-viral syndromes, 239–240
sickness behavior, 235–237
influenza A (H1N1) virus, 139–140

influenza viruses, 3
alcohol drinking and, 90
anxiety and depression during pandemics of, 219
disgust from, 18–19
escaped-from-a-lab conspiracies and, 139–140
major historical instances of, 6t
panic buying during, 87
infodemic, xvi, 116–117, 119–121
information exposure, 111–112, 121
Internet down-weighting, 146–147
interpersonal violence, 229–230
intimate partner violence, 229–230
intolerance of uncertainty, xvi, 202–203
introversion, 206–207
intuitive thinking, 122
invulnerability, illusion of, 190–191
Ireland, religious panic in, 1832, 186–187
irritability, 229

John of Ephesus, 96, 185
Justinian, Plague of, 27, 185

Kennedy, John F., 141–142
kissing, after end of pandemics, 270
Kraepelin, Emil, 240

labels, for diseases, 46–48
Lassa virus, 46
"last straw" events, 79–80
law of contagion, 182
law of similarity, 181–182
Le Bon, Gustave, 275
lifestyle management, 85
lockdown, xvi, 12, 39
"catch-and-release," 82
controversial alternatives to, 66–67
efficacy of, 62
emerging from, 270–271
fleeing from threats of, 104
historical shifts in, 61
intimate partner violence and, 229
objections to, 61
overcoming pandemic fatigue and, 257–259
for social distancing, 60
London, Great Plague of, 112, 163, 167
long COVID, xvi, 240–241
Lord Have Mercy broadsheets, 112

lurid rumors, 134
Luther, Martin, 106–107
Lyme disease, 46

Machiavelli, Niccolo, 185
magical thinking. See also superstitious behavior
  BIS and, 188
  concept of, 179
  conspiracy theories and, 143, 188
  law of contagion and, 181–182
  law of similarity and, 181–182
  omens and, 185–186
  prevalence of, 180–181
  shunning survivors and, 182–183
  superstitious behavior and, 179, 188
  sympathetic, 181–182
  talismans and, 183–184
  tempting fate and, 184–185
mail, fumigating, 174
maladaptive coping, 158–160
Mallon, Mary ("Typhoid Mary"), 13
mandates, 38
  during COVID-19 pandemic, 57
  vaccination pros and cons of, 58
  vaccine passports, 58
masks. See face masks
mass panic, risk communication and, 45
mass psychogenic illness (MPI), 247–248
measles vaccination hesitancy, 55
media. See news media; social media
media literacy, 120, 143
medical misdiagnosis, anchoring bias and, 123–124
memory distortion, hindsight bias and, 129
mental health, 22
  addictive behaviors and, 227–229
  anxiety and depression issues for, 215–219
  CBT for management of, 253–254
  Chengdu program for COVID-19 and, 256–257
  comprehensive management of, 256–257
  e-health for management of, 254–256
  fear and phobia issues for, 219–222
  interpersonal violence and, 229–230
  OCD and, 225–227
  online interventions for, 255–256
  overcoming pandemic fatigue and, 257–259
  pandemic-mitigation methods preserving, 40–41
  prolonged grief disorder and, 225
  PTSD and, 222–224
  social media and, 115
  stepped care for, 256
  stressors causing problems for, 215
  suicide and, 230–233
  telephone hotlines for, 254–255
MERS (Middle Eastern Respiratory Syndrome), xvi, 6t
methanol poisoning, 91
miasma theory, xvi
  germ theory compared to, 36–38
  pandemic-mitigation methods and, 37
  as proximal factor, 37
  on Russian flu pandemic, 37–38
Middle Eastern Respiratory Syndrome (MERS), xvi, 6t
misinformation, on social media, 114–115, 119–121
misinterpretations, health anxiety and, 154–156
mitigation methods. See pandemic-mitigation methods
Modi, Narendra, 14–15
monitoring cognitive style, 111–112
moon landing conspiracies, 141–142
moral injury
  burnout and, 260–261
  emotions associated with, 261
  HCW effects of, 261
morbid curiosity, 166–167
mortality salience, 163
  distal defenses and, 164–165
  politics and, 165
MPI (mass psychogenic illness), 247–248
mpox, disgust from, 18–19
myalgic encephalomyelitis (chronic fatigue syndrome), 241
myth-busting, 120–121

naming
  diseases, 46–48
  next pandemic, 48–49
  WHO guidelines for disease, 48
narcissism
  conspiracy theories and, 143
  nonadherence and, 209–210
nationalism, religious, 165–166

need for cognitive closure, 203–204
negative emotionality, 33–34, 84, 130, 199–200
negative social potency, of trolling, 146
negativity bias, law of contagion and, 182
Netherlands, 80
neuraminidase inhibitors, 53
neuroinvasive pathogens, 236–237
neuroticism, 199–200
New Orleans
    cholera in, 9–10
    yellow fever in, 9–10, 168, 177–178, 194
news media
    anxiety from, 100, 112–113
    attitude polarization and, 115–116
    dangers exaggerated by, 113–114
    debunking, myth-busting and, 120–121
    fake news and, 118–119
    infodemic and, 116–117, 119–121
    information exposure to, 111–112, 121
    media literacy for, 120
    sensationalism, 19
newsworthy diseases, 17
New York City
    rumors during cholera in, 135
    rumors during SARS in, 134
Nickerson, Raymond S., 124
nocebo effect, 250–251
nonadherence
    authoritarianism and, 207–208
    boredom proneness and, 209
    conscientiousness and, 210
    conspiracy theory belief and, 144
    distress provoked by addressing, 41
    to hygiene measures, 39–40
    narcissism, psychological entitlement and, 209–210
    personality traits and, 207–210
    psychological reactance and, 208
    to social distancing, 64
nostalgia, for coping, 95–96
nudges, xvi, 38
    during COVID-19 pandemic, 57
    examples of, 57
    impact of, 57–58
    text messages for, 57

obsessive-compulsive disorder (OCD), 225–227
omens, 185–186

online interventions, for mental health, 255–256
Operation Quack Hack, 92
Operation Warp Speed, 58
optimism bias, 189–190
oseltamivir (Tamiflu), 53
overestimation of threat, 201

pandemics. *See also* end of pandemics; psychology of pandemics; *specific pandemics*
    aging population and, 277–278
    animals, crowds, travel spreading, 12–13
    anxiety and, 8–9, 12
    causes of, 3
    climate change and, 277–278
    conflict lessons learned for, 287–288
    control lessons learned for, 286–287
    COVID-19 pandemic compared to past, 19–20
    definition of, 3
    disgust from, 18–19
    as dynamic events, 15
    as extended hazardous periods, 29–30
    extreme responses evoked by, 16–17
    false alarms and, 283–284
    fear and, 8–9, 17–19
    fear/anxiety lessons learned for, 285–286
    food insecurity from, 26–27
    forgetting past, 275–276
    frequency of, 276
    future scenarios, 279–283, *281t*
    global research on, xii
    human faces of, 9–11
    lessons learned from, 284–288
    major historical, 4–8, *4t, 6t, 7t*
    naming next, 48–49
    population growth and, 277–278
    prevalence of, xi
    psychological impact of, 8–9
    sequences of events in, 11–12
    societal change from, 273–274
    societal fault lines revealed by, 76–77
    societal strain of, 26–27
    spreading of, 12–15
    uncertainty lessons learned for, 285
    virus families causing, 3
    worst-case scenarios of, 283
    zoonotic spillover and, 276–277

pandemic fatigue, xvi, 12
  overcoming, 257–259
  from social distancing, 41, 65
  WHO on COVID-19, 65
pandemic-mitigation methods, xii–xiii
  contemporary, 38–40
  COVID-19 pandemic, countries with successful, 41–43
  germ theory and, 37–38
  goals of, 36, 40–41
  mental health preservation during, 40–41
  miasma theory and, 37
  psychological reactance and, 208
  psychology in, 3
  rise of modern, 36–38
  in Spanish flu pandemic, 40–41
  stress from, 17
  trust in government for, 74
pandemic-related stressors. See stressors
panic buying, xvi, 276
  for coping, 87–88
  price gouging and, 88
paramyxoviruses, 3
Parets, Miguel, 9, 27–28, 99, 102–103, 238
paroxetine, 160
Pepys, Samuel, 167
perfumes, health-promoting, 173–174
permanence of contamination, law of contagion and, 182
personal growth, end of pandemics and, 272–273
personality traits
  authoritarianism, 207–208
  boredom proneness, 209
  conscientiousness, 210
  distress vulnerability, 199–205, 210–211
  measuring, 199
  modifying, 210–211
  narcissism, psychological entitlement and, 209–210
  nonadherence and, 207–210
  psychological reactance, 208
  stress-buffering, 205–207
pessimism, anchoring bias and, 123
pharmaceutical industry conspiracy theories, 138–139
phobias, mental health issues with, 219–222
physical distancing. See social distancing
physical end of pandemic, 12, 267–268
PICS (post-intensive care syndrome), 239

placebo effects, hygiene theater and, 194–195
plague, xvii
  of Athens, 4t, 130, 140, 169–170, 238
  Barcelona, 1651, 9, 27–28
  bioweapon conspiracies during, 140–141
  church bell tolling during, 163
  dark humor during, 168
  death exposure during, 27–28
  delirium during, 238
  desperate pleasures during, 169
  disease-related stigma during, 32
  food insecurity during, 26–27
  Great Plague of London, 112, 163, 167
  immunity documentation during, 56
  in India, 1994, 100–101
  of Justinian, 27, 185
  major historical instances of, 4–8, 4t
  nonadherence to social distancing during, 64
  religious coping during, 93–94
  17th century costume for, 50
  societal change from, 273
Plandemic documentary, 119
poisonings, 90–92
polarization, xvii
  confirmation bias and, 125
  definition of, 16
  media use and attitude, 115–116
  need for cognitive closure causing, 204
  political, 75–76
  types of, 16
  vaccination hesitancy and, 54–55
political rallies, as superspreading events, 14–15
politics. See also government
  conspiracy theories promoted in, 145
  mortality salience and, 165
  polarization and, 75–76
  trust and, 72
population growth, 277–278
positive thinking, 84
post-intensive care syndrome (PICS), 239
post-traumatic stress disorder (PTSD)
  in contemporary disease outbreaks, 222–224
  historical record of, 224
  mental health and, 222–224
post-viral syndromes, 239–240
price gouging, panic buying and, 88

privacy, surveillance conflicts between safety and, 69
problem-focused coping, 84–85
Project PREDICT, 131
prolonged grief disorder, 225
protests
  cholera, 77
  COVID-19, 77–80
  diverse motivations of, 78–79
  economic hardship motivating, 79
  frustration, "last straw" events and, 79–80
  rumors, conspiracy theories and, 80–81
  social media organizing, 82
  as superspreading events, 14–15, 72–73
Protocols of the Elders of Zion, 138
proximal defenses, for death anxiety, 164
proximal factors, 37
psychogenic fever (stress-induced hyperthermia), 152
psychological entitlement, 209–210
psychological reactance, xvii, 208
psychology, applied, xi
psychology of COVID-19, xii, 19–21
psychology of pandemics, xi, xi–xi
  conflict and, 21
  control and, 20–21
  dynamic fluctuations in, 15
  fear and, 20
  future pandemic scenarios and, 279–283, 281t
  impact of, 8–9
  mitigation and, 3
  psychology of COVID-19 compared to, 19–21
  theories of, 21–22
  uncertainty and, 20
  variations over time, culture, and context, 278–279
psychopathic personality, of trolling, 146
psychotherapy, personal growth and, 272–273
PTSD. *See* post-traumatic stress disorder

quack cures, 89, 92
quality of life indicators, 42
quarantine, xvii, 39
  controversial alternatives to, 66–67
  historical shifts in, 61
  immunity documentation and, 56
  objections to, 62
  for social distancing, 60

racism. *See also* xenophobia
  anti-Asian, 177
  anti-Mexican, 176–177
  BIS triggering, 176–177
  COVID-19 conspiracy theories and, 144
  definition of, 176
reassurance-seeking, 160
religious coping, 92–94
religious nationalism, 165–166
religious panic in Ireland, 1832, 186–187
reopening progress indicators, 42
repetition-induced truth effect, 126–127
Republican Party, 75–76
resilience, xvii
  coping for, 98
  HCWs enhancing, 261–263
  strengthening personal, 259
  as stress-buffering trait, 205
Revolta Contra Vacina (Anti-Vaccination Revolts), 80
rhubarb, as folk remedy, 88–89
riots, 72–73. *See also* protests
  cholera, 77
  COVID-19, 77–80
risk communication, xvii, 38–39
  definition of, 44
  fear-evoking messages and, 45–46, 49
  importance of, 49
  mass panic and, 45
  naming diseases in, 46–48
  WHO guidelines for, 44–45
rituals, disrupted, 30–31
Rothkopf, David J., 116–117
ruminative thinking, 151
rumors. *See also* conspiracy theories
  cholera, gravediggers and, 135–136
  of cordon sanitaire, 145
  during COVID-19, 135
  definition of, 133
  as improvised news, 133–136
  lurid, 134
  managing, 146–148
  protests and, 80–81
  during SARS, 134
  social media spreading, 133–134
  superstitious behavior and, 188
Russian flu pandemic, 6t
  antipyrine and, 87, 91

Russian flu pandemic (*Continued*)
  anxiety and depression during, 219
  conspiracy theories during, 137
  disease concealment/under-reporting in, 73
  germ theory and miasma theory explaining, 37–38
  infodemic during, 117
  news media stoking anxieties of, 112–113
  over- and under-reactions to, 16–17
  panic buying during, 87
  quack cures during, 89
  suicide rate during, 230

sadism, trolling and, 146
safety. *See also* specific measures
  lack of boundaries between danger and, 17
  omens of, 185–186
  smells of, 173–175
  surveillance conflicts between privacy and, 69
Salkovskis, Paul M., 154
Salmonella typhi, 13
Sandman, Peter M., 283
SARS (Severe Acute Respiratory Syndrome), xvii
  in Beijing, 2003, 101
  bioweapon conspiracies during, 141
  disease concealment/under-reporting in, 73
  epidemic, 2002-2004, 6t
  folk remedies for, 88–89
  negative emotionality during, 200
  news media exaggerating danger of, 113
  personal growth and, 272
  PTSD related to, 222–223
  rumors during, 134
  suicide rate during, 230
  trait anxiety and harm avoidance during, 201
SARS-CoV-2, xvii, 140. *See also* COVID-19 pandemic
school closures, objections to, 62–64
security, false sense of, 195
selective attention, 157–158
self-help, for health anxiety, 160
Severe Acute Respiratory Syndrome. *See* SARS
sexually transmitted diseases
  fear of, 221–222
  naming, 46–47
shadowy elites, in conspiracy theories, 138
shunning survivors, 182–183
sickness, uncertainty of, 25
sickness behavior, 235–237
similarity, law of, 181–182
"sleeping sickness," 48–49, 242
smallpox pandemic and epidemics, 4t
  Brazil protests during, 80
  disgust from, 18–19
  vaccination hesitation in, 55
smells of danger and safety, 173–175
smoking
  for coping, 90
  as folk remedy, 191–192
  illusory correlations and, 192
Snowden, Frank M., 275–276
social distancing, xvii, 38–39. *See also* surveillance; test-trace-isolate approaches
  controversial alternatives to, 66–67
  lockdown for, 60
  nonadherence to, 64
  objections to closures and, 62–64
  overcoming pandemic fatigue and, 257–259
  pandemic fatigue from, 41, 65
  quarantine for, 60
  recurrent controversies with, 61–62
  temporal discounting and, 130
  uses of, 60
social end of pandemic, xvii, 12, 267–268
social media
  attitude polarization and, 115–116
  COVID-19 conspiracy theories on, 142
  debunking, myth-busting and, 120–121
  "doomsurfing/doomscrolling" and, 159
  fake news and, 118–119
  infodemic and, 116–117, 119–121
  information exposure to, 111–112, 121
  media literacy for, 120
  mental health and, 115
  misinformation on, 114–115, 119–121
  protests organized on, 82
  repetition-induced truth effect and, 126–127
  rumors spread on, 133–134
  sharing information on, 114
  users on, 114

social support, coping and, 85–86
"societal amnesia," 275–276
societal change, pandemics causing, 273–274
societal fault lines, pandemics revealing, 76–77
South Korea, test-trace-isolate approach of, 69, 70
Spanish flu pandemic, 6t
   anxiety and depression during, 219
   approach-avoidance conflicts during, 86–87
   aspirin poisoning and, 91–92
   bioweapon conspiracies during, 140–141
   conspiracy theories during, 136
   dark humor during, 168
   emerging from lockdown after, 270–271
   face mask backlash during, 51–52
   fear of infection during, 219–220
   food insecurity during, 26–27
   mass panic and risk communication during, 45
   mitigation measures in, 40–41
   naming, 47
   nonadherence to social distancing during, 64
   in North Carolina, 1918, 10–11
   over- and under-reactions to, 17
   panic buying during, 87
   PTSD and, 224
   quack remedies during, 89
   quarantine and lockdown for, 61
   smoking and illusory correlations during, 192
   societal change from, 273
   sulfur fad during, 96–97
   tobacco smoking and, 90
   vaccination during, 52
sporting events, as superspreading events, 15
stepped care, for mental health, 256
stigma, disease-related, 31–33
stress-buffering traits, 205–207
   hardiness, 205–206
   introversion, 206–207
   resilience, 205
stress-induced hyperthermia (psychogenic fever), 152
stressors
   death exposure as, 27–28
   definition of, xviii, 24
   disease-related stigma as, 31–33

   disrupted rituals as source of, 30–31
   immune system and, 33–34
   mental health problems from, 215
   from pandemic-mitigation methods, 17
   robust healthcare system dealing with, 34
   societal fault lines and distribution of, 77
   societal strain of pandemics and, 26–27
   traumatic, DSM-5 on, 29–30
   types of, 24
   uncertainty as, 24–26
   vaccination efficacy and, 34–35
stress reactions, xvii–xviii. *See also* immunization stress reactions
substance use, 227–228
suicide
   disease outbreaks and increase in, 230–231
   HCW, 232–233
   mental health and, 230–233
   mitigation methods for, 233
   motives and risk factors for, 231–232
sulfur fad, during Spanish flu, 96–97
superspreaders (people), xviii
   attributes of, 13
   historical instances of, 13
superspreading events, xviii
   conditions for, 14
   panic buying as, 88
   political rallies as, 14–15
   protests as, 14–15, 72–73
   sporting events as, 15
   venues for, 14
superstitious behavior, 22. *See also* magical thinking
   BIS and, 188
   coping and, 187–188
   illusory correlations and, 192
   magical thinking and, 179, 188
   omens and, 185–186
   religious panic in Ireland, 1832 and, 186–187
   rumors driving, 188
   talismans and, 183–184
   tempting fate and, 184–185
surveillance, 39
   China's health code system based on, 68–69
   creep, 70
   privacy and safety conflicts with, 69
   public acceptance of, 70

surveillance (*Continued*)
   in test-trace-isolate approaches, 67–68
survivors, shunning, 182–183
suspiciousness, conspiracy theories and, 143
swine flu pandemic, 6t
   anticipatory anxiety in, 8
   declaring end of, 268–269
   false alarm with, 283–284
   naming, 47
   news media exaggerating danger of, 113–114
   nonadherence to social distancing during, 64
   racism during, 176–177
sympathetic magic, 181–182
symptoms, misinterpretations of, 154–156
syphilis, naming, 46–47

Taiwan, Chinese trolling and, 145–146
talismans, 183–184
Tamiflu (oseltamivir), 53
Tanzania, 74–75
targeted isolation, in test-trace-isolate approaches, 67
Tedros Adhanom Ghebreyesus, 145
telephone hotlines, 254–255
temporal discounting, 130–131, 169
tempting fate, 184–185
terror management theory
   for death anxiety, 162–163
   mortality salience and, 163
   proximal defenses and, 164
testing, 38–39
test-trace-isolate approaches, xviii
   China's surveillance-based health code system and, 68–69
   of South Korea, 69, 70
   surveillance in, 67–68
   targeted isolation in, 67
text messages for nudges, 57
threat appraisal
   affect heuristic and, 128–129
   anchoring bias and, 123–124
   availability heuristic and, 125–126
   confirmation bias and, 124–125
   exponential growth bias and, 127–128
   hindsight bias and, 129
   repetition-induced truth effect and, 126–127
   temporal discounting and, 130–131

threat overestimation, 201
"three second rule," 192–193
Thucydides, 238
tobacco smoking, for coping, 90
trait anxiety, harm avoidance and, 200–201
traumatic stressors, DSM-5 on, 29–30
travel. *See also* fleeing
   pandemics spread by, 12–13
   restrictions, 105–106
trolling, conspiracy theories and, 145–146
Trump, Donald
   COVID-19 conspiracies and, 139
   dangerous methods suggested by, 91
   government mistrust and, 74–75
   superspreading events of, 14–15
trust
   disease concealment eroding, 73–74
   fleeing due to government and lack of, 104–105
   in government, 72, 74–75, 81–82
   uncertain end of pandemics and, 268
truth
   in conspiracy theories, 139
   repetition-induced truth effect and, 126–127
Tuskegee Syphilis Study, 138–139
"Typhoid Mary" (Mallon, Mary), 13

uncertainty, xii
   of death and sickness, 25
   disinfection and, 174–175
   in end of pandemic, 268–269
   intolerance of, xvi, 202–203
   long COVID and, 241
   pandemic lessons learned on, 285
   psychology of pandemics and, 20
   as stressor, 24–26
uncontrollable diseases, 17
under-reporting, by government, 73–74, 82
unfamiliar diseases, 17
United States (U.S.). *See also specific disease outbreaks*
   anti-Asian racism in, 177
   anti-Mexican racism in, 176–177
   China accused of disease concealment by, 73
   Christian nationalism in, 166
   COVID-19 and political polarization in, 75–76
   COVID-19 fear and anxiety in, 9

Ebola outbreak anxiety in, 8
firearm violence in, 229
HCW stigmatization in, 32
hero-worshiping for coping in, 95
measles vaccination hesitancy in, 55
naming diseases and misconceptions in, 47
news media exaggerating SARS danger in, 113
Operation Quack Hack, 92
Operation Warp Speed, 58
pandemic fatigue from social distancing in, 65
pandemic-related food insecurity in, 26
political rallies as superspreading events in, 14–15
Project PREDICT, 131
prolonged grief disorder due to COVID-19 in, 225
Trump and government mistrust in, 74–75
Tuskegee Syphilis Study, 138–139
vaccination hesitancy fluctuations in, 15
unpredictable diseases, 17
Urgency of Normal, 66
U.S. *See* United States

vaccination, 38–39, 50. *See also* immunization stress reactions
acute anxiety- and stress-reactions to, 246
authoritarianism and, 207
campaigns encouraging, 56
confirmation bias and, 125
during COVID-19 pandemic, 53, 196
functional neurological disorders from, 248–250
Guillain Barré syndrome risk of, 53
immune responses to, 33–34
mandate pros and cons for, 58
mass psychogenic illness triggered by, 247–248
nocebo effect and, 250–251
polarization and, 54–55
social media misinformation on, 115
during Spanish flu, 52
stressors and efficacy of, 34–35
vasovagal reactions to, 246–247
voluntary compared to mandatory, 55
vaccination hesitancy
ambiguity aversion and, 203

campaigns targeting, 56
causes of, 54
confirmation bias and, 125
conscientiousness and, 210
definition of, xviii, 54
immunization stress reaction implications for, 251–252
measles and, 55
polarization and, 54–55
smallpox and, 55
U.S. fluctuations in, 15
vaccine passports, 58
vasovagal reactions, 246–247
Vibrio cholerae, 4t
vicarious exposure, as traumatic stressor, 30
violence, interpersonal, 229–230
virus families, pandemics caused by, 3
volatile diseases, 17

wet markets, 276–277
"what-if" thinking, 150–151
White, Ryan, 32–33
WHO. *See* World Health Organization
workplace-related burnout, 260
workplace violence, against HCWs, 230
World Health Organization (WHO)
COVID-19 and face mask message inconsistency from, 25–26
end of pandemic declarations by, 268–269
future COVID-19 scenarios of, 279–283, 281t
on infodemic during COVID-19 pandemic, 117
naming disease guidelines of, 48
on pandemic fatigue during COVID-19, 65
on pandemic fatigue management, 258
risk communication guidelines of, 44–45
on workplace-related burnout, 260
worry
health-related, 150–151
proneness, 201–202
worst-case scenarios, 283

xenophobia, xviii. *See also* racism
BIS triggering, 175, 177–178
conspiracy theories and, 138
during COVID-19 pandemic, 94–95
immunity beliefs and, 177–178

yellow fever
  dark humor during, 168
  desperate pleasures during, 169
  disgust from, 18–19
  fumigating mail in, 174
  hygiene theater and, 194
  immunity documentation during, 56–57
  infodemic during, 117
  major historical instances of, 4–8, *4t*
  in New Orleans, 168, 177–178, 194
  in New Orleans, 1832-1833, 9–10
  PTSD and, 224
  xenophobia and immunity beliefs during, 177–178
Yersinia pestis, 4t, 141

Zika virus pandemic, *7t*
  naming, 46
  pharmaceutical industry conspiracy theories during, 138–139
  social media misinformation on, 114
zoonotic spillover, 276–277